A Practical Guide to Human Cancer Genetics

Shirley V. Hodgson • William D. Foulkes
Charis Eng • Eamonn R. Maher

A Practical Guide to Human Cancer Genetics

Fourth Edition

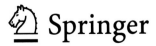 Springer

Shirley V. Hodgson
Cancer Genetics
St Georges Hospital
London
UK

Charis Eng
Genomic Medicine Institute
Cleveland Clinic
Cleveland, OH
USA

William D. Foulkes
Program in Cancer Genetics
Department of Human Genetics,
Medicine and Oncology
McGill University
Montreal
Québec
Canada

Eamonn R. Maher
Department of Medical Genetics
University of Cambridge
Cambridge
UK

Previous edition published by Cambridge University Press as
A Practical Guide to Human Cancer Genetics, 2007

ISBN 978-1-4471-2374-3   ISBN 978-1-4471-2375-0   (eBook)
DOI 10.1007/978-1-4471-2375-0
Springer London Heidelberg New York Dordrecht

Library of Congress Control Number: 2013954666

Printed on acid-free paper

Springer is part of Springer Science+Business Media (www.springer.com)

Foreword for the 4th Edition

Though cancer is essentially a genetic disease at the cellular level and mostly not clearly inherited, studies of familial cancers are not only interesting in their own right but have also made a major contribution to the identification of key genetic changes at the somatic level during cancer progression. The genetics of cancer at the germline level remains one of the most exciting and interesting developments in cancer research, if anything increasingly so with the enormous developments in the technology of DNA sequencing. This has made it possible to recognize the genetic basis of quite rare inherited conditions, sometimes based on only a few cases in only a single family. The new technologies have also made much more widespread testing of families for the presence of the commoner clearly inherited cancer susceptibilities economically feasible. Cancer genetics in this sense has thus become a major part of the workload of clinical genetics services.

Human genetics at the clinical level traditionally focused largely on congenital and pediatric problems. Cancer families, however, pose a completely different problem, since they mostly involve genetic susceptibilities with a late age of onset, offering in most cases the opportunity for effective intervention once individuals at risk have been identified. Such families can provide intriguing opportunities for testing the effectiveness of the removal of early cancers or precancerous growths.

The range of hereditary cancers is quite extraordinary, even though many are individually quite rare. They provide a unique source of material for understanding the carcinogenic process and a major challenge to the human and clinical geneticist.

This fourth edition of the book, originally published in 1992 by Shirley Hodgson and Eamonn Maher, is a substantial reworking of the first edition that takes into account the major developments over the last 20 years, with the addition of two new authors, William Foulkes and Charis Eng to the third and fourth editions. In addition to providing information on many new genes involving strong inherited susceptibility, there is increased coverage of lower-penetrance genes, possibilities for new therapies, and updated screening information. The new edition will be most valuable as an up-to-date account of cancer genetics with a comprehensive survey of a wide range of cancer predispositions, gathered together in a form that will be of great practical value to the clinician but also of great interest for the basic laboratory scientist.

May 27, 2013   Walter Bodmer, FRCPath, FRS
                                                       Cancer and Immunogenetics Lab.
                                            Weatherall Institute of Molecular Medicine
                                                            John Radcliffe Hospital
                                                            Oxford, OX39DS, UK

Preface

Since the third edition of this book, the rapid development in our understanding of inherited cancer susceptibility has continued apace. This edition is the first to be published by Springer, and the change in publisher has been accompanied by a thorough revision and updating on the whole book to reflect the numerous cancer gene discoveries since the last edition and the increasing relevance of genetic information for prognosis and management of individuals with or at risk of inherited cancers.

Although novel discoveries facilitated by technological advances (e.g., high-throughput second-generation sequencing) are often the most high-profile developments in cancer genetics, it remains true that improving the care of families affected by inherited cancers mainly uses information about highly penetrant genes and requires a well-coordinated multidisciplinary approach. Engaging families by sensitive counseling practices for predictive testing and awareness of psychosocial, insurance, and ethical issues remain fundamental to the delivery of an excellent clinical service. This edition of this book takes into account the many new developments in our understanding of cancer genetics – ranging from molecular pathways of oncogenesis to the translation of scientific knowledge into the development of novel clinical and diagnostic services. This edition reflects current clinical practice in Europe and North America and should therefore be of wide utility to those interested in clinical cancer genetics internationally.

Cancer genetics now accounts for at least half of the workload in most comprehensive genetics centers, and a knowledge of this discipline is now germane to an enormous range of specialties. Additionally, the increasing mainstreaming of cancer genetics means that clinicians from many disciplines will need to gain insight into details of cancer genetics. We therefore hope and believe that the popularity of previous editions of this book will sustain and enhance this edition and will be helpful to the many clinicians, laboratory scientists, and healthcare professionals who are faced with the ever-enlarging demand for knowledge of familial cancer risks.

London, UK   Shirley V. Hodgson
Montreal, QC, Canada   William D. Foulkes
Cleveland, OH, USA   Charis Eng
Cambridge, UK   Eamonn R. Maher

Acknowledgements

The authors are grateful to Dr. Julia Newton-Bishop for her contribution to the section on skin cancers and to Dr. Marc Tischkowitz for his help with the section on Fanconi Anemia and Dr. Andrew Shuen for his help with parts of chapter 6. They would also like to thank Prof. Gareth Evans, Prof. Diana Eccles, Prof. Doug Easton, and Prof. Ros Eeles for contributing tables, Prof. C. Mathew and Prof. Gill Birch for comments, and Prof. Patrick Morrison for illustrations. They also thank Virginia Manning for her help with the preparation of the manuscript.

Contents

Contributors

Charis Eng Genomic Medicine Institute, Cleveland Clinic, Cleveland, OH, USA

William D. Foulkes Program in Cancer Genetics, Department of Human Genetics, Medicine and Oncology, McGill University, Montreal, QC, Canada

Shirley V. Hodgson Cancer Genetics, St Georges Hospital, London, UK

Eamonn R. Maher Department of Medical Genetics, University of Cambridge, Cambridge, UK

Julia Newton-Bishop Department of Dermatology, University of Leeds, Leeds, UK

Marc Tischkowitz Department of Medical Genetics, University of Cambridge, Cambridge, UK

Andrew Shuen Department of Human Genetics, McGill University, Montreal, QC, Canada

Chapter 1
Central Nervous System

Primary central nervous system (CNS) neoplasms affect about 1 per 10,000 of the population. Although the incidence of brain tumors increases with advancing age, intracranial neoplasms are the most common cause of solid cancer in children. The distribution and histological type of brain tumor differ in children and in adults. In children, brain tumors most often arise in the posterior fossa, and the most frequent tumor types are medulloblastoma, spongioblastoma (including cerebellar astrocytoma and optic nerve glioma), and ependymomas. In adults, most tumors are supratentorial, and meningiomas and gliomas are the most frequent types. Familial brain tumors may occur as part of a rare specific inherited cancer syndrome (Table 1.1). Epidemiological studies have suggested that there is a small increased risk of cerebral neoplasms among relatives of brain tumor patients compared to controls: Choi et al. (1970) and Gold et al. (1994) found a ninefold increase in the incidence of brain tumor among relatives of patients with glioma compared to controls, whereas Burch et al. (1987) found a (statistically insignificant) sixfold increase among relatives of brain tumor patients. Nevertheless, the absolute risk to relatives is small, 0.6 % in the study by Choi et al. (1970). Miller (1971) found a ninefold increase in the expected number of sib pairs among children with brain tumors and a similar excess of families in which one child died of brain tumor and another of cancer of bone or muscle. Soft tissue sarcomas and brain tumors occur as part of the Li–Fraumeni syndrome. Mahaley et al. (1989) found a family history of cancer in 16–19 % of patients with brain tumors (similar to the expected incidence) but that the incidence was 30–33 % in patients with glioblastoma multiforme, malignant lymphoma, and neuroblastoma. A family history of neurofibromatosis was obtained in 1.6 % of cases. In a recent large joint Nordic study, 2.6 % of patients with nervous system cancer were familial. The SIR of brain tumors was 1.7 in offspring of affected parents, 2.0 in siblings, and 9.4 in families with a parent and sibling affected (Hemminki et al. 2010). As high-penetrance multiplex families with CNS tumors accounted for only a minority of cases, it has been suggested that most familial risks might be attributable to lower-penetrance genes (Hemminki et al. 2009). The familial risks for nervous system tumors do vary according to tumor histopathology (Hemminki et al. 2009), and the genetic implications of specific CNS tumors are described below.

S.V. Hodgson et al., *A Practical Guide to Human Cancer Genetics*,
DOI 10.1007/978-1-4471-2375-0_1, © Springer-Verlag London 2014

Table 1.1 Genetic disorders associated with tumors of the CNS

Neurofibromatosis type 1
Neurofibromatosis type 2
von Hippel–Lindau disease
Li–Fraumeni syndrome
Familial adenomatous polyposis
Turcot syndrome (including homozygous mismatch gene mutations)
Tuberose sclerosis
Gorlin syndrome
Ataxia telangiectasia
Werner syndrome
Blue rubber bleb nevus syndrome

Details of individual conditions are given in Chap. 11

Vestibular Schwannoma (Acoustic Neuroma)

This tumor accounts for around 8 % of all intracranial tumors and has an incidence of 13/million per year (Tos and Thomsen 1984). Although sometimes called acoustic neuromas, these are Schwann cell tumors. They usually arise from the vestibular nerve but can develop on the fifth cranial nerve and less often on the ninth and tenth nerves. Within the spinal canal, they usually arise on the dorsal spinal root. Familial and bilateral vestibular schwannomas are features of neurofibromatosis type 2 (NF2). About 4 % of vestibular schwannomas are bilateral, and all patients with bilateral tumors have NF2 (see p. 293). Sporadic vestibular schwannoma is typically seen in the fifth and sixth decades of life, which is about 20 years later than in patients with NF2. The clinical features and diagnostic criteria for NF2 are discussed on p. 293. Although vestibular schwannoma in NF2 is usually bilateral, it can be unilateral. Those mosaics for an *NF2* gene mutation may present with milder- and later-onset disease (see p. 294).

Multiple extracranial schwannomas (cutaneous and spinal) without vestibular schwannomas may be inherited as a dominant trait (Evans et al. 1997) and may be caused by germline mutations in *SMARCB1* (*see Nerve Root Tumors below*). Occasionally *SMARCB1* mutations have been described in individuals with unilateral vestibular schwannomas and multiple central and cutaneous schwannomas (Smith et al. 2011).

Choroid Plexus Tumor

Choroid plexus neoplasms are rare (0.5 % of all brain tumors) and are most frequent in infancy. The majority of choroid plexus tumors are benign papillomas, but up to 30 % are classified as carcinomas.

Childhood choroid plexus tumors in sibling pairs have been reported and autosomal recessive inheritance suggested (Zwetsloot et al. 1991). Tumors of the choroid plexus have been reported in the X-linked disorder Aicardi syndrome (Robinow et al. 1986). Germline *TP53* mutations are relatively frequent in children with choroid plexus tumors (Gozali et al. 2012). Though the family history may be suggestive of Li–Fraumeni syndrome in many cases, in others there may be no family history of cancer (Krutilkova et al. 2005; Tabori et al. 2010). The germline founder *TP53* mutation R337H occurs at high frequency in Brazil and can be detected in most children who develop choroid plexus carcinomas (Custodio et al. 2011).

Choroid plexus angiomas were reported in two out of four patients with Perlman syndrome (p. 298) reported by Henneveld et al. (1999).

Choroid plexus tumors should be differentiated from endolymphatic sac tumors, which are a feature of von Hippel–Lindau disease (p. 313).

Ependymoma

These glial cell tumors of the brain and spinal cord occur both sporadically and in association with cancer susceptibility syndromes. In children, the tumor usually presents as a posterior fossa mass. Ependymoma may be a feature of neurofibromatosis type 2 (see p. 293) and has rarely been reported as part of Turcot syndrome (Torres et al. 1997), multiple endocrine neoplasia type 1, and in association with a germline *P53* mutation. Familial ependymoma consistent with autosomal dominant inheritance with incomplete penetrance has also been described (Gilchrist and Savard 1989; Nijssen et al. 1994).

Gliomas (Including Astrocytoma and Glioblastoma)

Astrocytoma and glioblastoma account for about 4 % of brain tumors in childhood and 17 % in adults. Genetic conditions associated with a predisposition to glioma include neurofibromatosis type 1 (NF1) (p. 288), NF2, Li–Fraumeni syndrome (p. 271), tuberose sclerosis (p. 307), Gorlin syndrome (p. 252), Turcot syndrome (p. 311), and Maffucci syndrome (p. 274). The precise tumor type in some cases can be correlated with specific disorders, for example, in tuberose sclerosis a benign astrocytic tumor (subependymal nodule) is typically seen, although giant cell astrocytoma can occur. However, in NF1 and Turcot syndrome, both astrocytoma and glioblastoma multiforme may be seen. Kibirige et al. (1989) found that of 282 children with astrocytoma, 21 had neurofibromatosis and 4 had tuberose sclerosis, and there was evidence that a similar proportion might have had Li–Fraumeni syndrome.

Familial glioma not associated with the inherited syndromes described above occurs, but is uncommon. In a review by Vieregge et al. (1987), of 39 reports, most (60 %) were of affected siblings, and one-quarter was of affected twins or of individuals with affected relatives in two generations. There were three pairs of monozygotic twins with glioma. In most affected sibling cases, the onset in the second sibling was usually within 5 years of that of the first sibling. A high incidence of cerebral glioma was found in an isolated inbred community by Armstrong and Hanson (1969) and Thuwe et al. (1979). Glioblastoma multiforme is rare in children, but Duhaime et al. (1989) reported an affected sib pair aged 2 and 5 years with simultaneous onset of symptoms.

Rare families have been reported with a combination of melanoma and gliomas. In some families submicroscopic germline deletions of 9p21 have been identified which completely or partially involve *CDKN2A*±*CDKN2B* (Bahuau et al. 1998; Tachibana et al. 2000). The *CDKN2A* locus encodes two gene products, p14 and p16, and there is evidence that p14 loss is critical for this disorder (Randerson-Moor et al. 2001). Thus, in brain tumor–melanoma kindreds, deletion studies of this region may be warranted if clinical testing for *CDKN2A* mutations has been undertaken and is negative.

In general, candidate gene analysis in non-syndromic familial glioma cases has been largely unproductive. Thus, although a study from the Mayo Clinic of 15 brain cancer patients who had a family history of brain tumors found that one had a germline *TP53* mutation, and another had a germline hemizygous deletion of the *CDKN2A/CDKN2B* region (Tachibana et al. 2000), a more recent, larger analysis ($n = 101$) of familial glioma cases did not detect germline *CDKN2A* mutations and only one *TP53* mutation (Robertson et al. 2010).

In the light of the evidence that lower-penetrance genes might represent a major contribution to familial risks for nervous system tumors (Hemminki et al. 2009), large collaborations such as the GLIOGENE consortium have undertaken genomewide association studies and identified a number of polymorphic variants that predispose to glioma (Scheurer et al. 2010; Shete et al. 2011). Among the genes linked with susceptibility variants are *TERT, EGFR, CDKN2A/CDKIN2B*, and *PHLDB1*, but only a small part of familial risk can be explained by the linked variants (Shete et al. 2009, 2011).

Hemangioblastoma

These vascular tumors occur most frequently in the cerebellum followed by the spinal cord, brain stem, and, least frequently, supratentorially. Approximately 30 % of all cerebellar hemangioblastomas occur as part of von Hippel–Lindau (VHL) disease (see p. 313). Patients with multiple CNS hemangioblastomas satisfy the clinical diagnostic criteria for VHL disease. Hemangioblastoma is a benign tumor but may recur if surgical removal is not complete. In such cases the possibility of a new primary (and hence a diagnosis of VHL disease) should also be considered. The risk of VHL disease is highest in younger patients: the mean ages at diagnosis of cerebellar hemangioblastoma in this disease and in nonfamilial cases are 29 and 48 years, respectively (Maher et al. 1990). All patients with apparently sporadic hemangioblastomas should be screened for subclinical evidence of VHL disease. In addition, *VHL* mutation analysis is helpful, particularly in patients aged less than 50 years. Germline VHL gene mutations were detected in 4 % of apparently sporadic hemangioblastoma cases without clinical or radiological evidence of VHL disease (Hes et al. 2000). In view of the possibility of false-negative mutation analysis results (e.g., if mosaic), younger patients (less than 40 years) may be kept under review in case evidence of VHL disease develops later.

Hemangioma

Cavernous hemangiomas may occur sporadically or as a familial trait when they are inherited as a dominant trait with incomplete penetrance (Riant et al. 2010). Familial cases, which account for about 20 % of the total, frequently develop multiple cavernous hemangiomas, but these may be asymptomatic and only detected by magnetic resonance imaging (MRI) scanning. Retinal cavernous angiomas may be found in some patients (see p. 20).

Familial cavernous hemangiomas are genetically heterogeneous. The first gene to be mapped and identified was *CCM1/KRIT1* and accounts for about 40 % of all cases (Laberge-le Couteulx et al. 1999). Subsequently two further genes were described (*CCM2/MGC4607* and *CCM3/PDCD10*) which account for about 20 and 40 % of all familial cases, respectively (Dubovsky et al. 1995; Craig et al. 1998; Riant et al. 2010). There is a significant (40–60 %) mutation detection rate in sporadic individuals with multiple lesions, and some mutation negative cases might be mosaic (Riant et al. 2010).

Meningeal hemangioma and facial nevus flammeus constitute the Sturge–Weber syndrome, and cerebral vascular lesions occur in Rendu–Osler–Weber syndrome. Although the Sturge–Weber syndrome is sometimes designated the fourth phakomatosis, there is no evidence of a genetic basis and there is no predisposition to neoplasia.

Medulloblastoma

This tumor accounts for about 25 % of all brain tumors in children and has an incidence of approximately 1/100,000 per year. Medulloblastoma occurs predominantly in the first two decades of life, with a peak incidence between 3 and 5 years of age. Familial medulloblastoma appears to be uncommon, but has been reported in twins and siblings (Hung et al. 1990). Familial non-syndromic medulloblastoma occurs rarely (von Koch et al. 2002). Genetic disorders associated with medulloblastoma include Gorlin syndrome, familial adenomatous polyposis and Turcot syndrome, blue rubber bleb nevus syndrome, and ataxia telangiectasia (see p. 219). Gorlin syndrome is caused by germline mutations in the *PTCH* gene which encodes the sonic hedgehog receptor (see p. 252). In addition, germline and somatic mutations in another of the sonic hedgehog pathway, *SUFU* (encoding the human suppressor of fused), may be found in a subset of children with early-onset (before 3 years) medulloblastoma and can be dominantly inherited with incomplete penetrance (Taylor et al. 2002; Brugieres et al. 2010). Medulloblastoma may also occur in patients with homozygous *BRCA2* mutations (Fanconi Anaemia Type D1, see p. 249) (Offit et al. 2003; Hirsch et al. 2004).

Cancer genome analysis of medulloblastoma revealed that the most commonly altered genes were implicated in the Hedgehog, Wnt, and histone methylation pathways (Parsons et al. 2011).

Meningioma

The most common benign brain tumor, meningioma, accounts for about 15 % of all primary brain tumors. The frequency of meningioma increases with advancing age, and it is more common in women. Multiple or familial meningioma is associated with (a) neurofibromatosis type 2 (NF2), (b) pure familial meningioma, (c) constitutional chromosome 22 rearrangements, and (d) familial schwannomatosis and SMARCB1 mutations (see below). Meningioma also occurs with increased frequency in Werner syndrome (p. 318) and Gorlin syndrome (p. 252).

Multiple meningioma is frequent and occurs in about a third of patients with NF2 (see p. 293). Expression of NF2 is variable, so a careful search for evidence of NF2 and a detailed family history should be performed in all patients with multiple or familial meningioma, or with a young age at onset. Although many reports of familial meningioma may be variants of NF2, dominantly inherited meningioma with no evidence of NF2 does occur. However, signs of NF2 should be assiduously sought in all cases of familial meningioma as these may not be obvious. For example, Delleman et al. (1978) reported a family in which four members in two generations had meningiomas with no evidence of neurofibromatosis, but another relative had multiple meningiomas and bilateral vestibular schwannomas.

Rearrangements of chromosome 22 have been associated with meningioma: multiple tumors developed in the third decade in a mentally retarded patient with a ring chromosome 22 (breakpoints p12 and q13.3) (Arinami et al. 1986), and familial meningiomas associated with a Robertsonian chromosome 14;22 translocation have also been described. In addition, Pulst et al. (1993) reported exclusion of linkage to the NF2 kindred with familial meningioma.

Germline SMARCB1 mutations have been identified in patients with a combination of multiple meningiomas and schwannomatosis (van den Munckhof et al. 2012). However, among a cohort of patients with multiple meningiomas and no schwannomas, germline SMARCB1 mutations appeared to be rare (Hadfield et al. 2010) though Smith et al. (2013) described SMARCE1 mutations in kindreds with familial spinal meningiomas with clear cell histology.

Nerve Root Tumors

The commonest nerve root tumor is the benign schwannoma or neurolemmoma, and the most frequent site is the eighth cranial nerve (see vestibular schwannoma, p. 2). Multiple schwannomas are a feature of neurofibromatosis type 2 (NF2)

(p. 293), and schwannomas can occur in the Carney complex (p. 228), most commonly in the upper gastrointestinal tract and sympathetic nerve chains. Although familial extracranial schwannoma was initially postulated to be allelic with NF2, mutations in *SMARCB1* were demonstrated to cause autosomal dominantly inherited central and cutaneous familial schwannomas (Hulsebos et al. 2007). Subsequently *SMARCB1* mutations have been detected in about a half of familial patients and about 10 % of sporadic cases (higher in those with sporadic multiple schwannomas) (Rousseau et al. 2011; Smith et al. 2012). Although familial schwannomatosis was initially defined by the absence of vestibular schwannomas, *SMARCB1* mutations have been described in individuals with unilateral vestibular schwannomas and multiple central and cutaneous schwannomas (Smith et al. 2011). In addition, germline *SMARCB1* mutations have been reported in patients with a combination of multiple meningiomas and schwannomatosis (van den Munckhof et al. 2012). Germline mutations in *SMARCB1* can cause also cause rhabdoid tumor predisposition syndrome (see later), and very occasionally an *SMARCB1* mutation has been associated with both phenotypes (Eaton et al. 2011). It has been suggested that *SMARCB1* missense and splice site mutations are preferentially associated with schwannomatosis and deletions and truncating mutations with rhabdoid tumor predisposition.

Neuroblastoma

This tumor of postganglionic sympathetic neurons is the most common solid tumor in children. Most cases are sporadic; familial cases (in which predisposition to neuroblastoma is inherited as an autosomal dominant trait) account for less than 1 % of the total. However, in a statistical analysis of the age at onset of neuroblastoma, Knudson and Strong (1972) estimated that 22 % of neuroblastomas could result from a germinal mutation and follow a "single-hit" mutation model, as in inherited retinoblastoma (Knudson 1971). The mean age at diagnosis of familial cases is 9 months (60 % at less than 1 year) compared to 30 months (25 % at less than 1 year) in nonfamilial cases (Kushner et al. 1986), and familial tumors are frequently multiple (Robertson et al. 1991).

Neuroblastoma is occasionally seen in overgrowth disorders such as Beckwith–Wiedemann syndrome and hemihypertrophy and in disorders associated with abnormal neural crest differentiation such as NF1, Hirschsprung disease, and congenital central hypoventilation syndrome. Germline mutations in *PHOX2B* were initially demonstrated in congenital central hypoventilation syndrome and subsequently in patients with neuroblastoma in association with congenital central hypoventilation syndrome and/or Hirschsprung disease and in familial nonsyndromic neuroblastoma (Trochet et al. 2004). Although germline *PHOX2B* mutations may occasionally be found in patients with apparently sporadic neuroblastoma, overall it appears to be a rare cause of inherited neuroblastoma (Perri et al. 2005; McConville et al. 2006; Raabe et al. 2008).

Frequent somatic changes in neuroblastoma include *MYCN* amplification, chromosome 1p36 and 11q allele loss, and copy number gain at 17q. In addition copy number gain and activating mutations in the anaplastic lymphoma kinase (*ALK1*) proto-oncogene were found to be a common event (Chen et al. 2008; Janoueix-Lerosey et al. 2008; Mossé et al. 2008). Furthermore, germline *ALK1* mutations are an important cause of familial neuroblastoma (Janoueix-Lerosey et al. 2008; Mossé et al. 2008). Neuroblastoma susceptibility associated with *ALK1* missense mutations is inherited as an autosomal dominant trait with incomplete penetrance and often manifests with multiple tumors (Bourdeaut et al. 2012). Two *de novo ALK1* mutations have been associated with a novel syndrome of multifocal congenital neuroblastoma, encephalopathy, and abnormal brain stem morphology (de Pontual et al. 2011).

Genome-wide association studies have linked aggressive neuroblastoma susceptibility to common genomic variants at chromosome 6p22 and SNPs in *BARD1* (which interacts with BRCA1) (Maris et al. 2008; Capasso et al. 2009).

In familial neuroblastoma, screening by urinary catecholamine estimations from birth to age 6 years can be offered. However, although initially advocated, population screening of infants for neuroblastoma was not found to reduce mortality (Woods et al. 2002).

Pineal Tumor

Pineal tumors account for less than 1 % of all brain tumors. A proportion of children with bilateral retinoblastoma will develop a pineal tumor (the so-called trilateral retinoblastoma). Both familial pineoblastoma and familial pinealcytoma can occur but are very rare (Peyster et al. 1986; Gempt et al. 2012). Pineoblastoma has occasionally been reported in association with familial adenomatous polyposis coli. Extragonadal germ cell tumors may arise in the pineal gland and be associated with Klinefelter syndrome or 46XY gonadal dysgenesis. Pineoblastomas are also seen in carriers of *DICER1* mutations (Sabbaghian et al. 2012).

Primitive Neuroectodermal Tumors

Cerebral primitive neuroectodermal tumors (PNETs) can occur predominantly in childhood and arise most frequently in the posterior fossa, but can occur anywhere in the brain. Medulloblastoma (see above) is the most common form of PNET, but CNS malignant rhabdoid tumors are another subset. Germline mutations in *TP53*, *PTCH* (Gorlin syndrome), and *APC* may be associated with susceptibility to central PNETs. In contrast to the peripheral type, such as Ewing sarcoma, t(11;22)(q24;q12) is uncommon in the central type.

Rhabdoid tumors are rare aggressive neoplasms that can occur in a variety of locations including the kidney, central nervous system, and soft tissues. Taylor et al. (2000)

reported a kindred with two affected relatives with a posterior fossa brain tumor in infancy (cerebellar malignant rhabdoid tumor) and posterior fossa choroids plexus carcinoma and a germline *SMARCB1* (*hSNF5*) splice site mutation. Inheritance was autosomal dominant with incomplete penetrance, and mice heterozygous for an *Snf5* deletion developed T cell lymphomas and rhabdoid tumors (Roberts et al. 2002). Germline mutations in *SMARCB1* can cause familial schwannomatosis (see above) and rhabdoid tumor predisposition syndrome. Occasionally an *SMARCB1* mutation has been associated with both phenotypes (Eaton et al. 2011). Molecular analysis of sporadic rhabdoid tumors shows evidence of *SMARCB1* inactivation in most cases, and germline *SMARCB1* mutations have been reported to be frequent in patients with such apparently sporadic rhabdoid tumors(Bourdeaut et al. 2011; Eaton et al. 2011). Thus, Bourdeaut et al. (2011) detected mutations in about a quarter of these cases, with the highest frequency in the younger children (60 % in those aged <2 years) and those with multifocal disease. Germline *SMARCB1* mutations associated with rhabdoid tumors tend to be highly penetrant, and mean age at diagnosis of rhabdoid tumor was 6 months (Bourdeaut et al. 2011). However, non-penetrance and gonadal mosaicism have been reported (Eaton et al. 2011). It has been suggested that *SMARCB1* missense and splice site mutations are preferentially associated with schwannomatosis and deletions and truncating mutations with rhabdoid tumor predisposition. SMARCB1 is a member of the SWI/SNF chromatin-remodeling complex, and germline mutation in another member of this complex, the ATPase subunit *SMARCA4* (BRG1), was detected in two sisters with rhabdoid tumors (one brain and one renal) (Schneppenheim et al. 2010).

Supratentorial PNETs (sPNETs) are very rare and highly aggressive embryonal tumors of the cerebrum, pineal gland, and suprasellar region. sPNETs are associated with homozygous *PMS2* mutations (De Vos et al. 2004). Other features of recessively inherited *PMS2* mutations are café-au-lait lesions and susceptibility to hematological malignancies. A family history of colorectal cancer is often absent. Homozygous recessive mutations in *BRCA2* causing Fanconi anemia subtype D1 (see p. 249) predispose to solid tumors including medulloblastoma (Offit et al. 2003; Hirsch et al. 2004).

References

Arinami T, Kondo I, Hamaguchi H, Nakajima S. Multifocal meningiomas in a patient with a constitutional ring chromosome 22. J Med Genet. 1986;23:178–80.

Armstrong RM, Hanson CW. Familial gliomas. Neurology. 1969;19:1061–3.

Bahuau M, Vidaud D, Jenkins RB, Bièche I, Kimmel DW, Assouline B, Smith JS, Alderete B, Cayuela JM, Harpey JP, Caille B, Vidaud M. Germ-line deletion involving the INK4 locus in familial proneness to melanoma and nervous system tumors. Cancer Res. 1998;58:2298–303.

Bourdeaut F, Lequin D, Brugières L, Reynaud S, Dufour C, Doz F, André N, Stephan JL, Pérel Y, Oberlin O, Orbach D, Bergeron C, Rialland X, Fréneaux P, Ranchere D, Figarella-Branger D, Audry G, Puget S, Evans DG, Pinas JC, Capra V, Mosseri V, Coupier I, Gauthier-Villars M, Pierron G, Delattre O. Frequent hSNF5/INI1 germline mutations in patients with rhabdoid tumor. Clin Cancer Res. 2011;17(1):31–8.

Bourdeaut F, Ferrand S, Brugières L, Hilbert M, Ribeiro A, Lacroix L, Bénard J, Combaret V, Michon J, Valteau-Couanet D, Isidor B, Rialland X, Poirée M, Defachelles AS, Peuchmaur M, Schleiermacher

G, Pierron G, Gauthier-Villars M, Janoueix-Lerosey I, Delattre O. Comité Neuroblastome of the Société Francaise de Cancérologie. ALK germline mutations in patients with neuroblastoma: a rare and weakly penetrant syndrome. Eur J Hum Genet. 2012;20(3):291–7.

Brugieres L, Pierron G, Chompret A, Bressac-de Paillerets B, Di Rocco F, Varlet P, Pierre-Kahn A, Caron O, Grill J, Delattre O. Incomplete penetrance of the predisposition to medulloblastoma associated with germ-line SUFU mutations. J Med Genet. 2010;47:142–4.

Burch JD, Craib KJ, Choi BC, Miller AB, Risch HA, Howe GR. An exploratory case-control study of brain tumors in adults. J Natl Cancer Inst. 1987;78:601–9.

Capasso M, Devoto M, Hou C, Asgharzadeh S, Glessner JT, Attiyeh EF, Mosse YP, Kim C, Diskin SJ, Cole KA, Bosse K, Diamond M, Laudenslager M, Winter C, Bradfield JP, Scott RH, Jagannathan J, Garris M, McConville C, London WB, Seeger RC, Grant SF, Li H, Rahman N, Rappaport E, Hakonarson H, Maris JM. Common variations in BARD1 influence susceptibility to high-risk neuroblastoma. Nat Genet. 2009;41(6):718–23.

Chen Y, Takita J, Choi YL, Kato M, Ohira M, Sanada M, Wang L, Soda M, Kikuchi A, Igarashi T, Nakagawara A, Hayashi Y, Mano H, Ogawa S. Oncogenic mutations of ALK kinase in neuroblastoma. Nature. 2008;455(7215):971–4.

Choi NW, Schuman IM, Gullen WH. Epidemiology of primary central nervous system neoplasms. II. Case–control study. Am J Epidemiol. 1970;91:467–85.

Craig HD, Gunel M, Cepeda O, et al. Multilocus linkage identifies two new loci for a mendelian form of stroke, cerebral cavernous malformation, at 7p15–13 and 3q25.2–27. Hum Mol Genet. 1998;7(12):1851–8.

Custodio G, Taques GR, Figueiredo BC, Gugelmin ES, Oliveira Figueiredo MM, Watanabe F, Pontarolo R, Lalli E, Torres LF. Increased incidence of choroid plexus carcinoma due to the germline TP53 R337H mutation in southern Brazil. PLoS One. 2011;6(3):e18015.

de Pontual L, Kettaneh D, Gordon CT, Oufadem M, Boddaert N, Lees M, Balu L, Lachassinne E, Petros A, Mollet J, Wilson LC, Munnich A, Brugière L, Delattre O, Vekemans M, Etchevers H, Lyonnet S, Janoueix-Lerosey I, Amiel J. Germline gain-of-function mutations of ALK disrupt central nervous system development. Hum Mutat. 2011;32(3):272–6.

De Vos M, Hayward BE, Picton S, Sheridan E, Bonthron DT. Novel PMS2 pseudogenes can conceal recessive mutations causing a distinctive childhood cancer syndrome. Am J Hum Genet. 2004;74(5):954–64.

Delleman J, De Jong JGY, Bleeker GM. Meningiomas in five members of a family over two generations, in one member simultaneously with acoustic neurinomas. Neurology. 1978;28:567–70.

Dubovsky J, Zabramski JM, Kurth J, Spetzler RF, Rich SS, Orr HT, Weber JL. A gene responsible for cavernous malformations of the brain maps to chromosome 7q. Hum Mol Genet. 1995;4:453–8.

Duhaime AC, Bunin G, Sutton L, Rorke LB, Packer RJ. Simultaneous presentation of glioblastoma multiforme in siblings two and five years old: case report. Neurosurgery. 1989;24:434–9.

Eaton KW, Tooke LS, Wainwright LM, Judkins AR, Biegel JA. Spectrum of SMARCB1/INI1 mutations in familial and sporadic rhabdoid tumors. Pediatr Blood Cancer. 2011;56(1):7–15.

Evans DG, Mason S, Huson SM, Ponder M, Harding AE, Strachan T. Spinal and cutaneous schwannomatosis is a variant form of type 2 neurofibromatosis: a clinical and molecular study. J Neurol Neurosurg Psychiatr. 1997;62:361–6.

Gempt J, Ringel F, Oexle K, Delbridge C, Förschler A, Schlegel J, Meyer B, Schmidt-Graf F. Familial pineocytoma. Acta Neurochir (Wien). 2012;154:1413–6.

Gilchrist DM, Savard ML. Ependymomas in two sisters and a maternal male cousin. Am J Med Genet. 1989;45:A22.

Gold EB, Leviton A, Lopez R, Austin DF, Gilles FH, Hedley-Whyte ET, Kolonel LN, Lyon JL, Swanson GM, Weiss NS. The role of family history in risk of childhood brain tumors. Cancer. 1994;73:1302–11.

Gozali AE, Britt B, Shane L, Gonzalez I, Gilles F, McComb JG, Krieger MD, Lavey RS, Shlien A, Villablanca JG, Erdreich-Epstein A, Dhall G, Jubran R, Tabori U, Malkin D, Finlay JL. Choroid plexus tumors; management, outcome, and association with the Li-Fraumeni syndrome: the Children's Hospital Los Angeles(CHLA) experience, 1991–2010. Pediatr Blood Cancer. 2012;58(6):905–9.

Hadfield KD, Smith MJ, Trump D, Newman WG, Evans DG. SMARCB1 mutations are not a common cause of multiple meningiomas. J Med Genet. 2010;47(8):567–8.

Hemminki K, Tretli S, Sundquist J, Johannesen TB, Granström C. Familial risks in nervous-system tumours: a histology-specific analysis from Sweden and Norway. Lancet Oncol. 2009;10:481–8.

Hemminki K, Tretli S, Olsen JH, Tryggvadottir L, Pukkala E, Sundquist J, Granström C. Familial risks in nervous system tumours: joint Nordic study. Br J Cancer. 2010;102:1786–90.

Henneveld HT, van Lingen RA, Hamel BCJ, Stolte-Dijkstra I, van Essen AJ. Perlman syndrome: four additional cases and review. Am J Med Genet. 1999;86:439–46.

Hes FJ, McKee S, Taphoorn MJ, Rehal P, van Der Luijt RB, McMahon R, van Der Smagt JJ, Dow D, Zewald RA, Whittaker J, Lips CJ, MacDonald F, Pearson PL, Maher ER. Cryptic von Hippel-Lindau disease: germline mutations in patients with haemangioblastoma only. J Med Genet. 2000;37:939–43.

Hirsch B, Shimamura A, Moreau L, Baldinger S, Hag-alshiekh M, Bostrom B, Sencer S, D'Andrea AD. Association of biallelic BRCA2/FANCD1 mutations with spontaneous chromosomal instability and solid tumors of childhood. Blood. 2004;103:2554–9.

Hulsebos TJ, Plomp AS, Wolterman RA, Robanus-Maandag EC, Baas F, Wesseling P. Germline mutation of INI1/SMARCB1 in familial schwannomatosis. Am J Hum Genet. 2007;80(4):805–10.

Hung KL, Wu CM, Huang JS, How SW. Familial medulloblastoma in sib-lings: report in one family and review of the literature. Surg Neurol. 1990;33:341–6.

Janoueix-Lerosey I, Lequin D, Brugières L, Ribeiro A, de Pontual L, Combaret V, Raynal V, Puisieux A, Schleiermacher G, Pierron G, Valteau-Couanet D, Frebourg T, Michon J, Lyonnet S, Amiel J, Delattre O. Somatic and germline activating mutations of the ALK kinase receptor in neuroblastoma. Nature. 2008;455(7215):967–70.

Kibirige MS, Birch JM, Campbell RH, Cattamaneni HR, Blair VA. Review of astrocytoma in childhood. Pediatr Hematol Oncol. 1989;6:319–29.

Knudson AG. Mutation and cancer: statistical study of retinoblastoma. Proc Natl Acad Sci USA. 1971;68:820–3.

Knudson AG, Strong LC. Mutation and cancer: neuroblastoma and pheochromocytoma. Am J Hum Genet. 1972;24:514–32.

Krutilkova V, Trkova M, Fleitz J, Gregor V, Novotna K, Krepelova A, Sumerauer D, Kodet R, Siruckova S, Plevova P, Bendova S, Hedvicakova P, Foreman NK, Sedlacek Z. Identification of five new families strengthens the link between childhood choroid plexus carcinoma and germline TP53 mutations. Eur J Cancer. 2005;41(11):1597–603.

Kushner BH, Gilbert F, Helson L. Familial neuroblastoma: case reports, literature review, and etiologic considerations. Cancer. 1986;57:1887–93.

Laberge-le Couteulx S, Jung HH, Labauge P, Houtteville JP, Lescoat C, Cecillon M, Marechal E, Joutel A, Bach JF, Tournier-Lasserve E. Truncating mutations in CCM1, encoding KRIT1, cause hereditary cavernous angiomas. Nat Genet. 1999;23(2):189–93.

Mahaley MS, Mettlin C, Natarajan N, Laws ER, Peace BB. National survey of patterns of care for brain-tumor patients. J Neurosurg. 1989;71:826–36.

Maher ER, Yates JRW, Ferguson-Smith MA. Statistical analysis of the two-stage mutation model in von Hippel–Lindau disease and in sporadic cerebellar hemangioblastoma and renal cell carcinoma. J Med Genet. 1990;27:311–4.

Maris JM, Mosse YP, Bradfield JP, Hou C, Monni S, Scott RH, Asgharzadeh S, Attiyeh EF, Diskin SJ, Laudenslager M, Winter C, Cole KA, Glessner JT, Kim C, Frackelton EC, Casalunovo T, Eckert AW, Capasso M, Rappaport EF, McConville C, London WB, Seeger RC, Rahman N, Devoto M, Grant SF, Li H, Hakonarson H. Chromosome 6p22 locus associated with clinically aggressive neuroblastoma. N Engl J Med. 2008;358(24):2585–93.

McConville C, Reid S, Baskcomb L, Douglas J, Rahman N. PHOX2B analysis in non-syndromic neuroblastoma cases shows novel mutations and genotype-phenotype associations. Am J Med Genet A. 2006;140(12):1297–301.

Miller RW. Deaths from childhood leukemia and solid tumors among twins and other sibs in the United States, 1960–67. J Natl Cancer Inst. 1971;46:203–9.

Mossé YP, Laudenslager M, Longo L, Cole KA, Wood A, Attiyeh EF, Laquaglia MJ, Sennett R, Lynch JE, Perri P, Laureys G, Speleman F, Kim C, Hou C, Hakonarson H, Torkamani A, Schork NJ, Brodeur GM, Tonini GP, Rappaport E, Devoto M, Maris JM. Identification of ALK as a major familial neuroblastoma predisposition gene. Nature. 2008;455(7215):930–5.

Nijssen PC, Deprez RH, Tijssen CC, et al. Familial anaplastic ependymoma: evidence of loss of chromosome 22 in tumor cells. J Neurol Neurosurg Psychiatr. 1994;57(10):1245–8.

Offit K, Levran O, Mullaney B, Mah K, Nafa K, Batish SD, Diotti R, Schneider H, Deffenbaugh A, Scholl T, Proud VK, Robson M, Norton L, Ellis N, Hanenberg H, Auerbach AD. Shared genetic susceptibility to breast cancer, brain tumors, and Fanconi anemia. J Natl Cancer Inst. 2003;95:1548–51.

Parsons DW, Li M, Zhang X, Jones S, Leary RJ, Lin JC-H, Boca SM, Carter H, Samayoa J, Bettegowda C, Gallia GL, Jallo GI, and 35 others. The genetic landscape of the childhood cancer medulloblastoma. Science. 2011;331:435–9.

Perri P, Bachetti T, Longo L, Matera I, Seri M, Tonini GP, Ceccherini I. PHOX2B mutations and genetic predisposition to neuroblastoma. Oncogene. 2005;24(18):3050–3.

Peyster RG, Ginsberg F, Hoover ED. Computed tomography of familial pinealoblastoma. J Comput Assist Tomogr. 1986;10:32–3.

Pulst SM, Rouleau GA, Marineau C, Fain P, Sieb JP. Familial meningioma is not allelic to neurofibromatosis 2. Neurology. 1993;43(10):2096–8.

Raabe EH, Laudenslager M, Winter C, Wasserman N, Cole K, LaQuaglia M, Maris DJ, Mosse YP, Maris JM. Prevalence and functional consequence of PHOX2B mutations in neuroblastoma. Oncogene. 2008;27(4):469–76.

Randerson-Moor JA, Harland M, Williams S, Cuthbert-Heavens D, Sheridan E, Aveyard J, Sibley K, Whitaker L, Knowles M, Bishop JN, Bishop DT. A germline deletion of p14(ARF) but not CDKN2A in a melanoma-neural system tumor syndrome family. Hum Mol Genet. 2001;10:55–62.

Riant F, Bergametti F, Ayrignac X, Boulday G, Tournier-Lasserve E. Recent insights into cerebral cavernous malformations: the molecular genetics of CCM. FEBS J. 2010;277(5):1070–5.

Roberts CW, Leroux MM, Fleming MD, Orkin SH. Highly penetrant, rapid tumorigenesis through conditional inversion of the tumor suppressor gene Snf5. Cancer Cell. 2002;2:415–25.

Robertson CM, Tyrell JC, Pritchard J. Familial neural crest tumors. Eur J Pediatr. 1991; 150:789–92.

Robertson LB, Armstrong GN, Olver BD, Lloyd AL, Shete S, Lau C, Claus EB, Barnholtz-Sloan J, Lai R, Il'yasova D, Schildkraut J, Bernstein JL, Olson SH, Jenkins RB, Yang P, Rynearson AL, Wrensch M, McCoy L, Wienkce JK, McCarthy B, Davis F, Vick NA, Johansen C, Bødtcher H, Sadetzki S, Bruchim RB, Yechezkel GH, Andersson U, Melin BS, Bondy ML, Houlston RS. Survey of familial glioma and role of germline p16INK4A/p14ARF and p53 mutation. Fam Cancer. 2010;9(3):413–21.

Robinow M, Johnson GF, Minella PA. Aicardi syndrome, papilloma of the choroid plexus, cleft lip and cleft posterior palate. J Pediatr. 1986;104:404–5.

Rousseau G, Noguchi T, Bourdon V, Sobol H, Olschwang S. SMARCB1/INI1 germline mutations contribute to 10% of sporadic schwannomatosis. BMC Neurol. 2011;11:9.

Sabbaghian N, Hamel N, Srivastava A, Albrecht S, Priest JR, Foulkes WD. Germline DICER1 mutation and associated loss of heterozygosity in a pineoblastoma. J Med Genet. 2012;49(7):417–9.

Scheurer ME, Etzel CJ, Liu M, Barnholtz-Sloan J, Wiklund F, Tavelin B, Wrensch MR, Melin BS, Bondy ML, GLIOGENE Consortium. Familial aggregation of glioma: a pooled analysis. Am J Epidemiol. 2010;172(10):1099–107.

Schneppenheim R, Frühwald MC, Gesk S, Hasselblatt M, Jeibmann A, Kordes U, Kreuz M, Leuschner I, Martin Subero JI, Obser T, Oyen F, Vater I, Siebert R. Germline nonsense mutation and somatic inactivation of SMARCA4/BRG1 in a family with rhabdoid tumor predisposition syndrome. Am J Hum Genet. 2010;86(2):279–84.

Shete S, Hosking FJ, Robertson LB, Dobbins SE, Sanson M, Malmer B, et al. Genome-wide association study identifies five susceptibility loci for glioma. Nat Genet. 2009;41:899–904.

Shete S, Lau CC, Houlston RS, Claus EB, Barnholtz-Sloan J, Lai R, Il'yasova D, Schildkraut J, Sadetzki S, Johansen C, Bernstein JL, Olson SH, Jenkins RB, Yang P, Vick NA, Wrensch M, Davis FG, McCarthy BJ, Leung EH, Davis C, Cheng R, Hosking FJ, Armstrong GN, Liu Y, Yu RK, Henriksson R, Gliogene Consortium, Melin BS, Bondy ML. Genome-wide high-density SNP linkage search for glioma susceptibility loci: results from the Gliogene Consortium. Cancer Res. 2011;71(24):7568–75.

Smith MJ, Kulkarni A, Rustad C, Bowers NL, Wallace AJ, Holder SE, Heiberg A, Ramsden RT, Evans DG. Vestibular schwannomas occur in schwannomatosis and should not be considered an exclusion criterion for clinical diagnosis. Am J Med Genet A. 2011;158A:215–9.

Smith MJ, Wallace AJ, Bowers NL, Rustad CF, Woods CG, Leschziner GD, Ferner RE, Evans DG. Frequency of SMARCB1 mutations in familial and sporadic schwannomatosis. Neurogenetics. 2012;13(2):141–5.

Smith MJ, O'Sullivan J, Bhaskar SS, Hadfield KD, Poke G, Caird J, Sharif S, Eccles D, Fitzpatrick D, Rawluk D, du Plessis D, Newman WG, Evans DG. Loss-of-function mutations in SMARCE1 cause an inherited disorder of multiple spinal meningiomas. Nat Genet. 2013;45:295–8.

Tabori U, Shlien A, Baskin B, Levitt S, Ray P, Alon N, Hawkins C, Bouffet E, Pienkowska M, Lafay-Cousin L, Gozali A, Zhukova N, Shane L, Gonzalez I, Finlay J, Malkin D. TP53 alterations determine clinical subgroups and survival of patients with choroid plexus tumors. J Clin Oncol. 2010;28(12):1995–2001.

Tachibana I, Smith JS, Sato K, Hosek SM, Kimmel DW, Jenkins RB. Investigation of germline PTEN, p53, p16(INK4A)/p14(ARF), and CDK4 alterations in familial glioma. Am J Med Genet. 2000;92:136–41.

Taylor MD, Gokgoz N, Andrulis IL, Mainprize TG, Drake JM, Rutka JT. Familial posterior fossa brain tumors of infancy secondary to germline mutation of the hSNF5 gene. Am J Hum Genet. 2000;66:1403–6.

Taylor MD, Liu L, Raffel C, Hui CC, Mainprize TG, Zhang X, Agatep R, Chiappa S, Gao L, Lowrance A, Hao A, Goldstein AM, Stavrou T, Scherer SW, Dura WT, Wainwright B, Squire JA, Rutka JT, Hogg D. Mutations in SUFU predispose to medulloblastoma. Nat Genet. 2002;31(3):306–10.

Thuwe I, Lundstrom B, Walinder J. Familial brain tumor. Lancet. 1979;i:504.

Torres CF, Korones DN, Pilcher W. Multiple ependymomas in a patient with Turcot's syndrome. Med Pediatr Oncol. 1997;28:59–61.

Tos M, Thomsen J. Epidemiology of acoustic neuromas. J Laryngol Otol. 1984;98:685–92.

Trochet D, Bourdeaut F, Janoueix-Lerosey I, Deville A, de Pontual L, Schleiermacher G, Coze C, Philip N, Frébourg T, Munnich A, Lyonnet S, Delattre O, Amiel J. Germline mutations of the paired-like homeobox 2B (PHOX2B) gene in neuroblastoma. Am J Hum Genet. 2004;74(4):761–4.

van den Munckhof P, Christiaans I, Kenter SB, Baas F, Hulsebos TJ. Germline SMARCB1 mutation predisposes to multiple meningiomas and schwannomas with preferential location of cranial meningiomas at the falx cerebri. Neurogenetics. 2012;13(1):1–7.

Vieregge P, Gerhard L, Nahser HC. Familial glioma: occurrence within the 'familial cancer syndrome' and systemic malformations. J Neurol. 1987;234:220–32.

von Koch CS, Gulati M, Aldape K, Berger MS. Familial medulloblastoma: case report of one family and review of the literature. Neurosurgery. 2002;51(1):227–33.

Woods WG, Gao RN, Shuster JJ, Robison LL, Bernstein M, Weitzman S, Bunin G, Levy I, Brossard J, Dougherty G, Tuchman M, Lemieux B. Screening of infants and mortality due to neuroblastoma. N Engl J Med. 2002;346:1041–6.

Zwetsloot CP, Kros JM, Paz y Geuze HD. Familial occurrence of tumors of the choroid plexus. J Med Genet. 1991;28:492–4.

Chapter 2
Eye

The ocular tumors discussed in this section include retinoblastoma, hemangioblastoma, optic nerve glioma, meningioma, and melanoma. Ocular rhabdomyosarcoma is discussed with rhabdomyosarcoma of other sites. Genetic disorders associated with significant ocular manifestations (neoplastic and nonneoplastic) include neurofibromatosis type 1 (NF1) (p. 288), neurofibromatosis type 2 (NF2) (p. 293), von Hippel–Lindau (VHL) disease (p. 313), tuberous sclerosis (p. 307), and familial adenomatous polyposis coli (p. 241).

Retinoblastoma

Retinoblastoma is the commonest malignant ocular tumor of childhood and affects around 1 per 20,000 children. Survival rates in the USA approach 100 % though the rates are much lower in developing countries. The tumor is derived from primitive retinal cells (retinoblasts) and usually presents in early childhood (90 % before the age of 5 years). Less than 10 % of children with retinoblastoma have a positive family history (where inheritance is autosomal dominant), but new mutations are frequent and approximately 40 % of retinoblastoma patients have a genetic predisposition. Retinoblastoma holds a unique place in human cancer genetics as the subject of Al Knudson's pioneering work on the "two-hit model of tumorigenesis" and the paradigm of the tumor suppressor gene.

Retinoblastoma typically presents as leukocoria (white eye, cat's eye reflex) or strabismus. It is bilateral in about 30 % of cases, and these children have a younger age at diagnosis (mean 8 months) than those with unilateral tumor (mean 25 months). Bilateral or multifocal tumors occur in patients with germline mutations of the retinoblastoma (*RB1*) gene, but about 15 % of children with a single tumor will have a germline mutation. The 40 % of all children with retinoblastoma who carry a germline retinoblastoma gene mutation are at risk for secondary tumors, especially osteosarcoma and soft tissue sarcomas (see below). This predisposition is exacerbated in those who receive radiotherapy. A few individuals (less

S.V. Hodgson et al., *A Practical Guide to Human Cancer Genetics*,
DOI 10.1007/978-1-4471-2375-0_2, © Springer-Verlag London 2014

Table 2.1 Risk of retinoblastoma in relatives of a child with retinoblastoma and no family history

Retinoblastoma in proband	Relationship to proband	Risk of carrying *RB* mutation[a] (%)	Risk of developing retinoblastoma tumor[a] (%)	Risk of developing retinoblastoma tumor[b] (%)
Bilateral	Offspring	50	45	44
Bilateral	Sibling or dizygotic twin	5	2.7	2
Bilateral	Offspring of unaffected sibling	0.5	0.27	
Bilateral	First cousin	0.05	0.027	
Bilateral	Monozygotic twin	100	90	
Unilateral	Offspring	7.5	5.7	1
Unilateral	Sibling or dizygotic twin	0.8	0.4	1
Unilateral	Offspring of unaffected sibling	0.08	0.04	
Unilateral	First cousin	0.008	0.004	
Unilateral	Monozygotic twin	10	5.4	

[a]The calculated risks from Musarella and Gallie (1987) take into account the retinoblastoma mutation rate and assume that 90 % of individuals with a germline mutation will develop a tumor and 15 % of patients with unilateral retinoblastoma have a germline mutation
[b]The risks from Draper et al. (1992) for siblings relate to the first child, when there are further unaffected siblings the risk will be lower

than 2 %) with germline retinoblastoma gene mutations may develop a retinoma. These benign retinal lesions appear as focal translucencies with cottage-cheese-like calcification and underlying choroidal and retinal pigment epithelial disturbance. A retinoma is thought to result when a second *RB1* mutation occurs in a retinoblast which is almost differentiated. About 2 % of all patients with retinoblastoma also have an intracranial lesion, usually in the pineal gland. The association of pineal tumor and retinoblastoma is often termed trilateral retinoblastoma and occurs in patients with germline retinoblastoma mutations.

The retinoblastoma mutation is non-penetrant in approximately 10 % of obligate carriers. Although there is no detectable paternal age effect on new mutations for retinoblastoma, most new hereditary mutations develop in paternal germ cells (Zhu et al. 1989). An excess of males among patients with bilateral sporadic disease has been noted, and Naumova and Sapienza (1994) suggested the involvement of genomic imprinting effects. Although an excess of retinoblastoma cases was reported in a Netherlands cohort of children conceived by assisted reproductive technologies, this finding requires replication (Moll et al. 2003).

About 60 % of retinoblastomas result from somatic (acquired) mutations inactivating both alleles of the retinoblastoma gene. Such patients develop single tumors and there is no risk to their offspring. However, 15 % of patients with single tumors will have a germline mutation. Risk estimates for the relatives of isolated cases of retinoblastoma are given in Table 2.1. The later estimates of Draper et al. (1992) are lower in some cases than earlier estimates. Genetic counseling for the relatives of patients with isolated unilateral retinoblastoma is complicated by the possibility for mosaicism of a germline *RB1* mutation (Lohmann et al. 1997). Individuals with genetic retinoblastoma (germline mutation) are at increased risk for second tumors, but children with nonge-netic tumors are not. The risk of second primary neoplasms reflects a genetic predispo-sition to non-retinoblastoma tumors and the effects of treatment (e.g., radiation). Draper et al. (1986) estimated that the cumulative probability of a second primary neoplasm in genetic retinoblastoma patients at 18 years after diagnosis is 8.4 % for all tumors and 6 % for osteosarcoma. The risks for osteosarcoma outside and within the radiation fields were 2.2 and 3.7 %, respectively, and thus patients with genetic retinoblastoma may be more sensitive to radiation-induced oncogenesis. The most common site of osteosarcoma outside the radiation field is in the femur, and genetic retinoblastoma patients are at a 200–500-fold increased risk of this complication. Soft tissue sarcomas also occur with increased frequency in patients with genetic retinoblastoma. Studies of non-ocular cancer in relatives of retinoblastoma patients have demonstrated that reti-noblastoma mutation carriers are at increased risk of a variety of other cancers (overall relative risk 11.6) including cancer of the lung (relative risk 15), malignant melanoma, and bladder cancer (Sanders et al. 1988). Moll et al. (1996) estimated cumulative inci-dences of second primary tumors in hereditary retinoblastoma of 4 and 18 % at ages 10 and 35 years, respectively. Eng et al. (1993) reported a cumulative probability of death from a second primary neoplasm of 26 % at 40 years after bilateral retinoblastoma. The most common second primary tumors were bone and connective tissue neoplasms and malignant melanoma. Eng et al. (1993) also demonstrated that radiotherapy increased the risk of a second primary tumor and suggested that all patients with inherited reti-noblastoma should receive lifelong surveillance for second primary tumors. In a fol-low-up study of UK hereditary retinoblastoma cases, Fletcher et al. (2004) found a cumulative cancer incidence and mortality of 69 and 48 %, respectively. In contrast to patients treated by radiotherapy, sarcomas accounted for only a minority of tumors, and there was an increased mortality for lung cancer (standardized mortality ratio (SMR) = 7), bladder cancer (SMR = 26), and all other epithelial cancers combined (SMR = 3.3).

The retinoblastoma gene was initially assigned to chromosome 13 band q14 by reports of children with retinoblastoma and interstitial deletions of chromosome 13. About 3 % of children with retinoblastoma will have a cytogenetically visible chro-mosome 13 deletion or translocation. Retinoblastoma cases with constitutional chro-mosome deletion may have associated mental retardation, and most have reduced serum levels of esterase D (the gene for which maps close to the retinoblastoma gene (RB1)). The *RB1* gene spans 200 kb in 13q14 (Friend et al. 1986) and encodes a 110-kDa nuclear phosphoprotein with tumor suppressor activity (Huang et al. 1988).

The identification of the retinoblastoma gene has enabled the presymptomatic identification of individuals with germline mutations by a variety of techniques. Intragenic restriction fragment length polymorphisms (RFLPs) are informative in about 95 % of families and usually allow accurate presymptomatic diagnosis of at-risk relatives in families with two or more affected members but are unhelpful in families with only a single case (Wiggs et al. 1988). Mutation detection rates of

80 % or more were reported by Lohmann et al. (1996) and Houdayer et al. (2004) using a variety of molecular genetic techniques. Germline deletions are not infrequent, and an appropriate deletion scanning approach (e.g., multiplex ligation-dependent probe amplification (MLPA)) should be performed as part of the mutation detection strategy. *RB1* mutations are heterogeneous, and generally no clear genotype–phenotype associations have been described except that promoter mutations and some intragenic mutations with residual protein activity may display reduced penetrance (Kratzke et al. 1994; Cowell et al. 1996). The identification of a germline mutation in a unilateral sporadic case distinguishes those individuals with simplex retinoblastoma and a new germline mutation from nonhereditary cases. When a germline mutation is identified, other relatives can be tested. When histopathological material (formalin fixed paraffin embedded) from a deceased patient is available, mutation analysis can be undertaken on the tumor tissue and further investigations undertaken to determine if a characterized mutation is somatic or germline. Indeed, if tumor tissue is available, then this will be analyzed first to define the two *RB1* mutations. Constitutional DNA (e.g., blood) is then tested to determine if both are somatic or one is germline (as mosaicism is not uncommon, blood DNA testing must use methods sensitive enough to detect mosaic mutations). If two mutations are detected in the tumor and neither is detected in blood, then siblings do not require surveillance though there will still be a small risk to the patient's offspring (from mosaicism). A pathogenic mutation can be detected in blood DNA of ~95 % of patients with hereditary retinoblastoma. In patients who present with developmental delay and/or dysmorphic features, FISH or array CGH analysis to detect copy number variations is performed first.

Children with an *RB1* mutation should undergo an eye examination every 3–4 weeks until age 1 year and then every 2–3 months until age 5 years followed by annual examination for the rest of their lives (Lohmann et al. 2011). There are no specific guidelines for the detection of non-ocular second tumors, but complaints of bone pain or lumps should be investigated promptly.

In the absence of molecular genetic diagnosis, the parents and siblings of all children with retinoblastoma should undergo thorough ophthalmological assessment. Offspring and siblings of retinoblastoma patients should be followed up from birth, with complete retinal examination. For example, examination should be performed at birth and monthly until 3 months of age without anesthesia, then under general anesthetic every 3 months until the age of 2 years, then every 4 months until the age of 3 years. Thereafter, examinations without general anesthesia can be performed every 6 months until the age of 5 years, and then every 12 months until the age of 11 years (although the frequency and duration of screening can be modified according to the results of DNA analysis). Parents of children with apparently sporadic retinoblastoma must be examined to exclude a regressed tumor or retinoma because this would identify the child as having a germline *RB1* gene mutation. Children with retinoblastoma will require careful follow-up to detect new tumors or recurrence. New tumors occurred in 11 % of children studied by Salmonsen et al. (1979). Traditionally, all children with retinoblastoma are followed up with regular retinal examinations under general anesthesia. However, the application of DNA techniques to identify *RB1* gene mutations in tumors and constitutional DNA enables follow-up to be restricted to those shown to have germline *RB1* mutations. This not only enhances management of at-risk relatives but is also a cost-effective strategy (Noorani et al. 1996). Survivors of bilateral retinoblastoma (and unilateral retinoblastoma in those with germline retinoblastoma gene mutations) are at high risk of osteosarcoma in adolescence and of the occurrence of other cancers (see above).

Retinal Astrocytic Hamartoma

This benign, nonprogressive tumor is most commonly seen in patients with tuberous sclerosis and occurs in about 50 % of patients with this disorder. Retinal astrocytic hamartomas have also been described rarely in neurofibromatosis type 1 and type 2 (see p. 288 and p. 293) (Sachdeva et al. 2010; Martin et al. 2010). Sporadic retinal astrocytomas differ from those in tuberous sclerosis in that a proportion appear to be true neoplasms and may invade locally (Arnold et al. 1985).

Optic Glioma

Although rare, glioma is the commonest optic nerve tumor in childhood. Optic glioma is associated with neurofibromatosis type 1 (NF1) (see p. 288) in a third of cases. Approximately 15 % of patients with NF1 develop an optic glioma (which may be bilateral) though the frequency of symptomatic optic glioma is about 5 % (Lewis et al. 1984; Huson et al. 1988; Singhal et al. 2002). McGaughran et al. (1999) estimated an actuarial risk of optic glioma in NF1 patients of 3.7 % at age 10 years and 6.2 % at age 25 years. A potential association between mutations at the 5′ end of the *NF1* gene and the development of optic nerve gliomas has been reported (Sharif et al. 2011).

All patients with optic glioma, and their families, should be assessed for evidence of NF1. Histological appearance is of a low-grade (pilocytic) astrocytoma, spontaneous regression may occur, and many consider these tumors to be congenital hamartomas rather than acquired neoplasms (Riccardi and Eichner 1986). Optic gliomas usually originate in the optic nerves or chiasm, and presentation is usually with visual impairment and/or painless proptosis. Most NF1-associated optic gliomas are orbital. Computerized tomography (CT) or magnetic resonance image (MRI) scanning will demonstrate optic glioma and differentiate from optic nerve meningioma. The natural history of optic glioma is not well defined. Most are nonprogressive and conservative management is usually preferred. Treatment (surgery or radiotherapy) of optic nerve glioma is indicated for progressive visual loss associated with proptosis. Treatment of chiasmal lesions is more difficult, but again, most are nonprogressive and conservative management is pursued.

Ocular Choristoma

Ocular choristomas are congenital lesions, which are deposits of normal tissue in an abnormal location. They are the most common epibulbar and orbital tumors in children, with an incidence of about 1 per 5,000 (Mansour et al. 1989). Dermoid and epidermoid cysts are both included in this group. Ocular choristomas may be associated with Goldenhar syndrome (hemifacial microsomia) or epidermal nevus syndrome. In the latter disorder, choristomas are frequently bilateral and extensive. Goldenhar syndrome is usually sporadic but in rare cases can be familial (Tasse et al. 2007). Familial choristoma with dominant inheritance not associated with Goldenhar syndrome occurs rarely (Mansour et al. 1989).

Ciliary Body Medulloepithelioma

These very rare eye tumors have been reported to occur in children with DICER1 mutations (Slade et al. 2011).

Cavernous Hemangioma

This rare ocular tumor should be distinguished from retinal hemangioblastoma. Mean age at diagnosis is 23 years and less than 10 % are bilateral. Cavernous hemangioma is usually nonprogressive, and serious complications are uncommon. Retinal or optic disc cavernous hemangiomas are associated with cutaneous vascular lesions in about 28 % of patients and in some patients with intracranial cavernous hemangioma (Lewis et al. 1975). A triad of ocular, central nervous system, and cutaneous cavernous hemangiomas can be dominantly inherited with variable expression and incomplete penetrance (Brown and Shields 1985). Thus, the finding of retinal cavernous or choroidal hemangioma is an indication to search for features of systemic or familial disease (Sarraf et al. 2000). It has been estimated that about 5 % of patients with cerebral cavernous hemangiomas will have a retinal lesion (Labauge et al. 2006). Familial cerebral cavernous hemangioma (p. 5) is a genetically heterogeneous disorder and can be caused by mutations in *KRIT1* (*CCM1*), *CCM2*, or *PDCD10* (*CCM3*), and it appears that each of these subtypes may be associated with retinal lesions (Labauge et al. 2006).

Hemangioblastoma

Retinal hemangioblastoma (also called angioma) is the most common presentation of von Hippel–Lindau (VHL) disease (Maher et al. 1990). The exact proportion of patients with retinal hemangioblastoma who have this disease is unclear. The most frequent estimate is 40 %, but Neumann and Wiestler (1991) detected evidence of

Table 2.2 Estimated probability of underlying VHL disease in a patient with a solitary ocular angioma after careful ophthalmic screening

	Probability by age group (years)			
Other negative information	<20	21–40	41–60	>60
None	0.30	0.30	0.30	0.30
DNA	0.11	0.11	0.11	0.11
Systemic screening	0.27	0.13	0.06	0.02
Parent history	0.19	0.13	0.09	0.09
Parent history + systemic screening	0.17	0.05	0.02	0.01
DNA + parent history	0.06	0.04	0.03	0.03
DNA + systemic screening	0.10	0.04	0.02	0.01
DNA + systemic screening + parent history	0.06	0.01	0.00	0.00

Source: From Webster et al. (2000) – J Med Genet. 37:62–3

the disease in 86 % of their patients with retinal angiomatosis. All patients with retinal angioma should be investigated for subclinical manifestations of VHL disease (see p. 313). All patients with multiple retinal angiomas satisfy clinical diagnostic criteria for VHL disease, but in atypical cases, expert ophthalmological review is helpful to confirm that the lesions are hemangioblastomas and not other types of vascular lesion (e.g., Coat disease). Webster et al. (1998) investigated 17 cases with VHL-like solitary ocular angioma and found no evidence of other complications of this disease in themselves or in family members. They concluded that sporadic ocular angioma can occur in the absence of VHL disease. The tumors are similar in anatomical location, and cases are similar in age of presentation and degree of visual morbidity compared to those with the disease. Overall the risk of underlying VHL disease in a patient with a solitary ocular angioma was 30 %; this risk decreased with negative DNA and clinical screening and also with increasing age (Table 2.2) (Webster et al. 1999).

Histologically VHL-associated retinal hemangioblastomas resemble cerebellar hemangioblastomas with stromal cells surrounding capillary endothelial cells and glial cell admixed. Molecular studies demonstrate that loss of the wild-type VHL allele occurs in the stromal cells, and this leads to activation of HIF transcription factors and expression of vascular endothelial growth factor and other angiogenic factors (Chan et al. 2007).

Melanoma

Uveal melanoma is the most common primary intraocular malignancy in adults, with an incidence 6/million per year (lifetime risk 1 in 2,500) (Canning and Hungerford 1988). Familial cases are uncommon and account for about 0.6 % of all patients (Singh et al. 1996). Canning and Hungerford (1988) reviewed 14 kindreds with familial ocular melanoma. The mean age at diagnosis is significantly younger in familial than in sporadic cases (42 and 56 years, respectively), and inheritance can be autosomal dominant with incomplete penetrance. Intraocular melanoma may be associated with familial atypical mole-melanoma syndrome (p. 178), ocular melanocytosis, and neurofibromatosis type 1 (p. 288) (Singh et al. 1995). Though a few studies have suggested that uveal melanoma might be linked to breast cancer (in particular *BRCA2* mutations), this link does not appear to be a frequent cause of uveal melanoma (Harbour 2012).

The most commonly detected somatic mutations in uveal melanoma are missense mutations in *GNAQ* or *GNA11* genes (~80 % of cases) and inactivating mutations in *BAP1* (~50 % of cases) (van Raamsdonk et al. 2010; Harbour et al. 2010). Germline *BAP1* mutations can predispose to a multiple system-inherited cancer syndrome characterized by susceptibility to uveal melanoma and other tumors including cutaneous melanocytic tumors, malignant mesothelioma, lung adenocarcinoma, and abdominal adenocarcinoma (Testa et al. 2011; Abdel-Rahman et al. 2011). Familial uveal melanoma is now thought to account for 2–5 % of all cases (Harbour 2012).

Meningioma

Intraorbital meningioma is an uncommon tumor that may present at any age but predominantly occurs in middle-aged women. Most tumors are unilateral, but a small proportion of patients have bilateral involvement. Optic nerve sheath meningioma may complicate NF2 (see p. 293), when it is usually unilateral but can be bilateral (Jain et al. 2010).

References

Abdel-Rahman MH, Pilarski R, Cebulla CM, Massengill JB, Christopher BN, Boru G, Hovland P, Davidorf FH. Germline BAP1 mutation predisposes to uveal melanoma, lung adenocarcinoma, meningioma, and other cancers. J Med Genet. 2011 Dec;48(12):856–9.

Arnold AC, Hepler RS, Yee RW, Maggiano J, Eng LF, Foos RY. Solitary retinal astrocytoma. Surv Ophthalmol. 1985;30:173–81.

Brown GC, Shields JA. Tumors of the optic nerve head. Surv Ophthalmol. 1985;29:239–64.

Canning CR, Hungerford J. Familial uveal melanoma. Br J Ophthalmol. 1988;72:241–3.

Chan CC, Collins AB, Chew EY. Molecular pathology of eyes with von Hippel-Lindau (VHL) Disease: a review. Retina. 2007;27(1):1–7.

Cowell JK, Bia B, Akoulitchev A. A novel mutation in the promoter region in a family with a mild form of retinoblastoma indicates the location of a new regulatory domain for the RB1 gene. Oncology. 1996;12:431–6.

Draper GJ, Sanders BM, Kingston JE. Second primary neoplasms in patients with retinoblastoma. Br J Cancer. 1986;53:661–71.

Draper GJ, Sanders BM, Brownbill PA, Hawkins MM. Patterns of risk of hereditary retinoblastoma and applications to genetic counseling. Br J Cancer. 1992;66:211–9.

Eng C, Li FP, Abramson DH, et al. Mortality from second tumors among long-term survivors of retinoblastoma. J Natl Cancer Inst. 1993;85:1121–8.

Fletcher O, Easton D, Anderson K, Gilham C, Jay M, Peto J. Lifetime risks of common cancers among retinoblastoma survivors. Natl Cancer Inst. 2004;96(5):357–63.

Friend SH, Bernards R, Rogelj S, et al. A human DNA segment with properties of the gene that predisposes to retinoblastoma and osteosarcoma. Nature. 1986;323:643–6.

Harbour JW. The genetics of uveal melanoma: an emerging framework for targeted therapy. Pigment Cell Melanoma Res. 2012;25(2):171–81.

Harbour JW, Onken MD, Roberson ED, Duan S, Cao L, Worley LA, Council ML, Matatall KA, Helms C, Bowcock AM. Frequent mutation of BAP1 in metastasizing uveal melanomas. Science. 2010;330(6009):1410–3.

Houdayer C, Gauthier-Villars M, Laugé A, Pagès-Berhouet S, Dehainault C, Caux-Moncoutier V, Karczynski P, Tosi M, Doz F, Desjardins L, Couturier J, Stoppa-Lyonnet D. Comprehensive screening for constitutional RB1 mutations by DHPLC and QMPSF. Hum Mutat. 2004;23(2): 193–202.

Huang HS, Yeo J, Shaw Y, et al. Suppression of neoplastic phenotype by replacement of the RB gene in human cancer cells. Science. 1988;242:1563–6.

Huson SM, Harper PS, Compston DAS. Von Recklinghausen neurofibromatosis. Brain. 1988;111: 1355–81.

Jain D, Ebrahimi KB, Miller NR, Eberhart CG. Intraorbital meningiomas: a pathologic review using current World Health Organization criteria. Arch Pathol Lab Med. 2010;134(5):766–70.

Kratzke RA, Otterson GA, Hogg A, et al. Partial inactivation of the RB product in a family with incomplete penetrance of familial retinoblastoma and benign retinal tumors. Oncogene. 1994;9:1321–6.

Labauge P, Krivosic V, Denier C, Tournier-Lasserve E, Gaudric A. Frequency of retinal cavernomas in 60 patients with familial cerebral cavernomas: a clinical and genetic study. Arch Ophthalmol. 2006;124(6):885–6.

Lewis RA, Cohen MH, Wise GN. Cavernous hemangioma of the retina and optic disc. Br J Ophthalmol. 1975;59:422–4.

Lewis RA, Riccardi VM, Gerson LP, Whitford R, Axelson KA. Von Recklinghausen neurofibromatosis: II. Incidence of optic-nerve gliomata. Ophthalmology. 1984;91:929–35.

Lohmann DR, Brandt B, Hopping W, Passarge E, Horsthemke B. The spectrum of RB1 germ-line mutations in hereditary retinoblastoma. Am J Hum Genet. 1996;58:940–9.

Lohmann DR, Gerick M, Brandt B, et al. Constitutional RB1-gene mutations in patients with isolated unilateral retinoblastoma. Am J Hum Genet. 1997;61:282–94.

Lohmann D, Gallie B, Dommering C, Gauthier-Villars M. Clinical utility gene card for: retinoblastoma. Eur J Hum Genet. 2011;19. doi:10.1038/ejhg.2010.200.

Maher ER, Yates JRW, Harries R, et al. Clinical features and natural history of von Hippel–Lindau disease. Q J Med. 1990;77:1151–63.

Mansour AM, Barber JC, Reinecke RD, Wang FM. Ocular choristomas. Surv Ophthalmol. 1989; 33:339–58.

Martin K, Rossi V, Ferrucci S, Pian D. Retinal astrocytic hamartoma. Optometry. 2010; 81(5):221–33.

McGaughran JM, Harris DI, Donnai D, Teare D, MacLeod R, Westerbeek R, Kingston H, Super M, Harris R, Evans DG. A clinical study of type 1 neurofibromatosis in north west England. J Med Genet. 1999;36:197–203.

Moll AC, Imhof SM, Bouter LM, et al. Second primary tumors in patients with hereditary retinoblastoma: a register-based follow-up study, 1945–1994. Int J Cancer. 1996;67:15–9.

Moll AC, Imhof SM, Cruysberg JR, Schouten-van Meeteren AY, Boers M, van Leeuwen FE. Incidence of retinoblastoma in children born after in-vitro fertilisation. Lancet. 2003; 361(9354):309–10.

Musarella MA, Gallie BL. A simplified scheme for genetic counseling in retinoblastoma. J Pediatr Ophthalmol Strabismus. 1987;24:124–5.

Naumova A, Sapienza C. The genetics of retinoblastoma, revisited. Am J Hum Genet. 1994; 54:264–73.

Neumann HPH, Wiestler OD. Clustering of features of von Hippel–Lindau syndrome: evidence for a complex genetic locus. Lancet. 1991;337:1052–4.

Noorani HZ, Khan HN, Gallie BL, Detsky AS. Cost comparison of molecular versus conventional screening of relatives at risk for retinoblastoma. Am J Hum Genet. 1996;59:301–7.

Riccardi VM, Eichner JE. Neurofibromatosis: phenotype, natural history and pathogenesis. Baltimore: Johns Hopkins University Press; 1986.

Sachdeva R, Rothner DA, Traboulsi EI, Hayden BC, Rychwalski PJ. Astrocytic hamartoma of the optic disc and multiple café-au-lait macules in a child with neurofibromatosis type 2. Ophthalmic Genet. 2010;31(4):209–14.

Salmonsen PC, Ellsworth RM, Kitchen FD. The occurrence of new retinoblastoma after treatment. Ophthalmology. 1979;86:840–3.

Sanders BM, Draper CJ, Kingston JE. Retinoblastoma in Great Britain 1969–80: incidence, treatment, and survival. Br J Ophthalmol. 1988;72:576–83.

Sarraf D, Payne AM, Kitchen ND, Sehmi KS, Downes SM, Bird AC. Familial cavernous hemangioma: an expanding ocular spectrum. Arch Ophthalmol. 2000;118(7):969–73.

Sharif S, Upadhyaya M, Ferner R, Majounie E, Shenton A, Baser M, Thakker N, Evans DG. A molecular analysis of individuals with neurofibromatosis type 1(NF1) and optic pathway gliomas (OPGs), and an assessment of genotype-phenotype correlations. J Med Genet. 2011;48(4):256–60.

Singh AD, Shields CL, Shields JA, Eagle RC, De Potter P. Uveal melanoma and familial atypical mole and melanoma (FAM-M) syndrome. Ophthalmic Genet. 1995;16:53–61.

Singh AD, Wang MX, Donoso LA, Shields CL, De Potter P, Shields JA. Genetic aspects of uveal melanoma: a brief review. Semin Oncol. 1996;23:768–72.

Singhal S, Birch JM, Kerr B, Lashford L, Evans DG. Neurofibromatosis type 1 and sporadic optic gliomas. Arch Dis Child. 2002;87:65–70.

Slade I, Bacchelli C, Davies H, Murray A, Abbaszadeh F, Hanks S, Barfoot R, Burke A, Chisholm J, Hewitt M, Jenkinson H, King D, Morland B, Pizer B, Prescott K, Saggar A, Side L, Traunecker H, Vaidya S, Ward P, Futreal PA, Vujanic G, Nicholson AG, Sebire N, Turnbull C, Priest JR, Pritchard-Jones K, Houlston R, Stiller C, Stratton MR, Douglas J, Rahman N. DICER1 syndrome: clarifying the diagnosis, clinical features and management implications of a pleiotropic tumour predisposition syndrome. J Med Genet. 2011;48(4):273–8.

Tasse C, Majewski F, Bohringer S, Fischer S, Ludecke H-J, Gillessen-Kaesbach G, Wieczorek D. A family with autosomal dominant oculo-auriculo-vertebral spectrum. Clin Dysmorph. 2007;16:1–7.

Testa JR, Cheung M, Pei J, Below JE, Tan Y, Sementino E, Cox NJ, Dogan AU, Pass HI, Trusa S, Hesdorffer M, Nasu M, Powers A, Rivera Z, Comertpay S, Tanji M, Gaudino G, Yang H, Carbone M. Germline BAP1 mutations predispose to malignant mesothelioma. Nat Genet. 2011;43(10):1022–5.

Van Raamsdonk CD, Griewank KG, Crosby MB, Garrido MC, Vemula S, Wiesner T, Obenauf AC, Wackernagel W, Green G, Bouvier N, Sozen MM, Baimukanova G, Roy R, Heguy A, Dolgalev I, Khanin R, Busam K, Speicher MR, O'Brien J, Bastian BC. Mutations in GNA11 in uveal melanoma. N Engl J Med. 2010;363(23):2191–9.

Webster A, et al. An analysis of phenotypic variation in the familial cancer syndrome von Hippel-Lindau disease: evidence for modifier effects. Am J Hum Genet. 1998;63:1025–35.

Webster AR, Maher ER, Moore AT. Clinical characteristics of ocular angiomatosis in von Hippel-Lindau disease and correlation with germline mutation. Arch Ophthalmol. 1999;117:371–8.

Webster AR, Maher ER, Bird AC, Moore AT. Risk of multisystem disease in isolated ocular angioma (haemangioblastoma). J Med Genet. 2000;37:62–3.

Wiggs J, Nordenskjold M, Yandell D. Prediction of the risk of hereditary retinoblastoma, using DNA polymorphisms within the retinoblastoma gene. New Engl J Med. 1988;318:151–7.

Zhu X, Dunn JM, Phillips RA, et al. Preferential germline mutation of the paternal allele in retinoblastoma. Nature. 1989;340:312–4.

Chapter 3
Cardiorespiratory System and Thorax

Head and Neck Cancer

General

Squamous carcinomas of the head and neck (a grouping which includes tongue and mouth, nasopharynx, and larynx) are associated with cigarette smoking and alcohol ingestion (although the risk factors for different sites may differ). In addition, infection with human papillomavirus (HPV) is associated with cancers of the oropharynx (D'Souza et al. 2007). Specific head and neck cancers may be associated with familial cancer syndromes such as hereditary non-polyposis colon cancer syndrome and Li–Fraumeni syndrome (larynx) and Fanconi anemia (oral cancer). Foulkes et al. (1996) reported a relative risk of 3.7 for developing head and neck cancer in first-degree relatives of an affected case, but the relative risk was almost 8 if the index case had multiple primaries.

Exome resequencing studies of squamous carcinomas of the head and neck revealed that the most frequently mutated genes were *TP53,NOTCH1, CDKN2A, PIK3CA, FBXW7, IRF6, PTEN,* and *HRAS* (Agrawal et al. 2011; Stransky et al. 2011) and that HPV-associated cancers had a lower overall number of mutations per tumor. *TP53* mutations were not detected in HPV-associated tumors but were present in ~80 % of HPV-negative tumors (Agrawal et al. 2011). Overall, it was noteworthy that although head and neck squamous carcinomas are clinically categorized by anatomical location, at a molecular level the presence of *TP53* inactivation (through somatic mutation or HPV infection) appears to be a common feature (Stransky et al. 2011).

S.V. Hodgson et al., *A Practical Guide to Human Cancer Genetics*,
DOI 10.1007/978-1-4471-2375-0_3, © Springer-Verlag London 2014

Specific Sites

Nasopharynx

Cancers of the nasopharynx account for 0.1 % of all cancers and differ from tumors in other parts of the pharynx by not being associated with tobacco or alcohol. There is a high incidence (lifetime risk 1.6 %) of nasopharyngeal carcinoma among the southern Chinese (100-fold higher than that of European populations), and both environmental (high dietary intake of salted fish and, particularly, Epstein–Barr virus, EBV) and genetic factors have been implicated. Familial clustering of naso-pharyngeal carcinoma is well recognized (Zeng and Jia 2002).

Using meta-analysis, Burt et al. (1996) also demonstrated a significant associa-tion with HLA types in non-Chinese populations. This work has been followed up by more detailed studies, and *HLA-A* has been consistently shown to be associated with nasopharyngeal carcinoma susceptibility (Lu et al. 2005). A genome-wide association study confirmed the role of HLA and also identified novel associations at *MDS1-EVI1* (3q26), *CDKN2A/CDKN2B* (9p21), and *TNFRSF19* (13q12), impli-cating the TGF-β and JNK signaling pathways in susceptibility to nasopharyngeal carcinoma (Bei et al. 2010).

Larynx

Cancers of the larynx account for 1 % of all cancers and are associated with tobacco smoking and alcohol. Carcinoma of the larynx has been reported in families with HNPCC (Lynch syndrome) (p. 65), *BRCA2* mutations (p. 91), and in Muir–Torre (p. 286) and Li–Fraumeni syndromes (p. 271).

Tumors of the Thymus

Thymomas are rare tumors of the thymic epithelium that usually occur in adults (average age at onset of 48 years) and are usually sporadic. About 65 % are benign, but when they occur in children, they are more likely to be malignant. Familial occur-rence is rare, but a sibship has been described in which two of three siblings died of thymoma (Matani and Dristsas 1973). Malignant epithelial tumors of the thymus (thymic carcinoma and thymoma) have also been described in two members of a sib-ship (Wick et al. 1982). Nicodème et al. (2005) described a family harboring a con-stitutional translocation t(14;20)(q24;p12) in which 3 of 11 translocation carriers developed a thymoma (*RAD51L* and *BMP2* were suggested as candidate genes).

Other tumors that may involve the thymus are carcinoids, germ cell tumors, neuro-genic tumors, thymolipomas, and Hodgkin disease. About one-third of thymic carci-noids are associated with multiple endocrine neoplasia type 1 (MEN 1) (see p. 278). A possible genotype–phenotype association between thymic carcinoids and truncating *MEN1* mutations has been reported (Lim et al. 2006).

Tumors of the Lung

Lung (bronchial) cancer accounts for 14 % of all new cases of cancer in males and 11 % in females. The two most common histological types of lung cancer (small cell and squamous) are known to be strongly related to cigarette smoking. It is estimated that 90 % of lung cancer in males and 85 % in females is attributable to cigarette smoking. Adenocarcinoma (moderately associated with smoking) and alveolar cell carcinoma (not associated with smoking) account for 10 % of all lung cancer. In addition to smoking, other environmental agents such as asbestos, radiation, and air pollution have been associated with lung cancer. The most frequent somatic events in lung cancer are inactivation of *TP53* and mutations in *KRAS* or *EGFR* mutations (mainly in adenocarcinoma) and alterations in the CDKN2A/ARF/RB1 pathway (Brennan et al. 2011).

Familial clustering of lung cancer occurs, but as relatives of lung cancer patients are more likely than average to be smokers or passive smokers, careful studies are required to distinguish the effects of shared environment (e.g., asbestos exposure) and lifestyle (e.g., smoking) from that of genetic predisposition. Although studies of the familial incidence of smoking-related lung cancer should be interpreted cautiously, there is evidence for an increased risk of lung cancer among relatives of affected patients. Sellers et al. (1990) performed segregation analysis which allowed for variable age at onset and smoking history in affected patients. They concluded that familial clustering of lung cancer was consistent with Mendelian codominant inheritance of a rare autosomal gene with variable age at onset. It was estimated that at age 50 years, 69 % of lung cancer resulted from genetic factors acting in combination with smoking, but that at age 70 years, 72 % of lung cancer could be attributed to environmental factors alone. In a subsequent analysis, Sellers et al. (1994) provided further evidence that Mendelian factors may influence the occurrence of smoking-related cancers in the relatives of lung cancer probands. Schwartz et al. (1996) analyzed the family histories of nonsmokers with lung cancer and found a 7.2-fold increased risk of lung cancer in the first-degree relatives of nonsmokers who developed lung cancer aged 40–59 years. Risk of lung cancer was also increased in the offspring of nonsmoking cases. These findings suggest that a subset of relatives of early-onset, nonsmoking lung cancer cases is at increased genetic risk, and genetic factors have been particularly linked to early-onset cases (Cassidy et al. 2006).

Candidate gene lung cancer susceptibility studies have generally not been replicated by genome-wide association studies, though glutathione S transferase M1 (*GSTM1*) genotype has been associated with lung cancer risk in a meta-analysis, and the I157T *CHEK2* variant that has been reported to predispose to breast cancer has also been associated with a reduced risk of lung cancer (Brennan et al. 2011).

Genome-wide association studies have repeatedly demonstrated an association between lung cancer risk and common variants in the *CHRNA5-CHRNA3-CHRNB4* nicotinic acetylcholine receptor subunit gene cluster on chromosome 15q25 (relative risk ~1.3). However, it was unclear whether the association was direct or whether the link was indirect via susceptibility to cigarette smoking though recent data suggests the latter option (Wang et al. 2011). A locus for familial lung cancer susceptibility has been mapped to 6q23-25 and *RGS17* suggested as the possible candidate gene responsible (You et al. 2009). A *TERT* SNP histology on chromosome 5p15.33 has been associated with lung adenocarcinoma risk but not with other histologies (Landi et al. 2009). However, it has been estimated that <10 % of the familial risk of lung cancer can be explained by the susceptibility loci at 15q25, 5p14, and 6p21 (Brennan et al. 2011). The role of rare variants in lung cancer susceptibility remains to be fully investigated, but a germline *EGFR* variant (T790M) was detected in a family with multiple cases of non-small cell lung cancer (Bell et al. 2005). For a discussion of the genetics of the rare pediatric lung tumor pleuropulmonary blastoma, see page 294.

Mesothelioma

This cancer arises from the mesothelial cells that line the pleural, pericardial, and peritoneal surfaces. Although classically associated with asbestos exposure, familial clusters of mesothelioma may occur suggesting that genetic factors may influence susceptibility (Carbone et al. 2007). Testa et al. (2011) demonstrated that germline mutations in *BAP1* predisposed to mesothelioma, uveal melanoma (see p. 21), and possibly other cancer types, and it has been suggested that the occurrence of mesothelioma and melanoma in *BAP1* mutation carriers may depend on exposure to asbestosis and sunlight. The relative frequency of peritoneal to pleural mesothelioma appears to increase in inherited cases compared to sporadic cases.

Cardiac Tumors

Primary cardiac tumors are rare, being found in less than 0.1 % of autopsies. The most common tumor is myxoma, which accounts for up to 50 % of the total. Most myxomas are sporadic and occur in the over-50 years age group. However, familial myxoma has been described and may occur as a dominant trait. Familial myxomas are more frequently multiple and have an earlier age at diagnosis (20–40 years) than in sporadic cases.

Cardiac myxomas occur in the autosomal dominantly inherited Carney complex type 1 (NAME syndrome (Carney complex); p. 228), which is characterized by the occurrence of cardiac myxoma, spotty pigmentation and cutaneous myxomas, and pituitary and adrenocortical tumors (Carney 1995). Cardiac myxoma is the most serious complication of Carney complex, and all individuals at risk for familial cardiac myxoma should be screened regularly by echocardiography. Carney complex type 1 is caused by mutations in the protein kinase A regulatory subunit-1-alpha gene (*PRKAR1A*), and mutations in *PRKAR1A* have been described in familial cardiac myxoma without other features of Carney complex type 1 (Kirschner et al. 2000).

Cardiac rhabdomyomas are rare and most affected patients have tuberous sclerosis (see Part Three). These are usually asymptomatic, are most frequent in infants, and often involute with age.

Cardiac fibromas are a feature of Gorlin syndrome (p. 246), although they occur in only a small proportion (approximately 3 %) of patients with this disorder (Gorlin 1987, 1995).

References

Agrawal N, Frederick MJ, Pickering CR, Bettegowda C, Chang K, Li RJ, Fakhry C, Xie TX, Zhang J, Wang J, Zhang N, El-Naggar AK, Jasser SA, Weinstein JN, Treviño L, Drummond JA, Muzny DM, Wu Y, Wood LD, Hruban RH, Westra WH, Koch WM, Califano JA, Gibbs RA, Sidransky D, Vogelstein B, Velculescu VE, Papadopoulos N, Wheeler DA, Kinzler KW, Myers JN. Exome sequencing of head and neck squamous cell carcinoma reveals inactivating mutations in NOTCH1. Science. 2011;333(6046):1154–7.

Bei JX, Li Y, Jia WH, Feng BJ, Zhou G, Chen LZ, Feng QS, Low HQ, Zhang H, He F, Tai ES, Kang T, Liu ET, Liu J, Zeng YX. A genome-wide association study of nasopharyngeal carcinoma identifies three new susceptibility loci. Nat Genet. 2010;42(7):599–603.

Bell DW, Gore I, Okimoto RA, Godin-Heymann N, Sordella R, Mulloy R, Sharma SV, Brannigan BW, Mohapatra G, Settleman J, Haber DA. Inherited susceptibility to lung cancer may be associated with the T790M drug resistance mutation in EGFR. Nat Genet. 2005;37(12):1315–6.

Brennan P, Hainaut P, Boffetta P. Genetics of lung-cancer susceptibility. Lancet Oncol. 2011;12(4):399–408.

Burt RD, Vaughan TL, McKnight B, et al. Associations between human leukocyte antigen type and nasopharyngeal carcinoma in Caucasians in the United States. Cancer Epidemiol Biomark Prev. 1996;5:879–87.

Carbone M, Emri S, Dogan AU, Steele I, Tuncer M, Pass HI, Baris YI. A mesothelioma epidemic in Cappadocia: scientific developments and unexpected social outcomes. Nat Rev Cancer. 2007;7(2):147–54.

Carney JA. Carney complex; the complex of myxomas, spotty pigmentation. Endocrine overactivity and schwannomas. Semin Dermatol. 1995;14:90–8.

Cassidy A, Myles JP, Duffy SW, Liloglou T, Field JK. Family history and risk of lung cancer: age-at-diagnosis in cases and first-degree relatives. Br J Cancer. 2006;95(9):1288–90.

D'Souza G, Kreimer AR, Viscidi R, Pawlita M, Fakhry C, Koch WM, Westra WH, Gillison ML. Case-control study of human papillomavirus and oropharyngeal cancer. N Engl J Med. 2007;356(19):1944–56.

Foulkes WD, Brunet JS, Sieh W, Black MJ, Shenouda G, Narod SA. Familial risks of squamous cell carcinoma of the head and neck: retrospective case-control study. Br Med J. 1996;313:716–21.

Gorlin RJ. Nevoid basal-cell carcinoma syndrome. Medicine. 1987;66:98–113.

Gorlin RJ. Nevoid basal cell carcinoma syndrome. Dermatol Clin. 1995;13:113–25.

Kirschner LS, Carney JA, Pack SD, Taymans SE, Giatzakis C, Cho YS, Cho-Chung YS, Stratakis CA. Mutations of the gene encoding the protein kinase A type I-alpha regulatory subunit in patients with the Carney complex. Nat Genet. 2000;26:89–92.

Landi MT, Chatterjee N, Yu K, Goldin LR, Goldstein AM, Rotunno M, Mirabello L, Jacobs K, Wheeler W, Yeager M, Bergen AW, Li Q, Consonni D, Pesatori AC, Wacholder S, Thun M, Diver R, Oken M, Virtamo J, Albanes D, Wang Z, Burdette L, Doheny KF, Pugh EW, Laurie C, Brennan P, Hung R, Gaborieau V, McKay JD, Lathrop M, McLaughlin J, Wang Y, Tsao MS, Spitz MR, Wang Y, Krokan H, Vatten L, Skorpen F, Arnesen E, Benhamou S, Bouchard C, Metspalu A, Vooder T, Nelis M, Välk K, Field JK, Chen C, Goodman G, Sulem P, Thorleifsson G, Rafnar T, Eisen T, Sauter W, Rosenberger A, Bickeböller H, Risch A, Chang-Claude J, Wichmann HE, Stefansson K, Houlston R, Amos CI, Fraumeni Jr JF, Savage SA, Bertazzi PA, Tucker MA, Chanock S, Caporaso NE. A genome-wide association study of lung cancer identifies a region of chromosome 5p15 associated with risk for adenocarcinoma. Am J Hum Genet. 2009;85(5):679–91.

Lim LC, Tan MH, Eng C, Teh BT, Rajasoorya RC. Thymic carcinoid in multiple endocrine neo-plasia 1: genotype-phenotype correlation and prevention. J Intern Med. 2006;259(4):428–32.

Lu CC, Chen JC, Tsai ST, Jin YT, Tsai JC, Chan SH, Su IJ. Nasopharyngeal carcinoma-susceptibility locus is localized to a 132 kb segment containing HLA-A using high-resolution microsatellite mapping. Int J Cancer. 2005;115(5):742–6.

Matani A, Dristsas C. Familial occurrence of thymoma. Arch Pathol. 1973;95:90–1.

Nicodème F, Geffroy S, Conti M, Delobel B, Soenen V, Grardel N, Porte H, Copin MC, Laï JL, Andrieux J. Familial occurrence of thymoma and autoimmune diseases with the constitutional translocation t(14;20)(q24.1;p12.3). Genes Chromosomes Cancer. 2005;44(2):154–60.

Schwartz AG, Yang P, Swanson GM. Familial risk of lung cancer among non-smokers and their relatives. Am J Epidemiol. 1996;144:554–62.

Sellers TA, Bailey-Wilson JE, Elston RC, et al. Evidence for Mendelian inheritance in the patho-genesis of lung cancer. J Natl Cancer Inst. 1990;82(15):1272–9.

Sellers TA, Chen PL, Potter JD, Bailey-Wilson JE, Rothschild H, Elston R. Segregation analysis of smoking-associated malignancies: evidence for Mendelian inheritance. Am J Med Genet. 1994;52:308–14.

Stransky N, Egloff AM, Tward AD, Kostic AD, Cibulskis K, Sivachenko A, Kryukov GV, Lawrence MS, Sougnez C, McKenna A, Shefler E, Ramos AH, Stojanov P, Carter SL, Voet D, Cortés ML, Auclair D, Berger MF, Saksena G, Guiducci C, Onofrio RC, Parkin M, Romkes M, Weissfeld JL, Seethala RR, Wang L, Rangel-Escareño C, Fernandez-Lopez JC, Hidalgo-Miranda A, Melendez-Zajgla J, Winckler W, Ardlie K, Gabriel SB, Meyerson M, Lander ES, Getz G, Golub TR, Garraway LA, Grandis JR. The mutational landscape of head and neck squamous cell carcinoma. Science. 2011;333(6046):1157–60.

Testa JR, Cheung M, Pei J, Below JE, Tan Y, Sementino E, Cox NJ, Dogan AU, Pass HI, Trusa S, Hesdorffer M, Nasu M, Powers A, Rivera Z, Comertpay S, Tanji M, Gaudino G, Yang H, Carbone M. Germline BAP1 mutations predispose to malignant mesothelioma. Nat Genet. 2011;43(10):1022–5.

Wang Y, Broderick P, Matakidou A, Eisen T, Houlston RS. Chromosome 15q25(CHRNA3-CHRNA5) variation impacts indirectly on lung cancer risk. PLoS One. 2011;6(4):e19085.

Wick MR, Scheithauer BW, Dines DE, et al. Thymic neoplasia in 2 male sib-lings. Mayo Clin Proc. 1982;57:653–6.

You M, Wang D, Liu P, Vikis H, James M, Lu Y, Wang Y, Wang M, Chen Q, Jia D, Liu Y, Wen W, Yang P, Sun Z, Pinney SM, Zheng W, Shu XO, Long J, Gao YT, Xiang YB, Chow WH, Rothman N, Petersen GM, de Andrade M, Wu Y, Cunningham JM, Wiest JS, Fain PR, Schwartz AG, Girard L, Gazdar A, Gaba C, Rothschild H, Mandal D, Coons T, Lee J, Kupert E, Seminara D, Minna J, Bailey-Wilson JE, Amos CI, Anderson MW. Fine mapping of chromosome 6q23-25 region in familial lung cancer families reveals RGS17 as a likely candidate gene. Clin Cancer Res. 2009;15(8):2666–74.

Zeng YX, Jia WH. Familial nasopharyngeal carcinoma. Semin Cancer Biol. 2002;12(6):443–50.

Chapter 4
Endocrine System

Thyroid Tumors

The incidence of primary epithelial cancer of the thyroid is 0.7 per 100,000 in males and 1.9 per 100,000 in females in the UK. Overall, the annual incidence of thyroid cancer is between 0.9 and 5.2 per 100,000 people, with a ratio of women to men of 2–3:1. Thyroid cancer is the most rapidly rising incident cancer in women and the second most rapidly rising incident cancer in men in the USA. Whether the papillary or follicular histology is favored is dependent on the amount of dietary iodine in a particular region. Papillary thyroid carcinoma (PTC) accounts for more than 50 % of cases in the UK and USA, the next most common type of thyroid cancer being follicular thyroid carcinoma (FTC). Less frequent types are medullary thyroid carcinomas (MTC), anaplastic (undifferentiated) carcinomas, Hürthle cell carcinomas, and squamous cell carcinomas. Other non-epithelial malignancies that may be observed in the thyroid include lymphomas and sarcomas, but these are rare.

Papillary Thyroid Carcinoma (PTC)

Genetic susceptibility to PTC can be seen in familial adenomatous polyposis syndrome (FAP), Cowden syndrome (CS), possibly Carney complex (CNC), and in a familial site-specific syndrome. These syndromes are described in detail in the next section. Thyroid cancers can be detected in 2–25 % of FAP patients. It should be noted that there is evidence that what is commonly referred to as "PTC" in FAP is not identical to classic PTC (cPTC) nor its follicular variant of PTC (FvPTC). FAP-related thyroid cancer is of a distinct cribriform subtype, currently referred to as cribriform-morular variant (cmv) of PTC (Harach et al. 1994; Ito et al. 2011). In contrast to classic PTC, FAP-related thyroid cancers do not show the typical fir tree branching papillary pattern, and psammoma bodies are rare or nonexistent. This distinct architecture seen in APC-related thyroid carcinomas is very unusual in sporadic PTC (Harach et al. 1994). FAP-related cmv-PTC is often multifocal

S.V. Hodgson et al., *A Practical Guide to Human Cancer Genetics*,
DOI 10.1007/978-1-4471-2375-0_4, © Springer-Verlag London 2014

Table 4.1 Familial PTC

Syndrome	Chromosomal location	Comments
PTC with cell oxyphilia	TCO, 19p13.2	Oncocytic PTC
PTC without oxyphilia	19p13.2	
Multinodular goiter (MNG)	MNG1, 14q31	MNG and PTC
	MNG2, Xp22	MNG only
PTC and renal tumors	1q21	PTC, thyroid nodular disease, papillary renal cell carcinoma
PTC and clear cell renal cancer	t(3;8)(p14.2;q24.1)	
FNMTC	NMTC1, 2q21	Follicular variant of PTC

Reviewed in Eng (2000a, b, c)

compared to the rare sporadic cmv-PTC (Ito et al. 2011). Recent studies suggest that FAP-related cmv-PTC patients are predominantly female, and the great majority of the germline *APC* mutations occurred in exon 15, especially the 5′ portion of this exon (Cetta et al. 2000; Jarrar et al. 2011). Unlike the general population, PTC is underrepresented in CS-related thyroid carcinomas, especially in those with germline *PTEN* mutations (Harach et al. 1999). In contrast, however, pilot data suggest that PTC is overrepresented in individuals with CS who carry germline *SDHB/SDHD* variants of germline *KLLN* epimutation compared to those with germline *PTEN* mutations (Ni et al. 2008; Bennett et al. 2010). While thyroid tumors, for example, PTC, have been reported in CNC, it is currently unclear if PTC are true component cancers of CNC.

Several putative loci, but no genes, have been identified for non-syndromic familial PTC and are summarized in the Table 4.1. It is believed that the 14q31-related multinodular goiter gene is *DICER1* although it is unclear whether PTC is part of this newly described syndrome that most likely comprises multinodular goiter, Sertoli-Leydig cell tumor, and perhaps Wilms' tumor (Rio Frio et al. 2011). Previously, *DICER1* germline mutations are associated with the rare phenotypes of pleuropulmonary blastoma and familial cystic nephroma. Various low-penetrance germline variants, notably in pre-miR-146a (odds ratio = 1.6), have been reported (Jadziewski et al. 2009).

Sporadic PTC are characterized by somatic translocations between one of several genes and the intracellular domain of RET (at intron 11) termed RET/PTCn. The precise frequency is unknown but could range from 10 to 60 %. Typically, the 5′-translocation partner encodes a protein which can force dimerization of the kinase domain of RET, for example, leucine zippers (Lanzi et al. 1992; Sozzi et al. 1992; Bongarzone et al. 1993). It would appear that PTC tumors without RET/PTC translocations harbor a relatively high frequency of somatic gain-of-function *BRAF* mutations (Kimura et al. 2003; Soares et al. 2003). As somatic *BRAF* mutations and the presence of the RET/PTC translocation or *RAS* mutations are mutually exclusive, it is suggested that activation of the RAS-RAF-MAP kinase pathway is important in PTC development but that two insults to this pathway are not necessary.

Follicular Thyroid Carcinoma (FTC)

FTC is a proven component cancer in *PTEN*-related CS and Werner syndrome. In germline *PTEN* mutation-positive CS, FTC is the major component of thyroid cancer (Harach et al. 1999; Ni et al. 2008; Bennett et al. 2010). However, rarely, PTC and the follicular variant of PTC are also observed (Marsh et al. 1998). In Werner syndrome, thyroid carcinoma, mainly FTC, is more commonly observed in Japanese patients than those from elsewhere. Both syndromes are discussed in detail in the next section.

The molecular etiology of sporadic FTC remains unknown. A publication reporting a high frequency (50 %) of somatic *PAX8/PPARG* translocations in FTC initially suggested that this was the initiating event (Kroll et al. 2000). Subsequently, the frequency of this *PAX8/PPARG* translocation, which inactivates *PPARG* by a dominant negative mechanism, was found to be much less (10 %) in sporadic FTC (Aldred et al. 2003). Instead, loss of function by a haploinsufficient mechanism seems to occur more frequently and plays some role in FTC development (Aldred et al. 2003). Microarray expression strategies have been used to attempt to elucidate the molecular pathogenesis of sporadic FTC (Aldred et al. 2003).

Medullary Thyroid Carcinoma (MTC)

MTC, which is a carcinoma of the parafollicular C cells, is a proven component cancer of multiple endocrine neoplasia type 2 (MEN 2), caused by germline mutations in the *RET* proto-oncogene. This syndrome is detailed in the next section. While C cell hyperplasia was believed to be pathognomonic for MEN 2, once *RET* was identified as the MEN 2 susceptibility gene, it was discovered that this association no longer holds true, and indeed C cell hyperplasia can be found in truly sporadic MTC (Eng et al. 1995a, b; Marsh et al. 1996b).

The etiology of sporadic MTC is also not well known. Among all presentations of MTC, clinical epidemiological studies have shown that 25 % can be attributable to MEN 2. Occult germline mutations in the *RET* proto-oncogene can be found in 5–15 % of apparently sporadic MTC, that is, without obvious syndromic features or family history (Blaugrund et al. 1994; Eng et al. 1995a, b; Wohlik et al. 1996; Schuffenecker et al. 1997). Due to these accumulating data, the general recommendations, such as from the American Thyroid Association Management Guidelines, are to offer *RET* mutation analysis to all presentations of MTC regardless of age, presence of syndromic features, or family history (Kloos et al. 2009).

Somatic *RET* mutations have been reported to occur in 10–80 % of sporadic MTC (Eng et al. 1994, 1995a, b; Hofstra et al. 1994; Marsh et al. 1996a). The great majority of somatic *RET* mutations are M918T. Of note, somatic mutations have been found to occur in patches or subpopulations even within a single tumor (Eng et al. 1996a, b, 1998). Up to 80 % of sporadic MTC harbor at least one subpopulation with somatic

M918T mutation (Eng et al. 1996a, b). It remains controversial whether somatic M918T in the primary tumor portends a poor prognosis. Unfortunately, because some studies have used mixed primary and metastatic tumors (e.g., Schilling et al. 2001), and because of the presence of subpopulations and the varied mutation detection technologies employed, whether M918T status is associated with prognosis remains unknown. Nonetheless, one well-designed study did not show a difference in clinical outcome with or without somatic M918T (Marsh et al. 1996b). In general, MEN 2-associated MTC do not carry somatic intragenic *RET* mutation as a second genetic event (Eng et al. 1995a, b). However, there are rare instances of somatic M918T occurring in MEN 2-associated MTC (Marsh et al. 1996a). It is also believed that duplication of the mutated *REt al*lele in MEN 2A-associated MTC may contribute to carcinogenesis (Koch et al. 2001). A recent study of a relatively small series of sporadic MTC found that half of all somatic *RET* mutation-negative MTC harbored somatic mutations in *HRAS*, but not in other *RAS* family members (Moura et al. 2011).

Benign Neoplasia of the Thyroid

Benign thyroid neoplasia such as follicular adenomas, multinodular goiters, and hamartomas are components of CS (see below). Due to the risk of recurrence and the risk of thyroid cancer in CS patients or in those with a proven germline *PTEN* mutation, a total thyroidectomy should be performed if surgery is being considered for these benign thyroid lesions. Germline *DICER1* mutations have been described in individuals and families with multinodular goiter, usually accompanied by other features noted above and in the next chapter. At least in one study, benign thyroid nodules appear to be relatively common in individuals with FAP, although malignant disease was prevalent only in ~3 % (Jarrar et al. 2011).

Parathyroid Tumors

Parathyroid neoplasias are very common; however, familial hyperparathyroidism occurs at a frequency of about 0.14 per 10,000 and, for the most part, occurs as part of the multiple endocrine neoplasia syndromes (MEN; see p. 278 and 281), with chief cell hyperplasia as the usual histological change. The genetic differential diagnosis of parathyroid hyperplasia or parathyroid adenoma includes MEN 1, caused by germline *MEN1* mutations; MEN 2, caused by germline *RET* mutations; and hyperparathyroidism–jaw tumor syndrome (HPT-JT), caused by germline mutations in *HRPT2*. Familial site-specific hyperparathyroidism can be caused by germline *MEN1* mutations as well as due to HPT-JT (Teh et al. 1996; Kassem et al. 2000). Germline mutations in the calcium-sensing receptor gene have been identified in benign familial hypocalciuric hypercalcemia and, in homozygous form, cause neonatal severe hyperparathyroidism with parathyroid hyperplasia (Pollak et al. 1993). While parathyroid disease is very common in MEN 1 and often the first component neoplasia to manifest, hyperparathyroidism in MEN 2 occurs in 15–30 % of MEN 2A cases and likely manifests relatively later in life (Schuffenecker et al. 1998). Germline *RET* C634R is particularly associated with the development of hyperparathyroidism in MEN 2A (Mulligan et al. 1994; Eng et al. 1996a, b).

Parathyroid carcinoma is extremely rare, but it is an important component neoplasia of HPT-JT (Carpten et al. 2002). It is unclear, however, whether parathyroid carcinoma is a true component cancer of MEN 1 as well, but it does not appear to be so.

Somatic loss of heterozygosity (LOH) of markers on 11q13 and somatic *MEN1* mutations have been described in parathyroid hyperplasias (Friedman et al. 1992). Somatic mutations in *HRPT2* occur with a relatively high frequency in sporadic parathyroid carcinomas (Howell et al. 2003; Shattuck et al. 2003). Surprisingly, occult germline mutations in *HRPT2* were found in 3 of the 15 apparently sporadic patients with parathyroid carcinoma (Shattuck et al. 2003).

Those at risk for parathyroid hyperplasia and/or adenoma should undergo routine clinical surveillance. Management for parathyroid disease for MEN 2 is discussed in the chapter below.

Pituitary Tumors

Tumors of the pituitary gland rarely complicate genetic conditions other than MEN 1 (see section below). The most common pituitary tumor in MEN 1 is prolactinoma (Burgess et al. 1996), but there are several reports in the literature of familial pituitary adenomas without clinical evidence of MEN 1. Mostly, these are examples of familial acromegaly (Bergman et al. 2000; Gadelha et al. 2000; Tamura et al. 2002) and rarely of prolactinoma (Berezin and Karasik 1995). For over a decade, molecular genetic investigations have been used to argue for and against the hypothesis that familial acromegaly is allelic with *MEN1* (Bergman et al. 2000; Gadelha et al. 2000; Tamura et al. 2002). Recently, germline mutations in *AIP* were described as a predisposition gene for subsets of apparently sporadic and familial acromegaly (Vierimaa et al. 2006). The highest prevalence of germline *AIP* mutations were found in young patients with pituitary macroadenomas (Tichomirowa et al. 2011). Indeed, 20 % of the pediatric cases were found to have such mutations. Pituitary adenomas may occur in CNC and chromophobe adenomas may possibly have an increased frequency in Maffucci syndrome (see section below). No occult germline *PRKAR1A* mutations were found in a recent series of 74 pediatric presentations of pituitary adenomas/Cushing disease (Stratakis et al. 2010).

Both somatic tumor suppressor gene inactivation and oncogene activation have been implicated in the pathogenesis of pituitary tumors. Chromosome 11 allele loss (the *MEN1* gene maps to chromosome 11q13) is the most frequent event in sporadic pituitary adenomas, and chromosome 13 allele loss is also frequent. Accordingly, there exist somatic *MEN1* mutations in sporadic pituitary adenomas (Zhuang et al. 1997). Some growth-hormone-secreting pituitary tumors have been found to contain somatic mutations which inhibit the GTPase activity of a G-protein alpha chain and convert it to a putative oncogene *gsp* (Lyons et al. 1990). This results in activation of adenyl cyclase and bypasses the need for trophic-hormone-mediated activation. Similar mutations have been found in McCune–Albright syndrome (see below).

Adrenal Gland Tumors

Tumors of the adrenal glands arise from either the medulla or the cortex. Adrenal medullary tumors include neuroblastomas (p. 7), embryonal tumors, and pheochromocytomas.

Pheochromocytoma

Pheochromocytomas are derivatives of the neural crest and arise from adrenal chromaffin cells. Extra-adrenal (chromaffin) paragangliomas may be referred to as extra-adrenal pheochromocytomas. Medical textbooks have traditionally suggested that approximately 10 % of pheochromocytomas are heritable, 10 % are extra-adrenal, and 10 % are malignant. However, the frequency of heritable pheochromocytoma has been underestimated, and in one population-based study, 25 % of unrelated, apparently sporadic presentations of pheochromocytomas, without syndromic features or family history, were found to harbor germline mutations in one of four genes, *VHL, RET, SDHD,* or *SDHB* (Neumann et al. 2002). This frequency has been confirmed in referral series as well (Benn et al. 2006). Due to these and related findings, all presentations of pheochromocytomas, regardless of age, syndromic features, or family history, should considered for mutation analysis in the setting of cancer genetic consultation which includes genetic counseling. The genetic differential diagnosis of pheochromocytoma includes MEN 2 caused by germline mutations in the *RET* gene; von Hippel–Lindau (VHL) disease caused by *VHL* mutations; the pheochromocytoma–paraganglioma syndrome caused by germline mutations in the *SDHB, SDHC,* and *SDHD* genes; and, very rarely, NF 1 (Maher and Eng 2002; Eng et al. 2003; Neumann et al. 2004; Schiavi et al. 2005) (see below and section to follow). Familial site-specific pheochromocytomas are mainly attributable to germline mutations in *VHL, SDHD,* or *SDHB* (Woodward et al. 1997; Astuti et al. 2001a, b). Such families with pheochromocytomas as well as chemodectomas or glomus tumors are almost always due to germline mutations in *SDHB, SDHC,* or *SDHD* (Maher and Eng 2002; Neumann et al. 2004). Recently, germline mutations in *TMEM127* were described in rare familial adrenal pheochromocytoma cases (Yao et al. 2010). These cases were characterized by unilateral tumors diagnosed in the 40s. However, a subsequent registry-based study demonstrated that germline *TMEM127* mutations could also be associated with extra-adrenal disease, occurring in about 5 % of 48 individuals with paraganglioma but without mutations in the other predisposition genes (Neumann et al. 2011). Even more recently, germline *MAX* mutations were described in ~10 % of hereditary pheochromocytoma cases characterized by very early-onset and malignant disease (Comino-Mendez et al. 2011).

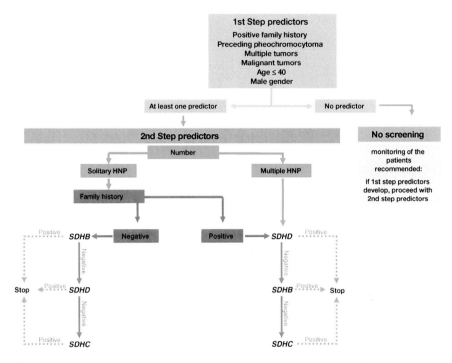

Fig. 4.1 Genetic testing algorithm for phaeochromocytoma presentations (Reproduced from AACR Journal paper, which is authored/coauthored by at least one of the authors of this book)

In general, like virtually all inherited neoplasias, the mean age at diagnosis for heritable pheochromocytoma is lower, and there will be a higher incidence of bilateral tumors and multifocal disease when compared to sporadic pheochromocytoma. Nonetheless, these clinical features, the clinical hallmarks of heredity, are syndrome dependent (and hence, dependent on susceptibility gene involved) (Neumann et al. 2004). For example, in the population-based study on non-syndromic pheochromocytomas, while the mean age at presentation in individuals without germline mutations (sporadic) was 44 years, the mean age was 36 years for those shown to carry a *RET* mutation (MEN 2), 18.3 years for VHL, and approximately 27 years for those found to have germline *SDHD/SDHB* mutations (Neumann et al. 2002). NF 1-related pheochromocytomas are usually diagnosed relatively older, around 40 years. Further, of those found to carry germline mutations, about one-third presented with multifocal disease compared to two-thirds with a solitary lesion (Neumann et al. 2002). Therefore, two algorithms were computed to help clinicians determine whether to offer germline gene testing in pheochromocytoma and paraganglioma presentations, and if so, then which genes to prioritize [Fig. 4.1 of Erlic and Fig. 4.2 of Neumann] (Erlic et al. 2009; Neumann et al. 2009).

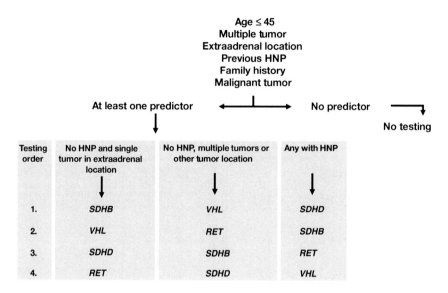

Fig. 4.2 Clinical algorithm to priorities whether genetic testing is warranted (first step predictors), and if so which gene(s) to prioritize (second step predictors) for pheochromocytoma presentations (Reproduced from AACR Journal paper, which is authored/coauthored by at least one of the authors of this book)

There has been scant information regarding somatic mutations in sporadic pheochromocytoma except for relatively low frequencies of somatic *VHL* mutations, somatic *RET* mutations, and somatic *SDHD* mutations (Eng et al. 1995a, b; Gimm et al. 2000; Astuti et al. 2001a, b). Interestingly, differential distributions of frequencies of LOH at 1p, 3p, and 22q exist between VHL-related pheochromocytomas and those of sporadic tumors (Bender et al. 2000). In VHL-related pheochromocytomas, almost all showed LOH of markers around *VHL* at 3p with LOH of markers at 1p and 22q being 15 and 21 %, respectively. In contrast, sporadic tumors showed LOH at 3p in only 21 % of samples but relatively high frequencies of 1p and 22q marker LOH (Bender et al. 2000). In MEN 2-related pheochromocytoma, it is believed that amplification of the mutant *REt al*lele could contribute to carcinogenesis in an unknown proportion of tumors (Huang et al. 2000). Despite genome-wide approaches, mainly of the transcriptome, clarity in regard to somatic alterations did not go beyond what was already known for 10 years. Recently, integrative genomic approaches utilizing 202 sporadic and 75 hereditary pheochromocytoma and paraganglioma tumors revealed that ~45 % carried some form of germline or somatic alteration, with 14 % harboring *VHL* or *RET* mutations (Burnichon et al. 2011). As found previously, transcriptome signatures were consistent with germline status and clearly distinguished *VHL*-related from *SDHx*-related tumors (Burnichon et al. 2011).

Individuals at risk for pheochromocytoma should be offered annual surveillance. The precise measures for clinical surveillance are dependent on the specific syndrome at risk for and the institution. In general, annual physical examination paying particular attention to the retinal examination and blood pressure measurements,

Table 4.2 Sample surveillance protocol for SDH mutation carrier

Proven *SDHB* mutation carrier
Annual 24-h urine for catecholamines and vanyllylmandelic acid measurements from age 5 years
Annual abdominal MRI scans from age 7 years (abdominal and thoracic every 3 years)
MRI neck age 20 years and every 3 years thereafter
Proven *SDHD* mutation carrier (paternally transmitted)
Annual 24-h urine for catecholamines and vanyllylmandelic acid measurements from age 5 years
Two yearly abdominal MRI scans from age 7 years (abdominal and thoracic every 5 years)
MRI neck age 20 years and every 1–2 years thereafter

especially with orthostatic maneuvers, and 24-h urinary catecholamines and vanyl-lylmandelic acid measurements are performed. Some centers advocate serum cate-cholamine, vanyllylmandelic acid, and chromogranin-A measurements as well. Further investigation may include MIBG and computerized tomography (CT) or magnetic resonance imaging (MRI) scans and selective venous sampling as appro-priate. Recently, positron emission tomography (PET) scanning is performed for surveillance in certain centers. Full details of screening protocols in VHL disease, NF1, and MEN 2 are described in the Chap. 11, and a sample screening protocol for *SDHB* and *SDHD* gene carriers is suggested in Table 4.2.

Adrenocortical Adenoma and Carcinoma

Adrenocortical tumors are rare (incidence approximately 0.2 per 100,000 per year) and may be benign or malignant. The most frequent presentation is with Cushing syndrome with or without associated virilization, sometimes with primary aldoste-ronism; estrogen-producing tumors are rare. Adrenocortical carcinomas are proven component cancers in Li–Fraumeni syndrome caused by germline *TP53* mutations (see below for complete discussion of this syndrome). Indeed, early-onset (under the age of 4 years) or bilateral disease carries a high likelihood of germline *TP53* muta-tion (Malkin et al. 1990; Eng et al. 1997). In a series of 14 patients with adrenocorti-cal carcinoma unselected for family history, 11 (82 %) carried a germline *TP53* mutation. Interestingly, the same two mutations (at codons 152 and 158) were pres-ent in 9 of the 11 mutation-positive cases. In another series of 36 cases of childhood adrenocortical carcinoma in southern Brazil, 35 carried an identical R337H muta-tion (Ribeiro et al. 2001). Some believe that adrenocortical carcinomas can be found at increased frequencies in Beckwith–Wiedemann syndrome (Wiedemann 1983).

A macroscopically and histologically distinctive type of adrenocortical hyperpla-sia called primary pigmented nodular adrenocortical disease (PPNAD) is a compo-nent neoplasia of CNC (NAME syndrome) and is discussed below. PPNAD can be clinically diagnosed by its paradoxical response to dexamethasone challenge (Stratakis et al. 1999). Benign adrenocortical lesions, usually nonfunctional, are reported in MEN 1 patients, some believe as frequently as 20–40 %. Adrenocortical nodular hyperplasia and rarely adenoma may be seen in McCune–Albright syndrome (see below). Hypercortisolism is often associated with macronodular hyperplasia of the adrenal cortex. Recently, germline variation in *PDE11* has been associated with macronodular hyperplasia of the adrenal cortex (Horvath et al. 2006).

Glomus Tumors (Non-chromaffin Paraganglioma)

Glomus tumors are benign tumors of the head and neck region derived from neural crest and are situated predominantly at the carotid bifurcation and jugular foramen. Glomus tumors, sometimes referred to as chemodectomas, are the most common type of paraganglioma in the head and neck region. They are non-chromaffin paragangliomas, that is, they do not secrete but instead are sensing organs. Glomus tumors have an incidence of approximately 1 in 30,000 and are usually sporadic and unilateral. However, about a third of multiple cases are familial, with an autosomal dominant inheritance pattern. Bilateral disease is significantly more frequent in familial (32–38 % of cases) than in nonfamilial (4–8 %) cases (Grufferman et al. 1980; Parry et al. 1982). Six percent of patients with familial chemodectomas develop second primary tumors, predominantly other paragangliomas. The inheritance of some instances of familial glomus tumors shows maternal imprinting: descendants of affected females who inherit the gene do not develop glomus tumors, but heterozygote descendants of affected males do. Two loci for familial glomus tumors in Dutch kindred have been mapped to the long arm of chromosome 11: PGL1 at 11q23.1 and PGL2 at 11q13 (Heutink et al. 1992; Mariman et al. 1995). Germline mutations in *SDHD* on 11q23.1 (PGL1) were described in families with glomus tumors with and without thoracic/adrenal paragangliomas (Baysal et al. 2000). In mutation-positive families, maternal imprinting was demonstrated. Perhaps because of maternal imprinting, occult germline *SDHD* mutations are evident in a relatively high frequency of apparently sporadic adrenal pheochromocytoma or paraganglioma patients (Gimm et al. 2000). Subsequently, germline mutations in *SDHB* (PGL4) in individuals and families with paraganglioma and/or pheochromocytomas were described (Astuti et al. 2001a, b). Interestingly, only two families with paragangliomas have been described with germline *SDHC* (PGL3) mutations (Niemann and Muller 2000). The gene on 11q13 underlying PGL2 eluded identification for many years, and only a single Dutch family is linked to this locus. Recently, *SDHAF2* (*hSdh5*) was identified as PGL2 (Hao et al. 2009). This gene rarely accounts for paraganglioma, and not surprisingly a single founder mutation Gly78Arg is the most common (Bayley et al. 2010). Initially thought only to predispose to pheochromocytoma, germline *TMEM127* has also been shown to predispose to paraganglioma (Yao et al. 2010; Neumann et al. 2011). Even more recently, germline *MAX* mutations were described in ~10 % of hereditary pheochromocytoma cases characterized by very early-onset and malignant disease (Comino-Mendez et al. 2011). Paragangliomas may occur in CNC (p. 228 – ex-176) or MEN 1 (p. 277).

In a population-based registry of head and neck paragangliomas, accrued without regard to clinical features, demographics, or family history, over 2/3 were due to germline *SDHD* mutations, 1/3 *SDHB* mutation, and, rarely, *SDHC* (Neumann et al. 2004; Schiavi et al. 2005; Peczkowska et al. 2007; Peczkowska et al. 2008). Unless there are other clinical features of or family histories, head and neck paragangliomas are rarely, if ever, associated with MEN 2 or VHL (Boedeker et al. 2009). Because there are multiple genes associated with head and neck paragangliomas, a clinically relevant algorithm was modeled which takes into account demographic, clinical, and gene-specific prevalence data to help prioritize which presentations should be offered genetic testing, and if so, which gene to prioritize. Using such an algorithm, a cost reduction of >50 % was achieved (Neumann et al. 2009).

Pancreatic Endocrine Tumors

Non-endocrine pancreatic tumors are described on page 52. Pancreatic endocrine tumors (islet cell adenomas such as gastrinoma, insulinoma, glucagonoma, VIPoma, somatostatinoma) may occur in up to 1.5 % of autopsies but are mostly asymptomatic. Pancreatic endocrine tumors are a feature of MEN 1 and VHL disease (see Chap. 11).

References

Aldred MA, Morrison CD, Gimm O, et al. Peroxisome proliferator-activated receptor gamma is frequently downregulated in a diversity of sporadic non-medullary thyroid carcinomas. Oncogene. 2003;22:3412–6.

Astuti D, Douglas F, Lennard TWJ, et al. Germline *SDHD* mutation in familial phaeochromocytoma. Lancet. 2001a;357:1181–2.

Astuti D, Latif F, Dallol A, et al. Mutations in the mitochondrial complex II subunit SDHB cause susceptibility to familial paraganglioma and pheochromocytoma. Am J Hum Genet. 2001b;69:49–54.

Bayley JP, Kunst HP, Cascon A, Sampietro ML, Gaal J, Korperschoek E, Hinojar-Guitierrez A, Timmers HJ, Hoefsloot LH, Hermsen MA, Suarez C, Hussain AK, Vriends AH, Hes FJ, Jansen JC, Tops CM, Corssmit EP, de Knijff P, Lenders JW, Cremers CW, Devilee P, Dinjens WN, de Krijger RR, Robledo M. SDHAF2 mutations in familial and sporadic paraganglioma and phaeochromocytoma. Lancet Oncol. 2010;11:366–72.

Baysal BE, Ferrell RE, Willett-Brozick JE, et al. Mutations in SDHD, a mitochondrial complex II gene, in hereditary paraganglioma. Science. 2000;287:848–51.

Bender BU, Gutsche M, Gläsker S, et al. Differential genetic alterations in sporadic and von Hippel–Lindau syndrome-associated pheochromocytomas. J Clin Endocrinol Metab. 2000;85:4568–74.

Benn DE, Gimenez-Roqueplo AP, Reilly JR, Bertherat J, Burgess J, Byth K, Croxson M, Dahia PL, Elston M, Gimm O, Henley D, Herman P, Murday V, Niccoli-Sire P, Pasieka JL, Rohmer V, Tucker K, Jeunemaitre X, Marsh DJ, Plouin PF, Robinson BG. Clinical presentation and penetrance of pheochromocytoma/paraganglioma syndromes. J Clin Endocrinol Metab. 2006;91:827–36.

Bennett KL, Mester J, Eng C. Germline epigenetic regulation of KILLIN in Cowden and Cowden-like syndrome. JAMA. 2010;304:2724–31.

Berezin M, Karasik A. Familial prolactinoma. Clin Endocrinol (Oxf). 1995;42:483–6.

Bergman L, Teh B, Cardinal J, et al. Identification of MEN1 gene mutations in families with MEN 1 and related disorders. Br J Cancer. 2000;83:1009–14.

Blaugrund JE, Johns MM, Eby YJ, et al. *RET* proto-oncogene mutations in inherited and sporadic medullary thyroid cancer. Hum Mol Genet. 1994;3:1895–7.

Boedeker CC, Erlic Z, Richard S, Kontny U, Gimenez-Roqueplo AP, Cascon A, Robledo M, deCampos JM, vanNedervenn FH, deKrijger RR, Burnichon N, Gaal J, Walter MA, Resch K, Wiech T, Weber J, Ruckauer K, Plouin PF, Darrouzet V, Giraud S, Eng C, Neumann HPH. Head and neck paragangliomas in von Hippel-Lindau syndrome and multiple endocrine neoplasia type 2. J Clin Endocrinol Metab. 2009;94:1938–44.

Bongarzone I, Monzini N, Borrello MG, et al. Molecular characterization of a thyroid tumor-specific transforming sequence formed by the fusion of *ret* tyrosine kinase and the regulatory subunit RI of cyclic AMP-dependent protein kinase A. Mol Cell Biol. 1993;13:358–66.

Burgess JR, Shepherd JJ, Parameswaran V, Hoffman L, Greenaway TM. Spectrum of pituitary disease in multiple endocrine neoplasia type 1 (MEN 1): clinical, biochemical, and radiological features of pituitary disease in a large MEN 1 kindred. J Clin Endocrinol Metab. 1996;81(7):2642–6.

Burnichon N, Vescovo L, Amar L, Libe R, de Reynies A, Venisse A, Jouanno E, Laurendeau I, Parfait B, Bertherat J, Plouin PF, Jeunemaitre X, Favier J, Gimenez-Roqueplo AP. Integrative genomic analysis reveals somatic mutations in pheochromocytoma and paraganglioma. Hum Mol Genet. 2011;20(20):3974–85.

Carpten JD, Robbins CM, Villablanca A, et al. HRPT 2, encoding parafibromin is mutated in hyperparathyroidism – jaw tumor syndrome. Nat Genet. 2002;32:676–80.

Cetta F, Montalto G, Gori M, Curia MC, Cama A, Olshwang S. Germline mutations of the APC gene in patients with familial adenomatous polyposis-associated thyroid carcinoma: results from a European cooperative study. J Clin Endocrinol Metab. 2000;85:286–92.

Comino-Mendez I, Gracia-Aznarez FJ, Schiavi F, Landa I, Leandro-Garcia LJ, Leton R, Honrado E, Ramos-Medina R, Caronia D, Pita G, Gomez-Grana A, de Cubas AA, Ingalda-Perez L, Maliszewska A, Taschin E, Bobisse S, Pica G, Loli P, Hernandez-Lavado R, Diaz JA, Gomez-Morales M, Gonzalez-Neira A, Roncador G, Rodriguez-Antona C, Benitez J, Mannelli M, Opocher G, Robledo M, Cascon A. Exome sequencing identifies MAX mutations as a cause of hereditary pheochromocytoma. Nat Genet. 2011;43:663–7.

Eng C. Familial papillary thyroid cancer – many syndromes, too many genes? J Clin Endocrinol Metab. 2000a;85:1755–7.

Eng C. Multiple endocrine neoplasia type 2 and the practice of molecular medicine. Rev Endocrinol Metab Dis. 2000b;1:283–90.

Eng C. Will the real Cowden syndrome please stand up: revised diagnostic criteria. J Med Genet. 2000c;37:828–30.

Eng C, Kiuru M, Fernandez MJ, Aaltonen LA. A role for mitochondrial enzymes in inherited neoplasia and beyond. Nat Rev Cancer 2003; 3:193–202.

Eng C, Smith DP, Mulligan LM, et al. Point mutation within the tyrosine kinase domain of the *RET* proto-oncogene in multiple endocrine neoplasia type 2B and related sporadic tumors. Hum Mol Genet. 1994;3:237–41.

Eng C, Mulligan LM, Smith DP, et al. Low frequency of germline mutations in the *RET* proto-oncogene in patients with apparently sporadic medullary thyroid carcinoma. Clin Endocrinol. 1995a;43:123–7.

Eng C, Mulligan LM, Smith DP, et al. Mutation in the *RET* proto-oncogene in sporadic medullary thyroid carcinoma. Genes Chromosomes Cancer. 1995b;12:209–12.

Eng C, Clayton D, Schuffenecker I, et al. The relationship between specific *RET* proto-oncogene mutations and disease phenotype in multiple endocrine neoplasia type 2: International *RET* Mutation Consortium analysis. J Am Med Assoc. 1996a;276:1575–9.

Eng C, Mulligan LM, Healey CS, et al. Heterogeneous mutation of the *RET* proto-oncogene in subpopulations of medullary thyroid carcinoma. Cancer Res. 1996b;56:2167–70.

Eng C, Schneider K, Fraumeni JF, Li FP. Third international workshop on collaborative interdisciplinary studies of *p53* and other predisposing genes in Li–Fraumeni syndrome. Cancer Epidemiol Biomark Prev. 1997;6:379–83.

Eng C, Thomas GA, Neuberg DS, et al. Mutation of the *RET* proto-oncogene is correlated with RET immunostaining in subpopulations of cells in sporadic medullary thyroid carcinoma. J Clin Endocrinol Metab. 1998;83:4310–3.

Erlic Z, Rybicki LA, Peczkowska M, Hohenberg W, Kann PH, Dralle H, Mussig K, Muresan M, Schaffler A, Reisch N, Schott M, Fassnacht M, Opocher G, Klose S, Fottner C, Forrer F, Plockinger U, Peterssen S, Januszwicz A, Waltz M, Eng C, Neumann HPH. Clinical predictors and algorithm for the genetic diagnosis of pheochromocytoma patients. Clin Cancer Res. 2009;15:6378–85.

Friedman E, deMarco L, Gejman PV, et al. Allelic loss from chromosome 11 in parathyroid tumors. Cancer Res. 1992;52:6804–9.

Gadelha MR, Une KN, Rohde K, Vaisman M, Kineman RD, Frohman LA. Isolated familial somato-tropinomas: establishment of linkage to chromosome 11q13.1–11q13.3 and evidence for a potential second locus at chromosome 2p16–12. J Clin Endocrinol Metab. 2000;85(2):707–14.

Gimm O, Armanios M, Dziema H, Neumann HPH, Eng C. Somatic and occult germline mutations in *SDHD*, a mitochondrial complex II gene, in non-familial pheochromocytomas. Cancer Res. 2000;60:6822–5.

Grufferman S, Gillman MW, Pasternak LR, Peterson CL, Young WG. Familial carotid body tumors: case report and epidemiologic review. Cancer. 1980;46:2116–22.

Hao HX, Khalimonchuk O, Schraders M, Dephoure N, Bayley JP, Kunst H, Devilee P, Cremers CW, Schiffman JD, Bentz BG, Gygi SP, Winge DR, Kremer H, Rutter J. SDH5, a gene required for flavination of succinate dehydrogease, is mutated in paraganglioma. Science. 2009;325: 1139–42.

Harach HR, Williams GT, Williams ED. Familial adenomatous polyposis associated thyroid carci-noma: a distinct type of follicular cell neoplasm. Histopathology. 1994;25:549–61.

Harach HR, Soubeyran I, Brown A, Bonneau D, Longy M. Thyroid pathologic findings in patients with Cowden disease. Ann Diagn Pathol. 1999;3(6):331–40.

Heutink P, van der Mey AGL, Sandkuijl LA, et al. A gene subject to genomic imprinting and responsible for hereditary paragangliomas maps to 11q23-qter. Hum Mol Genet. 1992;1:7–10.

Hofstra RMW, Landsvater RM, Ceccherini I, et al. A mutation in the *RET* proto-oncogene associ-ated with multiple endocrine neoplasia type 2B and sporadic medullary thyroid carcinoma. Nature. 1994;367:375–6.

Horvath A, Boikos S, Glatzakis C, Robinson-White A, Groussin L, Griffin KL, Stein E, Levine E, Delimpasi G, Hsiao HP, Keil M, Heyerdahl S, Matyakhina L, Libe R, Fratticci A, Kirschner LS, Cramer K, Gaillard RC, Bertagna X, Carney JA, Bertherat J, Bossis I, Stratakis CA. A genome-wide scan identifies mutations in the gene encoding phosphodies-terase 11A4 (PDE11A4) in individuals with adrenocortical hyperplasia. Nat Genet. 2006;38: 794–800.

Howell VM, Haven CJ, Kahnoski K, et al. *HRPT2* mutations are associated with malignancy in sporadic parathyroid tumors. J Med Genet. 2003;40:657–63.

Huang SC, Koch CA, Vortmeyer AO, et al. Duplication of the mutant *REt al*lele in trisomy 10 or loss of the wild-type allele in multiple endocrine neoplasia type 2-associated pheochromocy-toma. Cancer Res. 2000;60:6223–6.

Ito Y, Miyauchi A, Ishikawa H, Hirokawa M, Kudo T, Tomoda C, Miya A. Our experience of treat-ment of cribriform morular variant of papillary thyroid carcinoma; difference in clinicopatho-logical features of FAP-associated and sporadic patients. Endocr J. 2011;58(8):685–9.

Jadziewski K, Liyanarachchi S, Panchucki J, Ringel MD, Jarzab B, de la Chapelle A. Polymorphic mature micro-RNAs from passenger strand of miR-146a contribute to thyroid cancer. Proc Natl Acad Sci USA. 2009;106:1502–5.

Jarrar AM, Milas M, Mitchell J, Laguardia L, O'Malley M, Berber E, Siperstein A, Burke CA, Church JM. Screening for thyroid cancer in patients with familial adenomatous polyposis. Ann Surg. 2011;253:515–21.

Kassem M, Kruse TA, Wong FK, Larsson C, Teh BT. Familial isolated hyperparathyroidism as a variant of multiple endocrine neoplasia type 1 in a large Danish kindred. J Clin Endocrinol Metab. 2000;85:165–7.

Kimura ET, Nikiforova MN, Zhu Z, Knauf JA, Nikiforov YE, Fagin JA. High prevalence of BRAF mutations in thyroid cancer: genetic evidence for constitutive activation of the RET/PTC-RAS-BRAF signaling pathway in papillary thyroid carcinoma. Cancer Res. 2003;63:1454–7.

Kloos RT, Eng C, Evans DB, Francis GL, Gagel R, Gharib H, Moley JF, Pacini F, Ringel MD, Schlumberger M, Wells SA. Medullary thyroid carcinoma: management guidelines of the American Thyroid Association. Thyroid. 2009;19:565–612.

Koch CA, Huang SC, Moley JF, et al. Allelic imbalance of the mutant and wild-type *REt al*lele in MEN 2A-associated medullary thyroid carcinoma. Oncogene. 2001;20:7809–11.

Kroll TG, Sarraf P, Pecciarini L, et al. PAX8-PPARgamma1 fusion oncogene in human thyroid carcinoma. Science. 2000;289:1357–60.

Lanzi C, Borrello MG, Bongarzone I, et al. Identification of the product of two oncogenic forms of the ret proto-oncogene in papillary thyroid carcinomas. Oncogene. 1992;7:2189–94.

Lyons J, Landis CA, Harsh G, et al. Two G protein oncogenes in human endocrine tumors. Science. 1990;249:655–88.

Maher ER, Eng C. The pressure rises: update on the genetics of phaeochromocytoma. Hum Mol Genet. 2002;11:2347–54.

Malkin D, Li FP, Strong LC, et al. Germline p53 mutations in a familial syndrome of breast cancer, sarcomas, and other neoplasms. Science. 1990;250:1233–8.

Mariman ECM, van Beersum SEC, Cremers CWRJ, Struycken PM, Ropers HH. Fine mapping of a putatively imprinted gene for familial non-chromaffin paragangliomas to chromosome 11q13.1: evidence for genetic heterogeneity. Hum Genet. 1995;95:56–62.

Marsh DJ, Learoyd DL, Andrew SD, et al. Somatic mutations in the *RET* proto-oncogene in sporadic medullary thyroid carcinoma. Clin Endocrinol. 1996a;44:249–57.

Marsh DJ, Andrew SD, Eng C, et al. Germline and somatic mutations in an oncogene: RET mutations in inherited medullary thyroid carcinoma. Cancer Res. 1996b;6:1241–3.

Marsh DJ, Coulon V, Lunetta KL, et al. Mutation spectrum and genotype– phenotype analyses in Cowden disease and Bannayan–Zonana syndrome, two hamartoma syndromes with germline *PTEN* mutation. Hum Mol Genet. 1998;7:507–15.

Moura MM, Cavaco BM, Pinto AE, Leite V. High prevalence of RAS mutations in RET-negative sporadic medullary thyroid carcinomas. J Clin Endocrinol Metab. 2011;96:E863–8.

Mulligan LM, Eng C, Healey CS, et al. Specific mutations of the *RET* proto-oncogene are related to disease phenotype in MEN 2A and FMTC. Nat Genet. 1994;6:70–4.

Neumann HPH, Bausch B, McWhinney SR, Bender BU, Gimm O, Franke G, Schipper J, Klisch J, Altehoefer C, Zerres K, Januszewicz A, Eng C, Smith WM, Munk R, Manz T, Glaesker S, Apel TW, Treier M, Reineke M, Walz MK, Hoang-Vu C, Brauckhoff M, Klein-Franke A, Klose P, Schmidt H, Maier-Woelfle M, Peczkowska M, Szmigielski C, Eng C, The Freiburg-Warsaw-Columbus Pheochromocytoma Study Group. Germ-line mutations in nonsyndromic pheochromocytoma. N Engl J Med. 2002;346:1459–66.

Neumann HPH, Pawlu C, Pęczkowska M, Bausch B, McWhinney SR, Muresan M, Buchta M, Franke G, Klisch J, Bley T, Hoegerle S, Boedeker CC, Opocher G, Schipper J, Januszewicz A, Eng C. Distinct clinical features characterize paraganglioma syndromes associated with SDHB and SDHD mutations. JAMA. 2004;292:943–51.

Neumann HPH, Erlic Z, Boedeker CC, Rybicki LA, Robledo M, Hermsen M, Schiavi F, Falcioni M, Kwok P, Bauters C, Lampe K, Fischer M, Edelman E, Benn DE, Robinson BG, Wiegand S, Rasp G, Stuck BA, Ridder G, Hoffman MM, Sullivan M, Sevilla MA, Weiss MM, Peczkowska M, Kabaszek A, Pigny P, Ward RL, Learoyd D, Croxson M, Zabolotny D, Yaremchek S, Draf W, Muresan M, Lorenz RR, Knipping S, Strohm M, Dyckhoff G, Mattias C, Reisch N, Preuss SF, Esser D, Walter MA, Kaftan H, Stover T, Fottner C, Gorgulla H, Schipper J, Brase C, Glien A, Kuehnemund M, Koscielny S, Schwerdtfeger DT, Valimaki M, Szyfter W, Finckh U, Zerres K, Cascon A, Opocher G, Ridder G, Januszewicz A, Suarez C, Eng C. Clinical predictors for germline mutations in head and neck paraganglioma patients: cost reduction strategy in genetic diagnostic process as fall-out. Cancer Res. 2009;69:3650–6.

Neumann HPH, Sullivan M, Winter A, Malinoc A, Hoffmann MM, Boedeker CC, Bertz H, Walz MK, Moeller LC, Schmid KW, Eng C. Germline mutations of the TMEM127 gene in patients with paraganglioma of head and neck and extraadrenal abdominal sites. J Clin Endocrinol Metab. 2011;96:E1279–82.

Ni Y, Zbuk KM, Sadler T, Patocs A, Lobo G, Edelman E, Platzer P, Orloff MS, Waite KA, Eng C. Germline mutations and variants in the succinate dehydrogenase genes in Cowden and Cowden-like syndromes. Am J Hum Genet. 2008;83:261–8.

Niemann S, Muller U. Mutations in *SDHC* cause autosomal dominant paraganglioma. Nat Genet. 2000;26:141–50.

Parry DM, Li FP, Strong LC, et al. Carotid body tumors in humans: genetics and epidemiology. J Natl Cancer Inst. 1982;68:573–8.

Peczkowska M, Cascon A, Prejbisz A, Kubaszek A, Cwikla JB, Furmanek M, Erlic Z, Eng C, Januszewicz A, Neumann HPH. Metachronous extraadrenal and adrenal pheochromocytomas associated with a germline succinate dehydrogenase subunit C (*SDHC*) mutation. Nat Clin Pract Endocrinol Metab. 2007;4:111–5.

Peczkowska M, Erlic Z, Hoffman M, Furmanek M, Kubaszek A, Prejbisz A, Szutkowski Z, Kawaki A, Chojnowski K, Lewczuk A, Litwin M, Syfter W, Walter M, Sullivan M, Eng C, Januszewicz A, Neumann HPH. Screening *SDHD* Cys11X as a common mutation associated with paranganglioma syndrome type 1. J Clin Endocrinol Metab. 2008;93:4818–25.

Pollak MR, Brown EM, Chou YH, Hebert SC, Marx SJ, Steinmann B, Levi T, Seidman CE, Seidman JG. Mutations in the human Ca(2+)-sensing receptor gene cause familial hypocalciuric hypercalcemia and neonatal severe hyperparathyroidism. Cell. 1993;75(7):1297–303.

Ribeiro RC, Sandrini F, Figueiredo B, et al. An inherited p53 mutation that contributes in a tissue-specific manner to pediatric adrenal cortical carcinoma. Proc Natl Acad Sci USA. 2001; 98:9330–5.

Rio Frio T, Bahubeshi A, Kanellopoulou C, Hamel N, Niedziela M, Sabbaghian N, Pouchet C, Gilbert L, O'Brien PK, Serfas K, Broderick P, Houlston RS, Lesueur F, Bonora E, Muljo S, Schimke RN, Bouron-Dal Soglio D, Arseneau J, Schultz KA, Priest VH, Harach HR, Livingston DM, Foulkes WD, Tischkowitz M. DICER1 mutations in familial multinodular goiter with and without ovarian Sertoli-Leydig cell tumors. JAMA. 2011;305:68–77.

Schiavi F, Boedeker CC, Bausch B, Peçzkowska M, Fuentes-Gomez C, Strassburg T, Pawlu C, Buchta M, Saltzman M, Hoffman MM, Berlis A, Brink I, Cybulla M, Muresan M, Walter MM, Forer F, Välimäki M, Kawecki A, Szutkowski Z, Schipper J, Walz MK, Pigny P, Bauters C, Willet-Brozick JE, Baysal BE, Januszewicz A, Eng C, Opocher G, Neumann HPH. Predictors and prevalence of paraganglioma syndrome associated with mutations of the *SDHC* gene. JAMA. 2005;294:2057–63.

Schilling T, Burck J, Sinn HP, et al. Prognostic value of codon 918 (ATG->ACG) RET proto-oncogene mutations in sporadic medullary thyroid carcinoma. Int J Cancer. 2001;95:62–6.

Schuffenecker I, Ginet N, Goldgar D, et al. Prevalence and parental origin of *de novo RET* mutations in MEN 2A and FMTC. Am J Hum Genet. 1997;60:233–7.

Schuffenecker I, Virally-Monod M, Brohet R, et al. Risk and penetrance of primary hyperparathyroidism in MEN 2A families with codon 634 mutations of the *RET* proto-oncogene. J Clin Endocrinol Metab. 1998;83:487–91.

Shattuck TM, Valimaki S, Obara T, et al. Somatic and germ-line mutations of the HRPT2 gene in sporadic parathyroid carcinoma. New Engl J Med. 2003;349:1722–9.

Soares P, Trovisco V, Rocha AS, et al. BRAF mutations and RET/PTC rearrangements are alternative events in the etiopathogenesis of PTC. Oncogene. 2003;22:4578–80.

Sozzi G, Bongarzone I, Miozzo M, et al. A t(10;17) translocation creates the RET/ PTC2 chimeric transforming sequence in papillary thyroid carcinoma. Genes Chromosomes Cancer. 1992; 9:244–50.

Stratakis CA, Sarlis N, Kirschner LS, et al. Paradoxical response to dexamethasone in the diagnosis of primary pigmented nodular adrenocortical disease. Ann Int Med. 1999;131:585–91.

Stratakis CA, Tichomirowa MA, Boikos S, Azevdo MF, Lodish M, Martari M, Verman S, Daly AF, Raygada M, Keil MF, Papademetriou J, Drori-Herishanu L, Horvath A, Tsang KM, Nesterova M,

Franklin S, VanBellinghan JF, Bours V, Salvatori R, Beckers A. The role of germline AIP, MEN1, PRKAR1A, CDKN1B and CDKN2C mutations in causing pituitary adenomas in a large cohort of children, adolescents, and patients with genetic syndromes. Clin Genet. 2010;78:457–63.

Tamura Y, Ishibashi S, Gotoda T, et al. A Kindred of familial acromegaly without evidence for linkage to MEN 1 locus. Endocr J. 2002;49:425–31.

Teh BT, Farnebo F, Kristoffersson U, et al. Autosomal dominant primary hyper-parathyroidism and jaw tumor syndrome associated with renal hamartomas and cystic kidney disease: linkage to 1q21–q32 and loss of the wild type allele in renal hamartomas. J Clin Endocrinol Metab. 1996;81:4204–11.

Tichomirowa MA, Barlier A, Daly AF, Jaffrain-Rea ML, Ronchi CL, Yaneva M, Urban JD, Petrossians P, Elenkova AP, Tabarin A, Desailloud R, Maiter D, Schurmeyer T, Cozzi R, Theodoropoulou M, Sievers C, Benebeu I, LA N, Chabre O, Fajardo-Montanana C, Hana V, Halaby G, Delemer B, Labarta JI, Sonnet E, Ferrandez A, Hagelstein MT, Caron P, Stalla GK, Bours V, Zacharieva S, Spada A, Brue T, Beckers A. High prevalence of AIP gene mutations following focused screening in young patients with sporadic pituitary macroadenomas. Eur J Endocrinol. 2011;165(4):509–15.

Vierimaa O, Georgitsi M, Lehtonen R, Vahteristo P, Kokko A, Raitila A, Tuppurainen K, Ebeling TM, Salmela PI, Paschke R, Gundogdu S, DeMenis E, Makinen MJ, Launonen V, Karhu A, Aaltonen LA. Pituitary adenoma predisposition caused by germline mutations in the AIP gene. Science. 2006;312:1228–30.

Wiedemann H-R. Tumors and hemihypertrophy associated with Wiedemann–Beckwith syndrome. Eur J Pediatr. 1983;141:129.

Wohlik N, Cote GJ, Bugalho MMJ, et al. Relevance of RET proto-oncogene mutations in sporadic medullary thyroid carcinoma. J Clin Endocrinol Metab. 1996;81:3740–5.

Woodward ER, Eng C, McMahon R, Voutilainen R, Affara NA, Ponder BAJ, Maher ER. Genetic predisposition to pheochromocytoma: analysis of candidate genes GDNF, RET and VHL. Hum Mol Genet. 1997;6:1051–6.

Yao L, Schiavi F, Cascon A, Qin Y, Inglada-Perez L, King EE, Toledo RA, Ercolino T, Rappizzi E, Ricketts CJ, Mori L, Giacche M, Mendola A, Taschin E, Boaretto F, Loli P, Iaocobone M, Rossi GP, Biondi B, Lima-Junior JV, Kater CE, Bex M, Vikkula M, Grossman AB, Gruber SB, Barotini M, Persu A, Castellano M, Toledo SP, Maher ER, Manelli M, Opocher G, Robledo M, Dahia PLM. Spectrum and prevalence of FP/TMEM127 gene mutations in pheochromocytomas and paragangliomas. JAMA. 2010;304:2611–9.

Zhuang Z, Vortmeyer AO, Pack S, et al. Somatic mutations of the *MEN1* tumor suppressor gene in sporadic gastrinomas and insulinomas. Cancer Res. 1997;57:4682–6.

Chapter 5
Gastrointestinal System

Salivary Gland Tumors

Tumors at this site occur with a frequency of about 1 per 100,000 population. They are commoner in Spanish, Inuit, Indian, and Cantonese Chinese populations, but do not appear to have a strong genetic basis. Familial occurrence of mixed salivary tumors has been reported infrequently (Klausner and Handler 1994), and it is difficult to know whether the familial incidence is determined by hereditary or environmental factors. However, similarities in the epidemiology of nasopharyngeal carcinoma and salivary gland tumors suggest that they may have a similar etiology, perhaps involving Epstein–Barr virus (EBV) infection (Ponz de Leon 1994). Several Greenland Inuit families have been described with two or more siblings affected, and there was an increased risk of other cancers in these sibships (Merrick et al. 1986). Other studies from Greenland show that a significant fraction of all cases occurring among Greenland Inuit clusters in families (Albeck et al. 1993). Cancer incidence in this part of the world differs from that seen in more temperate climates: compared to the Caucasian population in Denmark (1973–1995), high standardized incidence ratios (SIRs) were found for cancers of the salivary gland and nasopharynx (EBV-related cancers), esophagus, stomach (probably related to a dried fish diet), and cervix (HPV-related). Low SIRs were seen for testis, bladder, prostate, breast, and hematological cancers (Friborg et al. 2003). In a further study in the same population, there was about an eightfold increased risk of salivary gland carcinoma in first-degree relatives of patients with nasopharyngeal carcinoma (none of the salivary gland carcinoma patients developed subsequent nasopharyngeal carcinoma in the follow-up period) (Friborg et al. 2005).

A single two-generation Inuit family from northern Quebec (Nunavik) that contained four family members of both sexes, all diagnosed with lymphoepithelioma of the parotid gland (without involvement of the nasopharynx), has been reported (Vu et al. 2008). Rare families with familial neuroendocrine carcinoma of the salivary glands and deafness and enamel hyperplasia (siblings) are described (Michaels et al. 1999).

S.V. Hodgson et al., *A Practical Guide to Human Cancer Genetics*,
DOI 10.1007/978-1-4471-2375-0_5, © Springer-Verlag London 2014

MALT lymphomas may occur in the lymphoid tissue of the salivary glands, often associated with a translocation t (14:18 [q.32;q.21]) (Streubel et al. 2003). MALT lymphomas may develop in benign lesions developing from long-standing Sjogren's syndrome. There has been a case report of a 3-year-old child with a plexiform neurofibroma involving the submandibular salivary gland that mimicked an intraglandular tumor (Bourgeois et al. 2001). There was a family history of neurofibromatosis.

Germline mutations in the *CYLD1* gene may cause Brooke–Spiegler syndrome, familial cylindromatosis, and multiple familial trichoepithelioma 1 (see p. 200). Salivary gland tumors (adenomas and adenocarcinomas) may be a feature of these disorders (Kakagia et al. 2004; Bowen et al. 2005).

Gastrointestinal System

Tumors of the gastrointestinal system are among the most common tumors in humans, and although environmental influences have been clearly implicated, heredity is recognized as being of major importance in their etiology.

Esophageal Tumors

The incidence of squamous cell carcinoma of the esophagus shows marked geographical variation, with a high frequency in the Caspian littoral of Iran, certain parts of the interior of China, and the Transkei region of South Africa. There is a low incidence in European and North American Caucasian populations. Oropharyngeal tumors are also commoner in areas with a high incidence of esophageal cancer. These findings are thought to be the result of differences in exposure to ingested carcinogens rather than of major genetic factors, although the at-risk individuals who develop this cancer in these high-risk areas are predominantly of Mongol or Turkic origin. The incidence of esophageal cancer in the UK is 6 per 100,000, and it is commoner in males. Almost all (98 %) of esophageal cancers are squamous carcinomas.

Early studies suggested that genetic factors do not play a major role in most cases of esophageal cancer as there did not appear to be an increased risk to relatives of index cases (Mosbech and Videbaek 1955), and recent studies in the United States have been in agreement (Dhillon et al. 2001). However other studies, particularly those in high-incidence regions, such as China, have come to the conclusion that the familial occurrence of esophageal cancer probably does have a Mendelian basis, with both autosomal dominant (Zhang et al. 2000; Guohong et al. 2010) and recessive models favored. A genome-wide search indicated that chromosome 13 could harbor such a gene, but sequence analysis of known candidate genes, such as *BRCA2*, has been inconclusive (Hu et al. 2002, 2004) (see below, however). Interestingly, gene expression studies indicate that true differences exist between familial and nonfamilial esophageal cancer, suggesting that there are susceptibility genes to be found (Su et al. 2003).

The autosomal dominant condition of late-onset tylosis (keratosis palmaris et plantaris), with hyperkeratosis of the palms and soles from late childhood to adolescence, is associated with a high incidence of esophageal cancer (p. 200; Shine and Alison 1966; Risk et al. 2002). Tylosis with onset in infancy does not seem to be associated with any such increased cancer risk. Thickening of the skin of the pressure areas on the soles of the feet is seen, and oral leukokeratosis and follicular hyperkeratosis occur. The risk of esophageal cancer reaches 95 % by 63 years of age, and the mean age at diagnosis of the cancer is 45 years of age. Prophylactic esophagectomy with interposition of a segment of colon has been suggested for affected individuals. If prophylactic esophagectomy has not been performed, then annual esophagoscopy is recommended, and immediate esophagectomy is advisable if dysplasia is detected. The gene for this condition was mapped to chromosome 17q, and a presumed gain-of-function mutation in *RHBDF2* has been reported as the cause (Hennies et al. 1995; Kelsell et al. 1996; Langan et al. 2004; Blaydon et al. 2012; Saarinen et al. 2012).

There is an increased risk of esophageal cancer in Fanconi anemia (Alter 1996; Rosenberg et al. 2003; see p. 249) and possibly also in epidermolysis bullosa (p. 195), dyskeratosis congenita (p. 194), and congenital abnormalities of the esophagus, such as strictures. In support of the earlier epidemiological data, mutations in genes in the Fanconi anemia pathway have been associated with esophageal cancer in Iran – most notably, *BRCA2 (FANCD1)*, where the p. Lys3326X mutation was present in 27 of 746 esophageal squamous cell cancer cases and in 16 of 1,373 controls (OR = 3.38, 95 % CI = 1.97–6.91, P = 0.0002) (Akbari et al. 2011). This is a notable finding because this particular *BRCA2* mutation is generally not thought to be a cause of breast cancer susceptibility.

The risk of esophageal cancer increases with celiac disease (p. 231) and is more common in the adult-onset form, but is probably uncommon when celiac disease is diagnosed and treated in childhood or infancy. There is an increased risk of esophageal cancer in achalasia. This condition is not usually genetic, but its familial occurrence has been described occasionally with some evidence of an autosomal recessive subgroup (Frieling et al. 1988; Gockel et al. 2010). Nevertheless it may occur rarely as part of a genetic condition (autosomal recessive), characterized by achalasia, alacrimia, and sensorimotor polyneuropathy (Achalasia–Addisonianism–Alacrimia syndrome, also known as Allgrove syndrome), and the responsible gene, *AAAS*, has been identified (Kasirga et al. 1996; Handschug et al. 2001).

There is also an increased risk of adenocarcinoma of the esophagus (possibly 10 %) in Barrett esophagus, in which columnar rather than squamous epithelium is found with chronic ulcerative esophagitis. Although this is usually sporadic, some familial cases have been described, and 70 families have recently been reported (Drovdlic et al. 2003). Importantly, there was no excess of extra-esophageal cancers in these families. In unselected individuals with Barrett esophagus, it is among older males that most familial cases are encountered (Chak et al. 2002). Germline mutations in *MSR1* have been reported in a small proportion of patients with Barrett esophagus/esophageal cancer (Orloff et al. 2011).

Management

In tylosis, annual esophagoscopy is recommended unless prophylactic esophagectomy has been performed, and because of the high risk of cancer in this disorder, immediate esophagectomy is advisable if dysplasia is detected. However, in other conditions in which the risk of carcinoma is less, the appropriate course of action if an abnormality is found may not be so clear, and results from an observational study of individuals undergoing surveillance for Barrett esophagus found that there was no impact on overall mortality (MacDonald et al. 2000). Nevertheless, those with a family history are likely to be screened by endoscopy even if they do not have long-segment disease. Screening for esophageal cancer by endoscopy with multiple biopsies to detect dysplasia is performed in some high-risk areas in China (Spigelman and Phillips 1991).

Gastric Tumors

Benign tumors of the stomach are uncommon. Polyploid adenomas occur in less than 1 % of the population and may occur in association with intestinal metaplasia. They predispose to carcinoma. Gastric polyps occur in familial adenomatous polyposis (in up to two-thirds of patients, but with a lower potential for malignant transformation than the colonic adenomas; see p. 241), in MUTYH-associated polyposis, in Peutz–Jeghers syndrome (p. 299), and in Cowden syndrome (p. 233). Gastric polyposis (with malignant potential) limited to the stomach has been described in three generations of a family (dos Santos and de Magalhes 1980). Recently three families with an autosomal dominantly inherited syndrome characterized by fundic gland polyposis and intestinal-type gastric cancer was described (gastric adenocarcinoma and proximal polyposis of the stomach (GAPPS)) (Worthley et al. 2012). Recommended diagnostic criteria for GAPPS were (1) gastric polyps restricted to the body and fundus without colorectal or duodenal polyposis, (2) >100 polyps carpeting the proximal stomach in the index case or >30 polyps in a first-degree relative of another case, (3) predominantly fundic gland polyps with regions of dysplasia or gastric adenocarcinoma, and (4) autosomal dominant inheritance. Earliest age at diagnosis of gastric cancer was 33 years of age. Relatives at high risk should be offered surveillance gastroscopy, and partial gastrectomy should be considered in affected cases.

Hyperplastic gastric polyps are five times as common as gastric polyps and have a much lower risk of malignancy. They are found with increased frequency in pernicious anemia and in familial adenomatous polyposis (Debinski et al. 1995) and the Peutz–Jeghers syndrome (Ushio et al. 1976; Williams et al. 1982). Carcinoids, lymphomas, sarcomas, and leiomyosarcomas may also arise in the stomach; a family with primary B cell gastric lymphoma in a father and his two daughters has been described (Hayoz et al. 1993).

Gastric Carcinoma

The incidence of gastric cancer (which is adenocarcinoma in 97 % of cases) shows marked geographical variation, being 88 per 100,000 males in Japan and 22 and 11 per 100,000 in the UK and USA, respectively. Women have about half the male incidence. There is a twofold to threefold excess risk of gastric cancer in the first-degree relatives of affected patients, particularly in cases diagnosed under the age of 50 years of age. Two major histological variants of gastric cancer are recognized: a diffuse type containing signet ring cells and intestinal-type gastric cancer which is associated with the presence of *H. pylori*. The latter is preceded by chronic gastritis, atrophy, and metaplasia. However, the diffuse histological type does not have recognized precursor changes (Correa and Shiao 1994). An association between blood group A and gastric cancer (particularly the diffuse type) has long been recognized. This could in part be due to the association of this blood group with pernicious anemia, which itself carries a higher than expected risk of gastric cancer (McConnell 1966). The risk of gastric cancer in relatives of index cases appears to be much more pronounced when the histological type in the index case is diffuse (seven times the risk in matched controls) rather than of the intestinal type (1.5 times higher than in control families) (Macklin 1960), but only a small proportion of diffuse gastric cancers occurs in families with an autosomal dominant gastric cancer susceptibility (reviewed in González et al. 2002).

The diffuse type of gastric carcinoma demonstrates a nearly equal sex ratio (compared with a male preponderance in the intestinal type), a younger patient age distribution, and little change with geographical migration, relative to the intestinal type. Chronic atrophic gastritis is found with increased frequency in relatives of index cases with pernicious anemia and gastric adenocarcinomas, but, specifically, it has been demonstrated to be more frequent in the relatives of index cases with diffuse spreading carcinoma than in controls; this has not been seen with other gastric cancer types (Kekki et al. 1987). Evidence suggests there may be an association between chronic *H. pylori* infection and intestinal-type chronic gastritis and cancer susceptibility: an increased frequency of infection with this organism has been reported in stomach cancer patients (Scott et al. 1990). Chronic gastritis may have a hereditary component, but the nature of this and its relationship to *Helicobacter* infection have not been clearly elucidated (Kekki et al. 1987). Ménétrier's disease is also associated with an increased risk (10 %) of gastric cancer – possibly because atrophic gastritis occurs in this etiologically obscure disease.

Most gastric cancers are sporadic, although up to 3 % occur in predisposed individuals. Nevertheless, there are many reports of families in which there is a strikingly high incidence of gastric cancer, following an autosomal dominant pattern of inheritance (Triantafillidis et al. 1993; Villanueva et al. 2010). Napoleon Bonaparte came from such a family (Creagan and Fraumeni 1973). Gastric cancer is a component of Lynch syndrome (see below). An increased incidence of stomach cancer has also been noted in the close relatives of women with the medullary or tubular histological types of breast cancer. Some of these families may have Li–Fraumeni syndrome (Burki et al. 1987), and gastric carcinoma has also been described in some families with p53 mutations (Varley et al. 1995). Lobular breast cancer is increased in families with germline *CDH1* mutations (see below).

Adenocarcinoma of the stomach is reported in familial adenomatous polyposis (Jagelman et al. 1988) and is also reported to be more frequent in ataxia telangiectasia (Haerer et al. 1969; see p. 219 Gylling et al. 2007; Ohue et al. 1996) and in patients with immune deficiency. IgA deficiency is associated with an increased risk of intestinal metaplasia and of gastric cancer. The inheritance of IgA deficiency is not clear-cut and may be multifactorial (Grundbacher 1972). Gastric cancer occurs with increased relative risk in carriers of germline BRCA2 mutations (Breast Cancer Linkage Consortium 1997; Jakubowska et al. 2002). Gastric carcinoma (particularly of the intestinal type) is also part of the spectrum of cancers found in Lynch syndrome and displays replication errors (RER) characteristic of the condition in such families. The average age at diagnosis of gastric carcinoma in Lynch syndrome has been reported to be 56 years of age (Arnio et al. 1997; Watson et al. 2008).

The International Gastric Cancer Linkage Consortium (IGCLC) defined hereditary diffuse gastric cancer (HDGC) as (a) families with two or more cases of diffuse gastric cancer in first- or second-degree relatives with one affected aged <50 years or (b) three cases or more cases of diffuse gastric cancer in first- or second-degree relatives at any age (Caldas et al. 1999; Pharoah et al. 2001). Overall, about 25–50 % of patients with HDGC will have germline *CDH1* mutations, and this rises to about 50 % in younger-onset cases (<50 years) with a positive family history (Gayther et al. 1998; Guilford et al. 1998; Richards et al. 1999). However isolated early-onset cases of diffuse gastric cancer are unlikely to have germline *CDH1* mutations (Brooks-Wilson et al. 2004). Recently, it was suggested that families meeting the HDGC criteria should be offered testing for *CDH1* mutations, and in addition, *CDH1* molecular genetic testing also should be considered in (a) families with two cases of gastric cancer in the family with one confirmed case of diffuse gastric cancer <50 years, (b) cases of diffuse gastric cancer aged <40 years, and (c) a personal or family history of diffuse gastric cancer and lobular breast cancer (with one diagnosed <50 years of age). About 4 % of *CDH1* mutation-positive families have exonic deletions.

The lifetime risk of gastric cancer in *CDH1* mutation carriers was originally estimated to be >80 %, and prophylactic gastrectomy should be offered to mutation carriers aged 20 years or older (Fitzgerald et al. 2010), and multiple foci of gastric cancer have been found in gastrectomy specimens from affected individuals (Huntsman et al. 2001). If gastrectomy is delayed, then intensive annual endoscopy with multiple biopsies should be performed, but the efficacy of such screening is uncertain, as multiple foci of gastric cancer have been detected in gastrectomy specimens from affected individuals previously screened in this way (Huntsman et al. 2001). Chromoendoscopic surveillance has also been advocated (Shaw et al. 2005), but is generally thought to be too insensitive to replace preventive surgery.

Further large-scale studies of penetrance are required as the long-term effects of total gastrectomy remain uncertain.

There is an increased risk of breast cancer, particularly lobular, in women with germline *CDH1* mutations, and it has been recommended that such women should have annual mammogram and breast MRI and biannual clinical breast examination from 25 years of age (Fitzgerald et al. 2010). In *CDH1* mutation-positive families with a history of colorectal cancer, mutation carriers might be offered colonoscopy from 40 years of age or, if younger, 10 years younger than the earliest age of onset of colorectal cancer in the family (Fitzgerald et al. 2010).

For individuals at risk for familial gastric cancer without *CDH1* mutations, endoscopy with eradication of *H. pylori* infection is performed as an initial step. Subsequent endoscopies may be performed annually.

Hepatic Tumors

Cancer of the liver typically occurs as hepatocellular carcinoma or intrahepatic bile duct cancer (cholangiocarcinoma) in adults and as hepatoblastoma in childhood.

Hepatoblastoma

This rare embryonal tumor originates from immature liver cells. It usually presents in children under 3 years of age, is more common in males than in females, and shows no association with hepatitis B infection or cirrhosis. The majority of cases of hepatoblastoma are sporadic, although familial cases occasionally occur (Hartley et al. 1990). Congenital abnormalities, particularly abnormalities of the urogenital system, are more common in children who develop hepatoblastoma. Syndromes associated with an increased susceptibility to hepatoblastoma development include Beckwith–Wiedemann syndrome and congenital hemihypertrophy, caused by dysregulation of the 11p15 growth region. Risk of neoplasia in children with this disorder is increased if hemihypertrophy is present, and children with BWS and loss of methylation at KvDMR1 appear to be at higher risk of hepatoblastoma than Wilms' tumor (Cooper et al. 2005). It is not a component of another overgrowth syndrome, Bannayan–Riley–Ruvalcaba syndrome. Hepatoblastoma may occur in children with familial adenomatous polyposis (Herzog et al. 2000) (p. 241). Hepatoblastoma surveillance for individuals at increased risk is controversial. Some clinicians advocate 3 monthly physical examinations, serum α-fetoprotein, and abdominal ultrasound until the age of 3 years and then 6 monthly until 6 years of age (Chitayat et al. 1990a, b; Clericuzio et al. 2003). However, there is little evidence for the efficacy of this screening program, and currently the potential benefits and risks are poorly understood.

Hepatocellular Carcinoma

Most cases of hepatocellular carcinoma occur in adults, appear to be sporadic, and are related to environmental carcinogens such as hepatitis B viral infections and aflatoxin. The marked geographical variations in the incidence of hepatocellular

Table 5.1 Genetic causes of liver cancer

Important causes	Less commonly associated
Hemochromatosis	Galactosemia
α_1-Antitrypsin deficiency	Hereditary fructose intolerance
Glycogen storage disease	Iron overload in thalassemia
Type I (hepatic)	Iron overload in hereditary hemorrhagic telangiectasia
Type IV	Acute intermittent porphyria
Tyrosinemia	Common bile duct atresia
Fanconi anemia	Neonatal hepatitis
Wilson disease	Cystic fibrosis
	De Toni–Fanconi syndrome
	Werner syndrome
	Familial cirrhosis
	Indian childhood cirrhosis
	Neonatal giant cell hepatitis
	Neonatal hemochromatosis
	Porphyria cutanea tarda

carcinoma (it is frequent in Africa and Asia, reaching an incidence of 40 per 100,000 males) are thought to be caused by environmental factors. The incidence in the UK is 1–1.6 per 100,000, and it is commoner in males. Familial clustering of hepatocellular cancer has occasionally been reported (Fernandez et al. 1994; Drinkwater and Lee 1995), and the relative risk of the cancer in the first-degree relatives of index cases with primary liver cancer has been assessed to be 2.4 (Fernandez et al. 1994). However, familial clustering of hepatitis B virus is common as a consequence of perinatal transmission, and this is regarded as the main cause of familial hepatocellular carcinoma in high-prevalence areas (Tai et al. 2002).

Liver cancer may occur as a complication of chronic liver disease and cirrhosis of a variety of causes (although it is rare in biliary cirrhosis), some of which have a genetic basis (see Table 5.1). In hemochromatosis, the incidence of hepatic carcinoma is usually only increased if cirrhosis has developed. Hemochromatosis is a common condition affecting about 1 in 300 individuals of Northern European descent. However, many cases are asymptomatic and women are less severely affected than men because of menstrual blood loss (Brind and Bassendine 1990). Hepatocellular carcinoma develops in up to one-third of cirrhotic cases, in whom the relative risk of hepatoma may be 200 (Edwards et al. 1982). Treatment by phlebotomy before cirrhosis develops appears to prevent malignancy (Niederau et al. 1985), although occasionally liver cancer has been reported in the absence of cirrhosis. The *HFE* gene is closely linked to the MHC class I gene cluster at 6p21 (Feder et al. 1996). The two common *HFE* mutations, p. C282Y and p. H63D, are readily screened. A diagnosis of hemochromatosis can be made in p. C283Y homozygotes and p. C282Y/H63D compound heterozygotes. Screening of at-risk relatives is important as early diagnosis allows treatment with prophylactic phlebotomy, and the prevention of cirrhosis from developing will reduce the risk of hepatocellular cancer (Harrison and Bacon 2005).

α-1 antitrypsin deficiency, particularly with the ZZ phenotype, predisposes to hepatocellular carcinoma (Eriksson et al. 1986). This is an autosomal recessive condition with a frequency of 1 in 2,000 births. α-1 antitrypsin is a serum protease inhibitor encoded by a gene on chromosome 14q31–q32. The phenotype (Pi type) is determined by isoelectric focusing of serum, and both parental alleles are expressed. PiMZ heterozygotes may also have an increased risk of hepatocellular cancer, but not those with the null–null phenotype. The commonest phenotype in the UK (PiM) is associated with normal levels of AAT, PiZ is associated with 15 % levels of serum AAT, and null variants are associated with no detectable levels. About 10 % of PiZZ individuals develop neonatal cholestatic jaundice, and 25 % of these develop cirrhosis. PiZ adults have a risk relative to the normal population of 7.4 for cirrhosis and 20 for hepatocellular carcinoma (higher in males) (Brind and Bassendine 1990; Perlmutter 1995).

Individuals with type 1 (hepatic) glycogen storage disease, an autosomal recessive condition due to deficiency of glucose-6-phosphatase, often develop liver adenomas, and hepatoblastomas and hepatocellular carcinomas have been described (Ito et al. 1987). Glycogen storage disease type IV (due to a glycogen debrancher enzyme defect) is also associated with cirrhosis and hepatic cancer.

Hepatoma is a significant cause of death in individuals suffering from the autosomal recessive condition of hereditary tyrosinemia (due to a defect in the fumarylacetoacetase gene on chromosome 15q; Sniderman King et al. 1993–2006; Rootwelt et al. 1996), consequent upon the progressive liver disease with cirrhosis in this condition. About a third of affected children develop liver cancer if they survive to 5 years of age.

Other inherited disorders (e.g., galactosemia, hereditary fructose intolerance) may result in chronic liver damage and so predispose to carcinoma of the liver. Wilson disease, an autosomal recessive copper storage disorder, can cause cirrhosis in the absence of successful therapy with chelating agents. The risk of intra-abdominal malignancy (hepatomas, cholangiocarcinomas, and poorly differentiated adenocarcinomas of unknown primary) is substantial in patients followed for > 10 years, and surveillance by abdominal ultrasound may be indicated (Walshe et al. 2003). Iron overload can produce cirrhosis of the liver in thalassemia, and hereditary hemorrhagic telangiectasia may occasionally predispose to liver carcinoma. The hepatic porphyrias can be associated with cirrhosis, and primary liver carcinoma (not always in the presence of cirrhosis) has been described in patients with acute intermittent porphyria. Common bile duct atresia, neonatal hepatitis, cystic fibrosis, and the De Toni–Fanconi syndrome are also associated with a risk of cirrhosis and potentially of liver cancer.

Hepatic carcinoma is described in Fanconi anemia (Alter 1996; Rosenberg et al. 2003) and may sometimes be secondary to androgen therapy for the pancytopenia (p. 249). Werner syndrome may also carry an increased risk for liver cancer (p. 318). Familial cases of cirrhosis without a known predisposing cause have been described, but this group is probably heterogeneous and often environmental in etiology. Indian childhood cirrhosis, with onset between 6 and 18 months of age, has been described with familial occurrence (in about 30 % of cases) in India, Pakistan, Sri Lanka, and Burma, but the clinical course is usually too rapid for liver cancer to have time to develop. Multifactorial inheritance has been suggested for this condition (Muller et al. 1999). Neonatal giant cell hepatitis is a rare autosomal recessive disorder or group of disorders (including neonatal hemochromatosis) in which primary hepatic cancer has occasionally been described.

There are occasional reports of familial hepatomas in the literature, occurring without cirrhosis, but these are rare. In one family, affected individuals also suffered from maturity onset diabetes mellitus of the young (MODY); Bluteau et al. (2002) demonstrated somatic and germline mutations in *TCF1* at 12q24 in patients with hepatic adenomas. MODY type 3 is caused by heterozygous germline mutations in the *TCF1* that encodes hepatocyte nuclear factor 1 (HNF1). Thus *TCF1* inactivation, with or without MODY3, is important in the pathogenesis of hepatic adenoma. The incidence of second malignancies in individuals with hepatocellular carcinoma has been reported to be high (9 %), and the second primaries were of the types seen in the cancer family syndrome, suggesting the involvement of a similar genetic predisposition in these conditions (Miyanaga et al. 1989). A specific mutation in *TP53* (a GC to TA transversion at codon 249) can be frequently demonstrated in sporadic cases of hepatocellular carcinoma and is probably related to the mutagenic action of aflatoxin B1 and possibly also the hepatitis virus.

Cholangiocarcinoma of the Liver

This liver tumor develops from the epithelial cells of the bile duct and occurs more often in males than females; it is 15 times less common than hepatocellular carcinoma. It occurs in individuals about 10 years older than those with hepatocellular carcinoma, and chronic liver disease is not such an important etiological feature. In patients with ulcerative colitis, the risk of biliary tract tumors is about ten times greater than in the general population and may be related to the duration and severity of the colitis. This association is particularly seen in patients of certain HLA haplotypes (HLA B8). Familial aggregation of biliary tract tumors is rarely reported. Periampullary cancers are seen in familial adenomatous polyposis (FAP) (p. 241), and bile duct cancers may also occur with congenital dilatation of the bile ducts or with congenital absence of the gallbladder and cystic ducts.

Hepatic Angiosarcoma

Hepatic angiosarcoma is a rare tumor (occurring in the 50–70-year age group) that may be associated with environmental exposure to agents such as vinyl chloride monomer, Thorotrast, and inorganic arsenic in up to 25 % of cases.

Tumors of the Gallbladder

Cancer of the gallbladder is relatively rare, with an incidence of 2 per 100,000. It is more common in females and has a peak incidence in the seventh decade. Most gallbladder cancers (95 %) are adenocarcinomas, and cholelithiasis appears to be the most important predisposing factor. The frequency is very high in North American aboriginals and commoner in the Japanese and in Caucasian than in negroid races. There is an increased relative risk of this cancer in the first-degree relatives of index cases of up to 14 (Fernandez et al. 1994). Familial clustering is very rare, but two families in which several cases of this disorder occurred were described in Hispanic Indians from New Mexico, perhaps reflecting a higher genetic risk for this cancer in this racial group (Devor and Buechley 1979). Developmental abnormalities of the pancreatobiliary ducts, including choledochal cysts, are associated with malignancy in situ, but these are rarely familial.

Biliary tract cancer appears to occur with increased frequency in Lynch syndrome (Aarnio et al. 1995; Watson et al. 2008, see p. 256).

Pancreatic Cancer

In recent years, the incidence of pancreatic cancer has been increasing in industrialized nations, and it now occurs with a frequency of 8–10 per 100,000 population and is more common in males. Pancreatic cancer accounts for about 5 % of all cancer deaths. Tumors of the endocrine pancreas are described on page 43.

Up to 6 % of individuals with pancreatic carcinoma may have a positive family history of the condition, and there is up to fivefold increased risk of this cancer in the first-degree relatives of index cases (Fernandez et al. 1994; Ghadirian et al. 2002). However, familial clustering is relatively rare, but the tumor may occur as part of the spectrum of malignancies in Lynch syndrome (p. 256), in hereditary cutaneous malignant melanoma families, (p. 180), in families segregating *BRCA1*, and especially *BRCA2* mutations (see below, and p. 91). It also occurs as part of Li–Fraumeni syndrome (p. 271), and occurs with increased frequency in Peutz–Jeghers syndrome (p. 299) and in ataxia telangiectasia (p. 219) (Flanders and Foulkes 1996; Lim et al. 2004; Beggs et al. 2010; Mehenni et al. 2006). The occurrence of pancreatic cancer in kindred with several cases of breast cancer is a significant predictor of a germline mutation in *BRCA2* (Ozcelik et al. 1997; see below). In addition, families have been reported in which several cases of cancer of the pancreas have occurred in a sibship, albeit with late age at onset. Although autosomal recessive inheritance has been suggested (Friedman and Fialklow 1976), there is evidence of autosomal dominant inheritance in most affected families (Ehrenthal et al. 1987; Bartsch et al. 2012; Lynch et al. 1990; Solomon et al. 2012; Evans et al. 1995), and dominant inheritance with incomplete penetrance would be a unifying explanation. The age at onset, histology, sex distribution, and survival of familial pancreatic cancer appear to be similar to those of nonfamilial cases. Mutations in *CDKN2A* (encoding p16) on chromosome 9p21 are present in some families with multiple cases of cutaneous malignant melanoma, and in some families, the risk of pancreatic cancer is very high, notably in individuals with the Dutch founder mutation (Goldstein et al. 1995a, b, 2004; Ghiorzo et al. 1999; Lynch et al. 2002; de Vos tot Nederveen Cappel et al. 2003; Bartsch et al. 2002; Vasen et al. 2000). By contrast, familial pancreatic cancer without other familial cases of melanoma is not associated with *CDKN2A* mutations (Lal et al. 2000; Bartsch et al. 2002).

Mutations in the breast cancer susceptibility gene, *BRCA2*, are found in some familial pancreatic cancer kindreds (Murphy et al. 2002; Hahn et al. 2003), although several of the mutations were *BRCA2:6174delT*, and studies that did not include a high proportion of Ashkenazi Jews tended to have lower *BRCA2* mutation frequencies. Nevertheless, there is an excess of pancreatic cancers in breast cancer families carrying *BRCA2* mutations, SIR 5.79 in individuals carrying the mutation, and there is also an increase in risk in carriers of mutations in *BRCA1*, SIR 4.11 (Mocci et al. 2013; Thompson and Easton 2002), although some recent data found a fourfold increased risk of pancreatic cancer in *BRCA2* mutation carriers but not in *BRCA1* mutation carriers (Moran et al. 2012). There also seems to be a small increased risk of pancreatic cancer in mutation-negative families with clustering of breast cancer (BRCAX), SIR 1.31 (Mocci et al. 2013).

Like *BRCA2, PALB2* is a pancreatic cancer susceptibility gene; although the lifetime risk is not known, it is likely to be at least 5 % in carriers of deleterious *PALB2* mutations (Axilbund and Wiley 2012). Notably, many of the families contain women affected by both breast and pancreatic cancer, and studies of both familial and sporadic pancreatic cancer have shown that these mutations are uncommon (reviewed in Tischkowitz and Xia 2010). Thus, sequencing isolated pancreatic cancer cases to look for *PALB2* mutations is likely to have a very low yield. There is some evidence, however, that such mutations could influence response to certain chemotherapeutic agents (Villarroel et al. 2011).

The gene responsible for ataxia telangiectasia (p. 219), *ATM*, has also been identified as a pancreatic cancer susceptibility gene, although as for *PALB2*, it is responsible for less than 5 % of very strongly familial pancreatic cancer families and only a very small proportion of all cases (Roberts et al. 2012).

The Fanconi anemia genes have been implicated in pancreatic cancer, but the true contribution of these genes is uncertain; *FANCA* mutations do not seem to be important overall (Rogers et al. 2004), although two truncating mutations in *FANCC*, both associated with loss of heterozygosity in the tumors, were seen in a series of 421 pancreatic cancer cases seen at the Mayo Clinic (Couch et al. 2005).

One family has been described with a specific form of hereditary pancreatic carcinoma, where there is clear architectural distortion within the pancreas, and a high incidence of dysplasia. In some cases, preventive pancreatectomy has been carried out, and incipient or early cancers were identified. The gene was linked to the telomeric regions of chromosome 4q (Eberle et al. 2002), and subsequently a missense mutation leading to a conserved proline to serine change at amino acid position 239 in the gene encoding palladin was identified in this single family (Pogue-Geile et al. 2006). This finding has not been universally accepted by other researchers in the field, however (Salaria et al. 2007; Slater et al. 2007; Zogopoulos et al. 2007; Klein et al. 2009).

To date, this has been the only family described with this gene mutation, and an interesting feature is precancerous dysplasia and prominent stromal fibrosis and so, early presentations include diabetes mellitus. Pancreatic cancer is reported to occur in familial adenomatous polyposis (p. 241), although the tumors usually actually arise from the ampulla of Vater.

There is an increased risk of adenocarcinoma of the pancreas in hereditary pancreatitis, a well-described but uncommon autosomal dominant condition associated with attacks from childhood of recurrent pancreatitis in affected family members (Kattwinkel et al. 1973). The condition has been mapped to chromosome 7q, and mutations in the cationic trypsinogen gene *PRSS1* have been detected in affected individuals (Whitcomb et al. 1996). One survey showed that among 112 families in 14 European countries (418 affected individuals), 58 (52 %) families carried a p. R122H mutation, 24 (21 %) had the p. N29I mutation, and 5 (4 %) had the p. A16V mutation. Other mutations were very rare, but 19 % of all families had no identified mutations in *PRSS1* (Howes et al. 2004). Other genetic causes of chronic pancreatitis, such as CFTR (Sharer et al. 1998; Pezzilli et al. 2003) or *SPINK1* (Witt et al. 2001) mutations, do not appear to frequent in individuals with pancreatic cancer (Malats et al. 2001; Pezzilli et al. 2003; Teich et al. 2003), but there could be instances where it would be worthwhile to look for specific mutations, such as p. EF508 in *CFTR* and p. N34S in *SPINK1* in individuals with pancreatic cancer in the context of chronic pancreatitis (Flanders and Foulkes 1996).

Pancreatic cancer has been described in a case of Williams syndrome, possibly secondary to hypercalcemia (Jensen et al. 1976). Pancreatoblastoma has been described in the BWS (Koh et al. 1986; see p. 221) and rarely, in familial adenomatous polyposis (Abraham et al. 2001). Overexpression of IGF2 may underlie these cancers in both conditions (Kerr et al. 2002).

Screening for pancreatic cancer is extremely difficult because minor abnormalities detected by screening may be difficult to interpret as there is no clear premalignant lesion, and there are no well-recognized protocols. However, abdominal and endoscopic ultrasonography and endoscopic retrograde cholangiopancreatography (ERCP) have been suggested as possible screening methods, although the latter is probably too invasive except for the most high-risk families, where structural abnormalities may be identified (Brentnall et al. 1999); serum CA 19.9 does not appear to be suitably sensitive, but islet amyloid polypeptide may detect early pancreatic cancer. MRI cholangiopancreatography and endoscopic ultrasound are likely to be the most acceptable choices, and a recent meeting of experts suggests that either or both are indicated for high-risk individuals (Canto et al. 2013). Interestingly, this expert group limited those suitable for screening to first-degree relatives (FDRs) of patients with pancreatic cancer from a familial pancreatic cancer kindred with at least two affected FDRs; patients with Peutz–Jeghers syndrome; and *CDKN2A*, *BRCA2*, and Lynch syndrome mutation carriers with ≥1 affected FDR (Verna et al. 2010; Giardiello and Trimbath 2006; de Vos tot Nederveen Cappel 2011; Brand et al. 2007; Canto et al. 2011; Harinck et al. 2010).

Somatic *KRAS* mutations are common in pancreatic carcinomas, and their detection in pancreatic juice may also be a helpful diagnostic marker; a combination of such indicators may be developed for use in screening for pancreatic cancer in time (Lynch et al. 1996; Urrita and DiMagno 1996), but as yet no clinically useful tests of this type have emerged. Next-generation sequencing has identified recurrent mutations in *GNAS* in pancreatic cysts that arise in intraductal papillary mucinous neoplasm (IPMN). These mutations may provide a helpful clue when deciding which pancreatic cysts to excise, as the same mutations were found in the associated invasive lesions (Wu et al. 2011).

Tumors of the Small Intestine

Benign tumors of the small gut are uncommon, the most frequent being leiomyomas and lipomas. Malignant small intestinal tumors are also rare, accounting for about 1 % of all intestinal neoplasms (incidence of 0.5 per 100,000 population in the UK). In order of decreasing frequency, these are adenocarcinomas, carcinoids, lymphomas, and leiomyosarcomas.

Gastric, duodenal, and jejunal adenomas have been reported in 8 %, 31 %, and 53 % of patients with familial adenomatous polyposis, respectively, and the total probability of adenomas developing in the duodenum in FAP is probably 50–90 % (see p. 241), with about 5 % risk of malignancy, and upper gastroenterological malignancy is the most common cause of death in individuals with familial adenomatous polyposis who have had a colectomy (Groves et al. 2002; Burt et al. 1994; De Pietri et al. 1995; Koornstra et al. 2008; Vasen et al. 2008; Bulow et al. 2004). Age is the most important risk factor; there is no clear association between mutation site and the development of duodenal polyposis. The severity of duodenal polyposis is assessed using the Spigelman classification, which classifies severity in five (0–IV) stages. Points are accumulated for number, size, histology, and severity of dysplasia of polyps. Stage I (1–4 points) indicates mild disease, whereas Stage III–IV (5–12 points) implies severe duodenal polyposis. Approximately 80 % of patients with duodenal polyposis have Stage I–III disease, and 10–20 % have Stage IV disease (Spigelman et al. 1989). The risk of developing cancer appears to be related to the Spigelman stage. In one study, 2 of 27 patients with Stage IV disease at the first endoscopy developed cancer compared with 2 of 339 with Stage 0–III. The overall cumulative risk of duodenal cancer at age 57 was 4.5 % (Bulow et al. 2004) and has been estimated at between 7–36 % in individuals with Stage I–IV disease. The rate of progression from adenoma to carcinoma is slow, although it appears that recurrence of adenomas after initial detection and removal of duodenal adenomas is high.

Adenocarcinoma of the small bowel has been reported in families with Lynch syndrome (p. 256), with a lifetime risk of about 4 % and a high relative risk (100–300) (Vasen et al. 1996), and individuals with Lynch syndrome present with small bowel cancer 10–20 years earlier than in the general population. Small bowel cancers may occur in individuals homozygous for MMR gene mutations (Herkert et al. 2011). A high proportion of small intestinal carcinomas (about 45 %) appear to demonstrate microsatellite instability in individuals with Lynch syndrome (Hibi et al. 1997). The cancers seem to be distributed evenly throughout the small bowel, and there is no clear genotype–phenotype correlation. Screening of the small bowel is not usually advocated in Lynch syndrome, but it has its advocates (Koornstra et al. 2008), and it is technically much easier to do this now that video capsule endoscopy is available. The rarity of small bowel cancer in Lynch families may, however, make this unfeasible in most centers.

Crohn's disease is associated with an increased risk of small intestinal carcinoma, usually in chronic cases (Fresko et al. 1982). Crohn's disease and ulcerative colitis are multifactorial conditions, but the familial contribution is becoming increasingly appreciated, with sibling relative risks of 30–40 for Crohn's and 10–20 for ulcerative colitis, and with the identification of a susceptibility locus, *NOD2/CARD2,* which is one of several susceptibility gene loci for this multifactorial condition (Mathew and Lewis 2004; Cooney et al. 2009).

Celiac disease in adults is associated with an increased risk of small bowel lymphoma and, less commonly, of carcinoma (Holmes et al. 1980). Small bowel lymphomas may develop as a complication of immune deficiency disorders.

Pancreatoduodenal endocrine tumors may occur in MEN1 and these require aggressive management (Bartsch et al. 2000). Hamartomatous polyps occur in the small intestine in Peutz–Jeghers syndrome (PJS) (p. 299), and there is a significant risk of malignant degeneration in these polyps, resulting in a 2–13 % lifetime risk of colorectal cancer (CRC) in affected individuals (Jenne et al. 1998; van Lier et al. 2011). The relative risk of small bowel cancer in PJS has been estimated as 520 (220 to 1,306), with a lifetime risk of 13 %, mean age at diagnosis 41.7 years of age, and age range of 21–84 years of age (Giardiello et al. 2000).

Other small bowel tumors are rare but may have genetic implications. Carcinoid tumors are rarely syndromic, hamartomatous polyposis of the upper gastrointestinal tract has been reported in Gorlin syndrome (p. 252), small intestinal neurofibroma may complicate NF1 (p. 288), and angiomas of the small gut occur in hereditary hemorrhagic telangiectasia. There have been rare reports of familial polyposis of the entire gastrointestinal tract, but these may be cases of FAP (Yonemoto et al. 1969). Gastrointestinal stromal tumors (GIST), leiomyomas, and leiomyosarcomas may occur, and germline c-kit mutations have been described in individuals with familial GISTs and hyperpigmentation (Robson et al. 2004). Leiomyoma of the small intestine has been described in neurofibromatosis type 1, but is uncommon (Chu et al. 1999).

Upper gastrointestinal surveillance is advocated for individuals with FAP from the age of 25–30 years of age, the frequency depending on the Spigelman score (Vasen et al. 2008). Individuals with Peutz–Jeghers syndrome should be offered a baseline upper GI endoscopy at 8 years followed by 3-yearly video capsule endoscopy (VCE) from 18 years of age (Beggs et al. 2011; van Lier et al. 2011; Cairns et al. 2010). If polyps were detected at 8 years of age, VCE should be performed 3 yearly from that age. Magnetic resonance enterography (MRE) and barium follow-through (BaFT) are reasonable alternatives in adult patients, but BaFT is not favored in children due to radiation exposure. Colonoscopy is also advised every 2–3 years from 40 years of age in individuals with PJS (Giardiello et al. 2005; Giardiello and Trimbath 2006).

Table 5.2 Conditions associated with gastrointestinal polyposis

1. *Adenomatous polyposis*
FAP (and variants such as Gardner and Turcot)
MUTYH-associated polyposis (MAP)
CMMRD[a] (biallelic mismatch repair gene mutations)
POLE
POLD1
2. *Hamartomatous polyposis*
Juvenile polyposis
Cowden disease
Ruvalcaba–Myhre–Smith syndrome
Peutz–Jeghers syndrome
Gorlin syndrome
McCune–Albright syndrome
Cronkhite–Canada syndrome
Tuberose sclerosis (few, rectal polyps)
Hereditary mixed polyposis syndrome
DICER1 syndrome (usually few in number)
3. *Inflammatory polyps*
Inflammatory bowel disease
Devon polyposis
4. *Ganglio/neurofibromata*
Neurofibromatosis type 1
MEN 2B
Cowden
5. Hyperplastic polyposis (now usually referred to as serrated polyposis)

[a]CMMRD – constitutional mismatch repair deficiency

Gastrointestinal Polyposis

Disorders associated with gastrointestinal polyposis may be classified according to the histological type of the polyps (Hodgson and Murday 1994; see Table 5.2). Adenomatous polyps occur in familial adenomatous polyposis (p. 241), Turcot syndrome (p. 311), MUTYH-associated polyposis (Sampson et al. 2009; Vogt et al. 2009; p. 287), in those with POLE or POLD1 mutations (Palles et al. 2013) and in Lynch syndrome and biallelic MMR mutation carriers (p. 232) and occasionally in Cowden syndrome (p. 233). Hamartomatous polyps occur in Peutz–Jeghers syndrome (p. 299), juvenile polyposis (p. 267) (Hyer et al. 2000; Zhou et al. 2001; Erdman and Barnard 2002), and the hereditary mixed polyposis syndrome (HMPS) (Whitelaw et al. 1997) caused by a single founder *GREM1* mutation (Jaeger et al. 2012), Cowden syndrome (p. 233) (Gentry et al. 1978; Eng et al. 2003), Ruvalcaba–Myhre syndrome (p. 221), McCune–Albright syndrome, and occasionally in Gorlin syndrome. The Cronkhite–Canada syndrome, characterized by hamartomatous (juvenile) polyps throughout the whole intestine and associated with alopecia, onychodystrophy, and abnormal pigmentation of adult onset, is probably not genetic (Daniel et al. 1982) but does predispose to CRC (Zugel et al. 2001).

Almost 50 % of cases of juvenile polyposis are due to germline mutations in *SMAD4* or *BMPR1A*, which encode proteins involved in TGF β signaling (Houlston et al. 1998; Howe et al. 2001; Sayed et al. 2002). There is a significant risk of colorectal malignancy in juvenile polyposis and Peutz–Jeghers syndrome. Ganglioneuromatous polyposis may occur in Cowden syndrome, and adenomas and hamartomas may also arise, with malignant potential (Trufant et al. 2011).

Hereditary mixed polyposis syndrome causes an autosomal dominant predisposition to colorectal polyps of varying histological type including sessile, hamartomatous, and adenomatous polyps and early-onset CRC. The locus for the susceptibility gene has been identified as CRAC1 on chromosome 15q in Ashkenazi Jewish families, and the responsible gene, *GREM1*, has now been identified. Thus far, only one founder mutation (in the AJ population) is known to exist (Jaeger et al. 2012).

Small rectal hamartomatous polyps have recently been described in tuberose sclerosis (p. 307), but these are thought to be of no clinical significance (Gould et al. 1990). Inflammatory polyps are associated with ulcerative colitis and Crohn's disease. Gastrointestinal hamartomatous polyps have been noted in those with germline *DICER1* mutations (Foulkes et al. 2011). Gastrointestinal polyps, predominantly neurofibromas, are found in NF1 (p. 288), possibly in up to 25 % of cases (Hochberg et al. 1974; Cooney and Jewell 2009). A diffuse ganglioneuromatosis of the gastrointestinal tract is described in MEN 2B (p. 281), with hyperplasia of the ganglion cells, leading to malfunction of the bowel (Fryns and Chrzanowska 1988). Rarely, autosomal dominant inheritance of intestinal neurofibromatosis has been described without other associated manifestations of neurofibromatosis (Heiman et al. 1988).

The juvenile polyps in individuals with McCune–Albright syndrome show some similarities to those seen in PJS, and activating mutations in *GNAS* have been detected in the polyps. Affected individuals may also have perioral freckling (Zacharin et al. 2011). The Cronkhite–Canada syndrome, characterized by hamartomatous (juvenile) polyps throughout the whole intestine and associated with alopecia, onychodystrophy, and abnormal pigmentation of adult onset, is probably not genetic, but does predispose to CRC (Zugel et al. 2001; Sweetser et al. 2012). Devon polyposis has been described in one family in which multiple inflammatory fibroid polyps were found in the upper gastrointestinal tract in members of three generations of a family from Devon, UK. There did not seem to be an increased risk of cancer in these individuals (Anthony et al. 1984; Allibone et al. 1992).

Tumors of the Colon and Rectum

Malignant disease of the large bowel is one of the commonest causes of cancer death, with an incidence of 32 per 100,000 population in the UK, but a much lower incidence in parts of Africa (2.5 per 100,000 in Nigeria) and in Asia. Almost all (98 %) large bowel cancers are adenocarcinomas. Adenomas of the colon are thought to have the potential to develop into malignancy and coexist in 75 % of cases in which more than one primary carcinoma is present in the colon; one or more adenomas are present in about a third of cases of colon carcinoma. It is thus probable that most

Table 5.3 Family history and risk of death from colon cancer: empiric risk estimates for counseling

Affected relatives	Relative risk of CRC	Lifetime risk of CRC
General population		1 in 50
One first-degree relative	×3 (OR 1.8)	1 in 17
One first degree aged <45 years	×5 (OR 3.7)	1 in 10
One first and one second degree		1 in 12
Both parents		1 in 8.5
Two first-degree relatives	(OR 5.7)	1 in 6
Three first-degree relatives		1 in 3

Odds ratio (OR) figures from St John et al. (1993); lifetime risks from Houlston et al. (1990)

carcinomas develop from adenomas (Morson 1966). The incidence of solitary colonic polyps in the general population is age-related, reaching 34 % in the sixth decade and 75 % in those over the age of 75 years (Lanspa et al. 1990; Dunlop 2002; Fletcher 2008). It has been calculated that the risk of invasive cancer in a single polyp is approximately 0.25 % per year, but for larger and/or villous polyps, the risks are up to 50 times higher (Eide 1986), indicating that screening guidelines need to be modified by the pathological findings at each colonoscopy. Inflammation is probably also a predisposing factor for bowel cancer, since ulcerative colitis and Crohn's disease are associated with an increased risk of colon carcinoma (Judge et al. 2002). The risk of colorectal cancer in these conditions is similar for a similar extent and duration of colonic involvement, and surveillance guidelines have been developed for individuals with inflammatory bowel disease (Eaden and Mayberry 2002; Cairns et al. 2010). Individuals with acromegaly also have an increased prevalence of colorectal adenomas and cancers, RR 7.4, prevalence 3.7 % overall (Jenkins and Besser 2001).

Genetic factors are important in the pathogenesis of cancer, and a comprehensive family history should be part of the assessment of all patients with CRC. Early age at diagnosis in the affected relative is an important predictor of risk. Empiric risk estimates based on the number of relatives affected by (and age at diagnosis of) CRC are given in Table 5.3 and indicate that risk increases with earlier age at diagnosis and increased numbers of affected relatives. Twin studies indicate that 35 % of CRCs are partly due to inherited factors (Lichtenstein et al. 2000). Identification of individuals at increased genetic risk of colon cancer is important because screening can be offered to high-risk individuals, and evidence is accumulating that this is likely to be effective in reducing morbidity and mortality from CRC.

It is estimated that about 5 % of CRCs occur in individuals with a dominantly inherited predisposition. Genetic conditions associated with colonic polyps carry an increased risk of CRC (Table 5.4). These include familial adenomatous polyposis (p. 241), juvenile polyposis (p. 267), and Peutz–Jeghers syndrome (p. 299). Familial adenomatous polyposis is characterized by the development of colorectal adenomas, whereas the latter conditions are characterized by gastrointestinal hamartomas, which are potentially premalignant although adenomas have more malignant potential. A rare familial syndrome of familial giant hyperplastic polyposis coli has been described which predisposes to CRC (Jeevaratnam et al. 1996;

Table 5.4 Conditions characterized by colorectal polyposis

Condition	Gene
Adenomatous polyposes	
Familial adenomatous polyposis (FAP)	*APC*
Attenuated polyposis/multiple adenomas	*APC, MUTYH, POLE, POLD1*, MMR genes
Hamartomatous polyposes	
Juvenile polyposis	*BMPR1A, SMAD4, ENG, STK11*
Peutz–Jeghers syndrome	*LKB1/STK11*
Cowden syndrome	*PTEN*
Hereditary mixed polyposis syndrome	*GREM1*

Sheikholeslami et al. 2004). More recently, the importance of some types of hyperplastic polyps, particularly as precursors of right-sided microsatellite unstable colon cancers, has been stressed (Jass et al. 2002). Conditions predisposing to gastrointestinal polyps are listed above (Ngeow et al. 2013; p. 62).

Germline *PTEN* mutations are also associated with hamartomatous gastrointestinal polyps, but unlike the genes listed above, mutation carriers (affected with Cowden or Ruvalcaba–Myhre–Smith syndromes) do not seem to have a greatly increased risk of CRC, but there may be some risk in specific families.

Familial adenomatous polyposis is the most common of these disorders but accounts for fewer than 1 % of all cases of colon cancer. A larger proportion of colon cancer (probably 2–3 %) is accounted for by Lynch syndrome (HNPCC) (Evans et al. 1997; Salovaara et al. 2000), an autosomal dominant inherited predisposition to CRC (p. 256), in which bowel cancers occur with high frequency at an early age (on average two decades earlier than sporadic cases). Mutations in one of several genes involved in the repair of DNA mismatch errors (*MLH1, MSH2, MSH6*, and *PMS2*) have been found to cause Lynch syndrome, and microsatellite instability (MSI) is seen, where multiple allelic changes are demonstrable in tumor DNA when compared to the constitutional DNA of the patient. The condition predisposes to early-onset tumors with increased proportion of right-sided colon cancers (65 % versus 25 % in sporadic cases), and a risk of multiple primary CRC. The risk of extracolonic cancers is higher in individuals with *MSH2* than *MLH1* mutations (Vasen et al. 2001; Bonadona et al. 2011), and *MSH6* mutations particularly predispose to endometrial cancer (Wijnen et al. 1999). These extracolonic malignancies comprise mainly endometrial, ovarian, pancreatic, gastric, and urinary tract cancers (Wijnen et al. 1999). Full details of Lynch syndrome are given on page 249. Muir–Torre syndrome is Lynch syndrome associated with sebaceous adenomas and other characteristic skin lesions, and they are allelic (i.e., due to mutations in the same gene), but Muir–Torre syndrome has generally been considered to be due to mutations in *MSH2* rather than *MLH1* (Lucci-Cordisco et al. 2003). Biallelic MMR mutation carriers are at significantly increased risk of very early-onset colorectal cancer (Herkert et al. 2011).

Germline mutations in *MLH3* and *EXO1* may account for a small proportion of CRC cases with MSI-positive tumors (Wu et al. 2001; Niessen et al. 2009; Liu et al. 2003; Laiho et al. 2002; Brassett et al. 1996; Sutter et al. 2004). Clinically important mutations in these genes are exceptionally rare.

Germline deletions of the last exons of *EPCAM*, the gene directly upstream of *MSH2*, result in loss of MSH2 expression by methylation of the promoter, and thus testing for *EPCAM* deletions is essential if IHC shows loss of MSH2, and yet no coding sequence or MLPA-identified mutation is found in *MSH2* (Kuiper et al. 2011). Interestingly, such mutations are associated with a lower risk of endometrial cancer (Ligtenberg et al. 2013; Charbonnier et al. 2002).

The estimated cumulative risks of colorectal cancer by 70 years of age in individuals with Lynch syndrome have recently been reported as 41 % (95 % confidence intervals [CI], 25–70 %) for *MLH1* mutation carriers, 48 % (95 % CI, 30–77 %) for *MSH2*, and 12 % (95 % CI, 8–22 %) for *MSH6* (Hampel et al. 2006). For endometrial cancer, corresponding risks were 54 % (95 % CI, 20–80 %), 21 % (95 % CI, 8–77 %), and 16 % (95 % CI, 8–32 %). For ovarian cancer, they were 20 % (95 % CI, 1–65 %), 24 % (95 % CI, 3–52 %), and 1 % (95 % CI, 0–3 %). The estimated cumulative risks by age 40 years did not exceed 2 % (95 % CI, 0–7 %) for endometrial cancer or 1 % (95 % CI, 0–3 %) for ovarian cancer. The estimated lifetime risks for other tumor types did not exceed 3 % with any of the gene mutations (Bonadona et al. 2011). These risks are lower than those published previously.

The term hereditary non-polyposis colon cancer (HNPCC) is something of a misnomer (Umar et al. 2004), since colonic adenomas do occur in patients with this condition; thus, the name Lynch syndrome has generally replaced HNPCC in common usage (Vasen et al. 1999). Although colonic adenomas are not more common in Lynch syndrome than in the general population, the adenomas progress more rapidly through the adenoma–carcinoma sequence than in normal individuals (Jass 1995a, b). This has implications for the frequency with which colonoscopic surveillance should be performed in these individuals. It is very rare for more than 50 polyps to develop in this condition, which distinguishes it from classical familial adenomatous polyposis in which there is a minimum of 100 colonic adenomas. There are, however, families with intermediate numbers of polyps that cannot easily be classified as Lynch syndrome or familial adenomatous polyposis (sometimes known as attenuated familial adenomatous polyposis, AFAP, or AAPC), and affected individuals in some such families may be demonstrated to have germline mutations in exons 3 or 4 of the *APC* gene (Spirio et al. 1993; Gismondi et al. 2002). Others may have MUTYH-associated polyposis, an autosomal recessive condition characterized by variable numbers of colonic adenomas and relatively early-onset CRC, with usually 30–100 adenomas (Halford et al. 2003; see p. 287). Very recently, rare mutations in *POLE* and *POLD1* have been identified in families with multiple colorectal adenomas and associated carcinomas. The families may resemble AFAP families in some respects (Palles et al. 2013). A subgroup of Lynch syndrome-related CRC may be distinguished by the occurrence of flat adenomas in the right hemicolon (Lynch et al. 1993), but it seems likely that this is merely another variant of Lynch syndrome. However, serrated adenomas are common in HMPS (hereditary mixed polyposis syndrome), characterized by colonic adenomas and hamartomas and early-onset CRC, caused by a single germline deletion in *GREM1* (Jaeger et al. 2012).

The prevalence of pathogenic *APC* and biallelic *MUTYH* mutations was 80 % and 2 %, respectively, among individuals with 1,000 or more adenomas, 56 % and 7 % among those with 100 to 999 adenomas, 10 % and 7 % among those with 20 to 99 adenomas, and 5 % and 4 % among those with 10 to 19 adenomas in a recent study, so *APC* mutations predominated in patients with classic polyposis, whereas prevalence of *APC* and *MUTYH* mutations was similar in attenuated polyposis (Grover et al. 2012).

A polymorphism in the *APC* gene, a T-A mutation germline mutation (predicted to result in a change from isoleucine to lysine position 1,307 of the protein; see familial adenomatous polyposis section, p. 241), confers an approximately twofold increase in the risk of CRC. The mechanism for this at a molecular level appears to be that the polymorphism, which converts an AAATAAAA sequence to $(A)_8$, predisposes to the development of somatic mutations in the *APC* gene (Laken et al. 1997). This mutation is common (about 6 %) in individuals of Ashkenazi Jewish origin, but is very rare in other ethnic groups. The relative risk or odds ratio for CRC in association with this mutation is about 1.5–1.8 (Gryfe et al. 1999), which is generally thought to be insufficient to warrant colonoscopic surveillance. The mutation is at least 2,200 years old (Niell et al. 2003) and has probably become frequent in this population by genetic drift.

There is possibly a slightly increased relative risk of colon cancer in individuals with germline *BRCA1* mutations, but this is accompanied by a decrease in risk for rectal cancer, and this increased risk has not been reported in men (Thompson and Easton 2002). Overall, the risks are probably not clinically important. In support of the absence of an effect, there is no apparent increased risk for CRC for Ashkenazi Jewish carriers of *BRCA1:185delAG* or *BRCA1:5382inC* (Ford et al. 1995; Struewing et al. 1997; Kirchhoff et al. 2004; Niell et al. 2004).

NAT2 (which alters the ability to acetylate N-acetyl transferase) and other metabolic gene variants may alter susceptibility to colonic adenomas and cancer in the general population and alter polyp density in FAP (Crabtree et al. 2002; Jass 2004), but are unlikely to cause a sufficiently increased CRC risk to be clinically important on their own. It may be that multiple variants in different genes including *MLH1*, *MSH2*, *APC*, *AXIN1*, and *CTNNB1* (beta catenin) can contribute to susceptibility to colonic adenomas and cancer (Fearnhead et al. 2004; Lammi et al. 2004), but none of these loci are clinically useful.

Identification of High-Risk Families

Efficient screening for Lynch syndrome requires that high-risk individuals are targeted for mutation testing. Approximately 10 % of patients with CRC have an affected first-degree relative, and 2 % have two affected first-degree relatives. However, the frequency of families that fulfill the "Amsterdam Criteria" (AC) for Lynch syndrome is less than 5 % of all cases (Stephenson et al. 1991; Peel et al. 1997). The Bethesda criteria are more sensitive but less specific (Umar et al. 2004). Most population-based mutation analysis studies start with individuals with microsatellite unstable cancers and then look for germline mutations in these cases only: these studies have found that between 1 and 4 % of all CRC is due to germline mutations in either *MLH1* or *MSH2* (Peel et al. 2000; Salovaara et al. 2000) (Table 5.5). Some patients with early-onset CRC with no family history still have germline mutations in the mismatch repair genes (Dunlop et al. 1997), and these may account for a substantial proportion of CRC in patients diagnosed below 35 years, but only a minority of older cases. Persons

Table 5.5   Frequency of germline MLH1 and MSH2 mutation carriers in early-onset CRC

		MLH1 mutation carriers		*MSH2* mutation carriers	
Age range (years)	Number of index cases	Number	%	Number	%
<30	50	7	14	7	14
<40	12	1	8.3	1	8.3
<45	38	1	2.6	2	5.3
<50	135	6	4.4	6	4.4

with CRC caused by germline *MSH6* mutations often do not fulfill either AC1 or AC2 (Sjursen et al. 2010).

In families not fulfilling the Amsterdam or Bethesda criteria for Lynch syndrome (see p. 258, Tables 11.4, 11.5, 11.6), pathological tumor analysis by immunohisto-chemical stains (IHC) gives a high specificity for the diagnosis of Lynch syndrome and indicates the gene which may be mutated in the germline, although MSH2 and MSH6 staining may both be lost in tumors in people with germline mutations in MSH2. Measurement of MSI in tumors is less specific because approximately 15 % of all CRCs may be MSI positive and does not indicate which gene is likely to be involved in the germline. Some cases, especially older women with MSI-high cancers, may have somatic MLH1 inactivation. The specificity of MSI for Lynch syndrome is increased considerably if two tumors from the same individual demonstrate MSI positivity (Vasen 2007; Lubbe et al. 2009; EGAPP Recommendation Statement 2009; Tresallet et al. 2012; Parsons et al. 2012).

In terms of identifying individuals at risk, it should be remembered that some patients with early-onset CRC without a family history of Lynch syndrome have germline mutations in mismatch repair genes (Dunlop et al. 1997; Hampel et al. 2005). If cases of CRC unselected for family history are studied for mismatch repair gene mutation analysis, the mutation detection rate is dependent on the age at diagnosis of CRC in the case (Mitchell et al. 2002; see Table 5.5). Familial clustering of CRC that does not fulfill the AC for a diagnosis Lynch syndrome is less likely to be due to germline *MLH1* or *MSH2* mutations. In early studies, only about 8 % of families not meeting the rather stringent AC1 had detectable mutations although some may have deletions or other gene rearrangements (Wijnen et al. 1997). This may be an underestimate, and detailed searches can find mutations in many more, as long as MSI-H is present in the CRC of the subject of the mutation analysis (Wagner et al. 2003), and would be considered to be very likely if MSH2 protein is absent, even if the family clustering in no way fulfills AC. In this context, looking for *BRAF* mutations (Davies et al. 2002) in the colorectal tumor may be a good step following MSI and IHC, as among MSI-H cancers that do not express MLH1, the presence of a *BRAF* mutation makes a germline *MLH1* mutation much less likely. Interestingly, loss of expression of MSH2 is rarely if ever associated with *BRAF* mutations (Wang et al. 2003; Koinuma et al. 2004; Domingo et al. 2004). More recent publications have presented improved algorithms for testing tumors in newly diagnosed cases of CRC, stratified by age at diagnosis and family history, and in general MSI analysis is performed initially, as it is more sensitive but less specific than IHC, and then IHC performed to indicate the most likely gene involved. IHC can be a first step in cases conforming to the Bethesda criteria for Lynch syndrome (Lubbe et al. 2009; Halbert et al. 2004; Hampel 2010; Hall 2010; Rodriguez-Bigas et al. 1997; Parsons et al. 2012; Steinhagen et al. 2012; Tresallet et al. 2012).

Pathological Features

Colorectal cancers with MSI-high features characteristically have increased mucin secretion, differentiation, and lymphocytic infiltrate. This is seen both in sporadic tumors and those arising in Lynch syndrome. There is now evidence that sporadic MSI-H cancers develop in adenomas with a somatic *BRAF* mutation and DNA methylation, particularly of *MLH1*, while those in Lynch syndrome arise in adenomas with somatic mutations in APC, beta catenin, and/or *KRAS*. This also translates into morphological differences, Lynch syndrome-associated cancers showing more tumor budding (de-differentiation), and sporadic tumors being more heterogeneous and displaying mucin secretion (Jass 2004; McGivern et al. 2004).

Molecular genetic studies of colon cancer have provided strong evidence for a multistep pathogenesis. This work started out with a simple linear model involving at least five genes (Fearon and Vogelstein 1990). Although this model is too simplistic, it has provided a framework for many other studies. *APC* mutations are thought to occur early in the process and may cause spindle aberrations via the interaction of APC with the kinetochore at mitosis through connections with the microtubules, leading to chromosome abnormalities (Powell 2002). Originally, it was thought that the critical factor is the accumulation of mutations rather than the particular order in which they occur, but more recent work, focusing on the idea of cell-type-specific "gatekeepers," suggests that there are genes which act as rate-limiting steps: it is likely that such genes are altered early in the carcinogenetic process. For example, in most CRC, biallelic *APC* mutations (or mutation plus loss of heterozygosity) occur at an early stage (Powell et al. 1992). These early alterations (such as the loss of sequences C-terminal to the beta catenin regulatory domain (Sidransky 1997)) could lead to a screening test for early CRC based on the detection of such mutations in stool. A stool test for *APC* mutations was developed (Traverso et al. 2002) but has not been taken up commercially, and it is not in widespread use. Other assays are based on multiple genes: for example, stool analysis of three gene markers (*TP53*, *BAT26*, and *KRAS*) detected 71 % of CRC patients and 92 % of those whose tumors actually had an alteration in these genes (Dong et al. 2001). Despite these and other encouraging findings, commercial molecular-based stool tests remain unadopted in the clinical setting.

Surveillance Strategies

Screening of patients at increased risk of colon cancer is likely to prevent early death, but large-scale studies are of course difficult to conduct. In Finland, one study has found that Lynch syndrome family members who undergo colonoscopy have a much lower CRC incidence rate, probably due to removal of adenomas. The overall death rates were 10 versus 26 subjects in the study and control groups ($P = 0.003$) and 4 versus 12 in mutation-positive subjects ($P = 0.05$) (Jarvinen et al. 2000). In addition, the benefits of a genetic register for ascertaining and coordinating the screening of individuals at risk for familial adenomatous polyposis are now well recognized (Kinzler and Vogelstein 1996; King et al. 2000; Vasen et al. 2008).

In a significant proportion (approximately 30 %) of families that meet the Amsterdam criteria, the results of the MSI and IHC analysis of the colorectal tumor(s) are negative. Clustering of CRC by chance or genetic factors other than Lynch syndrome may be responsible for the disease in these families, which are characterized by a more advanced age of onset of CRC than in families with Lynch syndrome, and the absence of endometrial cancer and multiple tumors. The risk of developing CRC in such families is increased only by a factor of 2.3, so a less-intensive colonoscopic surveillance program (e.g., colonoscopy every 5 years, starting 5–10 years before the first diagnosis of CRC or at 45 years) might be appropriate (Vasen et al. 2007, 2009; Järvinen et al. 2008). The close relatives of those found to have no evidence of Lynch syndrome, but where there is a family history of later-onset CRC, have a higher CRC risk where the CRC is microsatellite unstable (Aaltonen et al. 2007).

Predictive testing for Lynch syndrome is now available for the presymptomatic diagnosis of this condition in families in which the pathogenic mutation has been defined, so that it is becoming possible to target high-risk asymptomatic individuals for screening, as for familial adenomatous polyposis. Guidelines for screening individuals at risk for Lynch syndrome are regular colonoscopy (every 1–2 years) from the age of 25 years, and those with a family history that includes cancers at other sites, including endometrium, should be offered screening for other cancers as appropriate (Vasen et al. 2010a, b; see p. 256). In addition to detecting presymptomatic colonic carcinomas, such screening allows the endoscopic detection and removal of adenomas. It is presumed (but not proven) that most cancers in patients with Lynch syndrome arise from adenomas and that excision of the latter will prevent the development of colon cancer. Colonoscopy is the investigation of choice because of the preponderance of right-sided tumors in this condition (Vasen et al. 2013).

In familial CRC families without evidence for Lynch syndrome, surveillance for CRC should take into account the financial costs of screening and the possibility of adverse effects of screening by colonoscopy in particular and balance this with the individual's estimated risk of CRC (Johnson et al. 2008). Cairns et al. (2010) have published family history criteria for individuals at high–moderate and low–moderate risk of developing colorectal cancer based on the polygenic inheritance model and have advocated screening protocols based on these groupings. Briefly, individuals assessed as being at high–moderate risk may have three affected relatives at any age, in a first-degree kinship, or two affected relatives diagnosed below 60 years of age. Individuals at low–moderate risk would be those with one affected relative diagnosed before 50 years of age or two diagnosed over the age of 60 years of age. They advocated that the high–moderate risk group should have 5 yearly colonoscopies from 50 years of age and the low–moderate risk group one colonoscopy at 55 years of age, and no further investigations unless polyps were detected at the screening colonoscopy (Table 5.6). These guidelines for screening in those at moderately

Table 5.6 Screening guidelines for colon cancer in individuals with a moderate family history of CRC: a guide for the gastroenterologist and colorectal surgeon

CRC in 3 FDR in 1st-degree kinship, none diagnosed <50 years of age	Colonoscopy 5 yearly	From 50 to 75 years of age
CRC in 2 FDR in 1st-degree kinship, mean age <60 years of age	Colonoscopy 5 yearly	From 50 to 75 years of age
CRC in 2 FDR diagnosed >60 years of age	Single colonoscopy	Once at 55 years of age; no more if normal
CRC in 1 FDR diagnosed <50 years of age	Single colonoscopy	Once at 55 years of age; no more if normal
Other FH CRC unless diagnostic of Lynch	No screening	
Amsterdam criteria positive	Refer to genetics center	
Incident CRC cases diag. <50 years of age or MSI+, not Amsterdam criteria positive	Arrange MSI/IHC, consider referral to genetics center	
FAP/MUTYH polyposis	Refer to genetics center	

Adapted from Cairns et al. (2010)
FDR first-degree relative, SDR second-degree relative

increased risk of CRC as assessed by family history have been updated in the UK, commissioned by the British Society of Gastroenterology and the Association of Coloproctology for Great Britain and Ireland, based on literature review and expert opinion (Cairns et al. 2010). They take into account the fact that the risks of colonoscopy are small but significant (Williams and Fairclough 1991); in a population-based study, serious complications were recorded in 2 per 1,000 colonoscopies (Gatto et al. 2003). The 14-day death rate is around 5–10 % of the perforation rate, or 0.83 per 10,000 procedures (CI 0.025–3.69), and 3.9 per 10,000 (CI 1.1–8.8) after polypectomy (Anderson et al. 2000; Gatto et al. 2003). The perforation rate after polypectomy is quoted as 22 (CI 13.8–33.3) per 10,000, with post-polypectomy bleeding in a further 89 (CI 71.5–109.5) per 10,000 (Cairns et al. 2010; Zha et al. 2004; Imperiale et al. 2008).

Some newer forms of colonoscopic surveillance in Lynch syndrome have been advocated but are not yet in widespread use (Haanstra et al. 2013).

Chemoprophylaxis

There had been anecdotal evidence that COX-2 inhibitors could reduce the development of colonic neoplasia in susceptible individuals for some year, so aspirin and nonabsorbable starch were assessed in large-scale trials (the Concerted Action Polyp Prevention [CAPP] studies). In CAPP2, no preventive effect of starch was noted (Mathers et al. 2012). When individuals with Lynch syndrome were treated with 600 mg/day of aspirin for over 25 months, the risk of CRC was significantly reduced at almost 5 years follow-up (Burn et al. 2011a, b; Evans et al. 2012). No effect was seen for Lynch syndrome mutation carriers in an earlier analysis of the same study (Burn et al. 2008), suggesting that the preventive effect associated with aspirin use is delayed and prolonged. Larger trials are planned, and finding the optimal dose will be the next step. In FAP, the CAPP1 study showed that aspirin had a modest effect on polyp progression, but no effect on polyp number (Burn et al. 2011a, b) – but in view of the delayed effect seen in the later analysis of CAPP2, perhaps a long-term follow-up study will show benefit. Fish oils have long been thought to be protective against GI cancers, and a special formulation of eicosapentaenoic acid (EPA) was able to reduce polyp number and size (West et al. 2010).

References

Aaltonen L, Johns L, Järvinen H, Mecklin JP, Houlston R. Explaining the familial colorectal cancer risk associated with mismatch repair (MMR)-deficient and MMR-stable tumors. Clin Cancer Res. 2007;13(1):356–61.

Aarnio M, Mecklin J-P, Aaltonen LA, et al. Life-time risk of different cancers in hereditary nonpolyposis colorectal cancer (HNPCC) syndrome. Int J Cancer. 1995;64:430–3.

Abraham SC, Wu TT, Klimstra DS, Finn LS, Lee JH, Yeo CJ, Cameron JL, Hruban RH. Distinctive molecular genetic alterations in sporadic and familial adenomatous polyposis-associated pancreatoblastomas: frequent alterations in the APC/ beta-catenin pathway and chromosome 11p. Am J Pathol. 2001;159:1619–27.

Akbari MR, Malekzadeh R, Lepage P, Roquis D, Sadjadi AR, Aghcheli K, Yazdanbod A, Shakeri R, Bashiri J, Sotoudeh M, Pourshams A, Ghadirian P, Narod SA. Mutations in Fanconi anemia genes and the risk of esophageal cancer. Hum Genet. 2011;129(5):573–82.

Albeck H, et al. Familial clusters of nasopharyngeal carcinoma and salivary gland carcinomas in Greenland natives. Cancer. 1993;72(1):196–200.

Allibone RO, Nanson JK, Anthony PP. Multiple and recurrent inflammatory fibroid polyps in a Devon family ("Devon polyposis syndrome"): an update. Gut. 1992;33:1004–5.

Alter BP. Fanconi anaemia and malignancies. Am J Hematol. 1996;53:99–110.

Anderson ML, Pasha TM, Leighton JA. Endoscopic perforation of the colon: lessons from a 10-year study. Am J Gastroenterol. 2000;95:3418–22.

Anthony PE, Morris LS, Vowles KDJ. Multiple and recurrent inflammatory fibroid polyps in three generations of a Devon family. Gut. 1984;25:854–62.

Arnio M, Salovaara R, Aaltonen LA, et al. Features of gastric cancer in hereditary non-polyposis colorectal cancer syndromes. Int J Cancer. 1997;74:551–5.

Axilbund JE, Wiley EA. Genetic testing by cancer site: pancreas. Cancer J. 2012;18:350–4.

Bartsch DK, Langer P, Wild A, et al. Pancreatoduodenal endocrine tumors in multiple endocrine neoplasia type 1: surgery or surveillance? Surgery. 2000;128:958–60.

Bartsch DK, Sina-Frey M, Lang S, Wild A, Gerdes B, Barth P, Kress R, Grützmann R, Colombo-Benkmann M, Ziegler A, Hahn SA, Rothmund M, Rieder H. CDKN2A germline mutations in familial pancreatic cancer. Ann Surg. 2002;236(6):730–7.

Bartsch DK, Gress TM, Langer P. Familial pancreatic cancer – current knowledge. Nat Rev Gastroenterol Hepatol. 2012;9:445–53.

Beggs AD, Latchford AR, Vasen HF, Moslein G, Alonso A, Aretz S, Bertario L, Blanco I, Bülow S, Burn J, Capella G, Colas C, Friedl W, Møller P, Hes FJ, Järvinen H, Mecklin JP, Nagengast FM, Parc Y, Phillips RK, Hyer W, Ponz de Leon M, Renkonen-Sinisalo L, Sampson JR, Stormorken A, Tejpar S, Thomas HJ, Wijnen JT, Clark SK, Hodgson SV. Peutz-Jeghers syndrome: a systematic review and recommendations for management. Gut. 2010;59(7): 975–86.

Beggs AD, Bhate RD, Irukulla S, Achiek M, Abulafi AM. Straight to colonoscopy: the ideal patient pathway for the 2-week suspected cancer referrals? Ann R Coll Surg Engl. 2011;93(2):114–9. doi:10.1308/003588411X12851639107917.

Blaydon DC, Etheridge SL, Risk JM, Hennies HC, Gay LJ, Carroll R, Plagnol V, McRonald FE, Stevens HP, Spurr NK, Bishop DT, Ellis A, Jankowski J, Field JK, Leigh IM, South AP, Kelsell DP. RHBDF2 mutations are associated with tylosis a familial esophageal cancer syndrome. Am J Hum Genet. 2012;90(2):340–6. Epub 2012 Jan 19. PubMed PMID: 22265016. PubMed Central PMCID: PMC: 3276661.

Bluteau O, Jeannot E, Bioulac-Sage P, et al. Bi-allelic inactivation of TCFI in hepatic adenomas. Nat Genet. 2002;32:312–5.

Bonadona V, Bonaïti B, Olschwang S, Grandjouan S, Huiart L, Longy M, Guimbaud R, Buecher B, Bignon YJ, Caron O, Colas C, Noguès C, Lejeune-Dumoulin S, Olivier-Faivre L, Polycarpe-Osaer F, Nguyen TD, Desseigne F, Saurin JC, Berthet P, Leroux D, Duffour J, Manouvrier S, Frébourg T, Sobol H, Lasset C, Bonaïti-Pellié C, French Cancer Genetics Network. Cancer risks associated with germline mutations in MLH1, MSH2, and MSH6 genes in Lynch syndrome. JAMA. 2011;305(22):2304–10.

Bourgeois JM, et al. Plexiform neurofibroma of the submandibular salivary gland in a child. Can J Gastroenterol. 2001;15(12):835–7.

Bowen S, Gill M, Lee DA, Fisher G, Geronemus RG, Vasquez ME, Celebi JT. Mutations in the CYLD gene in Brooke-Spiegler syndrome, familial cylindromatosis, and multiple familial trichoepithelioma: lack of genotype-phenotype correlation. J Invest Derm. 2005;124:919–20.

Brand RE, Lerch MM, Rubinstein WS, Neoptolemos JP, Whitcomb DC, Hruban RH, Brentnall TA, Lynch HT, Canto MI. Advances in counselling and surveillance of patients at risk for pancreatic cancer. Gut. 2007;56:1460–9.

Brassett C, Joyce JA, Froggatt NJ, et al. Microsatellite instability in early onset and familial colorectal cancer. J Med Genet. 1996;33:981–5.

Breast Cancer Linkage Consortium. Pathology of familial breast cancer: differences between breast cancers in carriers of BRCA1 or BRCA2 mutations and sporadic cases. Lancet. 1997; 349:1505–10.

Brentnall TA, Bronner MP, Byrd DR, Haggitt RC, Kimmey MB. Early diagnosis and treatment of pancreatic dysplasia in patients with a family history of pancreatic cancer. Ann Int Med. 1999; 131:247–55.

Brind AM, Bassendine MF. Molecular genetics of chronic liver disease. Baillieres Clin Gastroenterol. 1990;4:233–53.

Brooks-Wilson AR, Kaurah P, Suriano G, et al. Germline E-cadherin mutations in hereditary diffuse gastric cancer: assessment of 42 new families and review of genetic screening criteria. J Med Genet. 2004;41(7):508–17.

Bulow S, Bjork J, Christensen IJ, et al. Duodenal adenomatosis in familial adenomatous polyposis. Gut. 2004;53:381–6.

Burki N, Gencik A, Torhost JKH, et al. Familial and histological analyses of 138 breast cancer patients. Breast Cancer Res Treat. 1987;10:159–67.

Burn J, Bishop DT, Mecklin JP, Macrae F, Möslein G, Olschwang S, Bisgaard ML, Ramesar R, Eccles D, Maher ER, Bertario L, Jarvinen HJ, Lindblom A, Evans DG, Lubinski J, Morrison PJ, Ho JW, Vasen HF, Side L, Thomas HJ, Scott RJ, Dunlop M, Barker G, Elliott F, Jass JR, Fodde R, Lynch HT, Mathers JC, CAPP2 Investigators. Effect of aspirin or resistant starch on colorectal neoplasia in the Lynch syndrome. N Engl J Med. 2008;359(24):2567–78. doi:10.1056/NEJMoa0801297. Erratum in: N Engl J Med. 2009 Apr.

Burn J, Gerdes AM, Macrae F, Mecklin JP, Moeslein G, Olschwang S, Eccles D, Evans DG, Maher ER, Bertario L, Bisgaard ML, Dunlop MG, Ho JW, Hodgson SV, Lindblom A, Lubinski J, Morrison PJ, Murday V, Ramesar R, Side L, Scott RJ, Thomas HJ, Vasen HF, Barker G, Crawford G, Elliott F, Movahedi M, Pylvanainen K, Wijnen JT, Fodde R, Lynch HT, Mathers JC, Bishop DT, CAPP2 Investigators. Long-term effect of aspirin on cancer risk in carriers of hereditary colorectal cancer: an analysis from the CAPP2 randomised controlled trial. Lancet. 2011a;378(9809):2081–7.

Burn J, Bishop DT, Chapman PD, Elliott F, Bertario L, Dunlop MG, Eccles D, Ellis A, Evans DG, Fodde R, Maher ER, Möslein G, Vasen HF, Coaker J, Phillips RK, Bülow S, Mathers JC, International CAPP Consortium. A randomized placebo-controlled prevention trial of aspirin and/or resistant starch in young people with familial adenomatous polyposis. Cancer Prev Res (Phila). 2011b;4:655–65.

Burt RW, Berenson MM, Lee RG, et al. Upper gastrointestinal polyps in Gardner's syndrome. Gastroenterology. 1994;86:295–301.

Cairns SR, Scholefield JH, Steele RJ, Dunlop MG, Thomas HJ, Evans GD, Eaden JA, Rutter MD, Atkin WP, Saunders BP, Lucassen A, Jenkins P, Fairclough PD, Woodhouse CR, British Society of Gastroenterology, Association of Coloproctology for Great Britain and Ireland. Guidelines for colorectal cancer screening and surveillance in moderate and high riskgroups (update from 2002). Gut. 2010;59(5):666–89.

Caldas C, Carneiro F, Lynch HT, Yokota J, Wiesner GL, Powell SM, Lewis FR, Huntsman DG, Pharoah PD, Jankowski JA, MacLeod P, Vogelsang H, Keller G, Park KG, Richards FM, Maher ER, Gayther SA, Oliveira C, Grehan N, Wight D, Seruca R, Roviello F, Ponder BA, Jackson CE. Familial gastric cancer: overview and guidelines for management. J Med Genet. 1999;36:873–80. Review.

Canto MI, Harinck F, Hruban RH, Offerhaus GJ, Poley JW, Fockens P, Kamel IR, Nio CY, Schulick RD, Bassi C, Kluijt I, Goggins MG, Bruno MJ. International consensus recommendations on the management of patients with increased risk for familial pancreatic cancer: Cancer of the Pancreas Screening Consortium (CAPS); 2011 Summit.

Canto MI, Harinck F, Hruban RH, Offerhaus GJ, Poley JW, Kamel I, Nio Y, Schulick RS, Bassi C, Kluijt I, Levy MJ, Chak A, Fockens P, Goggins M, Bruno M. International Cancer of Pancreas Screening (CAPS) Consortium. International Cancer of the Pancreas Screening (CAPS) Consortium summit on the management of patients with increased risk for familial pancreatic cancer. Gut. 2013;62(3):339–47.

Chak F, Lee A, Kinnard T, Brock MF, Faulx W, Willis A, Cooper J, Sivak Jr GS, Goddard KA. Familial aggregation of Barrett's esophagus, esophageal adenocarcinoma, and oesophagogastric junctional adenocarcinoma in Caucasian adults. Gut. 2002;51:323–8.

Charbonnier F, Olschwang S, Wang Q, Boisson C, Martin C, Buisine MP, Puisieux A, Frebourg T. MSH2 in contrast to MLH1 and MSH6 is frequently inactivated by exonic and promoter rearrangements in hereditary nonpolyposis colorectal cancer. Cancer Res. 2002;62:848–53.

Chitayat D, Friedman JM, Dimmick JE. Neuroblastoma in a child with Wiedemann–Beckwith syndrome. Am J Med Genet. 1990a;35:433–6.

Chitayat D, Rothchild A, Ling E, Friedman JM, Couch RM, Yong SL, Baldwin VJ, Hall JG. Apparent postnatal onset of some manifestations of the Wiedemann-Beckwith syndrome. Am J Med Genet. 1990b;36(4):434–9.

Chu MH, Lee HC, Shen EY, Wang NL, Yeung CY, Chen BE, Shih SL. Gastrointestinal bleeding caused by leiomyoma of the small intestine in a child with neurofibromatosis. Eur J Paed. 1999;158(6):460–2.

Clericuzio CL, Chen E, McNeil DE, O'Connor T, Zackai EH, Medne L, Tomlinson G, DeBaun M. Serum alpha-fetoprotein screening for hepatoblastoma in children with Beckwith-Wiedemann syndrome or isolated hemihyperplasia. J Pediatr. 2003;143(2):270–2.

Cooney R, Jewell D. The Genetic Basis of Inflammatory Bowel Disease. Dig Dis. 2009;27:428–42.

Cooney R, Cummings JR, Pathan S, Beckly J, Geremia A, Hancock L, Guo C, Morris A, Jewell DP. Association between genetic variants in myosin IXB and Crohn's disease. Inflamm Bowel Dis. 2009;15(7):1014–21.

Cooper WN, Luharia A, Evans GA, et al. Molecular subtypes and phenotypic expression of Beckwith–Wiedemann syndrome. Eur J Hum Genet. 2005;13:1025–32.

Correa P, Shiao YH. Phenotypic and genotypic events in gastric carcinogenesis. Cancer Res. 1994;54:1941s–3.

Couch FJ, Johnson MR, Rabe K, Boardman L, McWilliams R, de Andrade M, Petersen G. Germ line Fanconi anemia complementation group C mutations and pancreatic cancer. Cancer Res. 2005;65(2):383–6.

Crabtree MD, Tomlinson IP, Hodgson SV, et al. Explaining variation in familial adenomatous polyposis: relationship between genotype and phenotype and evidence for modifier genes. Gut. 2002;51:420–3.

Creagan ET, Fraumeni Jr JF. Familial gastric cancer and immunologic abnormalities. Cancer. 1973;1325–31.

Daniel ES, Ludvig SL, Levin KJ, Ruprecht RM, Rajachich GM, Schwabwe AD. The Cronkhite Canada syndrome. An analysis of clinical and pathologic features and therapy in 55 cases. Medicine. 1982;61:293–309.

Davies H, Bignell GR, Cox C, Stephens P, Edkins S, Clegg S, Teague J, Woffendin H, Garnett MJ, Bottomley W, Davis N, Dicks E, Ewing R, Floyd Y, Gray K, Hall S, Hawes R, Hughes J, Kosmidou V, Menzies A, Mould C, Parker A, Stevens C, Watt S, Hooper S, Wilson R, Jayatilake H, Gusterson BA, Cooper C, Shipley J, Hargrave D, Pritchard-Jones K, Maitland N, Chenevix-Trench G, Riggins GJ, Bigner DD, Palmieri G, Cossu A, Flanagan A, Nicholson A, Ho JW, Leung SY, Yuen ST, Weber BL, Seigler HF, Darrow TL, Paterson H, Marais R, Marshall CJ, Wooster R, Stratton MR, Futreal PA. Mutations of the BRAF gene in human cancer. Nature. 2002;417:949–54.

De Pietri S, Sassatelli R, Roncucci L, et al. Clinical and biological features of adenomatosis coli in northern Italy. Scand J Gastroenterol. 1995;30:771–9.

de Vos tot Nederveen Cappel WH. Magnetic resonance imaging surveillance detects early-stage pancreatic cancer in carriers of a p16-Leiden mutation. Gastroenterology. 2011;140:850–6.

de Vos tot Nederveen Cappel WH, Offerhaus GJ, van Puijenbroek M, Caspers E, Gruis NA, De Snoo FA, Lamers CB, Griffioen G, Bergman W, Vasen HF, Morreau H. Pancreatic carcinoma in carriers of a specific 19 base pair deletion of CDKN2A/p16 (p16-leiden). Clin Cancer Res. 2003;9(10 Pt 1):3598–605.

Debinski HS, Spigelman AD, Hatfield A, Williams CB, Phillips RK. Upper intestinal surveillance in familial adenomatous polyposis. Eur J Cancer. 1995;31A:1149–53.

Devor EJ, Buechley PW. Gallbladder cancer in Hispanic New Mexicans. II. Familial occurrence in two northern New Mexico kindreds. Cancer Cell Cytogenet. 1979;1:139–45.

Dhillon PK, Farrow DC, Vaughan TL, Chow WH, Risch HA, Gammon MD, Mayne ST, Stanford JL, Schoenberg JB, Ahsan H, Dubrow R, West AB, Rotterdam H, Blot WJ, Fraumeni Jr JF. Family history of cancer and risk of esophageal and gastric cancers in the United States. Int J Cancer. 2001;93:148–52.

Domingo E, Laiho P, Ollikainen M, Pinto M, Wang L, French AJ, Westra J, Frebourg T, Espin E, Armengol M, Hamelin R, Yamamoto H, Hofstra RM, Seruca R, Lindblom A, Peltomaki P, Thibodeau SN, Aaltonen LA, Schwartz Jr S. BRAF screening as a low-cost effective strategy for simplifying HNPCC genetic testing. J Med Genet. 2004;41:664–8.

Dong SM, Traverso G, Johnson C, Geng L, Favis R, Boynton K, Hibi K, Goodman SN, D'Allessio M, Paty P, Hamilton SR, Sidransky D, Barany F, Levin B, Shuber A, Kinzler KW, Vogelstein B, Jen J. Detecting colorectal cancer in stool with the use of multiple genetic targets. J Natl Cancer Inst. 2001;93:858–65.

dos Santos JG, de Magalhes J. Familial gastric polyposis: a new entity. J Genet Hum. 1980; 28:293–7.

Drinkwater NR, Lee G-H. Genetic susceptibility to liver cancer. Liver Regeneration and Carcinogenesis. San Diego: Academic Press; 1995. p. 301–21.

Drovdlic CM, Goddard KA, Chak A, Brock W, Chessler L, King JF, Richter J, Falk GW, Johnston DK, Fisher JL, Grady WM, Lemeshow S, Eng C. Demographic and phenotypic features of 70 families segregating Barrett's esophagus and esophageal adenocarcinoma. J Med Genet. 2003; 40:651–6.

Dunlop MG. Guidance on gastroenterological surveillance for hereditary non-polyposis colorectal cancer, familial adenomatous polyposis, juvenile polyposis and Peutz–Jeghers syndrome. Gut. 2002;51(Suppl V):v21–7.

Dunlop MG, Farrington SM, Carothers AD, Wyllie AH, Sharp L, Burn J, Liu B, Kinzler KW, Vogelstein B. Cancer risk associated with germline DNA mismatch repair gene mutations. Hum Mol Genet. 1997;6(1):105–10.

Eaden JA, Mayberry JF. Guidelines for screening and surveillance of asymptomatic colorectal cancer in patients with inflammatory bowel disease. Gut. 2002;51 Suppl 5:v10–2.

Eberle MA, Pfutzer R, Pogue-Geile KL, Bronner MP, Crispin D, Kimmey MB, Duerr RH, Kruglyak L, Whitcomb DC, Brentnall TA. A new susceptibility locus for autosomal dominant pancreatic cancer maps to chromosome 4q32–34. Am J Hum Genet. 2002;70:1044–8.

Edwards CQ, Dalone MM, Skolnick MH, et al. Hereditary hemochromatosis. Clin Haematol. 1982;11:411–36.

Ehrenthal D, Haeger L, Griffin T, et al. Familial pancreatic carcinoma in three generations: a case report and a review of the literature. Cancer. 1987;59:1661–4.

Eide TJ. Risk of colorectal cancer in adenoma-bearing individuals within a defined population. Int J Cancer. 1986;38:173–6.

Eng C, Kiuru M, Fernandez MJ, Aaltonen LA. A role for mitochondrial enzymes in inherited neoplasia and beyond. Nat Rev Cancer. 2003;3:193–202.

Erdman SH, Barnard JA. Gastrointestinal polyps and polyposis syndromes in children. Curr Opin Paeds. 2002;14:576–82.

Eriksson S, Carlson J, Velez R. Risk of cirrhosis and primary liver cancer in Alpha-1 antitrypsin deficiency. New Engl J Med. 1986;314:736–9.

Evaluation of Genomic Applications in Practice and Prevention (EGAPP) Working Group. Recommendations from the EGAPP Working Group: genetic testing strategies in newly diagnosed individuals with colorectal cancer aimed at reducing morbidity and mortality from Lynch syndrome in relatives. Genet Med. 2009;11(1):35–41.

Evans JP, Burke W, Chen R, et al. Familial pancreatic adenocarcinoma: association with diabetes and early molecular diagnosis. J Med Genet. 1995;32:330–5.

Evans DG, Walsh S, Jeacock J, Robinson C, Hadfield L, Davies DR, Kingston R. Incidence of hereditary non-polyposis colorectal cancer in a population-based study of 1137 consecutive cases of colorectal cancer. Br J Surg. 1997;84:1281–5.

Evans G, Maher ER, Bertario L, Bisgaard ML, Dunlop M, Ho JW, Hodgson S, Lindblom A, Lubinski J, Morrison PJ, Murday V, Ramesar R, Side L, Scott RJ, Thomas HJ, Vasen H, Gerdes AM, Barker G, Crawford G, Elliott F, Pylvanainen K, Wijnen J, Fodde R, Lynch H, Bishop DT, Burn J, CAPP2 Investigators. Long-term effect of resistant starch on cancer risk in carriers of hereditary colorectal cancer: an analysis from the CAPP2 randomised controlled trial. Lancet Oncol. 2012;13(12):1242–9. doi: 10.1016/S1470-2045(12)70475-8.

Fearnhead NS, Wilding JL, Winney B, et al. Multiple rare variants in different geness account for multifactorial inherited susceptibility to colorectal adenomas. Proc Natl Acad Sci U S A. 2004;101:15992–7.

Fearon ER, Vogelstein B. A genetic model for colorectal tumorigenesis. Cell. 1990;61:759–67.

Feder JN, Gnirke A, Thomas W, et al. A novel MHC class I-like gene is mutated in patients with hereditary haemochromatosis. Nat Genet. 1996;13:399–407.

Fernandez E, La Vecchia C, D'Avanzo B, et al. Family history and the risk of liver, gall bladder and pancreatic cancer. Cancer Epidemiol Biomark Prev. 1994;3:209–12.

Fitzgerald RC, Hardwick R, Huntsman D, Carneiro F, Guilford P, Blair V, Chung DC, Norton J, Ragunath K, Van Krieken JH, Dwerryhouse S, Caldas C, International Gastric Cancer Linkage Consortium. Hereditary diffuse gastric cancer: updated consensus guidelines for clinical management and directions for future research. J Med Genet. 2010;47(7):436–44.

Flanders TY, Foulkes WD. Pancreatic adenocarcinoma: epidemiology and genetics. J Med Genet. 1996;33:889–98.

Fletcher RH. Colorectal cancer screening on stronger footing. N Engl J Med. 2008;359(12):1285–7.

Ford D, Easton DF, Bishop DT, et al., Breast Cancer Linkage Consortium. Risks of cancer in BRCA1 mutation carriers. Lancet. 1995;343:692–5.

Foulkes WD, Bahubeshi A, Hamel N, Pasini B, Asioli S, Baynam G, Choong CS, Charles A, Frieder RP, Dishop MK, Graf N, Ekim M, Bouron-Dal Soglio D, Arseneau J, Young RH, Sabbaghian N, Srivastava A, Tischkowitz MD, Priest JR. Extending the phenotypes associated with DICER1 mutations. Hum Mutat. 2011;32(12):1381–4.

Fresko D, Lazarus SS, Dotan J, Reingold M. Early presentation of carcinoma of the small bowel in Crohn's disease ('Crohn's carcinoma'). Case reports and review of the literature. Gastroenterology. 1982;82:783–9.

Friborg J, et al. Cancer in Greenlandic Inuit 1973–1997: a cohort study. Int J Cancer. 2003;107(6):1017–22.

Friborg J, Wohlfahrt J, Koch A, Storm H, Olsen OR, Melbye M. Cancer susceptibility in nasopharyngeal carcinoma families–a population-based cohort study. Cancer Res. 2005;65(18):8567–72.

Friedman JM, Fialklow PJ. Familial carcinoma of the pancreas. Clin Genet. 1976;9:463–9.

Frieling T, Berges W, Borchard F, et al. Family occurrence of achalasia and diffuse spasm of the esophagus. Gut. 1988;29:1595–602.

Fryns JP, Chrzanowska K. Mucosal neuromata syndrome (MEN type IIb(III)). J Med Genet. 1988;25:703–6.

Gatto NM, Frucht H, Sundararajan V, Jacobson JS, Grann VR, Neugut AI. Risk of perforation after colonoscopy and sigmoidoscopy: a population-based study. J Natl Cancer Inst. 2003;95:230–6.

Gayther SA, Gorringe KL, Ramus SJ, et al. Identification of germ-line E-cadherin mutations in gastric cancer families of European origin. Cancer Res. 1998;58:4086–9.

Gentry Jr WC, Eskritt NR, Gorlin RJ. Multiple hamartomata syndrome (Cowden disease). Arch Dermatol. 1978;114:743–6.

Ghadirian P, Liu G, Gallinger S, Schmocker B, Paradis AJ, Lal G, Brunet JS, Foulkes WD, Narod SA. Risk of pancreatic cancer among individuals with a family history of cancer of the pancreas. Int J Cancer. 2002;97:807–10.

Ghiorzo P, Ciotti P, Mantelli M, Heouaine A, Queirolo P, Rainero ML, Ferrari C, Santi PL, De Marchi R, Farris A, Ajmar F, Bruzzi P, Bianchi-Scarra G. 1999.

Giardiello FM, Trimbath JD. Peutz–Jeghers syndrome and management recommendations. Clin Gastroenterol Hepatol. 2006;4:408e15.

Giardiello FM, Brensinger JD, Tersmette AC, et al. Very high risk of cancer in familial Peutz–Jeghers syndrome. Gastroenterology 2000;119:1447e53.

Giardiello FM, Hylind LM, Trimbath JD, Hamilton SR, Romans KE, Cruz-Correa M, Corretti MC, Offerhaus GJ, Yang VW. Oral contraceptives and polyp regression in familial adenomatous polyposis. Gastroenterology. 2005;128(4):1077–80.

Gismondi V, Bonelli L, Sciallero S, et al. Prevalence of the E1317Q variant of the APC gene in Italian patients with colorectal adenomas. Genet Test. 2002;6:313–7.

Gockel HR, Schumacher J, Gockel I, Lang H, Haaf T, Nöthen MM. Achalasia: will genetic studies provide insights? Hum Genet. 2010;128(4):353–64.

Goldstein AM, Fraser MC, Struewing JP, Hussussian CJ, Ranade K, Zametkin DP, Fontaine LS, Organic SM, Dracopoli NC, Clark Jr WH, et al. Increased risk of pancreatic cancer in melanoma-prone kindreds with p16INK4 mutations. N Engl J Med. 1995a;333(15):970–4.

Goldstein AM, Fraser MC, Struwing JR, et al. Increased risk of pancreatic cancer in melanoma-prone kindreds with p16INK4 mutations. New Engl J Med. 1995b;333:970–4.

Goldstein AM, Struewing JP, Fraser MC, Smith MW, Tucker MA. Prospective risk of cancer in CDKN2A germline mutation carriers. J Med Genet. 2004;41:421–4.

González CA, Sala N, Capellá G. Genetic susceptibility and gastric cancer risk. Int J Cancer. 2002;100(3):249–60.

Gould SR, Stewart JB, Temple DN. Rectal polyposis in tuberose sclerosis. J Ment Defic Res. 1990;34:465–73.

Grover S, Kastrinos F, Steyerberg EW, Cook EF, Dewanwala A, Burbidge LA, Wenstrup RJ, Syngal S. Prevalence and phenotypes of APC and MUTYH mutations in patients with multiple colorectal adenomas. JAMA. 2012;308(5):485–92. doi:10.1001/jama.2012.8780.

Groves C, et al. Duodenal cancer in patients with familial adenomatous polyposis (FAP): results of a 10 year prospective study. Gut. 2002;50:636–41.

Grundbacher FJ. Genetic aspects of selective IgA deficiency. J Med Genet. 1972;9:344–7.

Gryfe R, Di Nicola N, Lal G, Gallinger S, Redston M. Inherited colorectal polyposis and cancer risk of the APC I1307K polymorphism. Am J Hum Genet. 1999;64:378–84.

Guilford P, Hopkins J, Harraway J, et al. E-cadherin germline mutations in familial gastric cancer. Nature. 1998;392:402–5.

Guohong Z, Min S, Duenmei W, Songnian H, Min L, Jinsong L, Hongbin L, Feng Z, Dongping T, Heling Y, Zhicai L, Shiyong L, Quansheng G, Xiaoyun L, Yuxia G. Genetic heterogeneity of oesophageal cancer in high-incidence areas of southern and northern China. PLoS One. 2010;5(3):e9668.

Gylling A, Abdel-Rahman WM, Juhola M, Nuorva K, Hautala E, Järvinen HJ, Mecklin JP, Aarnio M, Peltomäki P. Is gastric cancer part of the tumour spectrum of hereditary non-polyposis colorectal cancer? A molecular genetic study. Gut. 2007;56(7):926–33.

Haanstra JF, Kleibeuker JH, Koornstra JJ. Role of new endoscopic techniques in Lynch syndrome. Fam Cancer. 2013;12(2):267–72. doi:10.1007/s10689-013-9610-6.

Haerer AF, Jackson JF, Evers CG. Ataxia telangiectasia with gastric adenocarcinoma. J Am Med Assoc. 1969;210:1884–7.

Hahn SA, Greenhalf B, Ellis I, Sina-Frey M, Rieder H, Korte B, Gerdes B, Kress R, Ziegler A, Raeburn JA, Campra D, Grutzmann R, Rehder H, Rothmund M, Schmiegel W, Neoptolemos JP, Bartsch DK. BRCA2 germline mutations in familial pancreatic carcinoma. J Natl Cancer Inst. 2003;95:214–21.

Halbert C, Lynch H, Lynch J, Main D, Kucharski S, Rustgi AK, Lerman C. Colon Cancer Screening Practices Following Genetic Testing for Hereditary Nonpolyposis Colon Cancer (HNPCC). Mutations. 2004;164(17):1881–7.

Halford SE, Rowan RJ, Lipton L, et al. Germline mutations but not somatic changes at the MYH locus contributes to the pathogenesis of unselected colorectal cancer. Am J path. 2003;162:1545–8.

Hall MJ. Counterpoint: implementing population genetic screening for Lynch Syndrome among newly diagnosed colorectal cancer patients–will the ends justify the means? J Natl Compr Canc Netw. 2010;8(5):606–11.

Hampel H. Point: justification for Lynch syndrome screening among all patients with newly diagnosed colorectal cancer. J Natl Compr Canc Netw. 2010;8(5):597–601.

Hampel H, Stephens JA, Pukkala E, Sankila R, Aaltonen LA, Mecklin JP, de la Chapelle A. Cancer risk in hereditary nonpolyposis colorectal cancer syndrome: later age of onset. Gastroenterology. 2005;129(2):415–21.

Hampel H, Frankel W, Panescu J, Lockman J, Sotamaa K, Fix D, Comeras I, La Jeunesse J, Nakagawa H, Westman JA, Prior TW, Clendenning M, Penzone P, Lombardi J, Dunn P, Cohn DE, Copeland L, Eaton L, Fowler J, Lewandowski G, Vaccarello L, Bell J, Reid G, de la Chapelle A. Screening for Lynch syndrome (hereditary nonpolyposis colorectal cancer) among endometrial cancer patients. Cancer Res. 2006;66(15):7810–7.

Handschug K, Sperling S, Yoon SJ, Hennig S, Clark AJ, Huebner A. Triple A syndrome is caused by mutations in AAAS, a new WD-repeat protein gene. Hum Mol Genet. 2001;10(3):283–90.

Harinck F, Poley JW, Kluijt I, Fockens P, Bruno MJ. Dutch Research Group of Pancreatic Cancer Surveillance in High-Risk I. Is early diagnosis of pancreatic cancer fiction? Surveillance of individuals at high risk for pancreatic cancer. Dig Dis. 2010;28:670–8.

Harrison SA, Bacon BR. Relation of hemochromatosis with hepatocellular carcinoma: epidemiology, natural history, pathophysiology, screening, treatment, and prevention. Med Clin North Am. 2005;89(2):391–409.

Hartley AL, Birch JM, Kelsey AM, et al. Epidemiological and familial aspects of hepatoblastoma. Med Pediatr Oncol. 1990;18:103–9.

Hayoz D, Extermann M, Odermatt BF, et al. Familial primary gastric lymphoma. Gut. 1993;34:136–40.

Heiman R, Verhest A, Verschraegen J, Grosjean W, Draps JP, Hecht F. Hereditary intestinal neurofibromatosis. Neurofibromatosis. 1988;1:26–32.

Hennies H-C, Hagedorn M, Rais A. Palmoplantar keratoderma in association with carcinoma of the esophagus maps to chromosome 17q distal to the keratin gene cluster. Genomics. 1995;29:537–40.

Herkert JC, Niessen RC, Olderode-Berends MJ, Veenstra-Knol HE, Vos YJ, van der Klift HM, Scheenstra R, Tops CM, Karrenbeld A, Peters FT, Hofstra RM, Kleibeuker JH, Sijmons RH. Paediatric intestinal cancer and polyposis due to bi-allelic PMS2 mutations: case series, review and follow-up guidelines. Eur J Cancer. 2011;47(7):965–82.

Herzog CE, Andrassy RJ, Eftekhari F. Childhood cancers: hepatoblastoma. Oncologist. 2000;5(6):445–53.

Hibi K, Kondo K, Akiyama S, et al. Frequent genetic instability in small intestinal carcinomas. Jpn J Cancer Res. 1997;86:357–60.

Hochberg FH, Dasilva AB, Galdabini J, Richardson Jr EP. Gastrointestinal involvement in Von Recklinghausen's neurofibromatosis. Neurology. 1974;24:1144–51.

Hodgson SV, Murday V. Other genetic conditions associated with gastro-intestinal polyps. In: Phillips RKS, Spigelman AD, Thomson JPS, editors. Familial Adenomatous Polyposis and Other Polyposis Syndromes. London: Edward Arnold; 1994. p. 215–27.

Holmes GKT, Dunn GI, Cockel R, Brookes VC. Adenocarcinoma of the upper small bowel complicating coeliac disease. Gut. 1980;21:1010–5.

Houlston RS, Murday V, Haracopos C, et al. Screening and genetic counselling for relatives of patients with colorectal cancer in a family cancer clinic. Br Med J. 1990;301:366–8.

Houlston R, et al. Mutations in DPC4 (SMAD4) cause juvenile polyposis syndrome but only account for a minority of cases. Hum Mol Genet. 1998;7:1907–12.

Howe JR, Blair JA, Sayed MG, et al. Germline mutations of BMPR1A in juvenile polyposis. Nat Genet. 2001;28:184–7.

Howes N, Lerch MM, Greenhalf W, Stocken DD, Ellis I, Simon P, Truninger K, Ammann R, Cavallini G, Charnley RM, Uomo G, Delhaye M, Spicak J, Drumm B, Jansen J, Mountford R, Whitcomb DC, Neoptolemos JP. Clinical and genetic characteristics of hereditary pancreatitis in Europe. Clin Gastroenterol Hepatol. 2004;2:252–61.

Hu N, Li G, Li WJ, Wang C, Goldstein AM, Tang ZZ, Roth MJ, Dawsey SM, Huang J, Wang QH, Ding T, Giffen C, Taylor PR, Emmert-Buck MR. Infrequent mutation in the BRCA2 gene in esophageal squamous cell carcinoma. Clin Cancer Res. 2002;8:1121–6.

Hu N, Wang C, Han XY, He LJ, Tang ZZ, Giffen C, Emmert-Buck MR, Goldstein AM, Taylor PR. Evaluation of BRCA2 in the genetic susceptibility of familial esophageal cancer. Oncogene. 2004;23:852–8.

Huntsman DG, Carneiro F, Lewis FR, MacLeod PM, Hayashi A, Monaghan KG, Maung R, Seruca R, Jackson CE, Caldas C. Early gastric cancer in young, asymptomatic carriers of germ-line E-cadherin mutations. New Engl J Med. 2001;344(25):1904–9.

Hyer N, Beveridge I, Domizio P, Phillips R. Clinical management of gastrointestinal polyps in children. J Paed Gastro Nutrit. 2000;21:469–72.

Imperiale TF, Glowinski EA, Lin-Cooper C, Larkin GN, Rogge JD, Ransohoff DF. Five-year risk of colorectal neoplasia after negative screening colonoscopy. N Engl J Med. 2008;359(12):1218–24.

Ito E, Sato Y, Kawauchi K, et al. Type 1a glycogen storage disease with hepatoblastoma in siblings. Cancer. 1987;59:1776–80.

Jaeger E, Leedham S, Lewis A, Segditsas S, Becker M, Cuadrado PR, Davis H, Kaur K, Heinimann K, Howarth K, East J, Taylor J, Thomas H, Tomlinson I. Hereditary mixed polyposis syndrome is caused by a 40-kb upstream duplication that leads to increased and ectopic expression of the BMP antagonist GREM1. Nat Genet. 2012;44(6):699–703.

Jagelman DG, DeCosse JJ, Bussey HJR, Group TLCP. Upper gastrointestinal cancer in familial polyposis coli. Lancet. 1988;i:1149–51.

Jakubowska A, Nej K, Huzarski T, Scott RJ, Lubiński J. BRCA2 gene mutations in families with aggregations of breast and stomach cancers. Br J Cancer. 2002;87(8):888–91.

Jarvinen HJ, Aarnio M, Mustonen H, Aktan-Collan K, Aaltonen LA, Peltomaki P, de La CA, Mecklin JP. Controlled 15-year trial on screening for colorectal cancer in families with hereditary nonpolyposis colorectal cancer. Gastroenterol. 2000;118:829–34.

Järvinen H, Mecklin JP, Møller P, Myrhøi T, Nagengast FM, Parc Y, Phillips R, Clark SK, de Leon MP, Renkonen-Sinisalo L, Sampson JR, Stormorken A, Tejpar S, Thomas HJ, Wijnen J. Guidelines for the clinical management of familial adenomatous polyposis (FAP). Gut. 2008;57(5):704–13.

Jass JR. Colorectal adenomas in surgical specimens from subjects with hereditary non-polyposis colorectal cancer. Histopathology. 1995a;27:263–7.

Jass JR. Colorectal adenoma progression and genetic change: is there a link? Ann Med. 1995b;27:301–6.

Jass JR. HNPCC and sporadic colorectal cancer: a review of the morphological similarities and differences. Fam Cancer. 2004;3(2):93–100.

Jass JR, Whitehall VL, Young J, Leggett BA. Emerging concepts in colorectal neoplasia. Gastroenterology. 2002;123:862–76.

Jeevaratnam P, Cottier DS, Browett PJ, et al. Familial giant hyperplastic polyposis pre-disposing to colorectal cancer: a new hereditary bowel cancer syndrome. J Pathol. 1996;179:20–5.

Jenkins PJ, Besser M. Clinical perspective, acromegaly and cancer: a problem. J Clin Endocrinol Metab. 2001;86:2935–41.

Jenne DE, Reimann H, Nezu J-I, et al. Peutz–Jeghers syndrome is caused by mutations in a novel serine threonine kinase. Nat Genet. 1998;18:38–44.

Jensen DA, Warburg M, Dupont A. Ocular pathology in the elfin face syndrome (the Fanconi–Schlesinger type of idiopathic hypercalcaemia of infancy). Ophthalmologica. 1976;172:434–44.

Johnson CD, Chen MH, Toledano AY, Heiken JP, Dachman A, Kuo MD, Menias CO, Siewert B, Cheema JI, Obregon RG, Fidler JL, Zimmerman P, Horton KM, Coakley K, Iyer RB, Hara AK, Halvorsen Jr RA, Casola G, Yee J, Herman BA, Burgart LJ, Limburg PJ. Accuracy of CT colonography for detection of large adenomas and cancers. N Engl J Med. 2008;359(12):1207–17.

Judge TA, Lewis JD, Lichtenstein GR. Colonic dysplasia and cancer in inflammatory bowel disease. Gastrointest Endosc Clin N Am. 2002;12:495–523.

Kakagia D, Alexiadis G, Kiziridou A, Lambropoulou M. Brooke-Spiegler syndrome with parotid gland involvement. Eur J Dermatol. 2004;14(3):139–41.

Kasirga E, Ozkinay F, Tutuncuoglu S, et al. Four siblings with achalasia, alacrimia and neurological abnormalities in a consanguineous family. Clin Genet. 1996;49:296–9.

Kattwinkel J, Lapey A, Di Sant Agnese PA, et al. Hereditary pancreatitis: 3 new kindreds and a critical review of the literature. Pediatrics. 1973;51:55–69.

Kekki M, Siurala M, Varis K, et al. Classification principles and genetics of chronic gastritis. Scand J Gastroenterol. 1987;22 Suppl 141:1–28.

Kelsell DP, Risk JM, Leigh IM, et al. Close mapping of the focal non-epidermolytic palmoplantar keratoderma (PPK) locus associated with esophageal cancer (TOC). Hum Mol Genet. 1996;5:857–60.

Kerr NJ, Chun YH, Yun K, Heathcott RW, Reeve AE, Sullivan MJ. Pancreatoblastoma is associated with chromosome 11p loss of heterozygosity and IGF2 overexpression. Med Pediatr Oncol. 2002;39:52–4.

King JE, Dozois RR, Lindor NM, et al. Care of patients and their families with familial adenomatous polyposis. Mayo Clin Proc. 2000;75:57–67.

Kinzler KW, Vogelstein B. Lessons from hereditary colorectal cancer. Cell. 1996;87:159–70.

Kirchhoff T, Satagopan JM, Kauff ND, et al. Frequency of BRCA1 and BRCA2 in unselected Ashkenazi Jewish patients with colorectal cancer. J Natl Cancer Inst. 2004;90:2–3.

Klausner RD, Handler SD. Familial occurrence of pleomorphic adenoma. Int J Pediatr Otorhinolaryngol. 1994;30:205–10.

Klein AP, Borges M, Griffith M, Brune K, Hong SM, Omura N, Hruban RH, Goggins M. Absence of deleterious palladin mutations in patients with familial pancreatic cancer. Cancer Epidemiol Biomarkers Prev. 2009;18(4):1328–30.

Koh THHG, Cooper JE, Newman CL, et al. Pancreatoblastoma in a neonate with Wiedemann–Beckwith syndrome. Eur J Pediatr. 1986;145:435–8.

Koinuma K, Shitoh K, Miyakura Y, Furukawa T, Yamashita Y, Ota J, Ohki R, Choi YL, Wada T, Konishi F, Nagai H, Mano H. Mutations of BRAF are associated with extensive hMLH1 promoter methylation in sporadic colorectal carcinomas. Int J Cancer. 2004;108:237–42.

Koornstra JJ, Kleibeuker JH, Vasen HF. Small-bowel cancer in Lynch syndrome: is it time for surveillance? Lancet Oncol. 2008;9(9):901–5.

Kuiper RP, Vissers LE, Venkatachalam R, Bodmer D, Hoenselaar E, Goossens M, Haufe A, Kamping E, Niessen RC, Hogervorst FB, Gille JJ, Redeker B, Tops CM, van Gijn ME, van den Ouweland AM, Rahner N, Steinke V, Kahl P, Holinski-Feder E, Morak M, Kloor M, Stemmler S, Betz B, Hutter P, Bunyan DJ, Syngal S, Culver JO, Graham T, Chan TL, Nagtegaal ID, van Krieken JH, Schackert HK, Hoogerbrugge N, van Kessel AG, Ligtenberg MJ. Recurrence and variability of germline EPCAM deletions in Lynch syndrome. Hum Mutat. 2011; 32(4):407–14.

Laiho P, Lainover V, Lahemo P, et al. Low level MSI in most colorectal cancers. Cancer Res. 2002;62:1166–70.

Laken SJ, Peterson GM, Gruber SB. Familial colorectal cancer in Ashkenazim due to a hypermutable tract in APC. Nat Genet. 1997;17:79–83.

Lal G, Liu L, Hogg D, Lassam NJ, Redston MS, Gallinger S. Patients with both pancreatic adenocarcinoma and melanoma may harbor germline CDKN2A mutations. Gene Chromosome Cancer. 2000;27:358–61.

Lammi L, et al. Mutations in AXIN2 cause familial tooth agenisis and predispose to colorectal cancer. Am J Hum Genet. 2004;74:1043–50.

Langan JE, Cole CG, Huckle EJ, Bryne S, McRonald FE, Rowbottom L, Ellis A, Shaw JM, Leigh IM, Kelsell DP, Dunham I, Field JK, Risk JM. Novel microsatellite markers and single nucleotide polymorphisms refine the tylosis with esophageal cancer t(TOC) minimal region on 17q25 to 42.5 kb: sequencing does not identify the causative gene. Hum Genet. 2004;114:534–40.

Lanspa SJ, Lynch HT, Smyrk TC, et al. Colorectal adenomas in the Lynch syndromes. Results of a colonoscopy screening program. Gastroenterology. 1990;98:1117–22.

Lichtenstein P, Holm NV, Verkasalo PK, Iliadou A, Kaprio J, Koskenvuo M, Pukkala E, Skytthe A, Hemminki K. Environmental and heritable factors in the causation of cancer – analyses of cohorts of twins from Sweden, Denmark, and Finland. New Engl J Med. 2000;343:78–85.

Ligtenberg MJ, Kuiper RP, Geurts van Kessel A, Hoogerbrugge N. EPCAM deletion carriers constitute a unique subgroup of Lynch syndrome patients. Fam Cancer. 2013;12(2):169–74. doi:10.1007/s10689-012-9591-x.

Lim W, Olschwang S, Keller JJ, et al. Relative frequency and morphology of cancers in STK11 mutation carriers. Gastroenterology. 2004;126:1788–94.

Liu HX, Zhou XL, Liu T, et al. The role of hMLH3 in familial colorectal cancer. Cancer Res. 2003;63:1894–9.

Lubbe SJ, Webb EL, Chandler IP, Houlston RS. Implications of familial colorectal cancer risk profiles and microsatellite instability status. J Clin Oncol. 2009;27(13):2238–44.

Lucci-Cordisco E, Zito I, Gensini F, Genuardi M. Hereditary nonpolyposis colorectal cancer and related conditions. Am J Med Genet. 2003;122A(4):325–34.

Lynch HT, Ens JA, Lynch JF. The Lynch syndrome II and urological malignancies. J Urol. 1990;143:24–8.

Lynch HT, Smyrk TC, Watson P, et al. Genetics, natural history, tumor spectrum and pathology of hereditary non-polyposis colorectal cancer: an updated review. Gastroenterology. 1993;104:1535–49.

Lynch HT, Smyrk T, Kern SE, et al. Familial pancreatic cancer: a review. Semin Oncol. 1996;23:251–75.

Lynch HT, Brand RE, Hogg D, Deters CA, Fusaro RM, Lynch JF, Liu L, Knezetic J, Lassam NJ, Goggins M, Kern S. Phenotypic variation in eight extended CDKN2A germline mutation familial atypical multiple mole melanoma-pancreatic carcinoma-prone families: the familial atypical mole melanoma-pancreatic carcinoma syndrome. Cancer. 2002;94:84–96.

MacDonald CE, Wicks AC, Playford RJ. Final results from 10 year cohort of patients undergoing surveillance for Barrett's esophagus: observational study. Br Med J. 2000;321:1252–5.

Macklin MT. Inheritance of cancer of the stomach and large intestine in man. J Natl Cancer Inst. 1960;24:551–71.

Malats N, Casals T, Porta M, Guarner L, Estivill X, Real FX. Cystic fibrosis transmembrane regulator (CFTR) DeltaF508 mutation and 5T allele in patients with chronic pancreatitis and exocrine pancreatic cancer. PANKRAS II Study Group. Gut. 2001;48:70–4.

Mathers JC, Movahedi M, Macrae F, Mecklin JP, Moeslein G, Olschwang S, Eccles D, Evans G, Maher ER, Bertario L, Bisgaard ML, Dunlop M, Ho JW, Hodgson S, Lindblom A, Lubinski J, Morrison PJ, Murday V, Ramesar R, Side L, Scott RJ, Thomas HJ, Vasen H, Gerdes AM, Barker G, Crawford G, Elliott F, Pylvanainen K, Wijnen J, Fodde R, Lynch H, Bishop DT, Burn J, CAPP2 Investigators. Long-term effect of resistant starch on cancer risk in carriers of hereditary colorectal cancer: an analysis from the CAPP2 randomised controlled trial. Lancet Oncol. 2012;13(12):1242–9. doi:10.1016/S1470-2045(12)70475-8. Epub 2012 Nov 7.

Mathew CG, Lewis CM. Genetics of inflammatory bowel disease: progress and prospects. Hum Mol Genet. 2004;13(13 spec no 1):R161–8.

McConnell RB. The Genetics of Gastrointestinal Disorders. Oxford: Oxford University Press; 1966.

McGivern A, Wynter CV, Whitehall VL. Promoter hypermethylation frequency and BRAF mutation distinguish hereditary non-polyposis colon cancer from sporadic MSI-H colon cancer. Fam Cancer. 2004;3:101–7.

Mehenni H, Resta N, Park JG, et al. Cancer risks in LKB1 germline mutation carriers. Gut. 2006;55:984–90.

Merrick Y, et al. Familial clustering of salivary gland carcinoma in Greenland. Cancer. 1986;57(10):2097–102.

Michaels L, et al. Family with low-grade neuroendocrine carcinoma of salivary glands, severe sensorineural hearing loss, and enamel hypoplasia. Am J Med Genet. 1999;83(3):183–6.

Mitchell RJ, Farrington SM, Dunlop MG, Campbell H. Mismatch repair genes hMLH1 and hMSH2 and colorectal cancer: a HuGE review. Am J Epidemiol. 2002;156:885–902.

Miyanaga O, Miyamoto Y, Shirahama M, Ishibashi H. A clinico-pathological study of hepatocellular carcinoma patients with other primary malignancies. Gan No Rinsho. 1989;35: 1729–34.

Mocci E, Milne RL, Yuste Méndez-Villamil E, Hopper JL, John EM, Andrulis IL, Chung WK, Daly MB, Buys SS, Malats N, Goldgar DE. Risk of pancreatic cancer in breast cancer families from the Breast Cancer Family Registry. Cancer Epidemiol Biomarkers Prev. 2013;22(5): 803–11. doi:10.1158/1055-9965.EPI-12-0195. Epub 2013 Mar 1.

Moran A, O'Hara C, Khan S, Shack L, Woodward E, Maher ER, Lalloo F, Evans DG. Risk of cancer other than breast or ovarian in individuals with BRCA1 and BRCA2 mutations. Fam Cancer. 2012;11:235–42.

Morson B. Factors influencing the prognosis of early cancer of the rectum. Proc R Soc Med. 1966;59:607–12.

Mosbech J, Videbaek A. On the aetiology of oesophageal carcinoma. J Natl Cancer Inst. 1955;15:1665–73.

Muller T, Schafer H, Rodeck B, Haupt G, Koch H, Bosse H, Welling P, Lange H, Krech R, Feist D, Muhlendahl KE, Bramswig J, Feichtinger H, Muller W. Familial clustering of infantile cirrhosis in Northern Germany: a clue to the etiology of idiopathic copper toxicosis. J Pediat. 1999;135:189–96.

Murphy KM, Brune KA, Griffin C, Sollenberger JE, Petersen GM, Bansal R, Hruban RH, Kern SE. Evaluation of candidate genes MAP2K4, MADH4, ACVR1B, and BRCA2 in familial pancreatic cancer: deleterious BRCA2 mutations in 17%. Cancer Res. 2002;62:3789–93.

Ngeow J, Heald B, Rybicki LA, et al. Prevalence of germline PTEN, BMPR1A, SMAD4, STK11 and ENG mutations in patients with moderate-load colorectal polyps. Gastroenterology. 2013;144(7):1402–9.

Niederau C, Fischer R, Sonnenberg A, et al. Survival and cause of death in cirrhotic and non-cirrhotic patients with primary haemochromatosis. New Engl J Med. 1985;313:1256–63.

Niell BL, Long JC, Rennert G, Gruber SB. Genetic anthropology of the colorectal cancer-susceptibility allele APC I1307K: evidence of genetic drift within the Ashkenazim. Am J Hum Genet. 2003;73:1250–60.

Niell BL, Rennert G, Bonner JD, et al. BRCA1 and BRCA2 founder mutations and the risk of colorectal cancer. J Natl Cancer Inst. 2004;96:15–21.

Niessen RC, Hofstra RM, Westers H, Ligtenberg MJ, Kooi K, Jager PO, de Groote ML, Dijkhuizen T, Olderode-Berends MJ, Hollema H, Kleibeuker JH, Sijmons RH. Germline hypermethylation of MLH1 and EPCAM deletions are a frequent cause of Lynch syndrome. Genes Chromosomes Cancer. 2009;48(8):737–44.

Ohue M, Tomita N, Monden T, et al. Mutations of the transforming growth factor b type II receptor gene and microsatellite instability in gastric cancer. Int J Cancer. 1996;68:203–6.

Orloff M, Peterson C, He X, Ganapathi S, Heald B, Yang YR, Bebek G, Romigh T, Song JH, Wu W, David S, Cheng Y, Meltzer SJ, Eng C. Germline mutations in MSR1, ASCC1, and CTHRC1 in patients with Barrett esophagus and esophageal adenocarcinoma. JAMA. 2011; 306(4):410–9.

Ozcelik H, Schmocker B, DiNicola N, et al. Germline BRCA2 6174del T mutations in Ashkenazi Jewish pancreatic cancer patients. Nat Genet. 1997;16:17–8.

Palles C, Cazier JB, Howarth KM, Domingo E, Jones AM, Broderick P, Kemp Z, Spain SL, Guarino E, Salguero I, Sherborne A, Chubb D, Carvajal-Carmona LG, Ma Y, Kaur K, Dobbins S, Barclay E, Gorman M, Martin L, Kovac MB, Humphray S; CORGI Consortium; WGS500 Consortium, Lucassen A, Holmes CC, Bentley D, Donnelly P, Taylor J, Petridis C, Roylance R, Sawyer EJ, Kerr DJ, Clark S, Grimes J, Kearsey SE, Thomas HJ, McVean G, Houlston RS, Tomlinson I. Nat Genet. 2013;45(2):136–44.

Parsons MT, Buchanan DD, Thompson B, Young JP, Spurdle AB. Correlation of tumour BRAF mutations and MLH1 methylation with germline mismatch repair (MMR) gene mutation status: a literature review assessing utility of tumour features for MMR variant classification. J Med Genet. 2012;49(3):151–7.

Peel D, Kolodner R, Li F, Anton-Culver H. Relationship between replication error (RER) and MSH2/MLH1 gene mutations in population-based HNPCC kindreds. Am J Hum Genet. 1997;61S:A208–1203.

Peel DJ, Ziogas A, Fox EA, Gildea M, Laham B, Clements E, Kolodner RD, Anton-Culver H. Characterization of hereditary nonpolyposis colorectal cancer families from a population-based series of cases. J Natl Cancer Inst. 2000;92:1517–22.

Perlmutter DH. Clinical manifestations of alpha 1-antitrypsin deficiency Gastroenterol. Clin North Am. 1995;24:27–43.

Pezzilli R, Morselli-Labate AM, Mantovani V, Romboli E, Selva P, Migliori M, Corinaldesi R, Gullo L. Mutations of the CFTR gene in pancreatic disease. Pancreas. 2003;27:332–6.

Pharoah PD, Guilford P, Caldas C. International Gastric Cancer Linkage Consortium. Incidence of gastric cancer and breast cancer in CDH1 (E-cadherin) mutation carriers from hereditary diffuse gastric cancer families. Gastroenterology. 2001;121(6):1348–53.

Pogue-Geile KL, Chen R, Bronner MP, Crnogorac-Jurcevic T, Moyes KW, Dowen S, Otey CA, Crispin DA, George RD, Whitcomb DC, Brentnall TA. Palladin mutation causes familial pancreatic cancer and suggests a new cancer mechanism. PLoS Med. 2006;3:e516.

Ponz de Leon M. Familial tumors of other organs. Recent result. Cancer Res. 1994;136:332–40.

Powell SM. Direct analysis for familial adenomatous polyposis mutations. Mol Biotechnol. 2002;20:197–207.

Powell SM, Zilz N, Beazer-Barclay Y, et al. APC mutations occur early during colorectal tumorigenesis. Nature. 1992;359:235–7.

Richards PM, McKee SA, Rajpar MH. Germline E-cadherin (CDH1) gene muta-tions predispose to familial gastric cancer and colorectal cancer. Hum Mol Genet. 1999;8:607–10.

Risk JM, Evans KE, Jones J, Langan JE, Rowbottom L, McRonald FE, Mills HS, Ellis A, Shaw JM, Leigh IM, Kelsell DP, Field JK. Characterization of a 500 kb region on 17q25 and the exclusion of candidate genes as the familial tylosis esophageal cancer (TOC) locus. Oncogene. 2002;21:6395–402.

Roberts NJ, Jiao Y, Yu J, Kopelovich L, Petersen GM, Bondy ML, Gallinger S, Schwartz AG, Syngal S, Cote ML, Axilbund J, Schulick R, Ali SZ, Eshleman JR, Velculescu VE, Goggins M, Vogelstein B, Papadopoulos N, Hruban RH, Kinzler KW, Klein AP. ATM mutations in patients with hereditary pancreatic cancer. Cancer Discov. 2012;2(1):41–6.

Robson ME, Glogowski E, Sommer G, et al. Pleomorphic characteristics of a germline KIT mutation in a large kindred with gastrointestinal stromal tumours, hyper-pigmentation, and dysphagia. Clin Cancer Res. 2004;10:1250–4.

Rodriguez-Bigas MA, Boland CR, Hamilton SR, et al. A National Cancer Institute workshop on hereditary non-polyposis colorectal cancer: meeting highlights and Bethesda guidelines. J Nat Cancer Inst. 1997;89:1758–62.

Rogers CD, Couch FJ, Brune K, et al. Genetics of the FANCA gene in familial pancreatic cancer. J Med Genet. 2004;41(12):e126.

Rootwelt H, Hoie K, Berger R, Kvittinger EA. Fumarylacetoacetase mutations in tyrosinaemia type I. Hum Mutat. 1996;7:239–43.

Rosenberg PS, Greene MH, Alter BP. Cancer incidence in persons with Fanconi anemia. Blood. 2003;101(3):822–6. Blood. 2003 Mar 15;101(6):2136.

Saarinen S, Vahteristo P, Lehtonen R, Aittomäki K, Launonen V, Kiviluoto T, Aaltonen LA. Analysis of a Finnish family confirms RHBDF2 mutations as the underlying factor in tylosis with esophageal cancer. Fam Cancer. 2012;11(3):525–8. doi:10.1007/s10689-012-9532-8.

Salaria SN, Illei P, Sharma R, Walter KM, Klein AP, Eshleman JR, Maitra A, Schulick R, Winter J, Ouellette MM, Goggins M, Hruban R. Palladin is overexpressed in the non-neoplastic stroma of infiltrating ductal adenocarcinomas of the pancreas, but is only rarely overexpressed in neoplastic cells. Cancer Biol Ther. 2007;6(3):324–8.

Salovaara R, Loukola A, Kristo P, Kaariainen H, Ahtola H, Eskelinen M, Harkonen N, Julkunen R, Kangas E, Ojala S, Tulikoura J, Valkamo E, Jarvinen H, Mecklin JP, Aaltonen LA, de La CA. Population-based molecular detection of hereditary nonpolyposis colorectal cancer. J Clin Oncol. 2000;18:2193–200.

Sampson JR, et al. MUTYH-associated polyposis. Best Pract Res Clin Gastroenterol. 2009; 23:209–18.

Sayed MG, et al. Germline SMAD4 or BMPR1A mutations and phenotype of juvenile polyposis. Ann Surg Oncol. 2002;9:901–6.

Scott N, Lansdown M, Diament R, et al. Helicobacter gastritis intestinal metaplasia in a gastric cancer family. Lancet. 1990;335:8691–728.

Sharer N, Schwarz M, Malone G, Howarth A, Painter J, Super M, Braganza J. Mutations of the cystic fibrosis gene in patients with chronic pancreatitis. New Engl J Med. 1998;339:645–52.

Shaw D, Blair V, Framp A, et al. Chromoendoscopic surveillance in hereditary diffuse gastric cancer: an alternative to prophylactic gastrectomy? Gut. 2005;54:461–8.

Sheikholeslami MR, Schaefer RF, Mukunyadzi P. Diffuse giant inflammatory polyposis: a challenging clinicopathologic diagnosis. Arch Pathol Lab Med. 2004;128:1286–8.

Shine I, Allison PR. Carcinoma of the esophagus with tylosis. Lancet. 1966;i:951–3.

Sidransky D. Nucleic acid-based methods for the detection of cancer. Science. 1997;278:1054–8.

Sjursen W, Haukanes BI, Grindedal EM, Aarset H, Stormorken A, Engebretsen LF, Jonsrud C, Bjørnevoll I, Andresen PA, Ariansen S, Lavik LA, Gilde B, Bowitz-Lothe IM, Maehle L, Møller P. J Med Genet. 2010;47(9):579–85.

Slater E, Amrillaeva V, Fendrich V, Bartsch D, Earl J, Vitone LJ, Neoptolemos JP, Greenhalf W. Palladin mutation causes familial pancreatic cancer: absence in European families. PLoS Med. 2007;4(4):e164.

Sniderman King L, Trahms C, Scott CR. Tyrosinemia Type 1. In: Pagon RA, Bird TD, Dolan CR, Stephens K, Adam MP, editors. GeneReviews™ Seattle (WA): University of Washington, Seattle; 1993–2006 Jul 24 [updated 2011 Aug 25].

Solomon S, Siddhartha Das BS, Brand R, et al. Inherited pancreatic cancer syndromes. Cancer J. 2012;18(6):485–91.

Spigelman AD, Phillips RKS. Screening for cancer and pre-cancer in the esophagus, stomach and duodenum. Hosp Update. 1991;17:220–8.

Spigelman AD, Williams CB, Talbot IC, et al. Upper gastrointestinal cancer in patients with familial adenomatous polyposis. Lancet. 1989;2:783–5.

Spirio L, Olschwang S, Groden J, et al. Alleles of the APC gene: an attenuated form of familial polyposis. Cell. 1993;75:951–7.

St John DVB, McDennett FT, Hopper VL, et al. Cancer risks in relatives with common colorectal cancer. Ann Int Med. 1993;118:785–90.

Steinhagen E, Shia J, Markowitz AJ, Stadler ZK, Salo-Mullen EE, Zheng J, Lee-Kong SA, Nash GM, Offit K, Guillem JG. Systematic immunohistochemistry screening for Lynch syndrome in early age-of-onset colorectal cancer patients undergoing surgical resection. J Am Coll Surg. 2012;214(1):61–7.

Stephenson BM, Finan PJ, Gascoyne J, et al. Frequency of familial colorectal cancer. Br J Surg. 1991;78:1162–6.

Streubel B, et al. T(14;18)(q32;q21) involving IGH and MALT1 is a frequent chromosomal aberration in MALT lymphoma. Blood. 2003;101(6):2335–9.

Struewing JP, Hartege P, Wacholder S, et al. The risk of cancer associated with specific mutations of BRCA1 and BRCA2 among Ashkenazi Jews. New Engl J Med. 1997;336:1401–8.

Su H, Hu N, Shih J, Hu Y, Wang QH, Chuang EY, Roth MJ, Wang C, Goldstein AM, Ding T, Dawsey SM, Giffen C, Emmert-Buck MR, Taylor PR. Gene expression analysis of esophageal squamous cell carcinoma reveals consistent molecular profiles related to a family history of upper gastrointestinal cancer. Cancer Res. 2003;63:3872–6.

Sutter C, Dallenbach-Hellweg G, Schmidt D. Molecular analysis of endometrial hyperplasia in HNPCC-suspicious patients may predict progression to endometrial carcinoma. Int J Gynecol Pathol. 2004;23(1):18–25.

Sweetser S, Ahlquist DA, Osborn NK, Sanderson SO, Smyrk TC, Chari ST, Boardman LA. Clinicopathologic features and treatment outcomes in Cronkhite-Canada syndrome: support for autoimmunity. Dig Dis Sci. 2012;57(2):496–502.

Tai DI, Chen CH, Chang TT, et al. Eight-year nationwide survival analysis in relatives of patients with hepatocellular carcinoma: role of vital infection. J Gastroenterol Hepatol. 2002;17:682–9.

Teich N, Schulz HU, Witt H, Bohmig M, Keim V. N34S, a pancreatitis associated SPINK1 mutation, is not associated with sporadic pancreatic cancer. Pancreatology. 2003;3:67–8.

Thompson D, Easton DF. Cancer incidence in BRCA1 mutation carriers. J Natl Cancer Inst. 2002;94:1358–65.

Tischkowitz M, Xia B. PALB2/FANCN: recombining cancer and Fanconi anemia. Cancer Res. 2010;70(19):7353–9.

Traverso G, Shuber A, Levin B, Johnson C, Olsson L, Schoetz Jr DJ, Hamilton SR, Boynton K, Kinzler KW, Vogelstein B. Detection of APC mutations in fecal DNA from patients with colorectal tumors. New Engl J Med. 2002;346:311–20.

Tresallet C, Brouquet A, Julié C, Beauchet A, Vallot C, Ménégaux F, Mitry E, Radvanyi F, Malafosse R, Rougier P, Nordlinger B, Laurent-Puig P, Boileau C, Emile JF, Muti C, Penna C, Hofmann-Radvanyi H. Evaluation of predictive models in daily practice for the identification of patients with Lynch syndrome. Int J Cancer. 2012;130(6):1367–77.

Triantafillidis JK, Kosmidis P, Kottaridis S. Familial stomach cancer. Am J Gastroenterol. 1993;88:1789–90.

Trufant JW, Greene L, Cook DL, McKinnon W, Greenblatt M, Bosenberg MW. Colonic ganglioneuromatous polyposis and metastatic adenocarcinoma in the setting of Cowden syndrome: a case report and literature review. Human Pathol. 2011;43:601–4.

Umar A, Boland CR, Terdiman JP, Syngal S, de La CA, Ruschoff J, Fishel R, Lindor NM, Burgart LJ, Hamelin R, Hamilton SR, Hiatt RA, Jass J, Lindblom A, Lynch HT, Peltomaki P, Ramsey SD, Rodriguez-Bigas MA, Vasen HF, Hawk E, Barrett JC, Freedman AN, Srivastava S. Revised Bethesda guidelines for hereditary nonpolyposis colorectal cancer (Lynch syndrome) and microsatellite instability. J Natl Cancer Inst. 2004;96:261–8.

Urrita R, DiMagno EP. Genetic markers: the key to early diagnosis and improved survival in pancreatic cancer? Editorial. Gastroenterology. 1996;110:306–10.

Ushio K, Sasagawa M, Doi H, et al. Lesions associated with familial polyposis coli. Studies of lesions of the stomach, duodenum, bones and teeth. Gastrointest Radiol. 1976;1:67.

van Lier MGF, Wagner A, Mathus-Vliegen EMH, Kuipers EJ, Steyerberg EW, van Leerdam ME. High cancer risk in Peutz-Jeghers syndrome: a systematic review and surveillance recommendations. Clin System Rev. 2011;105:1258–64.

Varley JM, McGowan G, Thorncroft M, et al. An extended Li–Fraumeni kindred with gastric carcinoma and a codon 175 mutation in TP53. J Med Genet. 1995;32:942–5.

Vasen HF. Review article: the Lynch syndrome (hereditary nonpolyposis colorectal cancer). Alim Pharmacol Ther. 2007;26 Suppl 2:113–26.

Vasen HF, Wijnen JT, Menko FH, et al. Cancer risk in families with hereditary nonpolyposis colorectal cancer diagnosed by mutation analysis. Gastroenterology. 1996;110:1020–7.

Vasen HFA, Watson P, Mecklin J-P, et al. New clinical criteria for hereditary non-polyposis colorectal cancer (HNPCC, Lynch syndrome) proposed by the inter-national collaborative group on HNPCC. Gastroenterology. 1999;116:1453–6.

Vasen HF, Gruis NA, Frants RR, van Der Velden PA, Hille ET, Bergman W. Risk of developing pancreatic cancer in families with familial atypical multiple mole melanoma associated with a specific 19 deletion of p16 (p16-Leiden). Int J Cancer. 2000;87(6):809–11.

Vasen HF, Stormorken A, Menko FH, Nagengast FM, Kleibeuker JH, Griffioen G, Taal BG, Moller P, Wijnen JT. Msh2 mutation carriers are at higher risk of cancer than Mlh1 mutation carriers: a study of hereditary nonpolyposis colorectal cancer families. J Clin Oncol. 2001;19(20):4074–80.

Vasen HFA, Möslein G, Alonso A, Bernstein I, Bertario L, Blanco I, Burn J, Capella G, Engel C, Frayling I, Friedl W, Hes FJ, Hodgson S, Mecklin J-P, Møller P, Nagengast F, Parc Y, Renkonen-Sinisalo L, Sampson JR, Stormorken A, Wijnen J. Guidelines for the clinical management of Lynch syndrome (hereditary non-polyposis cancer). J Med Genet. 2007;44:353–62. Gut, 59, 666–689.

Vasen HF, Möslein G, Alonso A, Aretz S, Bernstein I, Bertario L, Blanco I, Bülow S, Burn J, Capella G, Colas C, Engel C, Frayling I, Friedl W, Hes FJ, Hodgson S, Järvinen H, Mecklin JP, Møller P, Myrhøi T, Nagengast FM, Parc Y, Phillips R, Clark SK, de Leon MP, Renkonen-Sinisalo L, Sampson JR, Stormorken A, Tejpar S, Thomas HJ, Wijnen J. Guidelines for the clinical management of familial adenomatous polyposis (FAP). Gut. 2008;57(5):704–13. doi:10.1136/gut.2007.136127. Epub 2008 Jan 14.

Vasen HF, van der Meulen-de Jong AE, de Vos Tot Nederveen Cappel WH, Oliveira J, ESMO Guidelines Working Group. Familial colorectal cancer risk: ESMO clinical recommendations. Ann Oncol. 2009;20 Suppl 4:51–3. doi:10.1093/annonc/mdp127. Review.

Vasen HF, Abdirahman M, Brohet R, Langers AM, Kleibeuker JH, van Kouwen M, Koornstra JJ, Boot H, Cats A, Dekker E, Sanduleanu S, Poley JW, Hardwick JC, de Vos tot Nederveen Cappel WH, van der Meulen-de Jong AE, Tan TG, Jacobs MA, Mohamed FL, de Boer SY, van de Meeberg PC, Verhulst ML, Salemans JM, van Bentem N, Westerveld BD, Vecht J, Nagengast FM. One to 2-year surveillance intervals reduce risk of colorectal cancer in families with Lynch syndrome. Gastroenterology. 2010a;138(7):2300–6.

Vasen HF, Möslein G, Alonso A, Aretz S, Bernstein I, Bertario L, Blanco I, Bulow S, Burn J, Capella G, Colas C, Engel C, Frayling I, Rahner N, Hes FJ, Hodgson S, Mecklin JP, Møller P, Myrhøj T, Nagengast FM, Parc Y, de Leon Ponz M, Renkonen-Sinisalo L, Sampson JR, Stormorken A, Tejpar S, Thomas HJ, Wijnen J, Lubinski J, Järvinen H, Claes E, Heinimann K, Karagiannis JA, Lindblom A, Dove-Edwin I, Müller H. Recommendations to improve identification of hereditary and familial colorectal cancer in Europe. Fam Cancer. 2010b;9(2):109–15.

Vasen HFA, Möslein G, Alonso A, Bernstein I, Bertario L, Blanco I, Burn J. G Haanstra JF. Kleibeuker JH: Koornstra JJ. Role of new endoscopic techniques in Lynch syndrome. Fam Cancer; 2013 [Epub ahead of print].

Verna EC, Hwang C, Stevens PD, Rotterdam H, Stavropoulos SN, Sy CD, Prince MA, Chung WK, Fine RL, Chabot JA, Frucht H. Pancreatic cancer screening in a prospective cohort of high-risk patients: a comprehensive strategy of imaging and genetics. Clin CancerRes. 2010;16:5028–37.

Villanueva A, Newell P, Hoshida Y. Inherited hepatocellular carcinoma. Best Pract Res Clin Gastroenterol. 2010;24(5):725–34.

Villarroel MC, Rajeshkumar NV, Garrido-Laguna I, De Jesus-Acosta A, Jones S, Maitra A, Hruban RH, Eshleman JR, Klein A, Laheru D, Donehower R, Hidalgo M. Personalizing cancer treatment in the age of global genomic analyses: PALB2 gene mutations and the response to DNA damaging agents in pancreatic cancer. Mol Cancer Ther. 2011;10(1):3–8.

Vogt S, et al. Expanded extracolonic tumour spectrum in MUTYH-associated polyposis. Gastroenterology. 2009;137:1976–85.

Vu TT, Zeitouni AG, Tsinalis P, Foulkes WD, Hagr A. Familial clustering of parotid gland lymphoepithelioma in North America. J Otolaryngol Head Neck Surg. 2008;37(1):23–6.

Wagner A, Barrows A, Wijnen JT, van der KH, Franken PF, Verkuijlen P, Nakagawa H, Geugien M, Jaghmohan-Changur S, Breukel C, Meijers-Heijboer H, Morreau H, van Puijenbroek M, Burn J, Coronel S, Kinarski Y, Okimoto R, Watson P, Lynch JF, de La CA, Lynch HT, Fodde R. Molecular analysis of hereditary nonpolyposis colorectal cancer in the United States: high mutation detection rate among clinically selected families and characterization of an American founder genomic deletion of the MSH2 gene. Am J Hum Genet. 2003;72(5):1088–100.

Walshe JM, Waldenstrom E, Sams V, et al. Abdominal malignancies in patients with Wilson's disease. Q J Med. 2003;96:657–62.

Wang L, Cunningham JM, Winters JL, Guenther JC, French AJ, Boardman LA, Burgart LJ, McDonnell SK, Schaid DJ, Thibodeau SN. BRAF mutations in colon cancer are not likely attributable to defective DNA mismatch repair. Cancer Res. 2003;63:5209–12.

Watson P, Vasen HF, Mecklin JP, Bernstein I, Aarnio M, Järvinen HJ, Myrhøj T, Sunde L, Wijnen JT, Lynch HT. The risk of extra-colonic, extra-endometrial cancer in the Lynch syndrome. Int J Cancer. 2008;123(2):444–9.

West NJ, Clark SK, Phillips RK, Hutchinson JM, Leicester RJ, Belluzzi A, Hull MA. Eicosapentaenoic acid reduces rectal polyp number and size in familialadenomatous polyposis. Gut. 2010;59(7):918–25.

Whitcomb DC, Gorry MC, Preston RA, et al. Hereditary pancreatitis is caused by a mutation in the cationic trypsinogen gene. Nat Genet. 1996;14:141–5.

Whitelaw SC, Murday VA, Tomlinson IPM, et al. Clinical and molecular features of the hereditary mixed polyposis syndrome. Gastroenterology. 1997;112:327–34.

Wijnen J, Khan PM, Vasen H, et al. Hereditary nonpolyposis colorectal cancer families not complying with the Amsterdam criteria show extremely low frequency of mismatch-repair gene mutations. Am J Hum Genet. 1997;61:329–35.

Wijnen J, de Leew W, Nvasen H, et al. Familial endometrial cancer in female carriers of MSH6 germline mutations. Nat Genet. 1999;23:142–4.

Williams CB, Fairclough PD. Colonoscopy. Curr Opin Gastroenterol. 1991;7:55–65.

Williams CB, Goldblatt M, Delaney PV. Top and tail endoscopy and follow-up in Peutz–Jeghers syndrome. Endoscopy. 1982;14:22–34.

Winawer SJ, Zauber AG, O'Brien MJ, et al. Randomised comparison of surveillance intervals after colonoscopic removal of newly diagnosed adenomas. The National Polyp Study Workgroup. New Engl J Med. 1993;328:901–6.

Witt H, Luck W, Becker M, Bohmig M, Kage A, Truninger K, Ammann RW, O'Reilly D, Kingsnorth A, Schulz HU, Halangk W, Kielstein V, Knoefel WT, Teich N, Keim V. Mutation in the SPINK1 trypsin inhibitor gene, alcohol use, and chronic pancreatitis. J Am Med Assoc. 2001;285:2716–7.

Worthley DL, Phillips KD, Wayte N, Schrader KA, Healey S, Kaurah P, Shulkes A, Grimpen F, Clouston A, Moore D, Cullen D, Ormonde D, Mounkley D, Wen X, Lindor N, Carneiro F, Huntsman DG, Chenevix-Trench G, Suthers GK. Gastric adenocarcinoma and proximal polyposis of the stomach (GAPPS): a new autosomal dominant syndrome. Gut. 2012;61(5):774–9.

Wu Y, Berends MJ, Post JG, et al. Germline mutations in EXO1 gene in patients with hereditary non-polyposis colorectal cancer (HNPCC) and atypical HNPCC forms. Gastroenterology. 2001;120:1580–7.

Wu J, Matthaei H, Maitra A, Dal Molin M, Wood LD, Eshleman JR, Goggins M, Canto MI, Schulick RD, Edil BH, Wolfgang CL, Klein AP, Diaz Jr LA, Allen PJ, Schmidt CM, Kinzler KW, Papadopoulos N, Hruban RH, Vogelstein B. Recurrent GNAS mutations define an unexpected pathway for pancreatic cyst development. Sci Transl Med. 2011;3(92):92ra66.

Yonemoto RH, et al. Familial polyposis of the entire gastrointestinal tract. Arch Surg. 1969;99:427–34.

Zacharin M, Bajpai A, Chow CW, Catto-Smith A, Stratakis C, Wong MW, Scott R. Gastrointestinal polyps in McCune Albright syndrome. J Med Genet. 2011;48(7):458–61.

Zha S, Yegnasubramin V, Nelson WG, et al. Cyclooxygenases in cancer: progress and perspective. Cancer Lett. 2004;215:1–20.

Zhang W, Bailey-Wilson JE, Li W, Wang X, Zhang C, Mao X, Liu Z, Zhou C, Wu M. Segregation analysis of esophageal cancer in a moderately high-incidence area of northern China. Am J Hum Genet. 2000;67(1):110–9.

Zhou XP, Woodford-Richens K, Lehtonen R, et al. Germline mutations in BMPR1A/ALK3 cause a subset of juvenile polyposis syndrome and of Cowden and Bannayan–Riley–Ruvalcaba syndromes. Am J Hum Genet. 2001;69:704–11.

Zogopoulos G, Rothenmund H, Eppel A, Ash C, Akbari MR, Hedley D, Narod SA, Gallinger S. The P239S palladin variant does not account for a significant fraction of hereditary or early onset pancreas cancer. Hum Genet. 2007;121(5):635–7.

Zugel NP, Hehl JA, Jechart G, et al. Colorectal carcinoma in Cronkhite–Canada syndrome. Z Gastroenterol. 2001;39:365–7.

Chapter 6
Reproductive System

Breast Cancer

Background: Epidemiology and Family History

Breast cancer is the most common non-cutaneous cancer in women, accounting for 20 % of all new cases of cancer. The lifetime risk of breast cancer in the UK is one in nine females, with an annual incidence of <10 per 100,000 women aged <30 years, rising to 300 per 100,000 in women aged over 85 years. Similar, but slightly higher rates are seen in North America. It is rare in men (<1 per 100,000). Breast cancer incidence shows marked geographical variation: it is much less common in Asian than in Caucasian women and less frequent in South America and Spain than in Northern Europe, North America, and Australia. In India, the prevalence is lower (although rising) among most ethnic groups. In North America, the incidence of breast cancer appears to have increased in recent years; most of this increase is due to mammographic detection of ductal carcinoma in situ leading to early diagnosis of minimally invasive ductal carcinoma. It is notable that the rates of breast cancer to age 40 are fairly stable around the globe (Narod 2012a). Nearly all the differences in incidence from country to country occur in women diagnosed above this age, and it is even more noticeable in women diagnosed in the postmenopausal years (Leong et al. 2010), suggesting that nongenetic factors predominate in women diagnosed at older ages. Because the known highly penetrant breast cancer susceptibility genes cannot explain most of the diagnoses of breast cancer in women diagnosed under 40 years of age (they are clearly highly "genetic"), other genetic mechanisms must be at play.

In 1948, Penrose and colleagues observed that breast cancer may have a hereditary basis in some families (Penrose et al. 1948). A genetic influence on breast cancer susceptibility is suggested by twin studies, as the concordance for breast cancer in identical twins (0.28) is more than twice that in dizygotic twins (0.12). A statistically significant heritable factor of 27 % was observed for breast cancer (95 % confidence interval (CI): 4–41) in the three-country study of 44,788 pairs of twins (Lichtenstein et al. 2000). By contrast, the factor for prostate cancer was

S.V. Hodgson et al., *A Practical Guide to Human Cancer Genetics*,
DOI 10.1007/978-1-4471-2375-0_6, © Springer-Verlag London 2014

42 %, so clearly these percentages do not reflect the contribution of highly penetrant genes to these diseases.

There is an increased risk of breast cancer among female relatives of breast cancer patients and this increased relative risk (RR) is more pronounced when the index case has bilateral disease or early (premenopausal) age at onset. For patients 55 years of age or older at diagnosis, the RR of breast cancer in a first-degree female relative is approximately 1.8, increasing to 3–4 when more than one first-degree relative is affected. A large study (7,496 women with breast cancer and 7,438 controls) of the risks of breast cancer in women in relation to their family history found that, compared to women with no affected relative, the risk ratio for breast cancer was 1.80 (99 % CI 1.69–1.91), 2.93 (99 % CI 2.30–3.64), and 3.90 (2.03–7.49), respectively, for one, two, and three or more affected first-degree relatives ($P < 0.0001$ each) (Collaborative Group on Hormonal factors in breast cancer 2001). Risk ratios were greatest at young ages, and with younger age at diagnosis in the relative. For women with zero, one, or two or more first-degree affected relatives, the estimated cumulative risk of breast cancer up to age 50 years was 1.7, 3.7, and 8 %, respectively, corresponding to incidences up to age 80 of 7.8, 13.3, and 21.1 %, and death from breast cancer of 2.3, 4.2, and 7.6 %. There was no evidence for an autosomal recessive effect. An important finding was that other factors such as hormones and diet did not vary by family history.

Among women with one affected relative, the cumulative incidence of breast cancer between ages of 20 and 80 was 12.3 % if the relative was over 60, but 16.1 % if under 40. Another key finding was that most breast cancers in women with a family history of breast cancer were likely to occur after the age of 50, even if there were two affected relatives (Collaborative Group on Hormonal factors in breast cancer 2001).

For a woman aged 30 with a mother and a sister affected with breast cancer, the cumulative risk of breast cancer to age 70 has been found to be 17.4 %, significantly lower than the 43 % risk to be expected if all such familial clusters were due to highly penetrant mutations in susceptibility genes (Peto et al. 1996), suggesting that most such familial clusters are not due to these genes.

There is epidemiological evidence for overlap between breast and ovarian cancer susceptibility. The overall age-adjusted RR for ovarian cancer in first-degree relatives of women with breast cancer has been estimated to be 1.7 (and 2.1 for breast cancer), and first-degree relatives of index cases of ovarian cancer have RR of 1.6 and 2.8 for breast cancer and ovarian cancer, respectively. In one study, the RR for breast cancer in first-degree relatives of index cases ascertained because of colon cancer was estimated to be about 5, but in general, later studies of the risk of breast cancer after colorectal cancer, or colorectal cancer after breast cancer, have not supported this finding (Newschaffer et al. 2001). The only gene that might reasonably contribute to both breast and colorectal cancer in this context is *CHEK2* (Meijers-Heijboer et al. 2003), but this is probably only clinically relevant in the Netherlands and possibly Finland. It is possible that some "breast/colorectal" families are due to mutations in two genes, with one responsible for breast cancer, and the other for colorectal cancer (Thiffault et al. 2004). It should be noted that recent prospective studies have suggested an up to fourfold increase in breast cancer for patients

Table 6.1 RR estimates (95 % floated CI) for mutation carriers, in BRCA1 and BRCA2

Age group	*BRCA1*		*BRCA2*	
	Breast cancer	Ovarian cancer	Breast cancer	Ovarian cancer
20–29 years	18 (4.4–75)	1.0	19 (4.4–82)	1.0
30–39 years	36 (25–52)	38 (17–88)	16 (9.3–29)	1.0
40–49 years	31 (25–52)	61 (38–99)	9.5 (5.9–15)	6.3 (1.4–28)
50–59 years	16 (9.6–27)	30 (14–65)	11 (6.6–17)	19 (9.1–41)
60–69 years	11 (5.0–25)	48 (22–109)	9.2 (5.1–17)	7.3 (1.8–30)

Table based on country and cohort-specific background rates (Antoniou et al. 2003)

carrying germline mismatch repair gene mutations (Win et al. 2012) (see p. 256, Chap. 5 Lynch syndrome).

BRCA1 and BRCA2

The Genes and the Risks for Cancer

Twenty years after they were first discovered, *BRCA1* and *BRCA2* remain the two most important breast cancer susceptibility genes, by some considerable margin (Narod 2012b). *BRCA1* on chromosome 17q12–23 accounts for most families with inherited breast and ovarian cancer susceptibility and about 40 % of inherited breast cancer, particularly where the onset of breast cancer was at 45 years or younger (Figs. 6.1 and 6.2).

BRCA2, located on chromosome 13q, was identified a year later. Germline mutations in this gene confer a strong susceptibility to breast cancer and a smaller risk of ovarian cancer than with *BRCA1* mutations. Gene penetrance for lifetime risk of breast cancer in *BRCA2* mutation carriers is lower than in the case of *BRCA1* mutations and results in later-onset disease: in cases unselected for family history, the average cumulative risks for breast cancer in *BRCA1* mutation carriers by age 70 years was 65 % (95 % CI 44–78 %). In *BRCA2* carriers, the estimate was 45 % (31–56 %) (Figs. 6.1 and 6.2).

Relative risks (RR) are shown in Table 6.1, and age-dependent penetrance is shown in Fig. 6.1 (*BRCA1*) and Fig. 6.2 (*BRCA2*) (Mavaddat et al. 2013). Mutations in *BRCA2* predispose to a wider spectrum of other cancers than do mutations in *BRCA1*. These cancer sites include prostate, stomach, pancreatic, and male breast cancers (Couch et al. 1997). In this large international study, statistically significant increases in risks were observed for prostate cancer (Table 6.2) (estimated RR = 4.65; 95 % CI: 3.48–6.22), pancreatic cancer (RR = 3.51; 95 % CI: 1.87–6.58), gallbladder and bile duct cancer (RR = 4.97; 95 % CI: 1.50–16.52), stomach cancer (RR = 2.59; 95 % CI: 1.46–4.61), and malignant melanoma (RR = 2.58; 95 % CI: 1.28–5.17). The RR for prostate cancer for men below the age of 65 years was 7.33 (95 % CI: 4.66–11.52). There was a significant reduction in risks for women in earlier birth cohorts.

Fig. 6.1 Cumulative incidence of breast cancer (diamonds) and ovarian cancer (squares) in BRCA1-mutation carriers, to age 70. From Antoniou et al. 2003, with permission

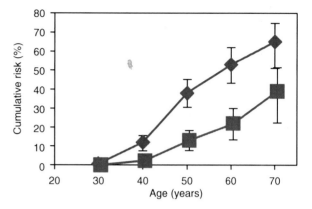

Fig. 6.2 Cumulative incidence of breast cancer (diamonds) and ovarian cancer (squares) in BRCA2-mutation carriers, to 70 age

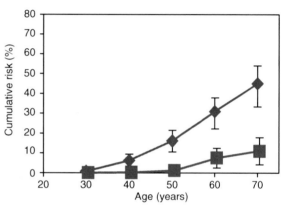

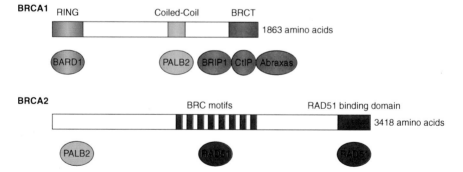

Fig. 6.3 BRCA1 and BRCA2 and binding partners (color-coded with corresponding interacting domain). BRCA1 consists of 1863 amino acids and contains three functionally important domains: a RING-finger domain which binds to BARD1 mediating ubiquitination of various proteins involved in chromosome stability, a coiled-coil domain which binds to PALB2 bridging it to BRCA2, and a BRCT domain which binds to phosphorylated proteins such as the protein complex, Abraxas-CtIP-BRIP1, regulating homologous repair. BRCA2 on the other hand is a larger 3418 amino acid protein that acts as a scaffold for the DNA recombinase, RAD51. It contains eight BRC motifs that bind RAD51 and another distinct RAD51-binding domain at its carboxyl end. BRCA2 mediates RAD51 loading on to single-stranded DNA, a critical step in the homologous repair of double-stranded DNA. Figure courtesy Andrew Shuen, MD

Table 6.2 Risks associated with BRCA2 mutations: non-breast/ovary sites by age of onset

Site	0–65 years of age		65–85 years of age	
	RR	95 % CI	RR	95 % CI
Buccal cavity + Pharynx	1.52	0.44–5.19	3.15	0.77–4.83
Stomach	2.57	1.13–5.84	1.93	0.77–4.83
Pancreas	5.54	2.72–11.32	1.61	0.45–5.72
Prostate	7.33	4.66–11.52	3.39	2.34–4.92
All except breast, ovary, prostate, pancreas	1.48	1.15–1.91	1.30	0.96–1.76

Breast Cancer Linkage Consortium, adapted from – Cancer risks in BRCA2 mutation carriers. J Natl Cancer Inst. 1999;91(15):1310–6

Particular mutations in *BRCA1* and *BRCA2* may confer higher RR of ovarian cancer than others, but currently this information is of limited clinical utility. Of course, men may transmit breast cancer susceptibility, but the mutation is usually non-penetrant for breast cancer in males. Among families with male breast cancer, 80 % are due to mutations in *BRCA2* and 20 % to *BRCA1*.

There is a high frequency of specific germline mutations in *BRCA1* and *BRCA2* in individuals of Ashkenazi Jewish origin (about 2 %; the *BRCA1* c.68_69delAG (also known as 185delAG or 187delAG) and c.5266dupC *BRCA1* (also known as 5382insC) and c.5946delT *BRCA2* (also known as 6174delT) mutations), and up to 30 % of breast cancer cases in women from this ethnic group diagnosed with breast cancer under the age of 40 years, 40 % of breast cancer families, and 60 % of breast/ovarian families carry one of these germline mutations. A high frequency of specific *BRCA1/2* mutations has been found in other ethnic groups, probably due to a founder effect, for example, the 999del5 *BRCA2* mutation in Iceland, detected in 0.6 % of the population, 7.7 % of female breast cancer patients, and 40 % of males with breast cancer. In one study from Poland, recurrent mutations were found in 33 (94 %) of the 35 families with detected mutations. Three *BRCA1* mutations – c.5266dupC, c.181T>G, and 4153delA – accounted for 51, 20, and 11 % of the identified mutations, respectively (Gorski et al. 2000). Mutations in *BRCA2* were rare. These observations simplify *BRCA1/2* genetic testing for individuals of Polish origin. Many other populations are known to have founder mutations in one or other of these two genes (Fackenthal and Olopade 2007).

The proportion of breast cancer attributable to *BRCA1* mutations was estimated at 5.3 % in women diagnosed below the age of 40 years to 1 % in those diagnosed over the age of 70 years (Easton et al. 1995), and subsequent mutation analysis studies have proved these estimates to be approximately accurate (Whittemore et al. 2004b).

BRCA *Protein Function*

BRCA1 and *BRCA2* are large genes with no known homology, containing 22 and 26 exons, respectively (Fig. 6.3). Many, but not all of the functions of the BRCA1 and BRCA2 proteins revolve around facilitating the repair of double-strand DNA breaks.

In addition, BRCA1 has functions that are not related to DNA repair. These roles include cell checkpoint control, protein ubiquitination, and chromatin remodeling, and BRCA1 may also have a role as transcription factor (Narod and Foulkes 2004) (for excellent more recent reviews focusing on the nexus between genome integrity, DNA repair, and BRCA1, see Li and Greenberg 2012; Silver and Livingston 2012). Recent developments in the understanding of the function of BRCA1, discussed in the reviews cited above, include the potential differential effect of some RING-finger *BRCA1* mutations on E3 ubiquitin ligase activity (which may be important clinically, in that some mutations could have differing clinical effects) and the finding that BRCA1 knockout or depletion in mouse models resulted in a decrease in the number of pericentric heterochromatic foci. Their morphology was also altered. This study, focused on the connection between BRCA1 and heterochromatin, is supported by previous work on both BRCA1-related and basal-like (but BRCA1-intact) breast cancer where there seems to be loss of maintenance of silencing of the inactive X-chromosome (Ganesan et al. 2005). Both these studies point to a broader role for BRCA1 in tumor suppression. The critical enigma of why female *BRCA1* mutation carriers are so prone to develop breast and ovarian cancer remains unresolved. Several hypotheses have been proposed, for example, that there is of a restricted period of time during breast development when estrogen-driven proliferation can be influenced by the level of BRCA1 protein (Elledge and Amon 2002; Scully and Livingston 2000), that allele loss rates at BRCA1 differ between tissues (Monteiro 2003), that there is a role for BRCA1 in breast stem cell regulation (Foulkes 2004) and, now most recently, that the involvement of BRCA1 in removal of bulky adducts (e.g., UV photoproducts) might extend to the removal of the products of estrogen metabolism, in the form of DNA adducts (Pathania et al. 2011). Moreover, this function may be impaired in cells heterozygous for *BRCA1* mutations, and thus the specificity for breast cancer is related to dependency of this cancer on estrogen (Pathania et al. 2011).

Cells defective in BRCA1 or BRCA2 are hypersensitive to agents that cross-link DNA strands or that break double-stranded DNA, such as cisplatin and mitomycin C (Yuan et al. 1999; Moynahan et al. 2001; Tassone et al. 2003). In these cells, double-strand breaks are repaired in an error-prone fashion (e.g., via nonhomologous end joining), and errors can lead to chromosomal rearrangements (Patel et al. 1998; Zhong et al. 1999). Notably, BRCA1 and BRCA2 function in a common pathway that is responsible for the integrity of the genome and the maintenance of chromosomal stability (Venkitaraman 2002). In the last few years, this commonality has been exploited therapeutically by several groups. Studies of patients with triple-negative cancers receiving neo-adjuvant cisplatin-based chemotherapy showed that complete clinical responses were much more likely to occur among BRCA1 mutation carriers than noncarriers (Silver et al. 2010). Similar effects were seen in uncontrolled studies of breast cancer arising in *BRCA1* mutation carriers (Byrski et al. 2008). Taken together, these studies suggest that *BRCA1* (and possibly *BRCA2* mutation) carriers may receive greater benefit from platinating compounds than other women with cancer. Definitive studies are underway. Because breast and ovarian cancers in women heterozygous for mutations in *BRCA1* or *BRCA2* mutation that carry a second somatic "hit" to BRCA1 or BRCA2 respectively will be rendered functionally null for the relevant protein and thus have impaired homologous DNA repair, PARP inhibitors (PARPi), which essentially convert single-strand breaks to double-strand breaks, were promoted as useful chemotherapeutic agents for breast and ovarian cancers in BRCA1/2 carriers affected by cancer. An extended Phase I study (Fong et al. 2009) and two Phase II clinical trials in *BRCA1/2* carriers showed promise in the treatment of both metastatic breast (Tutt et al. 2010) and ovarian cancers (Audeh et al. 2010), but most "triple-negative" breast cancers do not respond to PARP inhibition (Gelmon et al 2011). While the drugs are often initially effective in many mutation carriers, resistance often develops, by a number of different mechanisms, most notably revertant mutations that restore an open-reading frame resulting in the expression of a functional BRCA1 or BRCA2 protein (Swisher et al. 2008; Norquist et al. 2011; Edwards et al. 2008; Sakai et al. 2008). Perhaps because of such resistance, longer-term studies of PARP inhibitor treatment of ovarian cancer have not showed an improvement in overall survival (Ledermann et al. 2012).

As stated above, in the absence of underlying *BRCA1* or *BRCA2* mutations, most triple-negative breast cancers do not respond to PARPi, but a recent development suggests that PARPi-resistant triple-negative breast cancers might be converted to sensitivity to these drugs by the additions of PIK3CA inhibitors (Ibrahim et al. 2012; Pérez et al. 2012).

Other Genes Involved in Breast Cancer Susceptibility

A number of studies have now tested for *BRCA1* and *BRCA2* mutations in population-based series of breast cancer cases, and thus the contribution of these two genes to familial aggregation can be assessed. Peto et al. (1999) identified 30 *BRCA1/2* mutations in 617 breast cancer patients diagnosed before age 46. Interestingly, only five of their mothers or sisters had had breast cancer, compared with 64 in the relatives of the 587 noncarriers. After allowing for the number of breast cancers that would be expected at population rates, and assuming a mutation sensitivity of 64 %, this would equate to approximately 16 % of the observed familial risk being due to *BRCA1* and *BRCA2*. In a previous linkage study, over 80 % of families with six or more cases of breast cancer were found to be linked to either *BRCA1* or *BRCA2*, but the proportion fell to 40 % in families with four or five cases, leaving room for other genes (Ford et al. 1998).

In the last few years, four genes have emerged as strong candidate breast cancer susceptibility genes – *CHEK2, BRIP1, ATM,* and *PALB2* (Foulkes 2008) – and the candidacy of other so-called "moderate-penetrance" breast cancer susceptibility genes (such as *RAD50* and *NBS1*) have been advanced. It is important to recognize that identified mutations in all these genes are either too low in frequency or of too low penetrance to account for more than a small part of the remaining familial cases. In particular, *BRIP1* appears to have a very limited role (Seal et al. 2006; Wong et al. 2011), but has recently been associated with ovarian carcinoma (see below). In families with a strong family history of breast cancer, these moderate-risk alleles could be clinically useful (Byrnes et al. 2008). The same authors have suggested that the breast cancer penetrance for at least some *PALB2* alleles is as high as some *BRCA2* alleles (Erkko et al. 2008; Southey et al. 2010).

Approximately 50 % of women with Li–Fraumeni syndrome (see p. 271) develop breast cancer, particularly at young ages. The RR for breast cancer in women under 45 years of age in Li–Fraumeni syndrome families has been estimated at 17.9 (Garber et al. 1991). However, the proportion of cases of breast cancer overall is likely to be extremely small because fewer than 1 % of breast cancer cases can be demonstrated to have germline *TP53* mutations (Borresen et al. 1992), and even among early-onset breast cancer, *TP53* mutations have a minor role (Sidransky et al. 1992).

Other genes associated with a moderate to high penetrance for breast cancer include *PTEN* (Cowden Syndrome), *STK11* (Peutz–Jeghers syndrome), and *CDKN2A* (hereditary malignant melanoma). The contribution of mutations in all of these three genes to breast cancer incidence is negligible, but the risks for carriers can be as high as 50 %. Klinefelter syndrome (XXY) is also associated with an increased risk for breast cancer (p. 270).

Epidemiological data have demonstrated an increased RR of early-onset breast cancer in the female relatives of cases of ataxia telangiectasia (see p. 219), and the proportion of breast cancer due to heterozygosity for *ATM* mutations has been estimated to be 7 % overall, a smaller proportion at later ages at diagnosis than at earlier ages. Initial studies had suggested that a very small proportion of breast cancer cases, even in radiosensitive subjects, was attributable to mutations in this gene. One missense mutation, *ATM*7271T>G*, has been associated with a high risk of breast cancer in a few families (Chenevix-Trench et al. 2002), but it is not frequently implicated in hereditary breast cancer (Szabo et al. 2004). The most comprehensive genetic epidemiological study suggested that the RR for breast cancer in *ATM* carriers is 2.2 (95 % CI 1.2–4.3), but is nearly 5 for those diagnosed under 40 years of age (Thompson et al. 2005). This study was supported by a definitive molecular study which identified deleterious mutations in 12 of 443 probands from UK familial breast cancer pedigrees and in 2 in 521 controls, leading to an estimated RR of 2.37 (95 % CI, 1.51-3.78) (Renwick et al. 2006), a number remarkably similar to the estimate from epidemiological studies. This study also emphasized the need for very large studies when looking at rare alleles with moderate risks. The previous negative studies listed above were underpowered to detect relative risks as low as 2.4. RR between 2.0 and 5.0 and have been termed moderate-risk alleles, whereas those below this are generally grouped together as low-risk alleles.

A rare novel type of mutation resulting in somatic mosaicism has been uncovered by next-generation sequencing. Truncating somatic mutations in *PPM1D* have been identified in small percentage of breast and ovarian cancers, but interestingly, they appear not to be heritable. They are only present in lymphocytes and not in the tumors occurring in those carrying these mutations. Also, they are not present in the offspring of carriers thus far tested and identifying *PPM1D* mutation carriers will be a challenge. The relative risk for breast and ovarian cancer, however, is substantial (likely >20) and would warrant preventive intervention (Ruark et al. 2013).

Several score of low-risk breast cancer susceptibility alleles have been discovered through powerful genome-wide association studies (GWAS) (Easton et al. 2007), and there are probably hundreds more such alleles, but currently their usefulness in the clinic is very limited. In the future, it is hoped that risk calculation programs, such as BOADICEA (Antoniou et al. 2004), and perhaps BRCAPRO, will be able to incorporate these genotypes into the risk model. If so, low-risk alleles could be of considerable interest in planning screening protocols (Pharoah et al. 2008). Until that time, lower-risk alleles are more relevant to the clinician as modifiers of high-penetrance alleles. For example, SNPs at *ESR1*, *TOX3*, and one on 2q (not in a gene) have been found to modify breast cancer risk in *BRCA1* carriers. By contrast, so far 11 SNPs modify risk in *BRCA2*-related breast cancer. This is probably related to the fact that more SNPs are known to modify ER-positive breast cancer than are known to modify ER-negative breast cancer. Several alleles also modify risk for ovarian cancer in *BRCA1* or *BRCA2* mutation carriers (Barnes and Antoniou 2012). Clearly, many more such loci will be identified, and perhaps this will be of clinical use in the next decade or so, but currently the effect sizes are not large enough to warrant altering clinical recommendations for mutation carriers.

Histopathology of Breast Cancer and Its Relationship to Genetics

Breast cancers arising in *BRCA1* mutation carriers can often be distinguished from cancers occurring in *BRCA2* or non-*BRCA1/2* carriers on morphological (Lakhani et al. 1998), immunopathological (Lakhani et al. 2002), cytogenetic (Wessels et al. 2002), gene expression (Hedenfalk et al. 2001; Van't Veer et al. 2002; Sorlie et al. 2003), and mutational grounds (Nik-Zainal et al. 2012). *BRCA1*-related breast cancers are usually infiltrating ductal carcinomas of high grade. Although the term is seldom used now, studies have shown that an atypical medullary phenotype is more common in *BRCA1*-related breast cancer than in matched controls (Lakhani et al. 1998). *BRCA1*-related breast cancers are much more likely to be triple negative (TN) (ER, PR, and HER2 negative) than are other types of breast cancer (Schneider et al. 2008). Notably, some studies of *PALB2* mutation carriers have also noticed an excess of TN breast cancer, but comprehensive studies are required (Tischkowitz and Xia 2010). BRCA2-related cancers are usually ER positive, and unlike sporadic breast cancer, the percentage of tumors that are ER positive does not increase with age (Foulkes et al. 2004). It has been noted that HER2 positivity is commonly found in breast cancers arising in women with germline *TP53* mutations (Wilson et al. 2010; O'Shaughnessy et al. 2011), which could aid in selecting who to offer germline *TP53* testing.

Ductal carcinoma in situ (DCIS) and lobular carcinoma are underrepresented in *BRCA1* mutation carriers. Sequencing studies of women with DCIS have revealed a small percentage of *BRCA1* and *BRCA2* mutations (~1 and 2.5 %, respectively) (Claus et al. 2005).

Genetic Counseling

Genetic counseling for women with a family history of breast cancer requires an initial assessment of their lifetime risk of developing breast cancer on the basis of empirical data derived from taking a family history that includes information about cancer type and age at onset in all first-degree and second-degree relatives and as many more distant relatives as possible. It is important to try and confirm diagnoses if it will make a material difference to the clinical decisions made. Risk estimates can be obtained using epidemiological data, or with the help of computer programs which calculate risks using these data, and can be expressed as a lifetime risk or as a risk for developing cancer over a shorter time period, such as the ensuing 10 years (Antoniou et al. 2004). Programs such as IBIS and BRCAPRO can also calculate the probability of being a *BRCA1/2* mutation carrier, although IBIS is limited to unaffected women. Hand-scoring, non-Bayesian methods, such as the Manchester scoring system have the benefit of simplicity and user-friendliness, relying on a scoring system for the numbers of affected relatives. They avoid the need for a computer program (Evans et al. 2004). Screening guidelines based on family history and genetic testing are available on the NICE website, http://www.nice.org.uk/cg41: "Familial breast cancer: the classification and care of women at risk of familial breast cancer in primary, secondary and tertiary care (partial update of CG14)".

A woman whose mother has a germline breast cancer susceptibility mutation has a prior risk of 50 % of inheriting the susceptibility, so that her lifetime risk of developing breast cancer is about 40 % (assuming 80 % gene penetrance for breast cancer). However, if she remains healthy after the age of 50 years, her actual risk will have fallen because she has lived through a substantial amount of her risk period, with most hereditary breast cancer occurring at a younger age. The risk that the daughter of a gene carrier who remains unaffected at 50 years of age has inherited the susceptibility has fallen to approximately one-third, and if she remains healthy, it is less likely that she has inherited the susceptibility the older she becomes.

The probability that the family is segregating for a *BRCA1* or *BRCA2* germline mutation may be derived from family history data, in order to give an indication as to the likelihood that the consultant could be offered a predictive test for such a mutation. This chance is very dependent on age at diagnosis in the affected woman (there is a 17 % chance of a *BRCA1* mutation in breast cancer families with average age at diagnosis below 35 years, but a 1 % chance when the average age at diagnosis is over 59 years). A family history of ovarian cancer increases the chance of finding a *BRCA1* mutation, as does multiple primary breast or ovarian cancers in an affected woman of Ashkenazi Jewish origin (Couch et al. 1997).

The original model for counseling and genetic testing of women desiring and eligible for genetic testing includes a lengthy initial counseling, where the risks and benefits of genetic testing are fully discussed, with due attention being paid to all the implications of a positive or negative test result being discussed before testing, with offers of psychological support. Options for prophylactic and surveillance interventions should be discussed in detail before the test is undertaken, with additional discussions about insurance and employment issues. One of the premises of this model is that many potential psychological sequelae of predictive testing exist, particularly in relation to psychiatric morbidity. Additionally, any effect on uptake of surveillance and prophylactic measures required careful consideration (van Oostrom et al. 2003). These procedures were put in place partly because the detection of a germline *BRCA1* or *BRCA2* mutation in an affected woman can be of great psychological impact and was considered by some to be possibly equivalent to the shock of the original cancer diagnosis. In addition, detailed counseling would need to cover the possibility of identifying a germline mutation of uncertain significance, especially in population groups that have not been extensively sampled.

This traditional model is the most common context in which women receive genetic testing. More recently, however, population-based testing of unaffected women without detailed counseling has been carried out (Metcalfe et al. 2010). While long-term sequelae are not known, short-term data do not suggest harm (Metcalfe et al. 2012). Clearly, testing before a cancer diagnosis is optimal if the "risks of knowledge" and negative effects of surgical intervention (e.g., preventive oophorectomy) are outweighed by the decrease in cancer incidence. It will not be possible to know this without long-term follow-up. Nevertheless, if the initial treatment of women with breast cancer could be significantly and positively influenced by knowledge of mutation status at the time of diagnosis, then the benefit of rapid, low-cost, tailored genetic testing may be greater than the risks of harm resulting from a more limited pretest counseling. Early studies involving full counseling have suggested that affected women who learn they are carriers at time of diagnosis or soon afterwards tend to make different surgical decisions than those who find out later (Schwartz et al. 2004, 2005); thus, there is at least precedent for considering testing at time of diagnosis.

Screening and Prophylaxis

Screening for breast cancer is based upon the detection of early cancer and not of a premalignant lesion (Smith et al. 2000). Despite a meta-analysis that concluded that there is a reduction up to 18 % of the breast cancer mortality among 40–49 years old women following regular mammographic screening, the effectiveness of this tool for the surveillance of premenopausal women remains debatable. Indeed, after decades of research, the "mammography debate" continues with much vitriolic comment (Rogers 2003), and it seems unlikely that new data will help to resolve the issues easily (Goodman 2002).

The efficiency of screening should be higher if the women screened are at increased risk because of a family history of breast cancer, but as yearly mammography seems to be rather ineffective in *BRCA1/2* carriers (Brekelmans et al. 2001; Goffin et al. 2001; Tilanus-Linthorst et al. 2002), other screening modalities such as MRI have been found to be superior at detecting breast cancers.

Magnetic resonance imaging (MRI) is a non-ionizing imaging technique that has already been demonstrated to be sensitive for invasive breast cancer. Its sensitivity is less impaired than mammography by dense parenchyma. Preliminary results of a

German prospective nonrandomized pilot project (including 192 asymptomatic women proved or suspected to be *BRCA1/2* mutation carriers) demonstrated that the sensitivity and specificity of breast MRI was superior to conventional mammography and high-frequency breast ultrasound (Kuhl et al. 2000). Much larger studies in North America and Europe have confirmed that MRI is superior to mammography for the detection of breast cancers in *BRCA1/2* carriers (Kriege et al. 2004; Warner et al. 2004, 2011). It is not known if this will translate to a better long-term outcome but the data on medium-term survival are encouraging (Rijnsburger et al. 2010; Passaperuma et al. 2012). Interestingly, among those who develop an MRI-detected breast cancer, the survival for *BRCA1* mutation carriers may be inferior to *BRCA2* mutation carriers, and different screening regimens may be required for younger *BRCA* mutation carriers (Heijnsdijk et al. 2012).

For some women at very high risk of breast cancer (e.g., *BRCA1* or *BRCA2* mutation carriers, those with Cowden syndrome, Li–Fraumeni syndrome, or occasionally an undiagnosed dominant breast/ovarian cancer pedigree), preventive bilateral mastectomies may be the preferred option, but the women require careful counseling and a discussion of the residual risk of breast cancer following different types of surgical procedure (a subcutaneous mastectomy, leaving the nipple, may have a measurable residual risk, and a total mastectomy, with or without nipple-sparing, is probably the preferred option). Information is still accumulating about the efficacy of such prophylactic surgery, but so far, invasive breast cancers appear to be very rare after total mastectomy in *BRCA1/2* mutation carriers (Meijers-Heijboer et al. 2001; Rebbeck et al. 2004); by contrast, there are several reports of invasive breast cancer following subcutaneous mastectomy in *BRCA1* (Rebbeck et al. 2004) and *BRCA2* (Kasprzak et al. 2005) mutation carriers. Contralateral mastectomy should also be considered for women likely to be *BRCA1/2* mutation carriers who have had breast cancer because their risk of contralateral breast cancer is substantially increased to approximately 40 % at 10-year follow-up. Notably, the risk is reduced by tamoxifen and oophorectomy (Metcalfe et al. 2004). Testing at time of breast cancer diagnosis is likely to increase the frequency of initial contralateral mastectomy (Schwartz et al. 2004).

At present, many screening protocols for *BRCA1/2* carriers include ovarian cancer surveillance, but the true value, if any, of regular assessment with CA-125 and transvaginal ultrasound is unknown, and both case reports (e.g., Hebert-Blouin et al. 2002) and recent biological data (Berns and Bowtell 2012), combined with modeling (Brown and Palmer 2009), suggest that these cancers arise very quickly and are probably not amenable to any currently available form of screening.

The role of chemoprophylaxis is still unclear in women with a family history of breast cancer, but drugs such as tamoxifen may be considered for such at-risk women; the data are conflicting, but point towards a benefit even for women who are destined to develop an ER-negative breast cancer. Although tamoxifen was rarely prescribed for this purpose by US oncologists (Robson 2002), it has now been recommended that either tamoxifen or raloxifene should be offered for 5 years to postmenopausal women with a uterus and at high risk of breast cancer, unless they have a past history or may be at increased risk of thromboembolic disease or endometrial cancer, in the updated NICE guidelines, which also provide guidance on risk assessment and surveillance, at http://www.nice.org.uk/CG164.

Use of the oral contraceptive pill (OCP), even for relatively short periods, is protective against ovarian cancer in BRCA1/2 mutation carriers (Narod et al. 1998). The situation for breast cancer risk is less clear. There have been four major studies. A large case–control study showed that early use, use before 1975, and prolonged use (>5 years) was associated with significantly increased risks of breast cancer among *BRCA1*, but not *BRCA2* mutation carriers (Narod et al. 2002). By contrast, a population-based study found no evidence for increased risk and even some suggestion of a decreased risk for *BRCA1* carriers (Milne et al. 2005). A third study found no excess risk for women diagnosed with breast cancer under 50 for women using the OCP for one year; for *BRCA2*, there was a slightly increased risk for women who used the OCP for more than 5 years (Haile et al. 2006). The most recent, a retrospective cohort study of 1,593 *BRCA1/2* mutation carriers, found an increased risk of breast cancer for *BRCA1/2* mutation carriers who ever used oral contraceptives (adjusted hazard ratio [HR] = 1.47; 95 % CI, 1.16–1.87). HRs did not change when considering time since stopping use, age at start, or year of starting. Longer use was associated with an increased risk of breast cancer for both *BRCA1* and *BRCA2* mutation carriers, most notably among young women who used the OCP before their first full-term pregnancy (4 or more years of use before first full-term pregnancy was associated with a HR of 1.49 [95 % CI, 1.05–2.11] for *BRCA1* mutation carriers and HR = 2.58 [95 % CI, 1.21–5.49] for *BRCA2* mutation carriers) (Brohet et al. 2007). Thus, there is no consensus between the four studies. Perhaps, until larger prospective studies are completed, it might be prudent to avoid OCP use in young *BRCA1/2* mutation carriers (i.e., less than 25 years old) who have not had a full-term pregnancy. On the other hand, a decision to pursue genetic testing prior to considering OCP use in a young woman at known genetic risk who is not otherwise inclined to learn of her mutation status would need to be carefully considered.

Uterine Tumors

Tumors arising in the body of the uterus (for tumors of the uterine cervix, see later section) can arise from the endometrium or myometrium. The most common myometrial neoplasias are leiomyomas, while the most common endometrial tumors are endometrial carcinomas.

Uterine Leiomyoma

Leiomyomas are benign, smooth muscle tumors with some connective tissue elements. They are very common, occurring in about 20 % of women over the age of 35 years, and the incidence increases with advancing age. They occur more frequently in women of Afro-Caribbean origin. Uterine leiomyomas are probably more common in first-degree relatives of index cases than in the general population. Uterine leiomyomas are component neoplasias of at least two heritable neoplasia syndromes: hereditary leiomyoma–renal cell carcinoma syndrome (HLRCC), which is also known as multiple cutaneous uterine leiomyomatosis (MCUL), and

Cowden syndrome. HLRCC/MCUL is caused by germline heterozygous mutations in the gene encoding fumarate hydratase *(FH)* (Alam et al. 2001; Tomlinson et al. 2002). *FH* is a nuclear gene encoding a mitochondrial enzyme involved in electron transport and the Krebs cycle (Eng et al. 2003). While germline heterozygous *FH* mutations cause HLRCC, germline homozygous mutations cause severe neurodegeneration (Eng et al. 2003). Although searching for germline *FH* mutations in women with isolated leiomyomas is not justified, *FH* sequencing should be offered in rare cases where familial uterine leiomyomatosis is present, even in the absence of other features associated with *FH* mutations (Tolvanen et al. 2012). Although few somatic intragenic mutations in *FH* have been found in sporadic uterine leiomyomas, biallelic inactivation by both genetic and nongenetic mechanisms occur with some frequency in these sporadic tumors (Kiuru et al. 2002; Lehtonen et al. 2004).

Uterine leiomyomas are common in the general population which makes it difficult to establish that they are true components of Cowden syndrome, but have been associated in some studies (http://www.nccn.org/professionals/physician_gls/pdf/genetics_screening.pdf). Uterine leiomyomas were reported in a woman carrying heterozygous mutations in both *PTEN* and *SDHC* (Zbuk et al. 2007).

Carcinoma of the Uterus

This is the ninth most common malignancy in women with an incidence of 13 per 100,000 of population in the UK. In the USA, approximately 4 % of women will develop uterine cancer in a lifetime. The most common histological type is adenocarcinoma, and adenomatous hyperplasia (endometrial precancer, endometrial intraepithelial neoplasia) may be the premalignant lesion. Of all endometrial adenocarcinomas, the endometrioid histology is the most common. Squamous cell carcinomas, leiomyosarcomas, and mixed mesodermal tumors may occur, but are rare.

Epidemiological studies have shown a slight increase in RR for endometrial cancer in women with a family history of this cancer, leading to the conclusion that about 1 % of endometrial cancers may be explained by genetic factors. Endometrial adenocarcinoma is a component cancer of Lynch syndrome (previously known as hereditary non-polyposis colorectal cancer syndrome) and of Cowden syndrome (p. 256). In one large French study that attempted to control for ascertainment bias, the risk to age 70 for endometrial carcinoma among *MLH1* mutation carriers was 54 % (95 % CI 20–80 %), for *MSH2* it was 21 % (8–77 %), and 16 % (8–32 %) for *MSH6*. While the point estimates are of definite value, the confidence intervals are too broad to be useful in the clinic. In contrast, a recent review of 113 families with *MSH6* mutations gave a much higher estimate of a 44 % risk of endometrial cancer in mutation carriers to 80 years age (95 % CI = 30–58 %); and for any cancer associated with Lynch syndrome, and 47 % (95 % CI = 32–66 %) for men and 40 % (95 % CI = 32–52 %) and 65 % (95 % CI = 53–78 %) for women. Compared with incidence for the general population, female mutation carriers had a 26-fold increased incidence of endometrial cancer (HR = 25.5, 95 % CI = 16.8–38.7) and a sixfold increased incidence of other cancers associated with Lynch syndrome (HR = 6.0, 95 % CI = 3.4–10.7) (Baglietto et al 2010). This demonstrates some of the issues when comparing studies that focus on cancer-dense pedigrees, as often seen in the family cancer clinic, with those that are population based or that adjust for ascertainment bias in various ways.

In the French study, the risk of endometrial cancer by age 40 years for all three genes was two percent or lower, indicating that intensive early screening is probably not justified. In an international collaborative study, the 10-year cumulative risk of endometrial cancer for carriers of mismatch repair gene mutations (grouped together) who had not previously had cancer was approximately 10 % (95 % CI 3.5–26 %) (Win et al. 2012). In contrast, the same group reported that the 10-year cumulative risk of endometrial carcinoma was 23.4 % (95 % CI: 15–36 %) for women with mismatch repair gene mutations and a previous diagnosis of colorectal cancer. Roughly one-quarter of women diagnosed with a Lynch syndrome-associated colorectal cancer will develop endometrial cancer within 10 years of their diagnosis (Obermair et al. 2010). These findings should be taken into account when considering screening and preventive surgery options. Notably, there was no evidence that women with *MSH2* mutations were at higher risk of endometrial cancer than were female *MLH1* carriers, as previously suggested (Vasen et al. 2001). A retrospective study showed that prophylactic surgery is effective prevention for endometrial and ovarian cancer in MMR gene mutation carriers (Schmeler et al. 2006), but prospective studies have not been conducted. The risk of ovarian cancer was 3 % by age 50 in the French study (Bonadona et al. 2011) and was 3 % 10 years after identification of a MMR mutation in the Cancer Family Registry study (Win et al. 2012). Since the risk for *MLH1* and *MSH2* carriers in the French study increased rapidly after age 50 to reach 20–25 % by age 70, a strong case for peri- or postmenopausal hysterectomy with bilateral salpingo-oophorectomy can be made for MMR mutation gene carriers (NB fallopian tube cancer has been reported in Lynch syndrome patients) (Palma et al. 2008).

In terms of identifying Lynch syndrome in women with endometrial cancer, it has been pointed out that the difficulty in identifying MMR gene mutation carriers on clinical or morphological grounds justifies the use of immunohistochemistry for the four MMR proteins in all incident cases of endometrial cancers (Clarke and Cooper 2012). Nevertheless, it is clear that germline mutations would be found in a very small proportion of all such women tested.

Endometrioid endometrial carcinomas occur in women with Cowden syndrome, and a recent study estimated the lifetime risk for endometrial cancer to be 28 % (Tan et al. 2012), similar to the risk seen in *MSH2* mutation carriers. If confirmed, this would suggest preventive hysterectomy and enhanced surveillance might be indicated in *PTEN* mutation carriers. It is considered a major criterion for the clinical diagnosis of Cowden syndrome (p. 233) (http://www.nccn.org/professionals/physician_gls/pdf/genetics_screening.pdf).

Clinical surveillance for uterine malignancies in individuals at risk for endometrial cancers should be considered for all at-risk individuals. Indeed, the US-based National Comprehensive Cancer Network (NCCN) practice guidelines recommend annual uterine surveillance by blind repel biopsies of the endometrium from the age of 30 years for women with Lynch syndrome and from the age of 35–40 years for women with Cowden syndrome (www.nccn.org). After menopause, surveillance would change to annual endometrial (transabdominal or transvaginal) ultrasound with biopsy of suspicious lesions. These recommendations are similar to those put forward in 2006 by a group of European experts (Vasen et al. 2007), although since the value of surveillance is still unknown, the recommendation is that this should be offered to MMR mutation carriers from 35 to 40 years of age, preferably as part of a clinical trial (Vasen et al. 2013). Depending on their age, women who carry MMR gene mutations and have colorectal neoplasia should consider the option of concomitant prophylactic hysterectomy when they undergo bowel surgery for neoplasia.

Choriocarcinoma

Choriocarcinomas can follow pregnancy of any type. Hydatidiform mole, the precursor choriocarcinomas, is thought to result from the fusion of two male gametes (without the participation of an ovum). Invasive moles, choriocarcinomas, occur with a frequency of 1 in 15,000 pregnancies in the USA; there is marked geographical variation, with a 10-fold higher incidence in Southeast Asia and the Far East. Familial biparental hydatidiform mole (FBHM) is the only recessive condition that is only expressed in females. Heterogeneity occurs; one locus was mapped to 19q13, and the responsible gene at this locus, *NLRP7*, was identified as the first gene that predisposed to choriocarcinomas (Murdoch et al. 2006). The protein is involved in the intracellular regulation of bacterial-induced inflammation and is a negative regulation interleukins. A second gene, C6orf221 (*ECAT1*), was found to be mutated in three families with FBHM (Parry et al. 2011). The phenotypes of families with mutations in *ECAT1* and *NLRP7* appear to be indistinguishable.

Fallopian Tube Carcinoma

This cancer was considered to be extremely rare, and in women not carrying *BRCA1/2* mutations, this is still the case. Over the last decade, however, increasingly persuasive data have been produced to suggest that a significant proportion of high-grade serous carcinomas (HGSC), apparently arising in the ovary, actually have arisen from the fallopian tube (Colgan et al. 2001; Crum et al. 2007; Crum et al. 2012; Piek et al. 2001; Piek et al. 2008). The risk for fallopian tube cancer per se is clearly increased in *BRCA1/2* mutation carriers (Zweemer et al. 2000; Rutter et al. 2003), and up to 40 % of women with fallopian tube cancer carry *BRCA1/2* mutations (Vicus et al. 2010). It has even been suggested that perhaps distal salpingectomy in both average and higher-risk women might be a way to prevent HGSC (Tone et al. 2012). Fallopian tube carcinoma has also been reported in Lynch syndrome (Palma et al. 2008), but is very rare. In a recent next-generation sequencing study of 12 DNA repair-related cancer genes, of 31 patients with fallopian tube carcinoma, clearly deleterious mutations were seen in *BRCA1* in seven cases, in *BRCA2* in two cases, in *BARD1* in one case, and an unusual mosaic de novo missense mutation was seen in one case (Walsh et al. 2011). These findings suggest that exome sequencing, or panel-based screening for multiple genes, may soon replace the current labor-intensive and costly "gene-by-gene" approach (Table 6.3).

Ovarian Cancer

Ovarian tumors may develop from germ, epithelial, or granulosa/theca cells. Germ cell tumors include dermoid cysts, teratomas, and gonadoblastomas. Sex cord-stromal tumors may develop from the mesenchyme, may include granulosa cell tumors, and may be hormone secreting. Benign serous and mucinous fibromas and cystadenomas are also seen. Most ovarian tumors are serous and mucinous adeno-carcinomas. Carcinoma of the ovary is almost always derived from the epithelial cells and may originate more widely from coelomic epithelium (i.e., peritoneal carcinoma). Teratomas, embryonal carcinomas, sex cord–stromal tumors, choriocarcinoma, and dysgerminomas are much less common.

Ovarian Carcinoma

The incidence of ovarian carcinoma is about 15 per 100,000 females in the UK; the lifetime risk to age 70 years is about 1.5 % in the UK and North America, slightly less in Southern Europe, making it the fifth most common malignancy in females in Western Europe and North America. Ovarian cancer has a very high mortality and is the most frequent cause of death from gynecological malignancies in the Western world. Worldwide, one of the highest incidence for ovarian cancer is seen in Israeli Jewish women who were born in North America or Europe – these are highly likely to be Ashkenazi Jews (13.5 per 100,000, cumulative incidence, 1.55 % to 74 years of age). Interestingly, in Israeli non-Jews, these figures are 3.0 per 100,000 and 0.32, respectively. These observations fit with the finding that up to 30 % of unselected Ashkenazi Jewish women with ovarian cancer carry mutations (Moslehi et al. 2000). This is a much higher figure than that observed in other groups. Early data suggested that for *BRCA1* in unselected non-Ashkenazi women with ovarian cancer, between 4 and 9 % can be expected to carry a *BRCA1* mutation, and between 0 and 4 % will carry *BRCA2* mutations, although this figure will be higher in certain founder populations, such as Iceland. The most recent data, using more comprehensive mutation analysis, has suggested that in population unselected for ethnicity, about 15 % of women with ovarian cancer carry a mutation in *BRCA1* (10 %) or *BRCA2* (5 %). Notably, about 50 % of *BRCA2* carriers are diagnosed at over 60 years of age, whereas 90 % of *BRCA1* carriers are diagnosed below 60 years' age. Irrespective

Table 6.3 Genetic disorders associated with ovarian neoplasms

Syndrome	Gene	Proportion of hereditary predisposition to OC (%)	Risk of OC by age 70 (%)	Other clinical features
Hereditary breast–ovarian cancer	BRCA1	60	20–50	Breast, fallopian tube, peritoneal, pancreatic cancer
Hereditary breast–ovarian cancer	BRCA2	25	10–30	Breast, prostate, pancreatic cancer, melanoma
RAD51C-related susceptibility to ovarian cancer	RAD51C	<1	≤10	Fanconi anemia-like condition in biallelic mutation carriers
RAD51D-related susceptibility to ovarian cancer	RAD51D	<1	≤10	None reported yet
BRIP1-related susceptibility to ovarian cancer	BRIP1	<1	≤10	Breast, pancreatic, and rectal ca (moderate risk) Fanconi anemia in biallelic mutation carriers
HNPCC/Lynch syndrome	MLHH1, MSH2, MSH6, PMS2	10	≤10	Colon, endometrial, small bowel, urothelial, and pancreatic cancer
Peutz–Jeghers Syndrome	STK11	<1 (ovarian sex cord–stromal tumors)	<5	Mucocutaneous melanin spot, GI hamartomatous polyps, adenoma malignum of the uterine cervix, breast, GI, pancreatic cancer
Cowden disease	PTEN	<1	<3	Multiple hamartomas, mucocutaneous signs, breast, thyroid cancer
Nevoid basal cell carcinoma (Gorlin syndrome)	PTCH	<1	<2	Basal cell/nevi carcinoma, palmar/plantar pits, skeletal abnormalities, odontogenic keratocysts, medulloblastoma
DICER1-PPB multiple tumor syndrome	DICER1	<1 [ovarian sex cord–stromal (mainly) Sertoli–Leydig cell] tumor	<5	Pleuropulmonary blastoma, cystic nephroma, multinodular goiter, GI hamartomas, pituitary blastoma, other very rare manifestations
Multiple enchondromatosis (Ollier and Maffucci disease)	Somatic mosaic mutations in IDH1 and IDH2	<1	<2	Osteochondromatosis, hemangiomata
Epidermolytic palmoplantar keratoderma	KRT9	<1	<2	Epidermolytic hyperkeratosis

of family history, between 20 and 25 % of women diagnosed with ovarian cancer between the ages of 41 and 50 will carry a *BRCA1/2* mutation (Pal et al. 2005). These findings have important implications for referral guidelines to cancer genetics services. Among the Ashkenazim, these percentages are much higher, although some of the studies include selected cases. Overall, 25–30 % of all ovarian cancer in Ashkenazi Jewish women is attributable to one of the three founder mutations, with *BRCA1* mutation predominating at younger ages and *BRCA2* at older ages. Ovarian cancer is diagnosed at a significantly younger age in *BRCA1* carriers than in the general population. *BRCA2*-related ovarian cancers tend to be diagnosed at an older age than both the aforementioned groups.

Women with ovarian cancer (carcinoma) are more likely than expected to have a family history of ovarian neoplasia, and first-degree female relatives of patients with ovarian cancer are at increased risk. A collection of studies from around the world are summarized in Table 6.4; as can be seen, the odds ratios for ovarian cancer in association with a positive family history of ovarian cancer vary substantially, but are usually greater if the index case was diagnosed at a young age. The risk of death from ovarian cancer is very much greater if two first-degree relatives are affected. In this study, relatives of ovarian cancer cases also had significantly increased mortality from cancers of the stomach and rectum, but interestingly, the observed increased mortality from colon cancer, breast cancer, and pancreatic cancer failed to reach statistical significance.

Families in which there appears to be an autosomal, dominant susceptibility to ovarian cancer, with a high penetrance of the cancer in predisposed females have been recognized for years, and the identification of *BRCA1* and *BRCA2* has permitted more precise estimates of age-dependent cumulative incidence (i.e., penetrance). An analysis of 22 studies suggested that the risk of ovarian cancer among *BRCA1/2* carriers who were not selected on the basis of family history of breast or ovarian cancer is very low before age 40 (below 2 % for both genes), but rises substantially with age in the case of *BRCA1*, and is above 1 % per year from age 45 onwards, reaching 2.5 % per year by age 65. For *BRCA2*, the risks are lower, start to rise at later ages, and never reach 1 % per year (Antoniou et al. 2003).

The ovarian tumors arising in *BRCA1/2* carriers cases are carcinomas, with a predominance of serous papillary cystadenocarcinoma, and mucinous and borderline ovarian carcinoma are underrepresented.

The frequency of *BRCA* mutations in the general population is estimated to be about 1 in 800 for *BRCA1* and somewhat less for *BRCA2*, but it can vary significantly among some ethnic groups or geographic regions. Thus, the prevalence of the three *BRCA1/2* founder mutations among the Ashkenazim is approximately 1 in 50. The Icelandic population carries the founder *BRCA2* 999del5 mutation at a frequency of 0.4 %. The frequency of *BRCA1* and *BRCA2* mutations in unselected series of women with ovarian carcinoma has been extensively studied, particularly in the so-called founder populations. A founder effect can occur when a relatively small group is genetically isolated from the rest of the population, because of geographic conditions or religious belief. If an individual in that isolated population carries a rare genetic alteration, the frequency of this allele in the next generations could increase in the absence of selection. Specific *BRCA1* and *BRCA2* mutations have been identified in diverse populations, such as in Ashkenazi Jewish, Icelandic, Swedish, Norwegian, Austrian, Dutch, British, Belgian, Russian, Hungarian, French Canadian, and Polish families (summarized in Fackenthal and Olopade 2007). The knowledge of well-characterized founder mutations in individuals of particular ethnic origins can simplify genetic counseling and testing, as the mutation screening can be limited to specific panels of mutations.

The founder mutations (often referred to as *BRCA1* 185delAG and 5382insC in *BRCA1*, *BRCA2* 6174delT) have been identified in the Ashkenazi Jewish families of Eastern European ancestry. These mutations are carried by about 2.5 % of the Ashkenazi Jewish population. These founder mutations are particularly common in Ashkenazi Jewish women with ovarian cancer, even without a family history of breast/ovarian cancer (Table 6.4).

These results show that among women with ovarian cancer, *BRCA1* and *BRCA2* mutations are at least 3 times more likely to be found in Ashkenazi Jewish women than in non-Ashkenazi women. Interestingly, among otherwise unselected, very young-onset cases (under 30 years of age at diagnosis) *BRCA1/2* mutations have not been observed, even though from epidemiological studies, mutations in genes are likely to be playing an important role in susceptibility.

There is evidence for genotype–phenotype relationships for ovarian cancer in *BRCA1/2* mutation carriers. Mutations in the 3' portion of the *BRCA1* gene (exons 13–24) were initially associated with a higher frequency of breast cancer relative to ovarian cancer in a series of 32 European families. This observation has not been confirmed by most larger studies (Stoppa-Lyonnet et al. 1997; Ford et al. 1998), although one study provided nonsignificant evidence in favor of the original finding (Moslehi et al. 2000). In a series of 25 English breast/ovarian cancer families, ovarian cancer was more prevalent than breast cancer when *BRCA2* truncating mutations were located in a region of approximately 3.3 kb in exon 11 (the ovarian cancer cluster region (OCCR), nucleotides 3035–6629). Additional data from 45 *BRCA2* families ascertained outside the UK provided support for this clustering. The analysis of 164 families with *BRCA2* mutations, 67 of whom had mutations in the OCCR, has been reported (Thompson and Easton 2001). The odds ratio for ovarian versus breast cancer in families with mutations in the OCCR, relative to non-OCCR mutations was 3.9 ($P < 0.0001$), confirming the importance of the OCCR in terms of ovarian cancer risk, but the effect was lost when Ashkenazi Jewish cases were omitted (6174delT is an exon 11 mutation). Case reports of multiple-case ovarian cancer families with mutations outside the OCCR temper enthusiasm for the clinical utility of these observations (Al Saffar and Foulkes 2002).

The existence of a premalignant lesion for ovarian carcinoma is uncertain (Scully 2000). Careful histopathological analysis of prophylactic oophorectomy specimens among high-risk women, either because they have been identified as *BRCA1/2* mutation carriers or based on their family history, gave conflicting results regarding the presence of histological alterations that could evolve towards invasive carcinoma. A tiny carcinoma in situ was identified in an otherwise normal prophylactic oophorectomy specimen from a woman with a *BRCA1* mutation (Werness et al. 2000), but

Table 6.4 Risk of ovarian cancer in women with a family history of OC: studies prior to *BRCA1/2* identification

Relatives studied	Country	Age group (years)	Cases	Controls	Odds ratio (95 % CI)	References
Any	USA	All	150	300	"No positive association"	Wynder et al. (1969)
First + second degree	USA	<50	150	150	15.7 (0.9–278)	Casagrande et al. (1979)
First degree	USA	45–74	62	1,068	18.2 (4.8–69)	Hildreth et al. (1981)
First degree	USA	18–80	215	215	11.3 (0.6–211)	Cramer et al. (1983)
First degree	Greece	All	146	243	∞ (3.4–∞)	Tzonou et al. (1984)
First degree	Japan	N/A	110	220	∞ (0.1–∞)	Mori et al. (1988)
First degree	USA	20–54	493	2,465	3.6 (1.8–7.1)	Schildkraut and Thompson (1988)
Second degree					2.9 (1.6–5.3)	
First degree	USA	20–79	296	343	3.3 (1.1–9.4)	Hartge et al. (1989)
First degree + aunts	Canada	All	197	210	2.5 (0.7–11.1)	Koch et al. (1989)
First degree	Italy	25–74	755	2,023	1.9 (1.1–3.6)	Parazzini et al. (1992)
First degree	USA	N/A	883	Population	2.1 (1.0–3.4)	Goldgar et al. (1994)
First degree	USA	<65	441	2,065	8.2 (3.0–23)	Rosenberg et al. (1994)
First degree	USA	All	662	2,647	4.3 (2.4–7.9)	Kerber and Slattery et al. (1995)

carcinoma in situ is very rarely seen in ovarian tissue, and this finding has not been replicated. Perhaps the tumor arose from ectopic fallopian tube epithelium that had been implanted in the ovary. More recently, attention has become focused on the hypothesis that the origin for clinically diagnosed BRCA1/2-related ovarian carcinoma is the distal fallopian tube (see section on fallopian tube carcinoma, page 104).

The incidence of primary serous carcinoma of the peritoneum among *BRCA1/2* carriers after oophorectomy is thought to be 0.2 % per year (Finch et al. 2006). The protective effect of oophorectomy against high-grade serous cancer in this study was approximately 80 %, which was in agreement with a population-based study from Israel (Rutter et al. 2003). These two studies suggested substantially less protection than was seen in selected series (Rebbeck et al. 2002), implying that among women who have undergone prophylactic surgery, this cancer may become one of the major threats to health among *BRCA1/2* mutation carriers in their later years. Peritoneal cancer is indistinguishable histologically or macroscopically from ovarian cancer occurring among *BRCA1/2* mutation carriers and represents a major challenge in terms of prevention of cancer in mutation carriers. The potential increased risk of malignant transformation of the entire peritoneal surface is thought to reflect the common origin of the ovarian epithelium and peritoneum from embryonic meso-derm. However, the peritoneum on the surface of the ovary may be particularly vulnerable to malignant transformation as a result of repeated injury following ovu-lation and/or high levels of local estrogen exposure – or perhaps this leads to implan-tation of fimbrial epithelium that when internalized within the ovary, can undergo malignant change. Some peritoneal carcinomas may arise multifocally, particularly in the context of *BRCA1* mutations, and there may be a unique molecular pathogen-esis of *BRCA1*-related papillary serous carcinoma of the peritoneum (Schorge et al. 2000). It seems implausible that these cancers arise from the fallopian tube.

The natural history of ovarian cancer in *BRCA* mutation carriers is thought to be different from sporadic ovarian cancer. Forty-three serous ovarian adenocarcinomas (81 % of the total) had an actuarial median survival of 77 months, compared with 29 months for the age, stage, and histological type-matched control group who were believed not to have mutations in *BRCA1* on the basis of family history ($P<0.001$). This good prognosis was attributed partly to the relative youth of the patients (mean age 48 years) but was also thought to be directly related to the presence of a *BRCA1* mutation. This study was criticized on methodological grounds, but a second study using a historical cohort approach gave similar results (Boyd et al. 2000). Furthermore, the better survival in hereditary cases was particularly noted for those women receiving platinum-containing chemotherapy. Other more recent studies have supported the notion that the prognosis is better for *BRCA1/2*-related ovarian cancer, but the durability of this survival advantage (most evident at 5 years follow-ing diagnosis) remains in question.

Mutations in other genes can cause ovarian cancer (Table 6.3). Lynch syndrome is one of the most common autosomal conditions predisposing to cancer, account-ing for 3–4 % of all colorectal cancers (Moreira et al. 2012). Mutations in *MLH1* and *MSH2* are rare in ovarian cancers not selected on the basis of family history of cancer. The risk of developing ovarian cancer in MMR mutation carriers is about 8 %, with the highest risks in *MLH1* and *MSH2* mutation carriers and the lowest risk in *MSH6* mutation carriers (Walsh et al. 2011). Most symptomatic ovarian cancers (77–81 %) in Lynch syndrome are diagnosed at an early stage (FIGO stage I and II) and may have a relatively good prognosis (reviewed in Vasen et al. 2013). There may be an increased risk for ovarian cancer in Carney Complex (Stratakis et al. 2000), but the numbers are too small for accurate risk assessment.

A growing list of cancer predisposition alleles in the genes associated with the Fanconi anemia genetic pathway (Fanconi anemia-like) genes – *BRIP1* (Rafnar et al. 2011), *RAD51C* (Meindl et al. 2010), and *RAD51D* (Loveday et al. 2011) – have been shown to predispose to ovarian cancer. In addition, rare mutations in a number of genes involved in homologous repair, including *BARD1*, *CHEK1*, *MRE11A*, *NBN*, and *RAD50* have also been found in patients with ovarian cancer (Walsh et al. 2011).

Identifying patients with these mutations may have clinical importance because tumors with defects in the Fanconi anemia and homologous repair pathways are sensitive to platinum agents and PARP inhibition. The therapeutic effectiveness of PARP inhibitors for treating ovarian cancer in women with germline *BRCA* mutations has been acclaimed, but more recent trials have failed to confirm an overall survival benefit with such treatment (Ledermann et al. 2012), possibly because of the development of resistance (Barber et al. 2013).

Prevention of hereditary ovarian cancer is a major topic and is beyond the scope of this book; suffice to say that medically, the oral contraceptive pill is likely to offer significant (40 % of more) risk reduction (Narod et al. 1998; Whittemore et al. 2004a). Surgically, ovarian removal (Rutter et al. 2003) is an option. Prophylactic salpingo-oophorectomy is often offered to women with germline *BRCA1* or *BRCA2* mutations, as the evidence is that it very much reduces the risk of ovarian cancer and also reduces the risk of breast cancer to 50 % in premenopausal women (Rutter et al. 2003; Domchek et al. 2010). It may also be offered to women with Lynch syndrome (Schmeler et al. 2006). While surgery clearly is effective in preventing serous papillary cancers arising from the ovary, the peritoneum remains at risk (as above).

The early detection of carcinoma at a stage in which it might be surgically curable, or more amenable to chemotherapeutic agents, would have a significant impact on prognosis. The traditional screening methods for ovarian carcinoma are the measurement of the serum tumor marker, CA-125, transvaginal ultrasonography, and clinical examination. None of these methods alone achieve the required level of sensitivity; for example, CA-125 detects only about two-thirds of Stage 1 ovarian tumors. In the general population, clinical examination, transabdominal, transvaginal (van Nagell et al. 2000) ultrasound, and serum CA-125 screening tests either alone or in combination have all been assessed as potential screening tests in various settings. However, no test or combination of tests has yet proved to be effective for population screening. In a longer-term follow-up of their previous study, Jacobs and colleagues showed that although the median survival in the screened group was significantly better than for the control group, the number of deaths from an index cancer did not differ significantly between the two groups, with 18 deaths in 10 977 controls versus 9 in 10 958 screened women, RR 2.0 (95 % CI 0.78–5.13) (Jacobs et al. 1999). Long-term follow-up of this study is awaited.

For women at high risk of ovarian carcinoma, it has been recommended that they have an annual pelvic examination, vaginal ultrasonography, and serum CA-125 measurement every 6- or 12-month intervals from their mid-20s or 5 years less than the earliest age of onset of ovarian cancer in the family. However, data showing clear benefit of such screening remains unconvincing. In the absence of good supportive evidence, it is appropriate to restrict these tests to a research setting. A worrying feature of hereditary ovarian cancer is the possibility that high-grade cancers can arise in very small foci that would not be detectable by ultrasound. A case report of a case of ultimately fatal advanced ovarian cancer diagnosed in a woman referred for a prophylactic oophorectomy was an early suggestion that delaying surgery could be dangerous (Rose and Hunter 1994). Studies among proven *BRCA1/2* carriers have supported this finding. Three of 33 women with *BRCA1/2* mutations were found to have early ovarian cancers lesions on examination of prophylactic oophorectomy specimens. Notably, two of the three cases were bilateral at diagnosis, and both were only noted on histopathological review and not in the operating room (Lu et al. 2000). Similarly, high-risk lesions or frank cancers can be found in the fallopian tubes of *BRCA1/2* carriers at preventive oophorectomy (Leeper et al. 2002; Carcangiu et al. 2004; McEwen et al. 2004). In the latter study, 5 of 60 consecutive *BRCA1/2*-positive women undergoing preventive oophorectomy were found to have occult ovarian or fallopian cancer: one death had occurred at 4 years follow-up. In a similar study from the USA, 5 of 30 *BRCA1/2* carriers had cancer at surgery: one was a primary peritoneal cancer, three had tubal cancer, and one had ovarian adenofibroma with adjacent areas of low malignant potential carcinoma (Leeper et al. 2002). Taken together, these studies suggest that screening for ovarian cancer by ultrasound and CA-125 will prove to be insufficiently sensitive for routine use in *BRCA1/2* carriers, but definitive studies are awaited, and until such times as definitive benefit of screening has been demonstrated, it is appropriate to advocate consideration of prophylactic oophorectomy after childbearing age in high-risk women.

Other Ovarian Neoplasms

Non-epithelial ovarian tumors are found with increased frequency in Peutz–Jeghers syndrome (sex cord-stromal and granulosa cell tumors which are often hormone secreting) and Gorlin syndrome (ovarian fibroma), and Ollier disease and Maffucci syndrome have both been associated with ovarian granulosa cell tumors with precocious pseudopuberty. A family has been described in which ovarian germ cell tumors were found in two daughters of a woman who herself had had an ovarian tumor in childhood, and her third child had a soft tissue sarcoma, but the paucity of such case reports of familial female germ cell tumors suggests that most sporadic forms of ovarian germ cell tumors are not attributable to inherited mutations in cancer susceptibility genes (Giambartolomei et al. 2009). Teratomas are thought to be pathogenic, arising from a single female germ cell after the first meiotic division.

There is a single-case report of a mixed ovarian germ cell tumor occurring in a *BRCA2* carrier – interestingly, no LOH was seen and thus it is possible that this was an unrelated, chance finding (Hamel et al. 2007). Ovarian fibromas have been reported in a family in which the condition could have been inherited as an autosomal sex-limited dominant trait. Ovarian sex cord–stromal tumors can occur in *STK11* mutation carrier (usually with annular tubules) and more recently have been associated with germline *DICER1* mutations, particularly in the form of Sertoli–Leydig cell tumors (SLCT), when there may be associated androgenization (Rio Frio et al. 2011; Slade et al. 2011). In this context, SLCTs can be associated with goiter (Rio Frio et al. 2011) or other features of the DICER1-PPB syndrome (Schultz et al. 2011). SLCTs have also occasionally reported in STK11 mutation carriers (Hales et al. 1994; Howell et al. 2010).

Gonadoblastoma is a dysgenetic gonadoma that does not metastasize but which may be associated with dysgerminoma and other malignant germ cell elements. The overwhelming majority (96 %) of gonadoblastomas develop in dysgenetic gonads of 46XY individuals. Most patients with this tumor are phenotypic females, the rest are phenotypic males with abnormalities of the genitalia and undescended testes (Giambartolomei et al. 2009).

Cancer of the Cervix

Carcinoma of the uterine cervix affects about 1 % of women, with an incidence of 8 and 12.5 per 100,000 population in Canada and the UK, respectively, but much higher incidence rates in some countries such as 67 per 100,000 in Zimbabwe and 34 per 100,000 in Columbia. It is strongly linked to human papillomavirus (HPV), indeed infection with this virus is almost always a requirement for squamous cell carcinoma of the cervix. The E6 and E7 viral proteins are consistently retained and expressed in these tumors and can be demonstrated to bind to the p53 and Rb protein products, respectively. The viral proteins may thus interfere with the normal tumor suppressor function of the cellular proteins. Host factors may also have a role in the pathogenesis of cervical carcinoma as women with HLA-DQw3 appear to be at increased risk of developing this tumor. Other HLA haplotypes have also been associated with increased risk (Apple et al. 1995).

There is a documented increased incidence of cervical cancer in women who were exposed to diethylstilboestrol in utero. Although cervical cancer may occur as a complication of the genetic skin conditions ectodermal dysplasia and dyskeratosis congenita, a genetic predisposition to this cancer is rare.

Family history studies of women with cervical cancer have not shown a striking excess of cervical cancer in female relatives, although some familial aggregation has been observed (Ahlbom et al. 1997; Magnusson et al. 2000; Horn et al. 2002), as might be expected, especially if the HLA data are taken into consideration. A substantial fraction of the familial factors appear to be nongenetic, but this may depend on the relationship studied: in the Magnusson study, shared environments explained concordance between sisters, but not between concordant mothers and daughters. Similarly, cigarette smoking-associated cancers (lung, larynx, lip, and cervix) were inter-associated in one systematic study (Goldgar et al. 1994). Nevertheless, the Breast Cancer Linkage Consortium did identify an excess of cervical cancer in *BRCA1* mutation carriers (RR = 3.72, 95 % CI < 2.26–6.10, $P < 0.001$) (Thompson and Easton 2002), but there have been no follow-up studies.

Screening for cervical cancer is offered as part of the population-screening program in the UK, and no particular addition to this has been suggested for women families with hereditary cancer syndromes, except Peutz–Jeghers syndrome, where adenoma malignum of the cervix can sometimes arise in females with Peutz–Jeghers syndrome who have developed sex cord ovarian tumors with annular tubules, resulting in hyperestrogenization (Beggs et al. 2010). It is etiologically distinct from squamous cell carcinoma. Primary melanoma of the cervix is very rare and does not seem to be related to mutations in *CDKN2A* or *BRCA2*.

Embryonal tumors of the cervix include embryonal rhabdomyosarcoma (cERMS) (McClean et al. 2007) and primitive neuroectodermal tumors (Snijders-Keilholz et al. 2005); the latter have now been re-classified as Ewing tumors (Fletcher et al. 2002). Both types of cervical tumors are associated with germline *DICER1* mutations (Foulkes et al. 2011), and in the case of cERMS, somatic "second hits" in the RNase IIIb domain of *DICER1* have been identified (Heravi-Moussavi et al. 2012).

Other Tumors of the Female Reproductive System

Cancer of the female genital organs other than of the uterus, cervix, and ovary has an incidence of about 3.6 per 100,000.

Cancer of the External Genitalia

Cancer of the external genitalia is rare. Squamous cell carcinoma of the cervix and external genitalia may complicate dyskeratosis and congenital ectodermal dysplasia. Vulval carcinoma may complicate vulval lichen sclerosis (which can occur rarely as a familial condition, Vanin et al. 2002). Vulval neoplasia is generally "non-genetic" and is associated with HPV infection and smoking (Daling et al. 2002; Engelman et al. 2003). There is a possibility that genetic polymorphisms in genes altering susceptibility to cancer in smokers may also alter susceptibility to vulval and anal cancer. It can arise in Paget disease of the vulva and in Bowen disease of the vulva. Paget disease of the vulva is a rare intraepithelial cancer of the apocrine glands and is occasionally associated with an underlying adenocarcinoma (Tinari et al. 2002). Chromosomal 11p abnormalities have been described in the latter. Abnormalities of the *PRAD1* gene and *TP53* have been described in vulval carcinomas. Vulvar carcinoma occurs with increased frequency in Fanconi anemia (FA) and Morris syndrome. It appears that this increased prevalence in FA patients may be related to an increased susceptibility to HPV, and in FA patients an increased proportion of patients with FA and squamous cell carcinoma of the vulva are homozygous for Arg72, a p53 polymorphism that is thought to be associated with increased susceptibility to HPV infection (Kutler et al. 2003).

Primary malignant melanoma of the vulva is the second most common vulvar malignancy, an aggressive cancer, usually occurring on non-hairy skin, thus non-ultraviolet (UV) light associated (Ragnarsson-Olding 2004). A family history of cutaneous melanoma is found in 15 % of cases, and a germline mutation in the melanocortin type 1 receptor has been described in one case (Wechter et al. 2004).

Vaginal Carcinoma

An increased occurrence of this squamous cell cancer is associated with maternal ingestion of diethylstilboestrol during pregnancy. Invasive epithelial and in situ vaginal cancers have many of the same risk factors as cervical cancer, including a strong relationship to HPV infection (Daling et al. 2002). A vaginal intraepithelial neoplasia has been reported in a carrier of a deleterious *PALB2* mutation (K.A. Schrader, personal communication).

Rare types of cancer of the vagina that have been reported are Brenner tumors and leiomyomas. The latter has been reported to occur as part of a dominantly inherited syndrome of multiple adult-onset schwannomas, multiple nevi, and multiple vaginal leiomyomas. The nevi appear to be congenital in this condition. Giant hypertrophy of the labia minora and with neoplastic fibroblast and epithelial proliferation has been described in Ramon syndrome of arthritis, deafness, and pigmentary changes in the retina.

Primary vulval and vaginal extraosseous Ewing sarcoma and peripheral neuroectodermal tumor has been described (Vang et al. 2000).

Prostate Cancer

Prostate cancer is the most common cancer and the second most common cause of cancer death in North American men. Population prostate cancer risk is approximately 0.5 % by the age of 65 years and 2 % by the age of 75 years. The etiology of prostate cancer is unknown, but androgen stimulation is implicated by observations of a low incidence in males castrated before the age of 40 years, and a high-fat diet has also been implicated. Evidence for a genetic contribution was provided by genetic epidemiological studies in Mormon families that suggested that the heritability of prostate cancer was greater than that of breast or colorectal cancer. A case–control study by Steinberg et al. (1990) found 15 % of prostate cancer patients had an affected father or brother, compared to 8 % of controls (Table 6.5).

Furthermore, the RR increased: (1) with the number of affected relatives such that men with one, two, and three affected first-degree relatives were at twofold, fivefold, and 11-fold increased risk for developing prostate cancer, respectively, and (2) the younger the age at onset of prostate cancer in the proband. Meikle and Smith (1990) reported. A 17-fold increase in RR of prostate cancer has been reported in brothers of men developing prostate cancer between 45 and 50 years of age. Segregation analysis of the family histories of 740 prostate cancer patients suggested that familial clustering of the disease could be caused by a rare, highly penetrant, dominantly inherited predisposition gene. Under the most likely genetic model, 43 % of early-onset prostate cancer (in men <55 years) would occur in gene carriers, but only 9 % of cases in men aged <85 years. This proposed model of a rare dominant predisposing gene (or genes) was similar to that suggested for breast cancer. Johns and Houlston (2003) undertook a meta-analysis of 13 studies of prostate cancer risk in first-degree relatives. They found that the pooled RR in first-degree relatives was 2.5 and 3.5 in men with one or two affected relatives. Risks were also increased if the affected relative had early-onset disease (§60 years). Nieder et al. (2003) provided cumulative risks by age according to family history details and ethnicity (i.e., Table 6.5). The clinical course of familial and sporadic prostate cancer appears to be similar, although the disease may be more aggressive in African-Americans.

Multiple prostate cancer susceptibility loci have been mapped by family linkage studies (e.g., *CAPB*, *HPC1*, *HPC2*, *HPX*, *MSR1*, *PCAP*, *HPC20*, *RNASEL*), but none of these equate with major high-penetrance susceptibility genes present in many populations (as for *BRCA1* and *BRCA2* in familial breast cancer). Although mutations in three candidate prostate cancer susceptibility genes have been reported,

Table 6.5 Cumulative risks of prostate cancer according to ethnicity, age, and family history

Group	Cumulative risk of prostate cancer by age		
	50 years	60 years	70 years
White men			
No family history in (%)	0.2	2	7.5
One FDR in (%)	0.4	5.2	19
Two or more FDR in (%)	0.8	10	38
Black men			
No family history in (%)	0.4	3.6	10.6
One FDR in (%)	1.1	9.2	27.1
Two or more FDR in (%)	2.1	18	34

Adapted from Nieder et al. (2003)

FDR first-degree relative

RNASEL (*HPC1*, 1q24–q25), *MSR1* (8p22–p23), and *ELAC2* (*HPC2*, 17p11), in most cases these genes do not appear to represent rare highly penetrant loci and familial risks of prostate cancer may be explained better by a model of multiple interacting low-risk genetic variants. On the other hand, germline *BRCA2* mutations do account for a small but significant group (2–5 %) of familial prostate cancer clusters or early-onset cases (Edwards et al. 2002), and the relative risk of prostate cancer in carriers is increased significantly, higher at younger ages, in mutation carriers (RR 4.71) (Kirchhoff et al. 2004). The risk of prostate cancer is also increased in males with Lynch syndrome, highest in *MSH2* mutation carriers. Kaplan–Meier analysis suggested that cumulative risk by 70 years in MMR mutation carriers may be as high as 30 % (SE, 0.088) as compared to 8.0 % in the general population (Grindedal et al. 2009, see p. 262; Barrow et al. 2013).

The prognosis of prostate cancer in men with germline mutations in *BRCA2* appears to be worse than in the general population. Men who carry *BRCA2* mutations are more likely to develop early-onset prostate cancer (Grönberg et al. 2001; Willems et al. 2008; Tryggvadóttir et al. 2007; Mitra et al. 2008) and have a shorter survival time compared to *BRCA1* mutation carriers and to men in the general population (Narod et al. 2008; Edwards et al. 2010). In the latter study, the median survival in men with germline *BRCA2* mutation was 4.8 years, compared 8.5 years in controls (*P* = 0.002). Loss of heterozygosity was found in the majority of tumors of *BRCA2* mutation carriers and multivariate analysis confirmed that the poorer survival of prostate cancer in *BRCA2* mutation carriers is associated with the germline *BRCA2* mutation per se. Others have also suggested that the decreased survival in these men may be explained by the finding of an aggressive phenotype (Gleason score ≥8 and high T stage, ≥pT3) in the majority of tumors in the *BRCA2* carriers who die from prostate cancer (Thorne et al. 2011a, b). A strikingly worse outcome for prostate cancer has been reported in carriers of founder *BRCA2* mutations in Icelandic population (Sigurdsson et al. 1997; Tryggvadóttir et al. 2007). In addition, the Ashkenazi Jewish *BRCA2* founder mutation, c.5946delT (p. Ser1982fs), confers a 3-fold risk for prostate cancer, and carriers are more likely to develop high-grade prostate cancer than noncarrier (Gallagher et al. 2010).

Grönberg et al. (2001) reported a large family with a truncating *BRCA2* mutation which was responsible for hereditary prostate cancer in the father and four of his sons who developed early-onset disease. This mutation was also detected in three daughters diagnosed with breast cancer. All of the affected men with prostate cancer died of metastatic disease. Thus, more aggressive screening and treatment for prostate cancer may be justified, and an international study to this effect, known as IMPACT, is underway.

Fine-mapping by massively parallel sequencing of a previously identified susceptibility loci at 17q21–22 (Zuhlke et al. 2004) revealed a single mutation, *HOXB13* G84E, that co-segregated with the disease in four unrelated families and confirmed to be a risk allele in a large case–control population (Ewing et al. 2012). Independent analysis in an international sample of prostate cancer families validated G84E to be a disease-predisposing mutation, present among 5 % of prostate cancer families with an estimated odds ratio of 4.42 (Xu et al. 2013). Although in most Western populations the allele frequency is less than 1 per 1,000 men, the G84E variant has a much higher prevalence in Nordic populations and is found on a common haplotype block, suggesting presence of a founder effect originating in Finland; the missense variant appears to be very rare or absent among African-Americans and Asians (Gudmundsson et al. 2012). While it is unknown how the G84E variant predisposes to prostate cancer, the recurrent nature of the mutation and the lack of inactivating mutations suggest a gain-of-function mutation. Functional studies of the G84E variant are needed to clarify its role in cancer predisposition.

Men at increased risk of prostate cancer can be offered screening by annual measurement of prostate-specific antigen (PSA) and digital rectal examination from age 40 years. Male *BRCA1/BRCA2* mutation carriers are eligible for screening by annual PSA between 40 and 69 years with prostate biopsy if PSA > 3 mg/ml, under a research trial, IMPACT (Mitra et al. 2011).

Genome-wide association studies have discovered at least 50 separate loci that are associated with an increased risk for prostate cancer. All odds ratios are individually less than 1.5, but it is possible that combinations of alleles, and combining alleles with other established risk factors such as body mass index and family history could be of value n refining prostate cancer risk estimates. They could also be useful in modifying the risk of those carrying more highly penetrant alleles, such as *HOXB13* and *BRCA2* mutations.

Testicular Neoplasms

Testicular cancer accounts for only 1 % of all malignancy in males (with an incidence of 4 per 100,000 males), but is the most frequent carcinoma in the 15–35-year age group. Most tumors are of germ cell origin (seminoma, teratoma) but some arise from stromal cells (Sertoli cell), and gonadoblastoma contain germ cell and stromal elements.

Familial aggregation of testicular germ cell tumors accounts for up to 2 % of all adult cases. In a literature review, 24 father–son pairs, 45 pairs of non-twin brothers and 12 pairs of identical twins with testicular cancer were cited. Tumors are of the same histological type in 70 % of identical twin pairs, but were mostly of different histology in other degrees of relationship. Testicular tumors are bilateral in about 4 % of patients, which is suggestive of a genetic basis. In a Dutch single center study, RR of testicular cancer was increased 9- to 13-fold in brothers (Sonneveld et al. 1999). In an analysis of the Swedish Family-Cancer Database, familial risks were increased to 3.8-fold for fathers, 8.3-fold for brothers, and 3.9-fold for sons, and although seminomas showed a later age at onset than teratomas (30 versus 40 years), the familial risks were similar for the two tumor types (Dong et al. 2001). Forman et al. (1992) found that brothers of men with testicular cancer had a 2 % risk of developing testicular cancer by the age of 50 years, which corresponds to a 10-fold increase in RR. The mean age at diagnosis in familial cases was slightly younger than in sporadic cases (29.5 years versus 32.5 years).

Large families with a high incidence of testicular cancer have been described but are rare: Lynch and Walzak (1980) studied a large inbred Dutch kindred in which four individuals had histologically proven testicular cancers, and Goss and Bulbul (1990) reported a large cancer-prone family (including early-onset breast cancer) in which five males had testicular cancer. Nicholson and Harland (1995) and Heimdal et al. (1997) have suggested that familial clustering of testicular cancer might be attributable to a recessive gene. However, familial testicular cancer appears to be genetically heterogeneous, and an X-linked locus has been mapped (see below).

The principal risk factor for testicular cancer is cryptorchidism, which is associated with at least a 10-fold increase in risk, and orchidopexy should be performed in early childhood for boys with cryptorchidism if this risk is to be diminished. Genetic factors have been implicated in cryptorchidism because up to 14 % of cryptorchid males have an affected relative, but it is unclear to what extent this might explain the familial occurrence of testicular tumors. Patients with X-linked ichthyosis (steroid-sulfatase deficiency) appear to be at increased risk of cryptorchidism and testicular tumors. Testicular microcalcification is also a risk factor (Coffey et al. 2007).

Klinefelter syndrome has rarely been reported to predispose to testicular tumors, but in some cases this may be related to cryptorchidism. In one case, however, bilateral testicular teratoma occurred in a sib pair with Klinefelter syndrome. The risk of testicular cancer (seminoma, Sertoli cell, teratocarcinoma, and embryonal cell carcinoma) is unequivocally increased in patients with the testicular feminization syndrome, and prophylactic gonadectomy is usually performed after pubertal growth. Gonadoblastoma occurs in XY gonadal dysgenesis (see below), and also in patients with the WAGR syndrome (Wilms tumor–aniridia–genital abnormality–mental retardation, see p. 138). A subclass of Sertoli cell tumors (large cell calcifying) can be familial and can be associated with cardiac myxoma, endocrine activity, and pigmented skin lesions in Carney complex. Similar testicular lesions (intratubular large cell hyalinizing Sertoli cell tumors) are also seen in Peutz–Jeghers syndrome (http://www.uscap.org/site~/96th/SPECSURGH3v.htm) where they often present with gynecomastia (Ulbright et al. 2007).

Chromosomal analysis of germ cell testicular tumors has implicated isochromosome of 12p as a specific finding. Although various associations between HLA haplotypes and testicular cancer have been proposed, HLA class I analysis of affected sib pairs provided no evidence of a HLA-linked testicular cancer susceptibility gene. However, Rapley et al. (2000) mapped a locus for testicular germ cell tumors (TGCT1) to Xq27 using families compatible with X inheritance. Cases linked to Xq27 were more likely to have undescended testis and bilateral disease. There was clear evidence of locus heterogeneity and autosomal susceptibility loci are likely.

More recent data suggests that no one single locus can account for a significant fraction of familial testicular tumors (Crockford et al. 2006). Interestingly, a Y-chromosome locus involved in infertility known as the "gr/gr" deletion is a rare, low-penetrance susceptibility allele for testicle tumors (particularly seminomas) with a population frequency of n0.013 and an odds ratio of 3.0 for seminoma ($P = 0.0004$). Genome-wide association studies have identified low-penetrance variants in six loci, implicating *KITLG*, *SPRY4*, and *BAK1* (all involved in the KIT/KITL pathway), *TERT* and *ATF7IP* (both involved in telomerase regulation), and *DMRT1* (involved in sex determination) in tumorigenesis (Kanetsky et al. 2009; Rapley et al. 2009; Turnbull et al. 2010). The six loci, together with the "gr/gr" deletion account for less than 15 % of the familial risk of TGCT, which implies that potentially many more risk alleles remain to be identified. The clinical utility of testing for these alleles is therefore currently limited.

The occurrence of testicular tumors in high-risk individuals can be prevented by appropriate measures. Cryptorchidism should be corrected early to avoid an increased risk of testicular tumors. Nonfunctioning testes that present a significant risk for tumorigenesis (as in the testicular feminization syndrome or intersex states) should be removed. Individuals thought to be at high risk of familial testicular tumors can be monitored by regular self-examination and ultrasonography.

Testicular Tumors in Intersex States

Gonadoblastoma is a dysgenetic gonadoma that does not metastasize but which may be associated with dysgerminoma and other malignant germ cell elements. An overwhelming majority (96 %) of gonadoblastomas develop in dysgenetic gonads of 46XY individuals. Most patients with this tumor are phenotypic females, the rest are phenotypic males with abnormalities of the genitalia and undescended testes. The tumor is frequently bilateral, usually develops in the second decade, and may secrete estrogens or testosterone.

Germ cell tumors are rarely seen in individuals with gonadal dysgenesis who do not have any Y-chromosomal material present. Thus, girls with Turner syndrome with the chromosomal constitution 45,X;45,X/46,XX;46,X,del(Xp) or 46,X,del(Xq) are not at an increased risk of this tumor, but in cases of gonadal dysgenesis due to chromosomal mosaicism such as 45,X/46,XY, or where a Y fragment is present, gonadoblastomas are a significant risk in the dysgenetic gonads, perhaps occurring in up to 20 % of cases. However, in a population-based study of girls with Turner syndrome, analyzed by PCR to detect Y-chromosome material, Gravholt et al. (2000) reported that although the frequency of Y-chromosome material is high in Turner syndrome (12.2 %), the occurrence of gonadoblastoma among Y-positive patients was less than in previous estimates (7–10 %). Gonadal extirpation has been suggested for such patients unless they have an almost normal male phenotype with scrotal testes. Nevertheless, careful follow-up (perhaps including testicular biopsy) is needed. The report of an infant girl with Turner syndrome, gonadoblastoma and 46XY(del Yp) karyotype indicated that the genes on the Y-chromosome that induce gonadoblastoma are distinct from the sex-determining locus, and detailed mapping of the Y-chromosome gonadoblastoma susceptibility region close to the centromere has been undertaken and candidate genes proposed (Lau 1999).

There is probably no increased risk of gonadoblastoma in Klinefelter syndrome (47, XXY) or in the XYY syndrome. However, gonadoblastoma is associated with sex reversal caused by 9p deletion (Livadas et al. 2003) and WAGR syndrome caused by 11p13 deletion (see p. 138).

Single gene defects can also cause gonadal dysgenesis, and gonadal tumors are found in at least 30 % of XY cases. The tumors are gonadoblastomas or dysgerminomas, which arise in the second or third decade. Autosomal recessive forms of XX gonadal dysgenesis are probably not associated with an increased risk for gonadoblastomas, but XY gonadal dysgenesis (Swyer syndrome), is frequently complicated by this tumor. Affected individuals are of normal stature and do not have the features of Turner syndrome, but have streak gonads. H-Y antigen may or may not be positive. It has been suggested that the risk of gonadoblastoma and dysgerminoma is confined to the H-Y antigen-positive cases. XY gonadal dysgenesis may also occur as an autosomal recessive condition, and gonadal tumors frequently complicate the familial testicular dysgenesis syndrome, one of this group of conditions. Again, H-Y antigen-positive cases appear to be the ones susceptible to gonadoblastomas, with a 55 % incidence. Gonadoblastoma may be associated with renal impairment and gonadal dysgenesis in Frasier syndrome (see p. 252).

The incidence of gonadal neoplasia in true hermaphrodites (individuals with both testicular and ovarian tissue) appears to be low, although both ovarian and testicular tumors have been reported. Complete testicular feminization (X-linked recessive inheritance) is associated with an increased risk of testicular malignancy (about 5 %), most commonly seminoma. If malignancy develops, it is usually after the age of 25 years, so that orchidectomy can be delayed until after pubertal feminization. The risk of neoplasia in incomplete androgen-insensitivity states, including Reifenstein syndrome, is considered to be low.

In the syndromes of persistent Mullerian duct and pseudovaginal perineoscrotal hypoplasia, the abnormally situated testes are susceptible to the development of seminomas, choriocarcinomas, embryonal carcinomas, gonadoblastomas, or teratocarcinomas. The incidence of gonadal neoplasia may be slightly increased – to up to 4 % in 46XX cases and 10 % in 46XY cases.

In the conditions predisposing to gonadal tumors, it is advisable to remove the gonads prophylactically in the second decade.

Epididymal Tumors

Benign epididymal cystadenomas occur in von Hippel–Lindau disease, when they are frequently bilateral. Although scrotal ultrasound scan can be useful for demonstrating sub-clinical involvement, the presence of epididymal cysts alone does not represent a reliable criterion for identifying gene carriers in von Hippel–Lindau disease families.

References

Ahlbom BD, Yaqoob M, Larsson A, Ilicki A, Annerén G, Wadelius C. Genetic and linkage analysis of familial congenital hypothyroidism: exclusion of linkage to the TSH receptor gene. Hum Genet. 1997;99(2):186–90.

Al Saffar M, Foulkes WD. Hereditary ovarian cancer resulting from a non-ovarian cancer cluster region (OCCR) BRCA2 mutation: is the OCCR useful clinically? J Med Genet. 2002;39:e68.

Alam NA, Bevan S, Churchman M, et al. Localization of a gene (MCUL1) for multiple cutaneous leiomyomata and uterine fibroids to chromosome 1q42.3–q42. Am J Hum Genet. 2001;68:1264–9.

Antoniou A, Pharoah PD, Narod S, Risch HA, Eyfjord JE, Hopper JL, Loman N, Olsson H, Johannsson O, Borg A, Pasini B, Radice P, Manoukian S, Eccles DM, Tang N, Olah E, Anton-Culver H, Warner E, Lubinski J, Gronwald J, Gorski B, Tulinius H, Thorlacius S, Eerola H, Nevanlinna H, Syrjakoski K, Kallioniemi OP, Thompson D, Evans C, Peto J, Lalloo F, Evans DG, Easton DF. Average risks of breast and ovarian cancer associated with BRCA1 or BRCA2 mutations detected in case series unselected for family history: a combined analysis of 22 studies. Am J Hum Genet. 2003;72:1117–30.

Antoniou AC, Pharoah PP, Smith P, Easton DF. The BOADICEA model of genetic susceptibility to breast and ovarian cancer. Br J Cancer. 2004;91(8):1580–90.

Apple RJ, Becker TM, Wheeler CM, Erlich HA. Comparison of human leukocyte antigen DR-DQ disease associations found with cervical dysplasia and invasive cervical carcinoma. J Natl Cancer Inst. 1995;87(6):427–36.

Audeh MW, Carmichael J, Penson RT, Friedlander M, Powell B, Bell-McGuinn KM, Scott C, Weitzel JN, Oaknin A, Loman N, et al. Oral poly(ADP-ribose) polymerase inhibitor olaparib in patients with BRCA1 or BRCA2 mutations and recurrent ovarian cancer: a proof-of-concept trial. Lancet. 2010;376:245–51.

Baglietto L, Lindor NM, Dowty JG, White DM, Wagner A, Gomez Garcia EB, Vriends AH. Dutch Lynch Syndrome Study Group, Cartwright NR, Barnetson RA, Farrington SM, Tenesa A, Hampel H, Buchanan D, Arnold S, Young J, Walsh MD, Jass J, Macrae F, Antill Y, Winship IM, Giles GG, Goldblatt J, Parry S, Suthers G, Leggett B, Butz M, Aronson M, Poynter JN, Baron JA, Le Marchand L, Haile R, Gallinger S, Hopper JL, Potter J, de la Chapelle A, Vasen HF, Dunlop MG, Thibodeau SN, Jenkins MA. Risks of Lynch syndrome cancers for MSH6 mutation carriers. J Natl Cancer Inst. 2010;102(3):193–201.

Barber LJ, Sandhu S, Chen L, Campbell J, Kozarewa I, Fenwick K, Assiotis I, Rodrigues DN, Filho JS, Moreno V, Mateo J, Molife LR, De Bono J, Kaye S, Lord CJ, Ashworth A. Secondary mutations in BRCA2 associated with clinical resistance to a PARP inhibitor. J Pathol. 2013;229(3):422–9.

Barnes DR, Antoniou AC. Unravelling modifiers of breast and ovarian cancer risk for BRCA1 and BRCA2 mutation carriers: update on genetic modifiers. J Intern Med. 2012;271(4):331–43.

Barrow PJ, Ingham S, O'Hara C, et al. The spectrum of urological malignancy in Lynch syndrome. Fam Cancer. 2013;12(1):57–63.

Beggs AD, Latchford AR, Vasen HF, Moslein G, Alonso A, Aretz S, Bertario L, Blanco I, Bülow S, Burn J, Capella G, Colas C, Friedl W, Møller P, Hes FJ, Järvinen H, Mecklin JP, Nagengast FM, Parc Y, Phillips RK, Hyer W. Ponz de Leon M, Renkonen-Sinisalo L, Sampson JR, Stormorken A, Tejpar S, Thomas HJ, Wijnen JT, Clark SK. Hodgson SV. Peutz-Jeghers syndrome: a systematic review and recommendations for management. Gut. 2010;59(7):975–86.

Berns EM, Bowtell DD. The changing view of high-grade serous ovarian cancer. Cancer Res. 2012;72(11):2701–4.

Bonadona V, Bonaiti B, Olschwang S, Grandjouan S, Huiart L, Longy M, Guimbaud R, Buecher B, Bignon YJ, Caron O, Colas C, Nogues C, Lejeune-Dumoulin S, Olivier-Faivre L, Polycarpe-Osaer F, Nguyen TD, Desseigne F, Saurin JC, Berthet P, Leroux D, Duffour J, Manouvrier S, Frebourg T, Sobol H, Lasset C, Bonaiti-Pellie C. Cancer risks associated with germline mutations in MLH1, MSH2, and MSH6 genes in Lynch syndrome. JAMA. 2011;305(22): 2304–10.

Borresen AL, Andersen TI, Garber J, et al. Screening for germline TP53 mutations in breast cancer patients. Cancer Res. 1992;52:3234–6.

Boyd J, Sonoda Y, Federici MG, Bogomolniy F, Rhei E, Maresco DL, Saigo PE, Almadrones LA, Barakat RR, Brown CL, Chi DS, Curtin JP, Poynor EA, Hoskins WJ. Clinicopathologic features of BRCA-linked and sporadic ovarian cancer. J Am Med Assoc. 2000;283:2260–5.

Brekelmans CT, Seynaeve C, Bartels CC, Tilanus-Linthorst MM, Meijers-Heijboer EJ, Crepin CM, van Geel AA, Menke M, Verhoog LC, van den Ouweland A, Obdeijn IM, Klijn JG. Effectiveness of breast cancer surveillance in BRCA1/2 gene mutation carriers and women with high familial risk. J Clin Oncol. 2001;19:924–30.

Brohet RM, Goldgar DE, Easton DF, Antoniou AC, Andrieu N, Chang-Claude J, Peock S, Eeles RA, Cook M, Chu C, Nogues C, Lasset C, Berthet P, Meijers-Heijboer H, Gerdes AM, Olsson H, Caldes T, Van Leeuwen FE, Rookus MA. Oral contraceptives and breast cancer risk in the international BRCA1/2 carrier cohort study: a report from EMBRACE, GENEPSO, GEO-HEBON, and the IBCCS Collaborating Group. J Clin Oncol. 2007;25(25):3831–6.

Brown PO, Palmer C. The preclinical natural history of serous ovarian cancer: defining the target for early detection. PLoS Med. 2009;6(7):e1000114.

Byrnes GB, Southey MC, Hopper JL. Are the so-called low penetrance breast cancer genes, ATM, BRIP1, PALB2 and CHEK2, high risk for women with strong family histories? Breast Cancer Res. 2008;10(3):208.

Byrski T, Huzarski T, Dent R, Gronwald J, Zuziak D, Cybulski C, Kladny J, Gorski B, Lubinski J, Narod SA. Response to neoadjuvant therapy with cisplatin in BRCA1-positive breast cancer patients. Breast Cancer Res Treat. 2009;115(2):359–63.

Carcangiu ML, Radice P, Manoukian S, Spatti G, Gobbo M, Pensotti V, Crucianelli R, Pasini B. Atypical epithelial proliferation in fallopian tubes in prophylactic salpingo-oophorectomy specimens from BRCA1 and BRCA2 germline mutation carriers. Int J Gynecol Pathol. 2004;23:35–40.

Casagrande JT, Louie EW, Pike MC, Roy S, Ross RK, Henderson BE. "Incessant ovulation" and ovarian cancer. Lancet. 1979;2:170–3.

Chenevix-Trench G, Spurdle AB, Gatei M, Kelly H, Marsh A, Chen X, Donn K, Cummings M, Nyholt D, Jenkins MA, Scott C, Pupo GM, Dork T, Bendix R, Kirk J, Tucker K, McCredie MR, Hopper JL, Sambrook J, Mann GJ, Khanna KK. Dominant negative ATM mutations in breast cancer families. J Natl Cancer Inst. 2002;94:205–15.

Clarke BA, Cooper K. Identifying Lynch syndrome in patients with endometrial carcinoma: shortcomings of morphologic and clinical schemas. Adv Anat Pathol. 2012;19(4):231–8.

Claus EB, Petruzella S, Matloff E, Carter D. Prevalence of BRCA1 and BRCA2 mutations in women diagnosed with ductal carcinoma in situ. JAMA. 2005;293(8):964–9.

Coffey J, Huddart RA, Elliott F, Sohaib SA, Parker E, Dudakia D, Pugh JL, Easton DF, Bishop DT, Stratton MR, Rapley EA. Testicular microlithiasis as a familial risk factor for testicular germ cell tumor. Br J Cancer. 2007;97(12):1701–6.

Colgan TJ, Murphy J, Cole DE, Narod S, Rosen B. Occult carcinoma in prophylactic oophorectomy specimens: prevalence and association with BRCA germline mutation status. Am J Surg Pathol. 2001;25:1283–9.

Collaborative Group on Hormonal Factors in Breast Cancer. Familial breast cancer: collaborative reanalysis of individual data from 52 epidemiological studies including 58,209 women with breast cancer and 101,986 women without the disease. Lancet. 2001;358(9291):1389–99. Review.

Couch FJ, DeShano ML, Blackwood MA, et al. BRCA1 mutations in women attending clinics that evaluate the risk of breast cancer. New Engl J Med. 1997;336:1409–15.

Cramer DW, Hutchison GB, Welch WR, Scully RE, Ryan KJ. Determinants of ovarian cancer risk. I. Reproductive experiences and family history. J Natl Cancer Inst. 1983;71:711–16.

Crockford GP, Linger R, Hockley S, et al. Genome-wide linkage screen for testicular germ cell tumour susceptibility loci. Hum Mol Genet. 2006;15(3): 443–51.

Crum CP, Drapkin R, Kindelberger D, Medeiros F, Miron A, Lee Y. Lessons from BRCA: the tubal fimbria emerges as an origin for pelvic serous cancer. Clin Med Res. 2007;5(1):35–44.

Crum CP, McKeon FD, Xian W. BRCA, the oviduct, and the space and time continuum of pelvic serous carcinogenesis. Int J Gynecol Cancer. 2012;22 Suppl 1:S29–34.

Daling JR, Madeleine MM, Schwartz SM, et al. A population based study of squamous cell vaginal cancer: HPV and cofactors. Gynaecol Oncol. 2002;84:263–70.

Domchek SM, Friebel TM, Singer CF, Evans DG, Lynch HT, Isaacs C, Garber JE, Neuhausen SL, Matloff E, Eeles R, Pichert G, Van t.L. Tung N, Weitzel JN, Couch FJ, Rubinstein WS, Ganz PA, Daly MB, Olopade OI, Tomlinson G, Schildkraut J, Blum JL, Rebbeck TR. Association of risk-reducing surgery in BRCA1 or BRCA2 mutation carriers with cancer risk and mortality. JAMA. 2010;304(9):967–75.

Dong C, Lonnstedt I, Hemminki K. Familial testicular cancer and second primary cancers in testicular cancer patients by histological type. Eur J Cancer. 2001;37:1878–85.

Easton DE, Ford D, Bishop DT, The Breast Cancer Linkage Consortium. Breast and ovarian cancer incidence in BRCA1 mutation carriers. Am J Hum Genet. 1995;56:265–71.

Easton DF, Pooley KA, Dunning AM, Pharoah PD, Thompson D, Ballinger DG, Struewing JP, Morrison J, Field H, Luben R, Wareham N, Ahmed S, Healey CS, Bowman R, Luccarini C, Conroy D, Shah M, Munday H, Jordan C, Perkins B, West J, Redman K, Meyer KB, Haiman CA, Kolonel LK, Henderson BE, Le ML, Brennan P, Sangrajrang S, Gaborieau V, Odefrey F, Shen CY, Wu PE, Wang HC, Eccles D, Evans DG, Peto J, Fletcher O, Johnson N, Seal S, Stratton MR, Rahman N, Chenevix-Trench G, Bojesen SE, Nordestgaard BG, Axelsson CK, Garcia-Closas M, Brinton L, Chanock S, Lissowska J, Peplonska B, Nevanlinna H, Fagerholm R, Eerola H, Kang D, Yoo KY, Noh DY, Ahn SH, Hunter DJ, Hankinson SE, Cox DG, Hall P, Wedren S, Liu J, Low YL, Bogdanova N, Schurmann P, Dork T, Tollenaar RA, Jacobi CE, Devilee P, Klijn JG, Sigurdson AJ, Doody, MM, Alexander BH, Zhang J, Cox A, Brock IW, Macpherson G, Reed MW, Couch FJ, Goode EL, Olson JE, Meijers-Heijboer H, van den OA, Uitterlinden A, Rivadeneira F, Milne RL, Ribas G, Gonzalez-Neira A, Benitez J, Hopper JL, McCredie M, Southey M, Giles GG, Schroen C, Justenhoven C, Brauch H, Hamann U, Ko YD, Spurdle AB, Beesley J, Chen X, Aghmesheh M, Amor D, Andrews L, Antill Y, Armes J, Armitage S, Arnold L, Balleine R, Begley G, Beilby J, Bennett I, Bennett B, Berry G, Blackburn A, Brennan M, Brown M, Buckley M, Burke J, Butow P, Byron K, Callen D, Campbell I, Chenevix-Trench G, Clarke C, Colley A, Cotton D, Cui J, Culling B, Cummings M, Dawson SJ, Dixon J, Dobrovic A, Dudding T, Edkins T, Eisenbruch M, Farshid G, Fawcett S, Field M, Firgaira F, Fleming J, Forbes J, Friedlander M, Gaff C, Gardner M, Gattas M, George P, Giles G, Gill G, Goldblatt J, Greening S, Grist S, Haan E, Harris M, Hart S, Hayward N, Hopper J, Humphrey E, Jenkins M, Jones A, Kefford R, Kirk J, Kollias J, Kovalenko S, Lakhani S, Leary J, Lim J, Lindeman G, Lipton L, Lobb L, Maclurcan M, Mann G, Marsh D, McCredie M,

McKay M, Anne MS, Meiser B, Milne R, Mitchell G, Newman B, O'loughlin I, Osborne R, Peters L, Phillips K, Price M, Reeve J, Reeve T, Richards R, Rinehart G, Robinson B, Rudzki B, Salisbury E, Sambrook J, Saunders C, Scott C, Scott E, Scott R, Seshadri R, Shelling A, Southey M, Spurdle A, Suthers G, Taylor D, Tennant C, Thorne H, Townshend S, Tucker K, Tyler J, Venter D, Visvader J, Walpole I, Ward R, Waring P, Warner B, Warren G, Watson E, Williams R, Wilson J, Winship I, Young MA, Bowtell D, Green A, Defazio A, Chenevix-Trench G, Gertig D, Webb P, Mannermaa A, Kosma VM, Kataja V, Hartikainen J, Day NE, Cox DR, Ponder BA. Genome-wide association study identifies novel breast cancer susceptibility loci. Nature. 2007;447(7148):1087–93.

Edwards SM, Kote-Jarai Z, Meitz J, et al. Two percent of men with early-onset prostate cancer harbor germline mutations in the BRCA2 gene. Am J Hum Genet. 2002;72(1):1–12.

Edwards SL, Brough R, Lord CJ, Natrajan R, Vatcheva R, Levine DA, Boyd J, Reis-Filho JS, Ashworth A. Resistance to therapy caused by intragenic deletion in BRCA2. Nature. 2008;451:1111–5.

Edwards SM, Evans DG, Hope Q, Norman AR, Barbachano Y, Bullock S, Kote-Jarai Z, Meitz J, Falconer A, Osin P, Fisher C, Guy M, Jhavar SG, Hall AL, O'Brien LT, Gehr-Swain BN, Wilkinson RA, Forrest MS, Dearnaley DP, Ardern-Jones AT, Page EC, Easton DF, Eeles RA. UK Genetic Prostate Cancer Study Collaborators and BAUS Section of Oncology. Prostate cancer in BRCA2 germline mutation carriers is associated with poorer prognosis. Br J Cancer. 2010;103(6):918–24.

Elledge SJ, Amon A. The BRCA1 suppressor hypothesis: an explanation for the tissue-specific tumor development in BRCA1 patients. Cancer Cell. 2002;1(2):129–32.

Eng C, Kiuru M, Fernandez MJ, Aaltonen LA. A role for mitochondrial enzymes in inherited neoplasia and beyond. Nat Rev Cancer. 2003;3:193–202.

Engelman DE, Andrade LA, Vassallo J. Human papillomavirus infection and p53 protein expression vulvar intraepithelial neoplasia and invasive squamous cell carcinoma. Braz J Med Biol Res. 2003;36:1159–65.

Erkko H, Dowty JG, Nikkila J, Syrjakoski K, Mannermaa A, Pylkas K, Southey MC, Holli K, Kallioniemi A, Jukkola-Vuorinen A, Kataja V, Kosma VM, Xia B, Livingston DM, Winqvist R, Hopper JL. Penetrance Analysis of the PALB2 c.1592delT Founder Mutation. Clin. Cancer Res. 2008;14(14):4667–71.

Evans DG, Eccles DM, Rahman N, Young K, Bulman M, Amir E, Shenton A, Howell A, Lalloo F. A new scoring system for the chances of identifying a BRCA1/2 mutation outperforms existing models including BRCAPRO. J Med Genet. 2004;41:474–80.

Ewing CM, Ray AM, Lange EM, Zuhlke KA, Robbins CM, Tembe WD, Wiley KE, Isaacs SD, Johng D, Wang Y, Bizon C, Yan G, Gielzak M, Partin AW, Shanmugam V, Izatt T, Sinari S, Craig DW, Zheng SL, Walsh PC, Montie JE, Xu J, Carpten JD, Isaacs WB, Cooney KA. Germline mutations in HOXB13 and prostate-cancer risk. N Engl J Med. 2012;366(2):141–9.

Fackenthal JD, Olopade OI. Breast cancer risk associated with BRCA1 and BRCA2 in diverse populations. Nat Rev Cancer. 2007;7(12):937–48.

Finch A, Beiner M, Lubinski J, Lynch HT, Moller P, Rosen B, Murphy J, Ghadirian P, Friedman E, Foulkes WD, Kim-Sing C, Wagner T, Tung N, Couch F, Stoppa-Lyonnet D, Ainsworth P, Daly M, Pasini B, Gershoni-Baruch R, Eng C, Olopade OI, McLennan J, Karlan B, Weitzel J, Sun P, Narod SA. Salpingo-oophorectomy and the risk of ovarian, fallopian tube, and peritoneal cancers in women with a BRCA1 or BRCA2 Mutation. JAMA. 2006;296(2):185–92.

Fletcher CDM, Unni KK, Mertens F, editors. Pathology and genetics of tumors of soft tissue and bone. Lyon: IARC Press; 2002.

Fong P, Boss D, Yap T, Tutt A, Wu P. Inhibition of poly(ADP-ribose) polymerase in tumors from BRCA mutation carriers. N Engl J Med. 2009;361(2):123–34.

Ford D, Easton DF, Stratton M, Narod S, et al. Genetic heterogeneity and pene-trance analysis of the BRCA1 and BRCA2 genes in breast cancer families. Am J Hum Genet. 1998;62:676–89.

Forman D, Oliver RTD, Brett AR, et al. Familial testicular cancer: a report of the UK register, estimation of risk and HLA class I sib pair analysis. Br J Cancer. 1992;65:255–62.

Foulkes WD. BRCA1 functions as a breast stem cell regulator. J Med Genet. 2004;41(1):1–5.

Foulkes WD. Inherited susceptibility to common cancers. N Engl J Med. 2008;359(20):2143–53.

Foulkes WD, Metcalfe K, Sun P, Hanna WM, Lynch HT, Ghadirian P, Tung N, Olopade OI, Weber BL, McLennan J, Olivotto IA, Begin LR, Narod SA. Estrogen receptor status in BRCA1- and BRCA2-related breast cancer: the influence of age, grade, and histological type. Clin Cancer Res. 2004;10(6):2029–34.

Foulkes WD, Bahubeshi A, Hamel N, Pasini B, Asioli S, Baynam G, Choong CS, Charles A, Frieder RP, Dishop MK, Graf N, Ekim M, Bouron-Dal SD, Arseneau J, Young RH, Sabbaghian N, Srivastava A, Tischkowitz MD, Priest JR. Extending the phenotypes associated with DICER1 mutations. Hum Mutat. 2011;32(12):1381–4.

Gallagher DJ, Gaudet MM, Pal P, Kirchhoff T, Balistreri L, Vora K, Bhatia J, Stadler Z, Fine SW, Reuter V, Zelefsky M, Morris MJ, Scher HI, Klein RJ, Norton L, Eastham JA, Scardino PT, Robson ME, Offit K. Germline BRCA mutations denote a clinicopathologic subset of prostate cancer. Clin Cancer Res. 2010;16(7):2115–21.

Ganesan S, Richardson AL, Wang ZC, Iglehart JD, Miron A, Feunteun J, Silver D, Livingston DM. Abnormalities of the inactive X chromosome are a common feature of BRCA1 mutant and sporadic basal-like breast cancer. Cold Spring Harb Symp Quant Biol. 2005;70:93–7.

Garber JE, Goldstein AM, Kantor AF, et al. Follow-up study of twenty-four families with Li–Fraumeni syndrome. Cancer Res. 1991; 51: 6094–7.

Gelmon KA, Tischkowitz M, Mackay H, Swenerton K, Robidoux A, Tonkin K, Hirte H, Huntsman D, Clemons M, Gilks B, Yerushalmi R, Macpherson E, Carmichael J, Oza A. Olaparib in patients with recurrent high-grade serous or poorly differentiated ovarian carcinoma or triple-negative breast cancer: a phase 2, multicentre, open-label, non-randomised study. Lancet Oncol. 2011;12(9):852–61.

Giambartolomei C, Mueller CM, Greene MH, Korde LA. A mini-review of familial ovarian germ cell tumors: an additional manifestation of the familial testicular germ cell tumor syndrome. Cancer Epidemiol. 2009;33(1):31–6.

Goffin J, Chappuis PO, Wong N, Foulkes WD. Re: Magnetic resonance imaging and mammography in women with a hereditary risk of breast cancer. J Natl Cancer Inst. 2001;93:1754–5.

Goldgar DE, Easton DF, Cannon-Albright LA, Skolnick MH. Systematic population-based assessment of cancer risk in first-degree relatives of cancer probands. J Natl Cancer Inst. 1994;86:1600–8.

Goodman SN. The mammography dilemma: a crisis for evidence-based medicine? Ann Int Med. 2002;137:363–5.

Gorski B, Byrski T, Huzarski T, Jakubowska A, Menkiszak J, Gronwald J, Pluzanska A, Bebenek M, Fischer-Maliszewska L, Grzybowska E, Narod SA, Lubinski J. Founder mutations in the BRCA1 gene in Polish families with breast-ovarian cancer. Am J Hum Genet. 2000;66:1963–8.

Goss PE, Bulbul MA. Familial testicular cancer in five members of a cancerprone kindred. Cancer. 1990; 66:2044–6.

Gravholt CH, Fedder J, Naeraa RW, Muller J. Occurrence of gonadoblas-toma in females with Turner syndrome and Y chromosome material: a population study. J Clin Endocrinol Metab. 2000;85:3199–202.

Grindedal EM, Moller P, Eeles R, et al. Germ-line mutations in mismatch repair genes associated with prostate cancer. Cancer Epidemiol Biomarkers Prev. 2009;18(9):2460–7.

Grönberg H, Ahman AK, Emanuelsson M, Bergh A, Damber JE, Borg A. BRCA2 mutation in a family with hereditary prostate cancer. Genes Chromosomes Cancer. 2001;30(3):299–301.

Gudmundsson J, Sulem P, Gudbjartsson DF, Masson G, Agnarsson BA, Benediktsdottir KR, Sigurdsson A, Magnusson OT, Gudjonsson SA, Magnusdottir DN, Johannsdottir H, Helgadottir HT, Stacey SN, Jonasdottir A, Olafsdottir SB, Thorleifsson G, Jonasson JG, Tryggvadottir L, Navarrete S, Fuertes F, Helfand BT, Hu Q, Csiki IE, Mates IN, Jinga V, Aben KK, van Oort IM, Vermeulen SH, Donovan JL, Hamdy FC, Ng CF, Chiu PK, Lau KM, Ng MC, Gulcher JR, Kong A, Catalona WJ, Mayordomo JI, Einarsson GV, Barkardottir RB, Jonsson E, Mates D, Neal DE, Kiemeney LA, Thorsteinsdottir U, Rafnar T, Stefansson K. A study based on whole-genome sequencing yields a rare variant at 8q24 associated with prostate cancer. Nat Genet. 2012;44(12):1326–9.

Haile RW, Thomas DC, McGuire V, Felberg A, John EM, Milne RL, Hopper JL, Jenkins MA, Levine AJ, Daly MM, Buys SS, Senie RT, Andrulis IL, Knight JA, Godwin AK, Southey M, McCredie MR, Giles GG, Andrews L, Tucker K, Miron A, Apicella C, Tesoriero A, Bane A, Pike MC, Whittemore AS. BRCA1 and BRCA2 mutation carriers, oral contraceptive use, and breast cancer before age 50. Cancer Epidemiol Biomarkers Prev. 2006;15(10):1863–70.

Hales SA, Cree IA, Pinion S. A poorly differentiated Sertoli-Leydig cell tumor associated with an ovarian sex cord tumor with annular tubules in a woman with Peutz-Jeghers syndrome. Histopathology. 1994;25(4):391–3.

Hamel N, Wong N, Alpert L, Galvez M, Foulkes WD. Mixed ovarian germ cell tumor in a BRCA2 mutation carrier. Int J Gynecol Pathol. 2007;26(2):160–4.

Hartge P, Schiffman MH, Hoover R, McGowan L, Lesher L, Norris HJ. A case–control study of epithelial ovarian cancer. Am J Obstetr Gynecol. 1989;161:10–16.

Hebert-Blouin MN, Koufogianis V, Gillett P, Foulkes WD. Fallopian tube cancer in a BRCA1 mutation carrier: rapid development and failure of screening. Am J Obstet Gynecol. 2002;186(1):53–4.

Hedenfalk I, Duggan D, Chen Y, Radmacher M, Bittner M, Simon R, Meltzer P, Gusterson B, Esteller M, Kallioniemi OP, Wilfond B, Borg A, Trent J. Gene-expression profiles in hereditary breast cancer. New Engl J Med. 2001;344:539–48.

Heijnsdijk EA, Warner E, Gilbert FJ, Tilanus-Linthorst MM, Evans G, Causer PA, Eeles RA, Kaas R, Draisma G, Ramsay EA, Warren RM, Hill KA, Hoogerbrugge N, Wasser MN, Bergers E, Oosterwijk JC, Hooning MJ, Rutgers EJ, Klijn JG, Plewes DB, Leach MO, de Koning HJ. Differences in Natural History between Breast Cancers in BRCA1 and BRCA2 Mutation Carriers and Effects of MRI Screening-MRISC, MARIBS, and Canadian Studies Combined. Cancer Epidemiol Biomarkers Prev. 2012;21(9):1458–68.

Heimdal K, Olsson H, Tretli S, Fossa SD, Borresen AL, Bishop DT. A segregation analysis of testicular cancer based on Norwegian and Swedish families. Br J Cancer. 1997;75:1084–7.

Heravi-Moussavi A, Anglesio MS, Cheng SW, Senz J, Yang W, Prentice L, Fejes AP, Chow C, Tone A, Kalloger SE, Hamel N, Roth A, Ha G, Wan AN, Maines-Bandiera S, Salamanca C, Pasini B, Clarke BA, Lee AF, Lee CH, Zhao C, Young RH, Aparicio SA, Sorensen PH, Woo MM, Boyd N, Jones SJ, Hirst M, Marra MA, Gilks B, Shah SP, Foulkes WD, Morin GB, Huntsman DG. Recurrent somatic DICER1 mutations in nonepithelial ovarian cancers. N Engl J Med. 2012;366(3):234–42.

Hildreth NG, Kelsey JL, LiVolsi VA, Fischer DB, Holford TR, Mostow ED, Schwartz PE, White C. An epidemiologic study of epithelial carcinoma of the ovary. Am J Epidemiol. 1981;114:398–405.

Horn LC, Raptis G, Fischer U. Familial cancer history in patients with carcinoma of the cervix uteri. Eur J Obstet Gynecol Reprod Biol. 2002;101:54–7.

Howell L, Bader A, Mullassery D, Losty P, Auth M, Kokai G. Sertoli Leydig cell ovarian tumor and gastric polyps as presenting features of Peutz-Jeghers syndrome. Pediatr Blood Cancer. 2010;55(1):206–7.

Ibrahim Y, García-García C, Serra V, et al. PI3K Inhibition Impairs BRCA1/2 Expression and Sensitizes BRCA-Proficient Triple-Negative Breast Cancer to PARP Inhibition. Cancer Discov. 2012;2:1036–47.

Jacobs IJ, Skates SJ, MacDonald N, Menon U, Rosenthal AN, Davies AP, Woolas R, Jeyarajah AR, Sibley K, Lowe DG, Oram DH. Screening for ovarian cancer: a pilot randomised controlled trial. Lancet. 1999;353(9160):1207–10.

Johns LE, Houlston RS. A systematic review and meta-analysis of familial prostate cancer risk. BJU Int. 2003;91:789–94.

Kanetsky PA, Mitra N, Vardhanabhuti S, Li M, Vaughn DJ, Letrero R, Ciosek SL, Doody DR, Smith LM, Weaver J, Albano A, Chen C, Starr JR, Rader DJ, Godwin AK, Reilly MP, Hakonarson H, Schwartz SM, Nathanson KL. Common variation in KITLG and at 5q31.3 predisposes to testicular germ cell cancer. Nat Genet. 2009;41(7):811–5.

Kasprzak L, Mesurolle B, Tremblay F, Galvez M, Halwani F, Foulkes WD. Invasive breast cancer following bilateral subcutaneous mastectomy in a BRCA2 mutation carrier: a case report and review of the literature. World J Surg Oncol. 2005;3:52.

Kerber RA, Slattery ML. The impact of family history on ovarian cancer risk. The Utah Population Database. Arch Int Med. 1995;155:905–12.

Kirchhoff T, Kauff ND, Mitra N, et al. BRCA mutations and risk of prostate cancer in Ashkenazi Jews. Clin Cancer Res. 2004;10:2918–21.

Kiuru M, Lehtonen R, Arola J, et al. Few FH mutations in sporadic counterparts of tumor types observed in hereditary leiomyomatosis and renal cell cancer families. Cancer Res. 2002;62:4554–7.

Koch M, Gaedke H, Jenkins H. Family history of ovarian cancer patients: a case–control study. Int J Epidemiol. 1989;18:782–5.

Kriege M, Brekelmans CT, Boetes C, Besnard PE, Zonderland HM, Obdeijn IM, Manoliu RA, Kok T, Peterse H, Tilanus-Linthorst MM, Muller SH, Meijer S, Oosterwijk JC, Beex LV, Tollenaar RA, de Koning HJ, Rutgers EJ, Klijn JG, Magnetic Resonance Imaging Screening Study Group. Efficacy of MRI and mammography for breast-cancer screening in women with a familial or genetic predisposition. N Engl J Med. 2004;351(5):427–37.

Kuhl CK, Schmutzler RK, Leutner CC, Kempe A, Wardelmann E, Hocke A, Maringa M, Pfeifer U, Krebs D, Schild HH. Breast MR imaging screening in 192 women proved or suspected to be carriers of a breast cancer susceptibility gene: preliminary results. Radiology. 2000;215:267–79.

Kutler DI, Wreesmann VB, Goberdhan A. Human papillomavirus DNA and p53 polymorphisms in squamous cell carcinomas from Fanconi anaemia patients. J Natl Cancer Inst. 2003; 19:1718–21.

Lakhani SR, Jacquemier J, Sloane JP, et al. Multifactorial analysis of differences between sporadic breast cancers and cancers involving BRCA1 and BRCA2 mutations. J Natl Cancer Inst. 1998;90:1138–45.

Lakhani SR, van de Vijver MJ, Jacquemier J, Anderson TJ, Osin PP, McGuffog L, Easton DF. The pathology of familial breast cancer: predictive value of immuno-histochemical markers estrogen receptor, progesterone receptor, HER-2, and p53 in patients with mutations in BRCA1 and BRCA2. J Clin Oncol. 2002;20:2310–8.

Lau YF. Gonadoblastoma, testicular and prostate cancers, and the TSPY gene. Am J Hum Genetic. 1999;64:921–7.

Ledermann J, Harter P, Gourley C, Friedlander M, Vergote I, Rustin G, Scott C, Meier W, Shapira-Frommer R, Safra T, Matei D, Macpherson E, Watkins C, Carmichael J, Matulonis U. Olaparib maintenance therapy in platinum-sensitive relapsed ovarian cancer. N Engl J Med. 2012;366(15):1382–92.

Leeper K, Garcia R, Swisher E, Goff B, Greer B, Paley P. Pathologic findings in prophylactic oophorectomy specimens in high-risk women. Gynecol Oncol. 2002;87:52–6.

Lehtonen R, Kiuru MH, Vanharanta S, et al. Biallelic inactivation of fumarate hydratase (FH) occurs in nonsyndromic uterine leiomyomas but is rare in other tumors. Am J Pathol. 2004;164:17–22.

Leong SP, Shen ZZ, Liu TJ, Agarwal G, Tajima T, Paik NS, Sandelin K, Derossis A, Cody H, Foulkes WD. Is breast cancer the same disease in Asian and Western countries? World J Surg. 2010;34(10):2308–24.

Li ML, Greenberg RA. Links between genome integrity and BRCA1 tumor suppression. Trends Biochem Sci Trends Biochem Sci. 2012;37(10):418–24.

Lichtenstein P, Holm NV, Verkasalo PK, Iliadou A, Kaprio J, Koskenvuo M, Pukkala E, Skytthe A, Hemminki K. Environmental and heritable factors in the causation of cancer-analyses of cohorts of twins from Sweden, Denmark, and Finland. N Engl J Med. 2000;343(2):78–85.

Livadas S, Mavrou A, Sofocleous C, van Vliet-Constantinidou C, Dracopoulou M, Dacou-Voutetakis C. Gonadoblastoma in a patient with del(9)(p22) and sex reversal: report of a case and review of the literature. Cancer Genet Cytogenet. 2003;143:174–7.

Loveday C, Turnbull C, Ramsay E, Hughes D, Ruark E, Frankum JR, Bowden G, Kalmyrzaev B, Warren-Perry M, Snape K, Adlard JW, Barwell J, Berg J, Brady AF, Brewer C, Brice G, Chapman C, Cook J, Davidson R, Donaldson A, Douglas F, Greenhalgh L, Henderson A, Izatt L, Kumar A, Lalloo F, Miedzybrodzka Z, Morrison PJ, Paterson J, Porteous M, Rogers MT, Shanley S, Walker L; Breast Cancer Susceptibility Collaboration (UK), Eccles D, Evans DG,

Renwick A, Seal S, Lord CJ, Ashworth A, Reis-Filho JS, Antoniou AC, Rahman N. Germline mutations in RAD51D confer susceptibility to ovarian cancer. Nat Genet. 2011;43(9):879-82.

Lu KH, Garber JE, Cramer DW, Welch WR, Niloff J, Schrag D, Berkowitz RS, Muto MG. Occult ovarian tumors in women with BRCA1 or BRCA2 mutations undergoing prophylactic oophorectomy. J Clin Oncol. 2000;18(14):2728–32.

Lynch HT, Walzak MP. Genetics in urogenital cancer. Urol Clin North Am. 1980;7(3):815–29.

Magnusson PK, Lichtenstein P, Gyllensten UB. Heritability of cervical tumours. Int J Cancer. 2000;88:698–701.

Mavaddat N, Peock S, Frost D, et al. Cancer risks for BRCA1 and BRCA2 mutation carriers: results from prospective analysis of EMBRACE. JNCI. 2013;105(11):812–22.

McClean GE, Kurian S, Walter N, Kekre A, McCluggage WG. Cervical embryonal rhabdomyosarcoma and ovarian Sertoli-Leydig cell tumor: a more than coincidental association of two rare neoplasms? J Clin Pathol. 2007;60(3):326–8.

McEwen AR, McConnell DT, Kenwright DN, Gaskell DJ, Cherry A, Kidd AM. Occult cancer of the fallopian tube in a BRCA2 germline mutation carrier at prophy-lactic salpingo-oophorectomy. Gynecol Oncol. 2004;92:992–4.

Meijers-Heijboer H, van Geel B, van Putten WL, Henzen-Logmans SC, Seynaeve C, Menke-Pluymers MB, Bartels CC, Verhoog LC, van den Ouweland AM, Niermeijer MF, Brekelmans CT, Klijn JG. Breast cancer after prophylactic bilateral mastectomy in women with a BRCA1 or BRCA2 mutation. New Engl J Med. 2001;345:159–64.

Meijers-Heijboer H, Wijnen J, Vasen H, Wasielewski M, Wagner A, Hollestelle A, Elstrodt F, van den Bos R, de Snoo A, Fat GT, Brekelmans C, Jagmohan S, Franken P, Verkuijlen P, van den Ouweland A, Chapman P, Tops C, Moslein G, Burn J, Lynch H, Klijn J, Fodde R, Chapman P, Tops C, Moslein G, Burn J, Lynch H, Klijn J, Fodde R, Schutte M. The CHEK2 1100delC mutation identifies families with a hereditary breast and colorectal cancer phenotype. Am J Hum Genet. 2003;72:1308–14.

Meikle AW, Smith JA. Epidemiology of prostate cancer. Urol Clin North Am. 1990;17:709–18.

Meindl A, Hellebrand H, Wiek C, Erven V, Wappenschmidt B, Niederacher D, Freund M, Lichtner P, Hartmann L, Schaal H, Ramser J, Honisch E, Kubisch C, Wichmann HE, Kast K, Deissler H, Engel C, Müller-Myhsok B, Neveling K, Kiechle M, Mathew CG, Schindler D, Schmutzler RK, Hanenberg H. Germline mutations in breast and ovarian cancer pedigrees establish RAD51C as a human cancer susceptibility gene. Nat Genet. 2010;42(5):410–4.

Metcalfe K, Lynch HT, Ghadirian P, Tung N, Olivotto I, Warner E, Olopade OI, Eisen A, Weber B, McLennan J, Sun P, Foulkes WD, Narod SA. Contralateral breast cancer in BRCA1 and BRCA2 mutation carriers. J Clin Oncol. 2004;22:2328–35.

Metcalfe KA, Poll A, Royer R, Llacuachaqui M, Tulman A, Sun P, Narod SA. Screening for founder mutations in BRCA1 and BRCA2 in unselected Jewish women. J Clin Oncol. 2010;28(3):387–91.

Metcalfe KA, Mian N, Enmore M, Poll A, Llacuachaqui M, Nanda S, Sun P, Hughes KS, Narod SA. Long-term follow-up of Jewish women with a BRCA1 and BRCA2 mutation who underwent population genetic screening. Breast Cancer Res Treat. 2012;133(2):735–40.

Milne RL, Knight JA, John EM, Dite GS, Balbuena R, Ziogas A, Andrulis IL, West DW, Li FP, Southey MC, Giles GG, McCredie MR, Hopper JL, Whittemore AS. Oral contraceptive use and risk of early-onset breast cancer in carriers and noncarriers of BRCA1 and BRCA2 mutations. Cancer Epidemiol Biomarkers Prev. 2005;14(2):350–6.

Mitra A, Fisher C, Foster CS, Jameson C, Barbachanno Y, Bartlett J, Bancroft E, Doherty R, Kote-Jarai Z, Peock S, Easton D. IMPACT and EMBRACE Collaborators, Eeles R. Prostate cancer in male BRCA1 and BRCA2 mutation carriers has a more aggressive phenotype. Br J Cancer. 2008;98(2):502–7.

Mitra AV, Bancroft EK, Barbachano Y, Page EC, Foster CS, Jameson C, Mitchell G, Lindeman GJ, Stapleton A, Suthers G, Evans DG, Cruger D, Blanco I, Mercer C, Kirk J, Maehle L, Hodgson S, Walker L, Izatt L, Douglas F, Tucker K, Dorkins H, Clowes V, Male A, Donaldson A, Brewer C, Doherty R, Bulman B, Osther PJ, Salinas M, Eccles D, Axcrona K, Jobson I, Newcombe B, Cybulski C, Rubinstein WS, Buys S, Townshend S, Friedman E, Domchek S, Ramon YC,

Spigelman A, Teo SH, Nicolai N, Aaronson N, Ardern-Jones A, Bangma C, Dearnaley D, Eyfjord J, Falconer A, Gronberg H, Hamdy F, Johannsson O, Khoo V, Kote-Jarai Z, Lilja H, Lubinski J, Melia J, Moynihan C, Peock S, Rennert G, Schroder F, Sibley P, Suri M, Wilson P, Bignon YJ, Strom S, Tischkowitz M, Liljegren A, Ilencikova D, Abele A, Kyriacou K, van AC, Kiemeney L, Easton DF, Eeles RA. Targeted prostate cancer screening in men with mutations in BRCA1 and BRCA2 detects aggressive prostate cancer: preliminary analysis of the results of the IMPACT study. BJU Int. 2011;107(1):28–39.

Monteiro AN. BRCA1: the enigma of tissue-specific tumor development. Trends Genet. 2003;19(6):312–5.

Moreira L, Balaguer F, Lindor N, de la Chapelle A, Hampel H, Aaltonen LA, Hopper JL, Le ML, Gallinger S, Newcomb PA, Haile R, Thibodeau SN, Gunawardena S, Jenkins MA, Buchanan DD, Potter JD, Baron JA, Ahnen DJ, Moreno V, Andreu M, de Ponz LM, Rustgi AK, Castells A. Identification of Lynch syndrome among patients with colorectal cancer. JAMA. 2012;308(15):1555–65.

Mori M, Harabuchi I, Miyake H, Casagrande JT, Henderson BE, Ross RK. Reproductive, genetic, and dietary risk factors for ovarian cancer. Am J Epidemiol. 1988;128:771–7.

Moslehi R, Chu W, Karlan B, Fishman D, Risch H, Fields A, Smotkin D, Ben-David Y, Rosenblatt J, Russo D, Schwartz P, Tung N, Warner E, Rosen B, Friedman J, Brunet JS, Narod SA. BRCA1 and BRCA2 mutation analysis of 208 Ashkenazi Jewish women with ovarian cancer. Am J Hum Genet. 2000;66:1259–72.

Moynahan ME, Cui TY, Jasin M. Homology-directed DNA repair, mitomycin-c resistance, and chromosome stability is restored with correction of a Brca1 mutation. Cancer Res. 2001;61:4842–50.

Murdoch S, Djuric U, Mazhar B, Seoud M, Khan R, Kuick R, Bagga R, Kircheisen R, Ao A, Ratti B, Hanash S, Rouleau GA, Slim R. Mutations in NALP7 cause recurrent hydatidiform moles and reproductive wastage in humans. Nat Genet. 2006;38(3):300–2. Epub 2006 Feb 5.

Narod SA. Breast cancer in young women. Nat Rev Clin Oncol. 2012a;9(8):460–70.

Narod SA. The tip of the iceberg: A Countercurrents Series. Curr Oncol. 2012b;19(3):129–30.

Narod SA, Risch H, Moslehi R, Dorum A, Neuhausen S, Olsson H, Provencher D, Radice P, Evans G, Bishop S, Brunet JS, Ponder BA. Oral contraceptives and the risk of hereditary ovarian cancer. Hereditary Ovarian Cancer Clinical Study Group. New Engl J Med. 1998;339(7):424–8 [see comments].

Narod SA, Dube MP, Klijn J, et al. Oral contraceptives and the risk of breast cancer in BRCA1 and BRCA2 mutation carriers. J Natl Cancer Inst. 2002;94:1773–9.

Narod SA, Neuhausen S, Vichodez G, Armel S, Lynch HT, Ghadirian P, Cummings S, Olopade O, Stoppa-Lyonnet D, Couch F, Wagner T, Warner E, Foulkes WD, Saal H, Weitzel J, Tulman A, Poll A, Nam R, Sun P. Hereditary Breast Cancer Study Group, Danquah J, Domchek S, Tung N, Ainsworth P, Horsman D, Kim-Sing C, Maugard C, Eisen A, Daly M, McKinnon W, Wood M, Isaacs C, Gilchrist D, Karlan B, Nedelcu R, Meschino W, Garber J, Pasini B, Manoukian S, Bellati C. Rapid progression of prostate cancer in men with a BRCA2 mutation. Br J Cancer. 2008;99(2):371–4.

Newschaffer CJ, Topham A, Herzberg T, Weiner S, Weinberg DS. Risk of colorectal cancer after breast cancer. Lancet. 2001;357:837–40.

Nicholson PW, Harland SJ. Inheritance and testicular cancer. Br J Cancer. 1995;71(2):421–6.

Nieder AM, Taneja SS, Zeegens MP. Oshertt, genetic counselling for prostate can-cer risk. Clin Genet. 2003;63:169–76.

Nik-Zainal S, Alexandrov LB, Wedge DC, Van LP, Greenman CD, Raine K, Jones D, Hinton J, Marshall J, Stebbings LA, Menzies A, Martin S, Leung K, Chen L, Leroy C, Ramakrishna M, Rance R, Lau KW, Mudie LJ, Varela I, McBride DJ, Bignell GR, Cooke SL, Shlien A, Gamble J, Whitmore I, Maddison M, Tarpey PS, Davies HR, Papaemmanuil E, Stephens PJ, McLaren S, Butler AP, Teague JW, Jonsson G, Garber JE, Silver D, Miron P, Fatima A, Boyault S, Langerod A, Tutt A, Martens JW, Aparicio SA, Borg A, Salomon AV, Thomas G, Borresen-Dale AL, Richardson AL, Neuberger MS, Futreal PA, Campbell PJ, Stratton MR. Mutational processes molding the genomes of 21 breast cancers. Cell. 2012;149(5):979–93.

Norquist B, Wurz KA, Pennil CC, Garcia R, Gross J, Sakai W, Karlan BY, Taniguchi T, Swisher EM. Secondary Somatic Mutations Restoring BRCA1/2 Predict Chemotherapy Resistance in Hereditary Ovarian Carcinomas. J Clin Oncol. 2011;29:3008–15.

O'Shaughnessy J, Osborne C, Pippen JE, Yoffe M, Patt D, Rocha C, Koo IC, Sherman BM, Bradley C. Iniparib plus chemotherapy in metastatic triple-negative breast cancer. N Engl J Med. 2011;364(3):205–14.

Obermair A, Youlden DR, Young JP, Lindor NM, Baron JA, Newcomb P, Parry S, Hopper JL, Haile R, Jenkins MA. Risk of endometrial cancer for women diagnosed with HNPCC-related colorectal carcinoma. International. Journal.of. Cancer. 2010;127(11):2678–84.

Pal T, Permuth-Wey J, Betts JA, Krischer JP, Fiorica J, Arango H, LaPolla J, Hoffman M, Martino MA, Wakeley K, Wilbanks G, Nicosia S, Cantor A, Sutphen R. BRCA1 and BRCA2 mutations account for a large proportion of ovarian carcinoma cases. Cancer. 2005;104(12):2807–16.

Palma L, Marcus V, Gilbert L, Chong G, Foulkes WD. Synchronous occult cancers of the endometrium and fallopian tube in an MSH2 mutation carrier at time of prophylactic surgery. Gynecol Oncol. 2008;111(3):575–8.

Parazzini F, Negri E, La Vecchia C, Restelli C, Franceschi S. Family history of reproductive cancers and ovarian cancer risk: an Italian case–control study. Am J Epidemiol. 1992;135:35–40.

Parry DA, Logan CV, Hayward BE, Shires M, Landolsi H, Diggle C, Carr I, Rittore C, Touitou I, Philibert L, Fisher RA, Fallahian M, Huntriss JD, Picton HM, Malik S, Taylor GR, Johnson CA, Bonthron DT, Sheridan EG. Mutations causing familial biparental hydatidiform mole implicate c6orf221 as a possible regulator of genomic imprinting in the human oocyte. Am J Hum Genet. 2011;89(3):451–8.

Passaperuma K, Warner E, Causer PA, Hill KA, Messner S, Wong JW, Jong RA, Wright FC, Yaffe MJ, Ramsay EA, Balasingham S, Verity L, Eisen A, Curpen B, Shumak R, Plewes DB, Narod SA. Long-term results of screening with magnetic resonance imaging in women with BRCA mutations. British. Journal.of. Cancer. 2012;107(1):24–30.

Patel KJ, Yu VP, Lee H, Corcoran A, Thistlethwaite FC, Evans MJ, Colledge WH, Friedman LS, Ponder BA, Venkitaraman AR. Involvement of Brca2 in DNA repair. Mol Cell. 1998;1:347–57.

Pathania S, Nguyen J, Hill SJ, Scully R, Adelmant GO, Marto JA, Feunteun J, Livingston DM. BRCA1 is required for postreplication repair after UV-induced DNA damage. Mol Cell. 2011;44(2):235–51.

Penrose LS, Mackenzie HJ, Karn MN. A genetic study of human mammary cancer. Ann Eugen. 1948;14:234–66.

Pérez J, Rodón J, Cortés J, Ellisen LW, Scaltriti M, Baselga J. PI3K inhibition impairs BRCA1/2 expression and sensitizes BRCA-proficient triple-negative breastcancer to PARP inhibition. Cancer Discov. 2012;2(11):1036–47.

Peto J, Collins N, Barfoot R, Seal S, Warren W, Rahman N, Easton DF, Evans C, Deacon J, Stratton MR. Prevalence of BRCA1 and BRCA2 gene mutations in patients with early-onset breast cancer. J Nat Cancer Inst. 1999;91:943–9 [see comments].

Peto J, Easton DF, Matthews FE, et al. Cancer mortality in relatives of women with breast cancer: the OPCS study. Int J Cancer. 1996;65:275–8.

Pharoah PD, Antoniou AC, Easton DF, Ponder BA. Polygenes, risk prediction, and targeted prevention of breast cancer. N. Engl. J. Med. 2008;358(26):2796–803.

Piek JM, van Diest PJ, Zweemer RP, Jansen JW, Poort-Keesom RJ, Menko FH, Gille JJ, Jongsma AP, Pals G, Kenemans P, Verheijen RH. Dysplastic changes in prophylactically removed Fallopian tubes of women predisposed to developing ovarian cancer. J Pathol. 2001;195(4):451–6.

Piek JM, van Diest PJ, Verheijen RH. Ovarian carcinogenesis: an alternative hypothesis. Adv Exp Med Biol. 2008;622:79–87.

Rafnar T, Gudbjartsson DF, Sulem P, Jonasdottir A, Sigurdsson A, Jonasdottir A, Besenbacher S, Lundin P, Stacey SN, Gudmundsson J, Magnusson OT, le Roux L, Orlygsdottir G, Helgadottir HT, Johannsdottir H, Gylfason A, Tryggvadottir L, Jonasson JG, de Juan A, Ortega E, Ramon-Cajal JM, García-Prats MD, Mayordomo C, Panadero A, Rivera F, Aben KK, van Altena AM, Massuger LF, Aavikko M, Kujala PM, Staff S, Aaltonen LA, Olafsdottir K, Bjornsson J, Kong

A, Salvarsdottir A, Saemundsson H, Olafsson K, Benediktsdottir KR, Gulcher J, Masson G, Kiemeney LA, Mayordomo JI, Thorsteinsdottir U, Stefansson K. Mutations in BRIP1 confer high risk of ovarian cancer. Nat Genet. 2011;43(11):1104–7.

Ragnarsson-Olding BK. Primary malignant melanoma of the vulva-an aggressive tumour for modelling the genesis of non-UV light-associated melanoma. Acta Oncol. 2004;43:421–35.

Rapley EA, Crockford GP, Teare D, et al. Localization to Xq27 of a susceptibility gene for testicular germ-cell tumours. Nat Genet. 2000;24:197–200.

Rapley EA, Turnbull C, Al Olama AA, Dermitzakis ET, Linger R, Huddart RA, Renwick A, Hughes D, Hines S, Seal S, Morrison J, Nsengimana J, Deloukas P; UK Testicular Cancer Collaboration, Rahman N, Bishop DT, Easton DF, Stratton MR. A genome-wide association study of testicular germ cell tumor. Nat Genet. 2009;41(7):807–10. doi: 10.1038/ng.394.

Rebbeck TR, Lynch HT, Neuhausen SL, Narod SA, Van't Veer L, Garber JE, Evans G, Isaacs C, Daly MB, Matloff E, Olopade OI, Weber BL. Prophylactic oophorectomy in carriers of BRCA1 or BRCA2 mutations. New Engl J Med. 2002;346:1616–22.

Rebbeck TR, Friebel T, Lynch HT, Neuhausen SL, van Veer L, Garber JE, Evans GR, Narod SA, Isaacs C, Matloff E, Daly MB, Olopade OI, Weber BL. Bilateral prophylactic mastectomy reduces breast cancer risk in BRCA1 and BRCA2 mutation carriers: the PROSE Study Group. J Clin Oncol. 2004;22:1055–62.

Renwick A, Thompson D, Seal S, Kelly P, Chagtai T, Ahmed M, North B, Jayatilake H, Barfoot R, Spanova K, McGuffog L, Evans DG, Eccles D, Easton DF, Stratton MR, Rahman N. ATM mutations that cause ataxia-telangiectasia are breast cancer susceptibility alleles. Nat Genet. 2006;38(8):873–5.

Rijnsburger AJ, Obdeijn IM, Kaas R, Tilanus-Linthorst MM, Boetes C, Loo CE, Wasser MN, Bergers E, Kok T, Muller SH, Peterse H, Tollenaar RA, Hoogerbrugge N, Meijer S, Bartels CC, Seynaeve C, Hooning MJ, Kriege M, Schmitz PI, Oosterwijk JC, de Koning HJ, Rutgers EJ, Klijn JG. BRCA1-associated breast cancers present differently from BRCA2-associated and familial cases: long-term follow-up of the Dutch MRISC Screening Study. J Clin Oncol. 2010;28(36):5265–73.

Rio Frio T, Bahubeshi A, Kanellopoulou C, Hamel N, Niedziela M, Sabbaghian N, Pouchet C, Gilbert L, O'Brien PK, Serfas K, Broderick P, Houlston RS, Lesueur F, Bonora E, Muljo S, Schimke RN, Bouron-Dal SD, Arseneau J, Schultz KA, Priest JR, Nguyen VH, Harach HR, Livingston DM, Foulkes WD, Tischkowitz M. DICER1 mutations in familial multinodular goiter with and without ovarian Sertoli-Leydig cell tumors. JAMA. 2011;305(1):68–77.

Robson M. Tamoxifen for primary breast cancer prevention in BRCA heterozygotes. Eur J Cancer. 2002;38 Suppl 6:S18–9.

Rogers LF. Screening mammography: target of opportunity for the media. Am J Roentgenol. 2003;180:1.

Rose PG, Hunter RE. Advanced ovarian cancer in a woman with a family history of ovarian cancer, discovered at referral for prophylactic oophorectomy. A case report. J Repr Med. 1994;39:908–910.

Rosenberg L, Palmer JR, Zauber AG, Warshauer ME, Lewis JLJ, Strom BL, Harlap S, Shapiro S. A case–control study of oral contraceptive use and invasive epithelial ovarian cancer. Am J Epidemiol. 1994;139:654–61.

Ruark E, Snape K, Humburg P, Loveday C, Bajrami I, Brough R, Rodrigues DN, Renwick A, Seal S, Ramsay E, Duarte SV, Rivas MA, Warren-Perry M, Zachariou A, Campion-Flora A, Hanks S, Murray A, Pour NA, Douglas J, Gregory L, Rimmer A, Walker NM, Yang TP, Adlard JW, Barwell J, Berg J, Brady AF, Brewer C, Brice G, Chapman C, Cook J, Davidson R, Donaldson A, Douglas F, Eccles D, Evans DG, Greenhalgh L, Henderson A, Izatt L, Kumar A, Lalloo F, Miedzybrodzka Z, Morrison PJ, Paterson J, Porteous M, Rogers MT, Shanley S, Walker L, Gore M, Houlston R, Brown MA, Caufield MJ, Deloukas P, McCarthy MI, Todd JA, Turnbull C, Reis-Filho JS, Ashworth A, Antoniou AC, Lord CJ, Donnelly P, Rahman N. Mosaic PPM1D mutations are associated with predisposition to breast and ovarian cancer. Nature. 2013;493(7432):406–10.

Rutter JL, Wacholder S, Chetrit A, Lubin F, Menczer J, Ebbers S, Tucker MA, Struewing JP, Hartge P. Gynecologic surgeries and risk of ovarian cancer in women with BRCA1 and BRCA2

Ashkenazi founder mutations: an Israeli population-based case-control study. J Natl Cancer Inst. 2003;95:1072–8.

Sakai W, Swisher EM, Karlan BY, Agarwal MK, Higgins J, Friedman C, Villegas E, Jacquemont C, Farrugia DJ, Couch FJ, et al. Secondary mutations as a mechanism of cisplatin resistance in BRCA2-mutated cancers. Nature. 2008;451:1116–20.

Schildkraut JM, Thompson WD. Familial ovarian cancer: a population based case–control study. Am J Epidemiol. 1988;128:456–66.

Schmeler KM, Lynch HT, Chen LM, Munsell MF, Soliman PT, Clark MB, Daniels MS, White KG, Boyd-Rogers SG, Conrad PG, Yang KY, Rubin MM, Sun CC, Slomovitz BM, Gershenson DM, Lu KH. Prophylactic surgery to reduce the risk of gynecologic cancers in the Lynch syndrome. N Engl J Med. 2006;354(3):261–9.

Schneider BP, Winer EP, Foulkes WD, Garber J, Perou CM, Richardson A, Sledge GW, Carey LA. Triple-negative breast cancer: risk factors to potential targets. Clin Cancer Res. 2008;14(24):8010–8.

Schorge JO, Muto MG, Lee SJ, Huang LW, Welch WR, Bell DA, Keung EZ, Berkowitz RS, Mok SC. BRCA1-related papillary serous carcinoma of the peritoneum has a unique molecular pathogenesis. Cancer Res. 2000;60:1361–4.

Schultz KA, Pacheco MC, Yang J, Williams GM, Messinger Y, Hill DA, Dehner LP, Priest JR. Ovarian sex cord-stromal tumors, pleuropulmonary blastoma and DICER1 mutations: A report from the International Pleuropulmonary Blastoma Registry. Gynecol Oncol. 2011;122(2):246–50.

Schwartz MD, Lerman C, Brogan B, Peshkin BN, Halbert CH, DeMarco T, Lawrence W, Main D, Finch C, Magnant C, Pennanen M, Tsangaris T, Willey S, Isaacs C. Impact of BRCA1/BRCA2 counseling and testing on newly diagnosed breast cancer patients. J Clin Oncol. 2004;22(10):1823–9.

Schwartz MD, Lerman C, Brogan B, Peshkin BN, Isaacs C, DeMarco T, Halbert CH, Pennanen M, Finch C. Utilization of BRCA1/BRCA2 mutation testing in newly diagnosed breast cancer patients. Cancer Epidemiol Biomarkers Prev. 2005;14(4):1003–7.

Scully RE. Influence of origin of ovarian cancer on efficacy of screening. Lancet. 2000;355:1028–9 [see comments].

Scully R, Livingston DM. In search of the tumor-suppressor functions of BRCA1 and BRCA2. Nature. 2000;408(6811):429–32.

Seal S, Thompson D, Renwick A, Elliott A, Kelly P, Barfoot R, Chagtai T, Jayatilake H, Ahmed M, Spanova K, North B, McGuffog L, Evans DG, Eccles D, Easton DF, Stratton MR, Rahman N. Truncating mutations in the Fanconi anemia J gene BRIP1 are low-penetrance breast cancer susceptibility alleles. Nat Genet. 2006;38(11):1239–41.

Sidransky D, Tokino T, Helzlsouer K, Zehnbauer B, Rausch G, Shelton B, Prestigiacomo L, Vogelstein B, Davidson N. Inherited p53 gene mutations in breast cancer. Cancer Res. 1992;52:2984–6.

Sigurdsson S, Thorlacius S, Tomasson J, Tryggvadottir L, Benediktsdottir K, Eyfjörd JE, Jonsson E. BRCA2 mutation in Icelandic prostate cancer patients. J Mol Med (Berl). 1997;75(10):758–61.

Silver DP, Livingston DM. Mechanisms of BRCA1 Tumor Suppression. Cancer Discov. 2012;2(8):679–84.

Silver DP, Richardson AL, Eklund AC, Wang ZC, Szallasi Z, Li Q, Juul N, Leong CO, Calogrias D, Buraimoh A, Fatima A, Gelman RS, Ryan PD, Tung NM, De NA, Ganesan S, Miron A, Colin C, Sgroi DC, Ellisen LW, Winer EP, Garber JE. Efficacy of neoadjuvant Cisplatin in triple-negative breast cancer. J Clin Oncol. 2010;28(7):1145–53.

Slade I, Bacchelli C, Davies H, Murray A, Abbaszadeh F, Hanks S, Barfoot R, Burke A, Chisholm J, Hewitt M, Jenkinson H, King D, Morland B, Pizer B, Prescott K, Saggar A, Side L, Traunecker H, Vaidya S, Ward P, Futreal PA, Vujanic G, Nicholson AG, Sebire N, Turnbull C, Priest JR, Pritchard-Jones K, Houlston R, Stiller C, Stratton MR, Douglas J, Rahman N. DICER1 syndrome: clarifying the diagnosis, clinical features and management implications of a pleiotropic tumor predisposition syndrome. J Med Genet. 2011;48(4):273–8.

Smith TE, Lee D, Turner BC, Carter D, Haffty BG. True recurrence vs. new primary ipsilateral breast tumor relapse: an analysis of clinical and pathologic differences and their implications in natural history, prognoses, and therapeutic management. Int J Radiat Oncol Biol Phys. 2000;48(5):1281–9.

Snijders-Keilholz A, Ewing P, Seynaeve C, Burger CW. Primitive neuroectodermal tumor of the cervix uteri: a case report – changing concepts in therapy. Gynecol Oncol. 2005;98(3):516–9.

Sonneveld DJ, Sleijfer DT, Schrafford Koops H, Sijmons RH, van der Graaf WT, Sluiter WJ, Hoekstra HJ. Familial testicular cancer in a single-centre population. Eur J Cancer. 1999;35:1368–73.

Sorlie T, Tibshirani R, Parker J, Hastie T, Marron JS, Nobel A, Deng S, Johnsen H, Pesich R, Geisler S, Demeter J, Perou CM, Lonning PE, Brown PO, Borresen-Dale AL, Botstein D. Repeated observation of breast tumor subtypes in independent gene expression data sets. Proc Natl Acad Sci USA. 2003;100:8418–23.

Southey MC, Teo ZL, Dowty JG, Odefrey FA, Park DJ, Tischkowitz M, Sabbaghian N, Apicella C, Byrnes GB, Winship I, Baglietto L, Giles GG, Goldgar DE, Foulkes WD, Hopper JL. A PALB2 mutation associated with high risk of breast cancer. Breast Cancer Res. 2010;12(6):R109.

Steinberg GS, Carter BS, Beaty TH, Childs B, Walsh PC. Family history and the risk of prostate cancer. Prostate. 1990;17:337–47.

Stoppa-Lyonnet D, Laurent-Puig P, Essioux L, Pages S, Ithier G, Ligot L, Fourquet A, Salmon RJ, Clough KB, Pouillart P, Bonaiti-Pellie C, Thomas G. BRCA1 sequence variations in 160 individuals referred to a breast/ovarian family cancer clinic. Institute Curie Breast Cancer Group. Am J Hum Genet. 1997;60:1021–30 [see comments].

Stratakis CA, Papageorgiou T, Premkumar A, Pack S, Kirschner LS, Taymans SE, Zhuang ZP, Oelkers WH, Carney JA. Ovarian lesions in Carney complex: clinical genetics and possible predisposition to malignancy. J Clin Endocrinol Metab. 2000;85:4359–66.

Swisher EM, Sakai W, Karlan BY, Wurz K, Urban N, Taniguchi T. Secondary BRCA1 mutations in BRCA1-mutated ovarian carcinomas with platinum resistance. Cancer Res. 2008;68:2581–6.

Szabo CI, Schutte M, Broeks A, Houwing-Duistermaat JJ, Thorstenson YR, Durocher F, Oldenburg RA, Wasielewski M, Odefrey F, Thompson D, Floore AN, Kraan J, Klijn JG, van den Ouweland AM, Wagner TM, Devilee P, Simard J, Van't Veer LJ, Goldgar DE, Meijers-Heijboer H. Are ATM mutations 7271T–>G and IVS10–6T–>G really high-risk breast cancer-susceptibility alleles? Cancer Res. 2004;64(3):840–3.

Tan MH, Mester JL, Ngeow J, Rybicki LA, Orloff MS, Eng C. Lifetime cancer risks in individuals with germline PTEN mutations. Clin Cancer Res. 2012;18(2):400–40.

Tassone P, Tagliaferri P, Perricelli A, Blotta S, Quaresima B, Martelli ML, Goel A, Barbieri V, Costanzo F, Boland CR, Venuta S. BRCA1 expression modu-lates chemosensitivity of BRCA1-defective HCC1937 human breast cancer cells. Br J Cancer. 2003;88:1285–91.

Thiffault I, Hamel N, Pal T, McVety S, Marcus VA, Farber D, Cowie S, Deschenes J, Meschino W, Odefrey F, Goldgar D, Graham T, Narod S, Watters AK, MacNamara E, du SD, Chong G, Foulkes WD. Germline truncating mutations in both MSH2 and BRCA2 in a single kindred. Brit J Cancer. 2004;90(2):483–91.

Thompson D, Easton D. Variation in cancer risks, by mutation position, in BRCA2 mutation carriers. Am J Hum Genet. 2001;68:410–9.

Thompson D, Easton DF. Cancer incidence in BRCA1 mutation carriers. J Natl Cancer Inst. 2002;94:1358–65.

Thompson D, Duedal S, Kirner J, McGuffog L, Last J, Reiman A, Byrd P, Taylor M, Easton DF. Cancer risks and mortality in heterozygous ATM mutation carriers. J Natl Cancer Inst. 2005;97(11):813–22.

Thorne H, Willems AJ, Niedermayr E, Hoh IM, Li J, Clouston D, Mitchell G, Fox S, Hopper JL, Kathleen Cunningham Consortium for Research in Familial Breast Cancer Consortium, Bolton D. Decreased prostate cancer-specific survival of men with BRCA2 mutations from multiple breast cancer families. Cancer Prev Res (Phila). 2011a;4(7):1002–10.

Thorne H, et al. Decreased prostate cancer-specific survival of men with BRCA2 mutations from multiple breast cancer families. Cancer Prev Res. 2011b;4(7):1002–10.

Tilanus-Linthorst M, Verhoog L, Obdeijn IM, Bartels K, Menke-Pluymers M, Eggermont A, Klijn J, Meijers-Heijboer H, van der Kwast T, Brekelmans C. A BRCA1/2 mutation, high breast density and prominent pushing margins of a tumor independently contribute to a frequent false-negative mammography. Int J Cancer. 2002;102:91–5.

Tinari A, Pace S, Fambrini M, et al. Vulvar Pagets disease: review of the literature, considerations about histogenetic hypothesis and surgical approaches. Eur J Gynaecol Oncol. 2002;23:551–2.

Tischkowitz M, Xia B. PALB2/FANCN: recombining cancer and Fanconi anemia. Cancer Res. 2010;70(19):7353–9.

Tolvanen J, Uimari O, Ryynanen M, Aaltonen LA, Vahteristo P. Strong family history of uterine leiomyomatosis warrants fumarate hydratase mutation screening. Hum Reprod. 2012;27(6):1865–9.

Tomlinson IP, Alam NA, Rowan AJ, et al. Germline mutations in FH predispose to dominantly inherited uterine fibroids, skin leiomyomata and papillary renal cell caricinoma. Nat Genet. 2002;30:406–10.

Tone AA, Salvador S, Finlayson SJ, Tinker AV, Kwon JS, Lee CH, Cohen T, Ehlen T, Lee M, Carey MS, Heywood M, Pike J, Hoskins PJ, Stuart GC, Swenerton KD, Huntsman DG, Gilks CB, Miller DM, McAlpine JN. The role of the fallopian tube in ovarian cancer. Clin Adv Hematol Oncol. 2012;10(5):296–306.

Tryggvadóttir L, Vidarsdóttir L, Thorgeirsson T, Jonasson JG, Olafsdóttir EJ, Olafsdóttir GH, Rafnar T, Thorlacius S, Jonsson E, Eyfjord JE, Tulinius H. Prostate cancer progression and survival in BRCA2 mutation carriers. J Natl Cancer Inst. 2007;99(12):929–35.

Turnbull C, Rapley EA, Seal S, Pernet D, Renwick A, Hughes D, Ricketts M, Linger R, Nsengimana J, Deloukas P, Huddart RA, Bishop DT, Easton DF, Stratton MR, Rahman N; UK Testicular Cancer Collaboration. Variants near DMRT1, TERT and ATF7IP are associated with testicular germ cell cancer. Nat Genet. 2010;42(7):604–7.

Tutt A, Robson M, Garber JE, Domchek SM, Audeh MW, Weitzel JN, Friedlander M, Arun B, Loman N, Schmutzler RK, et al. Oral poly(ADP-ribose) polymerase inhibitor olaparib in patients with BRCA1 or BRCA2 mutations and advanced breast cancer: a proof-of-concept trial. Lancet. 2010;376:235–44.

Tzonou A, Day NE, Trichopoulos D, Walker A, Saliaraki M, Papapostolou M, Polychronopoulou A. The epidemiology of ovarian cancer in Greece: a case–control study. Eur J Cancer clin Oncol. 1984;20:1045–52.

Ulbright TM, Amin MB, Young RH. Intratubular large cell hyalinizing sertoli cell neoplasia of the testis: a report of 8 cases of a distinctive lesion of the Peutz-Jeghers syndrome. Am J Surg Pathol. 2007;31(6):827–35.

van Nagell J, DePriest PD, Reedy MB, Gallion HH, Ueland FR, Pavlik EJ, Kryscio RJ. The efficacy of transvaginal sonographic screening in asymptomatic women at risk for ovarian cancer. Gynecol Oncol. 2000;77:350–6.

van Oostrom I, Meijers-Heijboer H, Lodder LN, Duivenvoorden HJ, van Gool AR, Seynaeve C, van der Meer CA, Klijn JG, van Geel BN, Burger CW, Wladimiroff JW, Tibben A. Long-term psychological impact of carrying a BRCA1/2 mutation and prophylactic surgery: a 5-year follow-up study. J Clin Oncol. 2003;21(20):3867–74.

Van't Veer LJ, Dai HY, van de Vijver MJ, He YDD, Hart AAM, Mao M, Peterse HL, van der Kooy K, Marton MJ, Witteveen AT, Schreiber GJ, Kerkhoven RM, Roberts C, Linsley PS, Bernards R, Friend SH. Gene expression profiling predicts clinical outcome of breast cancer. Nature. 2002;415:530–6.

Vang R, Taubenberger JK, Mannion CM, et al. Primary vulvar and vaginal extraosseous Ewing's sarcoma/peripheral neuroectodermal tumour: diagnostic confirm-ation with CD99 immunostaining and reverse transcriptase-polymerase chain reaction. Int J Gynaecol Pathol. 2000;19:103–9.

Vanin K, Scurry J, Thorne H, et al. Overexpression of wild-type p53 in lichen sclerosus adjacent human papillomavirus-negative vulvar cancer. J Invest Dermatol. 2002;119:1027–33.

Vasen HF, Stormorken A, Menko FH, Nagengast FM, Kleibeuker JH, Griffioen G, Taal BG, Moller P, Wijnen JT. Msh2 mutation carriers are at higher risk of cancer than mlh1 mutation carriers: a study of hereditary nonpolyposis colorectal cancer families. J Clin Oncol. 2001;19(20):4074–80.

Vasen HF, Moslein G, Alonso A, Bernstein I, Bertario L, Blanco I, Burn J, Capella G, Engel C, Frayling I, Friedl W, Hes FJ, Hodgson S, Mecklin JP, Moller P, Nagengast F, Parc Y, Renkonen-Sinisalo L, Sampson JR, Stormorken A, Wijnen J. Guidelines for the clinical management of Lynch syndrome (hereditary non-polyposis cancer). J Med Genet. 2007;44(6):353–62.

Vasen HFA, Blanco I, Aktan K, Gopie JP, Alonso A, Aretz S, Bernstein I, Bertario L, Burn J, Capella G, Colas C, Engel C, Frayling IM, Genuardi M, Heinimann K, Hes FJ, Hodgson S, Karagiannis JA, Lalloo F, Lindblom A, Mecklin J-P, MØller P, Myrhoj T, Nagengast FN, Parc Y, Ponz de Leon M, Renkonen-Sinisalo L, Sampson JR, Stormorken A, Sijmons R, Tejpar S, Thomas HJW, Wijnen J, Järvinen H, Möslein G, (the Mallorca group). Revised guidelines for the clinical management of Lynch syndrome (HNPCC). Gut. 2013;62(6):812–23.

Venkitaraman AR. Cancer susceptibility and the functions of BRCA1 and BRCA2. Cell. 2002;108:171–82.

Vicus D, Finch A, Cass I, Rosen B, Murphy J, Fan I, Royer R, McLaughlin J, Karlan B, Narod SA. Prevalence of BRCA1 and BRCA2 germ line mutations among women with carcinoma of the fallopian tube. Gynecol Oncol. 2010;118(3):299–302.

Walsh T, Casadei S, Lee MK, Pennil CC, Nord AS, Thornton AM, Roeb W, Agnew KJ, Stray SM, Wickramanayake A, Norquist B, Pennington KP, Garcia RL, King MC, Swisher EM. Mutations in 12 genes for inherited ovarian, fallopian tube, and peritoneal carcinoma identified by massively parallel sequencing. Proc Natl Acad Sci USA. 2011;108(44):18032–7.

Warner E, Plewes DB, Hill KA, Causer PA, Zubovits JT, Jong RA, Cutrara MR, DeBoer G, Yaffe MJ, Messner SJ, Meschino WS, Piron CA, Narod SA. Surveillance of BRCA1 and BRCA2 mutation carriers with magnetic resonance imaging, ultrasound, mammography, and clinical breast examination. J Am Med Assoc. 2004;292(11):1317–25.

Warner E, Hill K, Causer P, Plewes D, Jong R, Yaffe M, Foulkes WD, Ghadirian P, Lynch H, Couch F, Wong J, Wright F, Sun P, Narod SA. Prospective study of breast cancer incidence in women with a BRCA1 or BRCA2 mutation under surveillance with and without magnetic resonance imaging. J Clin Oncol. 2011;29(13):1664–9.

Wechter ME, Gruber SB, Haefner HK, et al. Vulvar melanoma: a report of 20 cases and review of the literature. J Am Acad Dermatol. 2004;50:554–62.

Werness BA, Parvatiyar P, Ramus SJ, Whittemore AS, Garlinghouse-Jones K, Oakley-Girvan I, DiCioccio RA, Wiest J, Tsukada Y, Ponder BAJ, Piver MS. Ovarian carcinoma in situ with germline BRCA1 mutation and loss of heterozy-gosity at BRCA1 and TP53. J Natl Cancer Inst. 2000;92:1088–91.

Wessels LFA, van Welsem T, Hart AAM, Van't Veer LJ, Reinders MJT, Nederlof PM. Molecular classification of breast carcinomas by comparative genomic hybridization: a specific somatic genetic profile for BRCA1 tumors. Cancer Res. 2002;62:7110–7.

Whittemore AS, Balise RR, Pharoah PD, DiCioccio RA, Oakley-Girvan I, Ramus SJ, Daly M, Usinowicz MB, Garlinghouse-Jones K, Ponder BA, Buys S, Senie R, Andrulis I, John E, Hopper JL, Piver MS. Oral contraceptive use and ovarian cancer risk among carriers of BRCA1 or BRCA2 mutations. Br J Cancer. 2004a;91:1911–5.

Whittemore AS, Gongm G, John EM, McGuire V, Li FP, Ostrow KL, Dicioccio R, Felberg A, West DW. Prevalence of BRCA1 mutation carriers among US non-hispanic Whites. Cancer Epidemiol Biomarker Prev. 2004b;13:2078–83.

Willems AJ, Dawson SJ, Samaratunga H, De Luca A, Antill YC, Hopper JL, Thorne HJ. kConFab Investigators. Loss of heterozygosity at the BRCA2 locus detected by multiplex ligation-dependent probe amplification is common in prostate cancers from men with a germline BRCA2 mutation. Clin Cancer Res. 2008;14(10):2953–61.

Wilson JR, Bateman AC, Hanson H, An Q, Evans G, Rahman N, Jones JL, Eccles DM. A novel HER2-positive breast cancer phenotype arising from germline TP53 mutations. J Med Genet. 2010;47(11):771–4.

Win AK, Young JP, Lindor NM, Tucker KM, Ahnen DJ, Young GP, Buchanan DD, Clendenning M, Giles GG, Winship I, Macrae FA, Goldblatt J, Southey MC, Arnold J, Thibodeau SN,

Gunawardena SR, Bapat B, Baron JA, Casey G, Gallinger S, Le ML, Newcomb PA, Haile RW, Hopper JL, Jenkins MA. Colorectal and other cancer risks for carriers and noncarriers from families with a DNA mismatch repair gene mutation: a prospective cohort study. J Clin Oncol. 2012;30(9):958–64.

Wong MW, Nordfors C, Mossman D, Pecenpetelovska G, Avery-Kiejda KA, Talseth-Palmer B, Bowden NA, Scott RJ. BRIP1, PALB2, and RAD51C mutation analysis reveals their relative importance as genetic susceptibility factors for breast cancer. Breast Cancer Res Treat. 2011;127(3):853–9.

Wynder EL, Dodo H, Barber HR. Epidemiology of cancer of the ovary. Cancer. 1969;23:352–70.

Xu J, Lange EM, Lu L, Zheng SL, Wang Z, Thibodeau SN, Cannon-Albright LA, Teerlink CC, Camp NJ, Johnson AM, Zuhlke KA, Stanford JL, Ostrander EA, Wiley KE, Isaacs SD, Walsh PC, Maier C, Luedeke M, Vogel W, Schleutker J, Wahlfors T, Tammela T, Schaid D, McDonnell SK, DeRycke MS, Cancel-Tassin G, Cussenot O, Wiklund F, Grönberg H, Eeles R, Easton D, Kote-Jarai Z, Whittemore AS, Hsieh CL, Giles GG, Hopper JL, Severi G, Catalona WJ, Mandal D, Ledet E, Foulkes WD, Hamel N, Mahle L, Moller P, Powell I, Bailey-Wilson JE, Carpten JD, Seminara D, Cooney KA, Isaacs WB. International Consortium for Prostate Cancer Genetics. HOXB13 is a susceptibility gene for prostate cancer: results from the International Consortium for Prostate Cancer Genetics (ICPCG). Hum Genet. 2013;132(1):5–14.

Yuan SSF, Lee SY, Chen G, Song MH, Tomlinson GE, Lee EYHP. BRCA2 is required for ionizing radiation-induced assembly of rad51 complex in vivo. Cancer Res. 1999;59:3547–51.

Zbuk KM, Patocs A, Shealy A, Sylvester H, Miesfeldt S, Eng C. Germline mutations in PTEN and SDHC in a woman with epithelial thyroid cancer and carotid paraganglioma. Nat Clin Pract Oncol. 2007;4(10):608–12.

Zhong Q, et al. Association of BRCA1 with the hRad50–hMre11–p95 complex and the DNA damage response. Science. 1999;285(5428):747–50.

Zuhlke KA, Madeoy JJ, Beebe-Dimmer J, White KA, Griffin A, Lange EM, Gruber SB, Ostrander EA, Cooney KA. Truncating BRCA1 mutations are uncommon in a cohort of hereditary prostate cancer families with evidence of linkage to 17q markers. Clin Cancer Res. 2004;10 (18 Pt 1):5975–80.

Zweemer RP, van Diest PJ, Verheijen RH, Ryan A, Gille JJ, Sijmons RH, Jacobs IJ, Menko FH, Kenemans P. Molecular evidence linking primary cancer of the fallopian tube to BRCA1 germline mutations. Gynecol Oncol. 2000;76(1):45–50.

Chapter 7
Urinary System

Renal Neoplasms

Cancers of the kidney account for approximately 1.5 % of all cancers and cancer deaths (with an incidence of 5–8 per 100,000 population in the UK and commoner in males). Three main types of renal cancer are distinguished: (1) Wilms tumor, (2) renal cell carcinoma (RCC) (adenocarcinoma), and (3) medullary and transitional cell cancers of the renal pelvis.

Wilms Tumor

Wilms tumor is the most common solid tumor in children, with an incidence of approximately 10 per 100,000 live births and accounting for 8 % of all childhood cancers. Both sporadic and familial forms occur, although the latter is uncommon and only 1 % of Wilms tumor patients have a positive family history (Breslow et al. 1996). Median age at diagnosis of Wilms tumor is 3–4 years and 80 % of patients present by the age of 5 years. Approximately 5 % of cases have bilateral tumors. This subgroup has an earlier age at diagnosis (mean 30 months) and an increased incidence of renal blastemal rests and congenital abnormalities (Breslow and Beckwith 1982). In contrast to retinoblastoma, the age at onset and proportion of bilateral tumors are not significantly different in familial and sporadic cases. There are important associations between Wilms tumor and sporadic aniridia (see below), Beckwith–Wiedemann syndrome (p. 221), hemihypertrophy, genitourinary abnormalities (about 5 % of children with Wilms tumor have genitourinary abnormalities), Denys–Drash syndrome (p. 239), Frasier syndrome (p. 252), Perlman syndrome (p. 298), Simpson–Golabi syndrome (p. 306), and mosaic variegated aneuploidy. In addition, Wilms tumor has been associated occasionally with neurofibromatosis type 1, *BRCA1* mutations, and Bloom syndrome (Rahman et al. 1996). Familial Wilms tumor segregates as an autosomal dominant trait with incomplete penetrance.

S.V. Hodgson et al., *A Practical Guide to Human Cancer Genetics*,
DOI 10.1007/978-1-4471-2375-0_7, © Springer-Verlag London 2014

Wilms tumor is thought to be derived from a mesenchymal renal stem cell or metanephric blastema. Islands of cells resembling metanephric blastema (nephrogenic rests) may persist into infancy and are found in 1 % of normal infant kidneys but in up to 40 % of kidneys with unilateral Wilms tumor and in almost 100 % of bilateral cases (Beckwith et al. 1990). Nephrogenic rests have been categorized into perilobar and intralobar rests. It appears that tumors associated with intralobar rests have an earlier age at onset and higher frequency of associated congenital abnormalities than those associated with perilobar rests.

WAGR Syndrome (Wilms Tumour-Aniridia-Genital Abnormality-Mental Retardation) and the WT1 Gene

Most children with WAGR syndrome have cytogenetically visible chromosome 11 deletions involving band 11p13 and the combination of aniridia with Wilms' tumor results from the deletion of the *WT1* (Wilms Tumor 1) and *PAX6* (aniridia) genes that are ~700 kb apart. Aniridia is fully penetrant, but Wilms' tumor occurs in only 50 % of cases. For patients with sporadic aniridia, the risk of Wilms' tumor is about 15 % (Muto et al. 2002), but molecular cytogenetic and genetic analysis can determine the extent of a deletion and hence the risk of Wilms' tumor (Clericuzio et al. 2011).

WAGR Syndrome and the *WT1* Gene

There is a high risk of Wilms tumor in isolated cases of aniridia, particularly when the patient also has genitourinary abnormalities and learning disability (mental retardation), the so-called Wilms tumor–aniridia–genital abnormality–mental retardation (WAGR) syndrome. This represents a contiguous gene syndrome. Up to 2 % of Wilms tumor patients have aniridia, compared to 2 per 100,000 of the general population. Wilms tumor is associated with sporadic aniridia and not with familial aniridia. For patients with sporadic aniridia, the risk of Wilms tumor had been estimated to be as high as 1 in 3, but this appears to be an overestimate and the risk may be closer to 15 % (Muto et al. 2002). The association of Wilms tumor with aniridia results from a contiguous deletion of the aniridia (*PAX6*) and Wilms tumor 1 (*WT1*) genes. Though many patients with Wilms tumor and aniridia have a cytogenetically visible chromosome 11p13 deletion, Wilms tumor can also occur in those with submicroscopic deletions that involve *PAX6* and *WT1* – indeed it has been reported that the risk of Wilms tumor is actually higher in those with submicroscopic deletions (van Heyningen et al. 2007). Molecular cytogenetic and genetic analysis can determine the extent of a deletion and hence the risk of Wilms' tumor (Clericuzio et al. 2011). Patients with intragenic *PAX6* mutations are not at risk of Wilms tumor, but only about 50 % of patients with WT1 deletions develop Wilms tumor (Muto et al. 2002). Additional features of the WAGR complex include mental retardation, ambiguous genitalia and gonadoblastoma, and, in some cases, obesity (Gul et al. 2002). There is a high incidence of bilateral tumors (36 %) and a younger age at diagnosis in children with Wilms tumor and aniridia compared to non-WAGR children. In addition, children with WAGR syndrome have a significant risk of renal failure, albeit it less than in Denys–Drash syndrome (38 and 62 %, respectively, at 20 years) (Breslow et al. 2000).

The *WT1* gene encodes a zinc-finger protein that is primarily expressed in renal blastemal cells during a critical period in the development of the glomerulus. The *WT1* gene product has a critical role in normal genitourinary development (see Denys–Drash syndrome [see p. 239]). Somatic *WT1* mutations occur in less than 10 % of sporadic Wilms tumors, and *WT1* mutations are rare in familial Wilms tumor. Pelletier et al. (1991) reported a father–son pair with Wilms tumor (and hypospadias and cryptorchidism in the son) associated with a germline *WT1* mutation. However, the associated genitourinary developmental abnormalities seen in *WT1* mutation carriers reduce the chances of familial transmission. Severe genital developmental abnormalities are seen in Denys–Drash syndrome, which is associated with dominant negative-acting *WT1* mutations (see p. 239).

A second Wilms tumor gene (*WT2*) was mapped by loss of heterozygosity studies to chromosome 11p15 in the region of the Beckwith–Wiedemann locus (see p. 221). Chromosome 11p15.5 allele loss preferentially affects the maternal allele that is compatible with a genomic imprinting effect and would be consistent with *WT2* being a maternally expressed imprinted tumor suppressor gene. The *CDKN1C* (*p57KIP2*) gene is a candidate imprinted tumor suppressor gene that is mutated or silenced in many patients with Beckwith–Wiedemann syndrome but is apparently not mutated in sporadic Wilms tumors. Loss of *IGF2* imprinting associated with *IGF2* overexpression occurs in a subset of Beckwith–Wiedemann syndrome patients (Lim and Maher 2010) and in the majority of sporadic Wilms tumors.

Rahman et al. (1996) mapped a familial Wilms tumor gene (*FWT1*) to chromosome 17q12–21. Kindreds linked to *FWT1* demonstrate a later age at onset than unlinked familial cases and sporadic cases and do not have developmental anomalies (Rahman et al. 1998). In addition there is evidence of incomplete penetrance (15–26 %) in FWT1 kindreds suggesting that familial WT1 may be under-ascertained (Rahman et al. 2000). A further familial Wilms tumor locus (FWT2) was mapped to 19q13.3–q13.4, but there is evidence for further locus heterogeneity (Huff et al. 1997; Rapley et al. 2000). Wilms tumor may also occur in children with biallelic *BRCA2* mutations (Fanconi anemia Type D1 see p. 249).

Cystic nephroma, a benign kidney tumor with differentiated septa but without blastemal elements, along with pleuropulmonary blastoma and ovarian Sertoli-Leydig cell tumors is associated with *DICER1* mutations (Hill et al. 2009). In addition, Wilms tumor has also been shown to be a component of the tumor spectrum associated with *DICER1* mutations (Foulkes et al. 2011).

All children at increased risk of Wilms tumor (e.g., with sporadic aniridia, hemihypertrophy, and Beckwith–Wiedemann syndrome) should be followed up carefully. A typical surveillance program would include 3-monthly renal ultrasound from birth to the age of 8 years. Nevertheless, Wilms tumor may develop between ultrasound scans, and it has been suggested that parents should also be taught how to perform abdominal palpation. The exact risk threshold for offering Wilms tumor surveillance is not universally agreed. Scott et al. (2006a, b) suggested that screening should only be offered to those children with a 5 % or greater risk of developing Wilms' tumor and should only be offered to children with hemihypertrophy and paternal uniparental disomy 11p15 or isolated *H19* hypermethylation. In contrast, Clericuzio and Martin (2009) recommended that abdominal ultrasound screening should be offered to all children with idiopathic hemihypertrophy.

Renal Cell Carcinoma (Adenocarcinoma, Hypernephroma)

Renal cell carcinoma (RCC) accounts for almost 90 % of malignant renal tumors. Familial cases of RCC are infrequent and are estimated to account for about 3 % of all cases. McLaughlin et al. (1984), in a population-based case–control study, found a family history of RCC in 2.4 % of affected patients, compared to 1.4 % of controls. Sporadic RCC is histopathologically heterogeneous. The most common form is clear cell (conventional RCC) which accounts for 75–80 % of all cases. The most frequent non-clear cell histopathology is papillary RCC (~15 % of all cases) which can be divided into types 1 and 2. Chromophobe RCC and oncocytomas and other rare forms of RCC make up the remainder. In some cases, there is a good correlation between genetic causes of familial RCC and histopathological appearance. Thus, von Hippel–Lindau (VHL) disease (see p. 313) is the most frequent syndromic cause of renal carcinoma susceptibility, and RCC in VHL disease invariably has a clear cell appearance. Germline mutations in the *MET* proto-oncogene cause type 1 papillary RCC, while RCC in hereditary leiomyomatosis patients with germline fumarate hydratase mutations (see p. 201) is usually classified as type 2 papillary or collecting duct RCC. However, in Birt–Hogg–Dube syndrome although the characteristic tumor is that of a mixed chromophobe–oncocytoma appearance, other types of RCC, including clear cell, can occur (see p. 224). Similarly, the histological subtype of RCC associated with germline *SDHB* mutations is also variable (Maher 2010).

Familial RCC is characterized by (1) an early age at onset compared to sporadic cases, (2) frequent bilateralism, and (3) multicentricity. In addition, features of a susceptibility syndrome (e.g., VHL disease, hereditary leiomyomatosis and RCC syndrome or Birt–Hogg–Dube syndrome, germline succinate hydrogenase subunit gene mutation) may be present. Mean age at diagnosis in familial cases is about 45 years, more than 15 years earlier than for sporadic cases (Maher et al. 1990).

In addition to the major RCC susceptibility syndromes described above, familial clear cell RCC may be associated with constitutional translocations, characteristically but not exclusively, involving chromosome 3. The first such kindred was reported by Cohen et al. (1979) and contained ten affected patients in three generations. In this family, RCC segregated with a t(3:8)(p14.2:q24.1), and it was estimated that each translocation carrier had an 87 % risk of developing this cancer by 60 years of age. Subsequently an increased risk of thyroid cancer was also reported in the family. At least 10 other chromosome 3 translocation-RCC families have been described, but the breakpoints and partner chromosome are heterogeneous. In the original t(3:8)(p14.2:q24.1) kindred, the 3p breakpoint occurred at the fragile site and disrupts the fragile histidine triad (*FHIT*) tumor suppressor gene. However, the precise role of *FHIT* (and the chromosome 8 gene *TRC8*) in RCC is unclear, and it has been suggested that instability of the translocated chromosome may be an important factor in this and other chromosome 3 translocation-RCC kindreds. All patients with possible RCC susceptibility should be examined for constitutional translocations. Adult translocation carriers in kindreds with chromosome 3 translocations and RCC should be offered regular renal surveillance (e.g., annual renal MRI or ultrasound scans). However, incidentally discovered chromosome 3 translocation carriers do not appear to require follow-up for RCC unless there is a personal or family history of RCC (or unless a translocation appears to disrupt a RCC suppressor gene) (Woodward et al. 2010).

Clinical and molecular genetic evidence of von Hippel–Lindau disease (see p. 313) should be sought in all cases of potential inherited clear cell RCC (e.g., familial, young onset, or multiple RCC).

Familial non-VHL clear cell RCC without evidence of a specific syndrome is generally characterized by autosomal dominant inheritance of susceptibility to RCC only (Teh et al. 1997; Woodward et al. 2000). It can be helpful to consider familial non-syndromic RCC according to the histopathology of the renal tumors (see above), e.g., the presence of type 1 papillary RCC would be an indication for *MET* gene analysis and non-clear cell RCC would exclude VHL disease. In a series of patients presenting with features suggestive of inherited non-syndromic RCC (mostly clear cell type), germline mutations in *SDHB* and *FLCN* (Birt–Hogg–Dube gene) were each detected in about 5 % of cases (Ricketts et al. 2008; Woodward et al. 2008). Hence, a preferred method for investigating potential inherited RCC is to test for mutations in a panel of inherited RCC genes (e.g., *VHL, FLCN, SDHB, SDHD, MET, FH*).

Renal tumors (consisting of a mixture of epithelial and stromal elements) may occur in hyperparathyroidism–jaw tumor syndrome (see p. 266) and rarely in tuberous sclerosis (although the most common renal tumor in this disease is angiomyolipoma) (see p. 307). Renal tumors may be seen in patients with Cowden syndrome or Cowden-like syndrome, particularly the subgroup in whom germline epimutations (promoter methylation of *KLLN* has been described) are found (see p. 233). Strategies for RCC are discussed in the sections on the relevant syndromes.

Cancer of the Ureter and Renal Pelvis

Carcinoma of the renal pelvis accounts for approximately 10 % of all malignant renal tumors. Environmental causes of carcinoma of the renal pelvis include occupational exposure (as for bladder cancer) and prolonged excessive phenacetin ingestion.

Examples of familial ureteric and renal pelvis transitional cell carcinoma are rare. Lynch et al. (1979) described two families with a predisposition to carcinoma of the bladder and renal pelvis, and familial ureteric cancer (mother and son) was observed by Burkland and Juzek (1966). Cancer of the ureter and renal pelvis is a feature of hereditary non-polyposis colorectal cancer (HNPCC) syndrome (Lynch syndrome, see p. 256), and urothelial cancers may cluster in some HNPCC families. It has been suggested that the presence of an inverted growth pattern (endophytic) in urothelial carcinomas of the upper urinary tract may serve as a marker for identifying tumors with a higher frequency of microsatellite instability and thus help identify patients who should be offered testing for HNPCC (Hartmann et al. 2002).

Renal medullary carcinomas are very rare, highly aggressive tumors that occur in young patients with sickle cell trait or disease (Noguera-Irizarry et al. 2003).

Bladder Cancer

Carcinoma of the bladder accounts for 4 % of all cancers (with an incidence in men of 30 per 100,000 and in women of 10 per 100,000 in the UK), is the fifth most common cancer in men, and has a peak prevalence in the seventh decade. Environmental factors, including tobacco, amine compounds used in the manufacture of dyes, and schistosomiasis, have been clearly implicated in bladder tumorigenesis, but genetic factors may also be relevant. Ninety percent of bladder tumors are transitional cell carcinomas, which may contain elements of squamous carcinoma or adenocarcinoma. Less commonly, sarcoma, melanoma, or small cell undifferentiated carcinoma may occur.

Familial clusters of bladder cancer were reported by Fraumeni and Thomas (1967) and McCullough et al. (1975). In these reports, bladder cancer affected a total of ten individuals from two-generation families. Lynch et al. (1979) also described two families showing a predisposition to transitional cell carcinoma of the bladder and renal pelvis. One individual developed bladder cancer at the age of 24 years. Familial clustering of bladder cancer could reflect shared exposure to environmental hazards or genetic susceptibility. A role for genetic factors is indicated by the association of bladder and other urothelial cancers with Lynch (HNPCC) syndrome and by the increased risk of bladder cancer in patients with germline *RB1* mutations. However, the most important contribution of genetic factors to bladder cancer risk is probably in determining individual susceptibility to environmental carcinogens, such as tobacco or occupational exposure to aromatic amine compounds. Hence, research into genetic susceptibility to bladder cancer has focused predominantly on the identification low-penetrance susceptibility genes, and large numbers of SNPs that convey small increases in relative risks have been identified. These SNPs are linked to genes implicated in detoxification of carcinogens, control of the cell cycle, and apoptosis and maintenance of DNA integrity (Golka et al. 2011).

Bladder tumors are frequently synchronous or metachronous. However, while these features are classical indicators of genetic susceptibility, molecular studies have suggested that multicentricity does not reflect a high incidence of multiple primary tumors but rather that a single primary transformation event may seed other tumors by spread across the urothelium. Individuals who are at increased risk of bladder cancer should be screened by 6-monthly urinalysis and urinary cytology, with cystourethroscopy when these tests are abnormal. Analysis of urine sediment for microsatellite DNA markers may provide a novel method for monitoring bladder cancer recurrence (Steiner et al. 1997).

References

Beckwith JB, Kiviat NB, Bonadio JF. Nephrogenic rests, nephroblastomatosis and the pathogenesis of Wilms tumor. Pediatr Pathol. 1990;10:1–36.

Breslow NE, Beckwith JB. Epidemiological features of Wilms' tumor: results of the national Wilms' tumor study. J Natl Cancer Inst. 1982;68:429–36.

Breslow NE, Olson J, Moksness J, Beckwith JB, Grundy P. Familial Wilms' tumor: a descriptive study. Med Pediatr Oncol. 1996;27:398–403.

Breslow NE, et al. Renal failure in the Denys-Drash and Wilms' tumor-aniridia syndromes. Cancer Res. 2000;60(15):4030–2.

Burkland CE, Juzek RH. Familial occurrence of carcinoma of the ureter. J Urol. 1966;96:697–701.

Clericuzio CL, Martin RA. Diagnostic criteria and tumor screening for individuals with isolated hemihyperplasia. Genet Med. 2009;11(3):220–2.

Clericuzio C, Hingorani M, Crolla JA, van Heyningen V, Verloes A. Clinical utility gene card for: WAGR syndrome. Eur J Hum Genet. 2011;19(4).

Cohen AJ, Li FP, Berg S, et al. Hereditary renal cell carcinoma associated with a chromosomal translocation. N Engl J Med. 1979;301:592–5.

Foulkes WD, Bahubeshi A, Hamel N, Pasini B, Asioli S, Baynam G, Choong CS, Charles A, Frieder RP, Dishop MK, Graf N, Ekim M, Bouron-Dal Soglio D, Arseneau J, Young RH, Sabbaghian N, Srivastava A, Tischkowitz MD, Priest JR. Extending the phenotypes associated with DICER1 mutations. Hum Mutat. 2011;32:1381–4.

Fraumeni JF, Thomas LB. Malignant bladder tumors in a man and his three sons. J Am Med Assoc. 1967;201:507–9.

Golka K, Selinski S, Lehmann ML, Blaszkewicz M, Marchan R, Ickstadt K, Schwender H, Bolt HM, Hengstler JG. Genetic variants in urinary bladder cancer: collective power of the "wimp SNPs". Arch Toxicol. 2011;85(6):539–54.

Gul D, et al. Third case of WAGR syndrome with severe obesity and constitutional deletion of chromosome (11)(p12p14). Am J Med Genet. 2002;107(1):70–1.

Hartmann A, et al. Frequent microsatellite instability in sporadic tumors of the upper urinary tract. Cancer Res. 2002;62(23):6796–802.

Hill DA, Ivanovich J, Priest JR, Gurnett CA, Dehner LP, Desruisseau D, Jarzembowski JA, Wilkenheiser-Brokamp KA, Suarez BK, Whelan AJ, Williams G, Bracamontes D, Messinger Y, Goodfellow PJ. DICER1 mutations in familial pleuropulmonary blastoma. Science. 2009;325:965.

Huff V, Amos CI, Douglass EG, et al. Evidence for genetic heterogeneity in familial Wilms' tumor. Cancer Res. 1997;57:1859–62.

Lim DH, Maher ER. Genomic imprinting syndromes and cancer. Adv Genet. 2010;70:145–75.

Lynch HT, Walzak MP, Fried R, et al. Familial factors in bladder cancer. J Urol. 1979;122:458–61.

Maher ER. Genetics of familial renal cancers. Nephron Exp Nephrol. 2010;118(1):e21–6.

Maher ER, Yates JRW, Ferguson-Smith MA. Statistical analysis of the two stage mutation model in von Hippel–Lindau disease and in sporadic cerebellar haeman-gioblastoma and renal cell carcinoma. J Med Genet. 1990;27:311–4.

McCullough DL, Lamma DL, McLaughlin AP, et al. Familial transitional cell carcinoma of the bladder. J Urol. 1975;113:629–35.

McLaughlin JK, Mandel JS, Blot WJ, Schuman LM, Mehl ES, Fraumeni JF. A population-based case–control study of renal cell carcinoma. J Natl Cancer Inst. 1984;72:275–84.

Muto R, et al. Prediction by FISH analysis of the occurrence of Wilms tumor in aniridia patients. Am J Med Genet. 2002;108(4):285–9.

Noguera-Irizarry WG, Hibshoosh H, Papadopoulos KP. Renal medullary carcinoma: case report and review of the literature. Am J Clin Oncol. 2003;26:489–92.

Pelletier J, Bruening W, Li FP, Haber DA, Glaser T, Housman DE. WT1 mutations contribute to abnormal genital system development and hereditary Wilms' tumour. Nature. 1991;353:431–4.

Rahman N, Arbour L, Tonin P, et al. Evidence for a familial Wilms' tumour gene (FWT1) on chromosome 17q12–q21. Nat Genet. 1996;13:461–3.

Rahman N, et al. Confirmation of FWT1 as a Wilms' tumour susceptibility gene and phe-notypic characteristics of Wilms' tumour attributable to FWT1. Hum Genet. 1998;103(5):547–56.

Rahman N, et al. Penetrance of mutations in the familial Wilms tumor gene FWT1. J Natl Cancer Inst. 2000;92(8):650–2.

Rapley EA, Crockford GP, Teare D, et al. Localization to Xq27 of a susceptibility gene for testicular germ-cell tumours. Nat Genet. 2000;24:197–200.

Ricketts C, Woodward ER, Killick P, Morris MR, Astuti D, Latif F, Maher ER. Germline SDHB mutations and familial renal cell carcinoma. J Natl Cancer Inst. 2008;100(17):1260–2.

Scott RH, Stiller CA, Walker L, Rahman N. Syndromes and constitutional chromosomal abnormalities associated with Wilms tumour. J Med Genet. 2006a;43(9):705–15.

Scott RH, Walker L, Olsen ØE, Levitt G, Kenney I, Maher E, Owens CM, Pritchard-Jones K, Craft A, Rahman N. Surveillance for Wilms tumour in at-risk children: pragmatic recommendations for best practice. Arch Dis Child. 2006b;91(12):995–9.

Steiner G, Schoenberg MP, Linn JF, Mao L, Sidransky D. Detection of bladder cancer recurrence by microsatellite analysis of urine. Nat Med. 1997;3:621–4.

Teh BT, McArdle J, Chan SP, et al. Clinicopathologic studies of thymic carcinoids in multiple endocrine neoplasia type 1. Medicine. 1997;76:21–9.

van Heyningen V, Hoovers JM, de Kraker J, Crolla JA. Raised risk of Wilms tumour in patients with aniridia and submicroscopic WT1 deletion. J Med Genet. 2007;44:787–90.

Woodward ER, et al. Familial clear cell renal cell carcinoma (FCRC): clinical features and mutation analysis of the VHL, MET, and CUL2 candidate genes. J Med Genet. 2000;37(5):348–53.

Woodward ER, Ricketts C, Killick P, Gad S, Morris MR, Kavalier F, Hodgson SV, Giraud S, Bressac-de Paillerets B, Chapman C, Escudier B, Latif F, Richard S, Maher ER. Familial non-VHL clear cell (conventional) renal cell carcinoma: clinical features, segregation analysis, and mutation analysis of FLCN. Clin Cancer Res. 2008;14(18):5925–30.

Woodward ER, Skytte AB, Cruger DG, Maher ER. Population-based survey of cancer risks in chromosome 3 translocation carriers. Genes Chromosomes Cancer. 2010;49(1):52–8.

Chapter 8
Blood and Lymph

Leukemia

Leukemia is responsible for approximately 2 % of all cancers, with an incidence of about 8 per 100,000 in the UK. Acute myeloid and lymphoblastic leukemia (AML and ALL) account for about 1 % of all cancers and 1.5 % of cancer deaths. The age incidence of leukemia shows two peaks, in childhood and in the elderly. Genetic factors are not considered to have a prominent role in the pathogenesis of acute leukemia or in chronic myeloid leukemia, but have been implicated in chronic lymphocytic leukemia. Gunz et al. (1975) studied the incidence of leukemia in relatives of 909 patients with leukemia. The overall incidence of leukemia in first-degree relatives was three times higher than expected although only 2 % of patients had a first-degree relative with leukemia. Among the main subtypes of leukemia, an increased risk to relatives was most marked in chronic lymphocytic leukemia, less so in acute leukemia and absent in chronic myeloid leukemia. When familial clusters of leukemia have been reported, the type of leukemia in individual relatives is not always concordant. Familial leukemia does not necessarily indicate a genetic cause, and shared exposure to an environmental leukemogen also needs to be considered, particularly in childhood acute leukemia. In Western countries, leukemia affects approximately 1–2 % of the population. B cell chronic lymphocytic leukemia (CLL) is the most common form of leukemia, accounting for around 30 % of all cases. The incidence rate of CLL increases logarithmically from age 35, with a median age of diagnosis at 65 years Acute myeloid and lymphoblastic leukemia (AML and ALL) account for about 1 % of all cancers and 1.5 % of cancer deaths. The age incidence of leukemia shows two peaks, in childhood and in the elderly. Genetic factors are not considered to have a prominent role in the pathogenesis of acute leukemia or chronic myeloid leukemia, but genes are being identified which do play a role in leukemia susceptibility, particularly chronic lymphocytic leukemia. Among the main subtypes of leukemia, an increased risk to relatives is most marked in chronic lymphocytic leukemia and less so in acute leukemia, but when familial clusters of leukemia have been reported, the type of leukemia in individual

Table 8.1 Genetic disorders associated with leukemia

Ataxia telangiectasia
Blackfan–Diamond syndrome
Bloom syndrome
Fanconi anemia
Biallelic mismatch repair gene mutations
Immune deficiency diseases (e.g., severe combined immunodeficiency, common variable immunodeficiency)
Incontinentia pigmenti
Kostmann syndrome
Li–Fraumeni syndrome
Lynch syndrome
N syndrome
Neurofibromatosis type 1
Seckel syndrome
Shwachman syndrome
Trisomy 21
Wiskott–Aldrich syndrome

relatives is not always concordant. An increased relative risk of leukaemia is found in the siblings, especially twins, of cases of childhood ALL suggesting a significant contribution of genetic factors. Exposure to environmental factors may also play a part, particularly in childhood acute leukemia, where an infectious etiology has been suggested to account for increased numbers of cases in areas where there has been a sudden influx of people to a town with increased population mixing, a possible contributing cause for increased cases seen in areas around certain nuclear sites (Kinlen 2011; Bithell et al. 2008). Recent genome-wide association studies have identified loci which may contribute small alterations in relative risk of leukemia, especially CLL (Brown 2008).

Genetic disorders that have been associated with a predisposition to leukemia are shown in Table 8.1 and discussed in detail in Chap. 11. Genetic disorders are ought to account for only 3 % of childhood leukemia.

Acute Lymphoblastic Leukemia (ALL)

The most common malignancy in childhood, ALL accounts for 80 % of leukemia in the pediatric age group. ALL is less common in adults, in whom it constitutes approximately 15 % of acute leukemia. ALL is caused by the malignant proliferation of lymphoblasts which are the precursor cells of B and T lymphocytes. ALL is a heterogeneous disorder, and various criteria have been used for subclassification, for example, morphological (e.g., French–American–British classification), immunophenotyping (e.g., T cell, B cell, and various precursor B cell subtypes) or cytogenetic criteria (e.g., t(9;22), t(4;11), t(1;19), and t(12;21)). Immunological classification can be refined by the molecular characterization of immunoglobulin heavy and light chain gene arrangements to define further the cell of origin of ALL.

Childhood leukemia is associated with genetic abnormalities in about 3 % and radiation exposure in less than 8 % of cases, so that the vast majority of cases are unexplained, although an infective (e.g., viral) origin has been postulated. Gunz et al. (1975) found that only 2 % of patients with acute leukemia had a first-degree relative with leukemia, and Till et al. (1975) observed that only 1.4 % of children with ALL had a close relative with leukemia or lymphoma. However, there is a significant risk of childhood leukemia in twins, particularly monozygotic. Thus Miller (1971) estimated that acute leukemia in an identical twin under 6 years of age is associated with a 1 in 6 risk that the co-twin will develop leukemia. The risk of leukemia in the unaffected twin is highest in infancy, decreases with age, and appears to be linked to a shared placental circulation. Thus, it is suggested that the leukemia lineage arises in utero in one twin and migrates to the other (Ford et al. 1993).

Familial clustering of adult ALL has been reported infrequently and might reflect shared environmental and/or genetic factors. De Moor et al. (1988) found 5 of 74 adult patients with ALL had a relative with acute leukemia or lymphoma and that this subgroup of patients with familial leukemia had a greater than expected incidence of HLA-Cw3 antigen. Horwitz et al. (1996) noted evidence of anticipation in familial leukemia, but for ALL this was based on only four pedigrees, each containing two affected individuals. In contrast to childhood ALL, twin-risks are not high in adult acute leukemia. Specific genetic disorders associated with ALL include Down syndrome, chromosome breakage syndromes (ataxia telangiectasia, Bloom syndrome), Li–Fraumeni syndrome, and immune deficiency disorders (severe combined, Bruton agamma-globulinemia, adenosine deaminase deficiency). Germ-line mutations in *PAX5* have recently been identified in familial pre-cell B-ALL (Shah et al. 2013).

Acute Myeloid (Myelogenous) Leukemia

Whereas ALL is the most common form of acute leukemia in children, AML predominates in adults. The overall incidence of AML is 2.5 cases/100,000 per year, with the highest incidence in those over the age of 60 years. Genetic disorders which have been associated with a predisposition to AML include Down syndrome, Fanconi anemia, neurofibromatosis type 1 (NF1), and Kostmann syndrome and DNA repair defects (see Chap. 11). An autosomal dominant syndrome of cerebellar ataxia, hypoplastic anemia, and predisposition to AML (associated with monosomy 7 in bone marrow cells) has been described (Daghistani et al. 1990). Bone marrow monosomy 7 is a frequent finding in chronic myeloproliferative disorders and AML, and only a small proportion of pediatric cases will have the ataxia pancytopenia syndrome. Monosomy 7 is the most common abnormality seen in familial cases of AML, and familial clustering of AML with monosomy 7 may indeed occur (Kwong et al. 2000).

Inherited susceptibility to acute myeloid leukemia (AML) is rare apart from the conditions listed above (Horwitz et al. 1997). True nonsyndromic familial AML includes autosomal recessive disorders with myelodysplasia and monosomy 7, and some large pedigrees demonstrating autosomal dominant inheritance have been reported (Horwitz et al. 1996/1997). An autosomal dominant condition character-ized by thrombocytopenia and platelet dense granule storage pool deficiency, plate-let dysfunction, with a strong predisposition to acute myeloid leukemia and lymphoma, is well recognized, where the underlying genetic defect is a germline mutation in the RUNX1 (runt-related transcription factor 1) (AML1, CBFA2) gene (Dowton et al. 1985; Ganly et al. 2004). *RUNX1* was first identified as the gene on chromosome 21 that is rearranged in the somatic translocation t(8:21)(q22;q22.12) detected in patients with AML. The RUNX1 protein complexes with the core-bind-ing transcription factor (CBF) which regulates many genes involved in hematopoi-esis. Other families have been described with familial AML associated with an inactivating germline *CEBPA* (CCAAT enhancer-binding protein) mutation, the gene encoding the granulocyte differentiating factor C/EBPα. There were latent periods of 10–30 years before the onset of overt leukemia in three affected patients in a family (Smith et al. 2004). Homozygous or monoallelic germline inactivating mutations in *EZH2* (a histone methyltransferase) have recently been found in about 12 % of a series of patients with myelodysplastic and myeloproliferative disorders (Ernst et al. 2011).

Davies et al. (2003) reported an increased risk of myeloid leukemia (40-fold), but not other cancers, in individuals with Prader–Willi syndrome.

Evidence of anticipation in familial AML has been noted such that of 79 indi-viduals in nine families transmitting the disease, the mean age at onset in the grand-parental generation was 57 years, compared to 32 years in the parental generation and 13 years in the youngest generation.

A rare form of AML, erythroleukemia (FAB-M6), may be familial (Di Guglielmo syndrome) in a minority of cases. Familial erythroleukemia is a leukemic or preleu-kemic state in which red cell proliferation is the predominant feature. Hematologic characteristics include ineffective and hyperplastic erythropoiesis with megaloblas-tic components accompanied by myeloblastic proliferation of varying degree (Park et al. 2002). A possible link between a missense mutation in the erythropoietin receptor (EPOR) and erythroleukemia has been reported (Le Couedic et al. 1996), but the role of the *EPOR* mutation in erythroleukemia is unclear.

Chronic Myeloid Leukemia

Chronic myeloid leukemia results from the malignant transformation of a pluripo-tent bone marrow stem cell. Typically, the disease has a triphasic course with an initial chronic phase (median duration 3.5 years) followed by an accelerated phase and then, after 3–12 months, an acute blastic phase associated with a poor response to therapy. The hallmark of chronic myeloid leukemia is the Philadelphia chromosome (Ph), which was the first consistent chromosomal aberration to be associated with human malignancy (Nowell and Hungerford 1960). It is now recognized that the Ph chromosome is present in more than 90 % of patients with chronic myeloid leukemia and that a proportion of apparently Ph-negative chronic myeloid leukemia have a variant Ph translocation not visible by cytogenetic techniques (Kurzrock et al. 1988). The Ph chromosome is not specific for chronic myeloid leukemia, and it is also found (and is associated with a poor prognosis) in a small proportion of patients with ALL (20 % of adults, 5 % children) and AML (2 % of adults). The classic Ph_3 chromosome results from a translocation involving chromosomes 9 and 22, (t(9; 22)(q34; q11)). The breakpoint on chromosome 9 involves the Abelson oncogene (*ABL*), and on chromosome 22, the breakpoints occur within a small region that was originally designated the breakpoint cluster region (BCR). The BCR is a central segment within a 90-kb gene, now named the *BCR* gene (Laurent et al. 2001). The 9;22 translocation results in the juxtaposition of proximal 5′ *BCR* gene exons (1, 2, and 3) and *ABL* sequences (exons 2–11, exons 1a and 1b).

Environmental agents associated with chronic myeloid leukemia include irradiation and chemical (e.g., benzene) exposure (Jacobs 1989), but there is relatively little evidence for a genetic predisposition. Familial chronic myeloid leukemia has been reported, and abnormal hematological investigations (evidence of a myeloproliferative disorder) have been observed in the healthy close relatives of cases. Nevertheless, familial cases of chronic myeloid leukemia appear to be rare.

Chronic Lymphocytic Leukemia

This is the most common form of leukemia accounting for >30 % of all cases and occurs particularly in the elderly, with a peak incidence between 60 and 80 years of age. Most cases are B cell type. This type of leukemia has the highest familial risk of all leukemias, with relatives of cases at significantly increased risk for CLL RR = 7.52 (3.63–15.56), for non-Hodgkin lymphoma RR 1.45 (0.98–2.16), and Hodgkin lymphoma RR 2.35 (1.08–5.08) (Goldin et al. 2010; Yuille et al. 2000). Moreover, approximately 13 % of apparently healthy relatives of patients with familial CLL have a monoclonal blood B lymphpocyte population detectable by cell flow analysis (3 % in controls).

In contrast to the acute leukemia and chronic myeloid leukemia, there is abundant evidence for a role of genetic factors in chronic lymphocytic leukemia. An association between disordered immune function and lymphoreticular malignancy is suggested by the finding that in some reports of familial chronic lymphocytic leukemia, autoimmune or immunological disorders have been noted among unaffected relatives. There is a fourfold excess of hematoproliferative malignancies among siblings of patients with chronic lymphocytic leukemia. Case–control studies have revealed relative risks in relatives ranging from 2.3 to 5.7 (reviewed by

Houlston et al. 2003). Among familial cases of chronic lymphocytic leukemia, the mean age at onset was >10 years earlier than in sporadic cases, and an increased risk of second primary tumors was noted (Ishibe et al. 2001). Among 18 affected individuals from seven pedigrees with dominantly inherited chronic lymphocytic leukemia, Horwitz et al. (1996) described evidence for anticipation in most cases, and this has been confirmed by others. The age at diagnosis in the offspring appears to be >20 years earlier than in affected parents.

Rawstron et al. (2002) detected subclinical levels of chronic lymphocytic leukemia-like cells in 14 % of relatives compared to about 1 % of normal controls suggesting that although the lifetime risk of chronic lymphocytic leukemia in familial cases is 20–30 %, there may be a significant incidence of subclinical disease.

The relative risks of lymphoproliferative disease in first-degree relatives of CLL cases have been found to be 1.8 for B cell NHL, 2.2 for indolent B cell NHL, 1.6 for follicular lymphoma, 3.3 for hairy cell leukemia, and 4 % for LPL/Waldenstroms macroglobulinemia (Goldin et al. 2010).

Rare high-penetrance and more common lower-penetrance susceptibility alleles are thought to be implicated in familial chronic lymphocytic leukemia. Recent genome-wide association studies have found several low-penetrance risk alleles for CLL (DiBernardo et al. 2008; Crowther-Swanepoel et al. 2010) and ALL each conferring small relative risks of disease (1.2–1.7 per allele), which act independently, such that the 2 % of the population who carry 13 or more risk alleles would have an eightfold increased risk of disease. Interestingly, these variants are involved in lymphoid cell development (Houlston 2010).

Germline mutations in *DAPK1*, a Ca2+/calmodulin-dependent serine/threonine kinase that acts as a positive regulator of apoptosis in part via phosphorylation of *p53* causing loss or reduced expression of DAPK1, cause an inherited susceptibility to CLL (Lynch et al. 2002, 2008b; Raval et al. 2007). *DAPK1* expression of the CLL allele may be downregulated due to increased HOXB7 binding, and promotor methylation results in additional loss of *DAPK1* expression.

Somatic inactivation of the ataxia-telangiectasia gene (*ATM*, see p. 219) occurs in >20 % of chronic lymphocytic leukemia cases, and in some cases. a germline mutation is also present. However while heterozygous *ATM* mutations may confer an increased risk of chronic lymphocytic leukemia, it seems likely that germline *ATM* mutations do not make a major contribution to familial cases of chronic lymphocytic leukemia (Houlston et al. 2003). Wiley et al. (2002) reported that a loss-of-function polymorphism in the cytolytic P2X7 receptor gene was overrepresented in patients with chronic lymphocytic leukemia compared to controls. However in another study, the P2X7 SNP was associated with survival in, but not risk of chronic lymphocytic leukemia (Thunberg et al. 2002).

Familial clustering (sibling or parent–child pairs) of hairy cell leukemia, an uncommon subtype of chronic lymphocytic leukemia with a prevalence of 1 per 150,000, has been reported in at least 30 cases (Colovic et al. 2001; Cetiner et al. 2003). Linkage to specific HLA haplotype has been suggested, but the influence of genetic and environmental factors in familial cases is unclear.

The first-degree relative of an affected person may have an eightfold increased risk of developing CLL themselves, and a 2.6 relative risk of any other lymphopro-liferative disorder, but considering the population risk of these conditions is low, the absolute risk is low, and early detection of CLL is not likely to affect outcome, therefore surveillance would not be recommended.

Other subtypes of leukemia which may occur commonly in certain genetic con-ditions include juvenile myelomonocytic leukemia (JMML), where about 10 % of cases arise in children with neurofibromatosis type 1 (NF1), and in Noonan syn-drome (see p. 297), a condition due to germline gain of function mutations in one of the oncogenes in the RAS signaling pathway, including *PTPN11*, *SOS1*, *RAF1*, *KRAS* and *CBL* (Pandit et al. 2007). Children with Noonan syndrome (NS) are at increased risk of developing juvenile myelomonocytic leukemia or a myeloprolif-erative disorder associated with NS (MPD/NS) resembling JMML in the first weeks of life. JMML constitutes about 30 % of childhood cases of myelodysplastic syn-drome and 2 % of leukemia. Whereas JMML is an aggressive disorder requiring hematopoietic stem cell transplantation, MPD/NS may resolve without treatment, and cases with spontaneous remission have also been reported (Bastida et al. 2011).

CBL is an E3 ubiquitin protein ligase responsible for the inactivation of protein tyrosine kinases by tagging them for degradation. Somatic mutations in this gene, as with *PTPN11*, *KRAS*, and *NRAS*, are well characterized in a variety of leukemia, particularly Juvenile myelomonocytic leukemia (JMML) and CML. Germline mutations in the *CBL* gene have been identified in a very small proportion of Noonan syndrome patients with a predisposition to JMML (Niemeyer et al. 2010). These children have impaired growth, developmental delay, and cryptorchidism.

Legius syndrome, due to germline mutations in the *SPRED1* gene, is a syndrome characterized by café-au-lait macules, axillary and inguinal freckling, and neurofi-bromas and schwannomas. There is an increased risk of JMML in this condition also.

In Down syndrome, there is a 500-fold increased risk of acute megakaryoblastic leukemia, with an overall risk of developing leukemia of about 2 %, and about 10 % of DS patients have transient myeloproliferative disorder (TMD) at birth. TMD is the clonal proliferation of myeloid blasts, usually with megakaryoblastic features and presents almost exclusively in DS patients (Klusmann et al. 2007; Izraeli et al. 2007). The symptoms vary from asymptomatic leukocytosis to severe disease caus-ing multiorgan failure. The disorder regresses in about 80 % cases, but about 20 % of cases will develop AML, usually by 5 years of age (Rabin and Whitlock 2009). TMD is a preleukemic state, and additional mutations of genes regulating the pro-liferation of the megakaryocyte progenitors such as *GATA-1* and *RUNX-1* need to occur for disease progression (Izraeli 2005). *GATA1* mutations are almost univer-sally found in the AML of children with DS, and these may arise very early in the child's life.

Children with DS are also predisposed to ALL but much less so than to acute megakaryocytic leukemia. Twenty to thirty-three percent of DS ALL cases are found to have a point mutation in exon 14 of *JAK2*, compared to 0 out of 41 *JAK2* mutations in non-DS ALL patients (Kearney et al. 2009). Patients with a *JAK2* mutation usually present earlier and with a higher WBC count than other ALL patients (Tigay 2009). *JAK2* mutations confer a cell advantage by promoting cell growth via the JAK/STAT signaling pathway (Mulligan 2008), and the mutations found in DS patients appear to be specific for DS ALL (Bercovich et al. 2008; Rabin and Whitlock 2009).

In non-DS patients, the most common genetic association seen in ALL is the *TEL-AML1* translocation between chromosomes 12 and 21, which accounts for about 25 % of childhood ALL (Armstrong and Look 2005). The mechanism by which the fusion protein formed by this translocation causes leukemogenesis is unclear, but the roles of both *TEL* and *AML1* have been shown to be vital in hematopoiesis. The translocation disrupts parts of *AML1* known as the core-binding factor, causing disruption of normal differentiation of B cell progenitors (Ford et al. 2009). The translocation can be found in the blood cells of patients at birth, which is many years before the age at which ALL patients typically present, as it takes so many years for the disease to develop sufficiently to present clinically (Armstrong and Look 2005).

Polycythemia

Increased red cell mass may be a primary abnormality, as in polycythemia rubra vera, or secondary to a variety of causes including hypoxia, renal cysts or tumors, and genetic disorders (benign primary familial polycythemia or familial erythrocytosis), such as inherited hemoglobin variants (e.g., hemoglobin Chesapeake), familial disorders of erythropoietin regulation (Kralovics et al. 1998), and recessive von Hippel–Lindau (*VHL*) gene mutations as in Chuvash polycythemia (Ang et al. 2002). However, there is evidence for further loci for autosomal dominant primary familial polycythemia (Jedlickova et al. 2003).

Polycythemia rubra vera is an uncommon myeloproliferative disorder (five new cases/million per year) in which increased red cell mass is usually associated with increased white cell and platelet counts. Polycythemia rubra vera usually pursues a chronic course, but there is a significant risk of an acute leukemic transformation occurring. Clonal cytogenetic abnormalities, such as del(20q), trisomy 8 and 9, del(13q), and dupl(1q), have been reported in a minority of patients with polycythemia rubra vera but are present in most patients with leukemic transformation (Heim and Mitelman 1987). More than 95 % of individuals with polycythemia vera and 50–60 % of individuals with essential thrombocythemia have an acquired activating point mutation in the cytoplasmic tyrosine kinase gene *JAK2, V617F*, which appears to be the underlying somatic mutation leading to clonal expansion of myeloid progenitor cells. In the remaining cases, there may be other mutations in the *JAK2* gene. Somatic mutations in the *TET2* gene have also been found in cases of polycythemia vera. Familial polycythemia rubra vera is rare, but the relative risk of the disorder in first-degree relatives of index cases is three to fourfold in individuals carrying the same haplotype block including the 3′ portion of *JAK2* (Campbell 2009). This must be distinguished from the more common benign familial polycythemia which is not associated with leukemia. Inheritance of this appears to be autosomal dominant with incomplete inheritance (Kralovics et al. 2003).

MPL mutations may be detected in patients with myeloproliferative disorders without demonstrable mutations in *JAK2* (Ma et al. 2011).

Trisomy 8 and 9, del(13q) and dupl(1q), have been reported in a minority of patients with polycythemia rubra vera but are present in most patients with leukemic transformation (Heim and Mitelman 1987). More than 95 % of individuals with polycythemia vera and 50–60 % of individuals with essential thrombocythemia have an acquired activating point mutation in the cytoplasmic tyrosine kinase gene *JAK2*, V617F, which appears to be the underlying somatic mutation leading to clonal expansion of myeloid progenitor cells. In the remaining cases there may be other mutations in the *JAK2* gene, familial polycythemia rubra vera is rare, but the relative risk of the disorder in first-degree relatives of index cases is three to fourfold in individuals carrying the same haplotype block including the 3′ portion of *JAK2* (reviewed by Campbell 2009). This must be distinguished from the more common benign familial polycythemia which is not associated with leukemia.

Inheritance of this appears to be autosomal dominant with incomplete inheritance (Kralovics et al. 2003).

MPL mutations may be detected in patients with Myelofroliferative disorders without demonstrable mutations in *JAK2* (Ma et al. 2011).

Thrombocythemia

Primary or essential thrombocythemia is a myeloproliferative disorder characterized by megakaryocyte hyperplasia and elevated platelet count. The main complications are bleeding and thrombotic events, and occasionally, acute leukemic transformation can occur. Familial essential thrombocythemia has been reported. Familial cases may be inherited as an autosomal dominant trait and may be caused by mutations in the thrombopoetin gene (*THPO*) on chromosome 3, or its receptor c-Mpl on chromosome 1p34 (Ding et al. 2004; Kondo et al. 1998). Large families with multiple generations involved (and male-to-male transmission in some cases) have been described (Schlemper et al. 1994; Kikuchi et al. 1995, van Dijken et al.1996). Activating mutations in the *MPL* gene, which encodes the receptor for the major hormone driving platelet production, may be seen in 5 % of patients with thrombocythemia, and 50–60 % cases have a somatic point mutation in *JAK2* (Scott et al. 2007). Somatic mutations in the *TET2*, *ASXL1*, and *SH2B3* genes have also been found.

Lymphoma

The two major categories of malignant lymphoma are Hodgkin disease (which accounts for just under half of the total) and non-Hodgkin lymphoma. The latter is a heterogeneous group of disorders, most are of monoclonal B cell origin, and a lesser number are of T cell or non-T non-B type. Genetic disorders that predispose to malignant lymphoma are listed in Table 8.2 and discussed in Chap. 11. Clearly,

Table 8.2 Genetic disorders predisposing to lymphoma

Ataxia telangiectasia
Chediak–Higashi syndrome
Common variable immunodeficiency
HyerIgM syndrome
Hypogammaglobulinemia
Severe combined immunodeficiency
Wiskott–Aldrich syndrome
X-linked lymphoproliferative disease

there is a strong association between genetic disorders that cause clinical immuno-deficiency and the development of malignant lymphoma. Furthermore, the incidence of lymphoproliferative disorders is increased among patients with immunodeficiency secondary to therapeutic immunosuppression or human immu-nodeficiency virus (HIV) infection. Although many lymphomas in immune-deficient individuals are of B cell origin, some are derived from other cells such as T lympho-cytes (Baumler et al. 2003).

Tumors, especially lymphoproliferative disorders, are the second leading cause of death in immunodeficiency disorders, and it is estimated that 15–25 % of patients with the three major immunodeficiency syndromes (Wiskott–Aldrich syndrome, AT and common variable immunodeficiency) develop cancer. Approximately 60 % of cancers reported in patients with immunodeficiency disorders are lymphomas, and non-Hodg-kin lymphoma is about six times as frequent as Hodgkin disease in these patients.

There is a slight increase in risk of lymphoma in the relatives of patients with hemopoietic malignancy (Chang et al. 2005; Altieri et al. 2006).

In patients with childhood onset of colonic adenocarcinoma, lymphoma, and brain tumors, (Menko et al. 2004; Poley et al. 2007) homozygous germline muta-tions in the *MSH6* gene have been identified, and in other patients, biallelic germ-line mutations in other genes involved in repair of microsatellite errors in DNA have been detected. Leukemia is thus a feature of the homozygous state for germline mutations in the "MMR" genes, which in heterozygous individuals cause Lynch syndrome (constitutional mismatch repair deficiency, p. 232).

A subset of patients with lymphoma have been found to have germline mutations in the perforin gene. Patients with biallelic mutations in this gene may have familial hemophagocytic lymphohistiocytosis (HLH), but a few such patients have been found to have Hodgkin or non-Hodgkin lymphoma. (Clementi et al. 2005).

Hodgkin Disease

This has an incidence of 2–3 per 100,000 population in the UK. Analysis of the age at onset of Hodgkin disease reveals a bimodal distribution, with one peak around the age of 25 years, then decreasing to a plateau in middle age, after which rates increase with advancing age for the second peak. The disease is more common in males than in females, in people of higher socioeconomic status, and in smaller families. The etiology of Hodgkin disease is unknown, but an infective agent has been suggested, particularly in the younger age group and in the nodular sclerosis subtype. An association between familial clustering of multiple sclerosis and young-adult-onset Hodgkin lymphoma (HL) has been reported and suggests that the two conditions share environmental and/or constitutional factors (Hjalgrim et al. 2004; Shugart et al. 2000).

Ferraris et al. (1997) reviewed the literature on familial Hodgkin disease. They confirmed an excess of males in familial cases, that the male-to-female ratio (1.5:1) was similar in familial and sporadic cases, and that the age distribution of familial cases shows a single major peak between 15 and 34 years of age. Both genetic and environmental (e.g., viral infections) factors have been implicated in familial clustering of Hodgkin disease. Analysis of 432 sets of twins affected by Hodgkin disease revealed that 0 of 187 dizygotic twins were concordant for Hodgkin disease, compared to 10 of 179 monozygotic twins – expected cases >0.1 for each group (Mack et al. 1995). The higher concordance in monozygotic twins compared to dizygotic twins clearly implicates genetic factors in familial clustering of Hodgkin disease in young adults. In a study of Hodgkin disease in Sweden, Shugart et al. (2000) estimated the heritability to be 28 % and suggested that there was significant evidence for anticipation in parent–child pairs with Hodgkin disease (mean difference 14 years). The relative risk of HL in relatives of cases is about 3.1, and there is also an increased relative risk for chronic lymphatic leukemia and non-Hodgkin lymphoma, and these relative risks are higher in relatives of young-onset cases (Goldin et al. 2004).

Epidemiological evidence suggests that Hodgkin disease may be a rare outcome of a specific infective agent, possibly Epstein–Barr virus (EBV). However EBV infection is common and often asymptomatic suggesting that additional factors, such as inherited immune response variants, might be implicated in susceptibility to Hodgkin disease. Hence a number of groups have investigated the associations between Hodgkin disease and HLA loci. Linkage studies in multiple-case families have confirmed an association with a susceptibility gene at the HLA locus and are consistent with a recessive gene which would account for a twofold increase in relative risk for siblings of patients with Hodgkin disease (Chakravarti et al. 1986). Linkage to the HLA class II region has also been demonstrated (Klitz et al. 1994); in particular, alleles at the HLA-DPB1 locus have been implicated specific histological subtypes, and an association with EBV-positive cases has been suggested (Taylor et al. 1999; Alexander et al. 2001). A recent assessment suggests that HL A determinants contribute additively with one or more other genes to susceptibility to Hodgkin's (Shugart and Collins 2000). There is an increased incidence of Hodgkin disease in immunodeficient patients, and it accounts for about 10 % of tumors associated with primary immunodeficiency disorders. The mean age at diagnosis of Hodgkin disease in immunodeficient patients is 10.9 years, although there was a wide range, from less than 1–73 years (Kersey et al. 1988). Compared to pediatric patients with Hodgkin disease and no immunodeficiency disorder, there is an excess of mixed cellularity and lymphocyte depletion subtypes. However, most lymphomas that occur in immunodeficient individuals are categorized as non-Hodgkin lymphoma. The recent finding of chromosomal rearrangements involving *JAK2*, t(4;9)(q21;p24) *JAK2* rearrangements, including the novel *SEC31A-JAK2* fusion, which are recurrent in classical Hodgkin lymphoma, is of importance; the t(4;9)(q21;p24) leads to a novel *SEC31A-JAK2* fusion which is oncogenic in vitro and acts as a constitutively activated tyrosine kinase that is sensitive to JAK inhibitors (Van Roosbroeck et al. 2011).

Germline mutations in *NPAT* (nuclear protein ataxia-telangiectasia locus) have been found to segregate with nodular lymphocyte predominant Hodgkin's lymphoma in a family and have also been detected in sporadic cases of the disease, suggesting that these mutations confer an increased risk (OR = 4.11) of this condition (Saarinen et al. 2011a, b).

Non-Hodgkin Lymphoma

This is a heterogeneous group of disorders with a wide range of histological, immunological, and cytogenetic subtypes. Non-Hodgkin lymphoma is the most frequent tumor to complicate the primary immunodeficiency syndromes (see Table 8.2) and may also occur in families of patients with chronic lymphocytic leukemia.

The most frequent causes of non-Hodgkin lymphoma complicating primary immunodeficiency are ataxia telangiectasia, Wiskott–Aldrich syndrome, common variable immunodeficiency, and severe combined immunodeficiency (see Chap. 11. Kersey et al. 1988), and it is the predominant malignancy in each of these disorders. Mean age at diagnosis is 7 years (from range less than 1–75 years), and the brain and gastrointestinal tract are frequent presenting sites. Compared to non-Hodgkin lymphoma in non-immunodeficient patients, lymph node involvement is less common. Most non-Hodgkin lymphoma in primary immunodeficient children is of B cell origin, but the lymphomas in ataxia telangiectasia are very heterogeneous, with all the major histological sub-groups represented. There appears to be no relationship between the severity of immunodeficiency and the risk of malignancy (Kersey et al. 1988).

A tendency for familial aggregations of hematolymphoproliferative cancers is recognized. Pottern et al. (1991) found 4.5 % of patients with non-Hodgkin lymphoma had at least one sibling and 3.3 % had a parent with a hematoproliferative cancer, while only 1.7 % of controls had an affected sibling and 2.2 % had a parent with a hematoproliferative cancer. There is a fourfold excess of leukemia and lymphomas among first-degree relatives of patients with non-Hodgkin lymphoma. When familial aggregations of hematoproliferative cancers occur, there is often no particular pattern of tumor type, so that although concordant cancers may occur, so may seemingly diverse cell types. A history of hemopoietic malignancy in any first-degree relative has been found to be associated with an increased risk of all non-Hodgkin's lymphoma (OR = 1.8), more pronounced in siblings than in parent–child relationships (Chang et al. 2005). Familial clustering of lymphoma is uncommon, but Lynch et al. (1989) reported a single exceptional family with seven cases of malignant lymphoma (six non-Hodgkin lymphoma and one Hodgkin lymphoma) in three generations with autosomal dominant inheritance. However most family clusters are small. In familial clusters of non-Hodgkin lymphoma with vertical transmission, evidence for anticipation has been reported (Wiernik et al. 2000; Shugart et al. 2001).

Wiernik et al. (2000) analyzed 11 published reports of multigenerational familial non-Hodgkin lymphoma (NHL) and 18 previously unreported families with familial NHL for evidence of anticipation. The median age of onset in the child and parent generations of all families (48.5 and 78.3 years, respectively) and in the selected pairs (52.5 and 71.5 years, respectively) was significantly different. A significant difference was observed between the ages of onset between the child generation and that of the SEER population but not between the parent generation and the SEER population. They thus concluded that anticipation in familial NHL is a genuine phenomenon.

Using the Swedish Family-Cancer Database, Altieri et al. (2005) calculated standardized incidence ratios (SIRs) for histopathology-specific subtypes of NHL in 4,455 offspring with NHL whose parents or sibs were affected with different types of lymphoproliferative malignancies. SIRs for affected patients with a parental history of NHL were significantly increased for NHL (1.8) and diffuse large B cell lymphoma (2.3). SIRs for affected patients with a sib history of NHL were significantly increased for NHL (1.9), follicular lymphoma (2.3), and B cell lymphoma not otherwise specified (3.4). With a parental history of histopathology-specific concordant cancer, familial risks were significantly increased for diffuse large B cell lymphoma, follicular NHL, plasma cell myeloma, and chronic lymphocytic leukemia (SIRs of 11.8, 6.1, 2.5, and 5.9, respectively).

Clementi et al. (2005) reported 4 patients with non-Hodgkin lymphoma with features of hemophagocytic lymphohistiocytosis who had mutations in the perforin gene.

Diffuse large B cell lymphoma (DLBCL) is the most common form of non-Hodgkin lymphoma, accounting for 30–40 % of cases. Survival of the malignant cells is dependent on constitutive activation of the nuclear factor-κB (NF-κB) signaling pathway. In normal B cells, antigen receptor-induced NF-κB activation requires CARD11, a cytoplasmic scaffolding protein. Missense mutations in *CARD11* have been demonstrated in about 10 % of LBCL biopsies, all within exons encoding the coiled-coil domain. Such experimental *CARD11* mutants cause constitutive NF-κB activation and enhanced NF-κB activity upon antigen receptor stimulation (Lenz et al. 2008; Davis et al. 2010).

Follicular lymphoma susceptibility has been associated with a SNP on chromosome 6p21.33 (Skibola et al. 2009).

Myeloma

Reports of sibling pairs with multiple myeloma (MM) suggest that occasionally, genetic factors may predispose to myeloma, and Hemminki (2002) reported that offspring of multiple myeloma cases had a fourfold increased risk of disease. Horwitz et al. (1985) reviewed 30 families with two affected siblings and a further nine families with three affected siblings. In two reports of twins with multiple myeloma (Judson et al. 1985; Comotti et al. 1987), one emphasized the contribution of shared environment and the other genetic factors. A 2 % incidence of plasma cell disorders in siblings of myeloma patients has been reported, but this may not be excessive (Horwitz et al. 1985). There have been a few families described with several cases of MM, although these are rare (Lynch et al. 2008b). Lynch et al. (2001) described a large kindred with familial multiple myeloma in three cases and a monoclonal gammopathy of unknown significance in two further relatives. Although there is no case for routine screening of relatives of myeloma patients, when familial myeloma is found, first-degree relatives should be screened (by blood and urine electrophoresis) and those with benign monoclonal gammopathy kept under surveillance. There is evidence for an increased relative risk of multiple myeloma in relatives of MM cases (SIR 2.45), chronic lymphatic leukemia (2.45), and non-Hodgkin lymphoma (1.34) (Altieri et al. 2005). A hereditary predisposition to B cell proliferative diseases has been established, and IgG/A and IgM disorders may occur together in families, where enhanced B cell responsiveness may be found in healthy subjects clustered around cases (Steingrimsdottir et al. 2011).

Waldenstrom Macroglobulinemia

Familial occurrences of Waldenstrom macroglobulinemia, a rare subtype of non-Hodgkin lymphoma, are uncommon but well described (Renier et al. 1989; Blattner et al. 1980). It has been suggested that 4 % of relatives of affected persons have a monoclonal IgM component (Kalff and Hijmans 1969). In the family of Blattner et al. (1980), all four affected relatives had a common HLA haplotype (A2, B8, DRw3). However, in the other two reports, no consistent HLA associations were found. The monoclonal IgM light chain type may differ between relatives with familial Waldenstrom macroglobulinemia, as occurred in monozygotic twins with Waldenstrom macroglobulinemia (Fine et al. 1986). Autoimmune disorders and immunoglobulin abnormalities are frequent in relatives of patients with familial Waldenstrom macroglobulinemia, suggesting that in these families Waldenstrom macroglobulinemia may be one manifestation of a genetic predisposition to abnormal immunoglobulin synthesis control mechanisms (McMaster 2003). Linkage of WM to chromosome 4q has been described (McMaster et al. 2006). Only 4 of 200 healthy controls (2 %) were found to be carriers of paratarg-7 (pP-7), whereas pP-7 carrier state was associated with a significantly increased risk (odds ratio=6.2; P=.001) for developing IgM-MGUS/Waldenstrom macroglobulinemia. The pP-7 carrier state is inherited as a dominant trait. After IgA/IgG-MGUS and multiple myeloma, IgM-MGUS/WM is the second neoplasia associated with pP-7 carrier state (Grass et al. 2011).

Histiocytoses

This is a heterogeneous group of disorders characterized by abnormal proliferation of histiocytes, and nonmalignant histiocytic disorders are subdivided into two major types: (1) Langerhans' cell histiocytosis (including histiocytosis X, eosinophilic granuloma, Letterer–Siwe disease, and Hand–Schuller–Christian disease and are characterized by the presence of the Birbeck granule) and (2) hemophagocytic syndromes (which include familial erythrophagocytic lymphocytosis, also known as familial lymphohistiocytosis or familial reticuloendotheliosis).

Langerhans cell histiocytosis (LCH) is considered a nonhereditary disorder but rarely may be familial (Arico et al. 1999). Most such cases are in monozygotic twins and the concordance rate is 85 % (this does not necessarily indicate genetic factors as in utero spread via intraplacental anastomosis cannot be excluded).

A hereditary predisposition to B cell proliferative diseases has been established, and IgG/A and IgM disorders may occur together in families, where enhanced B cell responsiveness may be found in healthy subjects clustered around cases (Steingrimsdottir et al. 2011).

Familial hemophagocytic lymphohistiocytosis is a rare autosomal recessive disorder (1.2 cases/million children each year), which usually presents in early childhood (80 % by the age of 2 years) with failure to thrive, fever, anemia and hepatosplenomegaly and, histologically, multisystem (liver, spleen, lymph nodes, bone marrow, central nervous system) lymphohistiocytic infiltrates. Without treatment the prognosis is very poor. Familial hemophagocytic lymphohistiocytosis is a heterogeneous disorder. Mutations in the perforin gene account for >30 % of cases, and about 10 % are linked to the chromosome 9 FHL1 locus (Goransdotter Ericson et al. 2001). Recently mutations in hMunc13-4, a member of the Munc13 family of proteins involved in vesicle priming function, were identified in a further subset of familial hemophagocytic lymphohistiocytosis (FHL3). Inactivation of hMunc13-4 causes defective exocytosis of perforin containing lytic granules (Feldmann et al. 2003). Other genes that may be involved in different families include *RAG1* and *RAG2*, the syntaxin-11 gene, and syntaxin-binding protein 2.

An autosomal recessive form of histiocytosis associated with sensorineural deafness and joint contractures, Faisalabad histiocytosis, has been mapped to 11q25. Further genetic heterogeneity in familial hemophagocytic lymphohistiocytosis was suggested by a study in which FHL in 2 unrelated Canadian families with affected first cousins was not linked to 9q21.3-q22 or 10q21-q22 (Graham et al. 2000).

References

Alexander FE, Jarrett RF, Cartwright RA, Armstrong AA, Gokhale DA, Kane E, Gray D, Lawrence DJ, Taylor GM. Epstein-Barr Virus and HLA-DPB1-*0301 in young adult Hodgkin's disease: evidence for inherited susceptibility to Epstein-Barr Virus in cases that are EBV(+ ve). Cancer Epidemiol Biomark Prev. 2001;10(6):705–9.

Altieri A, Bermejo JL, Hemminki K. Familial risk for non-Hodgkin lymphoma and other lymphoproliferative malignancies by histopathologic subtype: the Swedish Family-Cancer Database. Blood. 2005;106:668–72.

Altieri A, Chen B, Bermejo JL, Castro F, Hemminki K. Familial risks and temporal incidence trende of multiple myeloma. Eur J Cancer. 2006;42(11):1661–70.

Ang SO, Chen H, Hirota K, Gordeuk VR, Jelinek J, Guan Y, Liu E, Sergueeva AI, Miasnikova GY, Mole D, Maxwell PH, Stockton DW, Semenza GL, Prchal JT. Disruption of oxygen homeostasis underlies congenital Chuvash polycythemia. Nat Genet. 2002;32:614–21.

Arico M, Nichols K, Whitlock JA, Arceci R, Haupt R, Mittler U, Kuhne T, Lombardi A, Ishii E, Egeler RM, Danesino C. Familial clustering of Langerhans cell histiocytosis. Br J Haematol. 1999;107:883–8.

Armstrong SA, Look AT. Molecular genetics of acute lymphoblastic leukemia. J Clin Oncol. 2005;23(26):6306–15.

Bastida P, García-Miñaúr S, Ezquieta B, Dapena JL, Sanchez de Toledo J. Myeloproliferative disorder in Noonan syndrome. J Pediatr Hematol Oncol. 2011;33(1):e43–5.

Baumler C, Duan F, Onel K, et al. Differential recruitment of caspase 8 to cFlip confers sensitivity or resistance to Fas-mediated apoptosis in a subset of familial lymphoma patients. Leuk Res. 2003;27:841–51.

Bercovich D, Ganmore I, Scott LM, Wainreb G, Birger Y, Elimelech A, Shochat C, Cazzaniga G, Biondi A, Basso G, Cario G, Schrappe M, Stanulla M, Strehl S, Haas OA, Mann G, Binder V, Borkhardt A, Kempski H, Trka J, Bielorei B, Avigad S, Stark B, Smith O, Dastugue N, Bourquin JP, Tal NB, Green AR, Izraeli S. Mutations of JAK2 in acute lymphoblastic leukemia associated with Down syndrome. Lancet. 2008;372(9648):1484–92.

Bithell JF, Keegan TJ, Kroll ME, Murphy MF, Vincent TJ. Childhood leukaemia near British nuclear installations: methodological issues and recent results. Radiat Prot Dosim. 2008;132:191–7.

Blattner WA, Garber JE, Mann DL, et al. Waldenstrom's macroglobulinaemia and autoimmune disease in a family. Ann Int Med. 1980;93:830–2.

Brown J. Inherited predisposition to chronic lymphatic leukemia. Expert Rev Haematol. 2008;1(1):51–61.

Campbell PJ. Somatic and germline genetics at the JAK2 locus. Nat Genet. 2009;41:385–6.

Cetiner M, Adiguzel C, Argon D, Ratip S, Eksioglu-Demiralp E, Tecimer T, Bayik M. Hairy cell leukemia in father and son. Med Oncol. 2003;20(4):375–8.

Chakravarti A, Halloran SL, Bale SJ, Tucker MA. Etiological heterogeneity in Hodgkin's disease: HLA linked and unlinked determinants of susceptibility independent of histological concordance. Genet Epidemiol. 1986;3:407–15.

Chang ET, Smedby KE, Hjalgrim H, et al. Family history of haematopoietic malignancy and risk of lymphoma. JNCI. 2005;97:1466–74.

Clementi R, Locatelli F, Dupre L, Garaventa A, Emmi L, Bregni M, Cefalo G, Moretta A, Danesino C, Comis M, Pession A, Ramenghi U, Maccario R, Arico M, Roncarolo MG. A proportion of patients with lymphoma may harbor mutations of the perforin gene. Blood. 2005;105:4424–8.

Colovic MD, Jankovic GM, Wiernik PH. Hairy cell leukemia in first cousins and review of the literature. Eur J Haematol. 2001;67(3):185–8.

Comotti B, Bassan R, Buzzeti M, Finazzi G, Barbui T. Multiple myeloma in a pair of twins. Br J Haematol. 1987;65:123–4.

Crowther-Swanepoel D, Broderick P, Di Bernardo MC, Dobbins SE, Torres M, Mansouri M, Ruiz-Ponte C, Enjuanes A, Rosenquist R, Carracedo A, Jurlander J, Campo E, Juliusson G, Montserrat E, Smedby KE, Dyer MJ, Matutes E, Dearden C, Sunter NJ, Hall AG, Mainou-Fowler T, Jackson GH, Summerfield G, Harris RJ, Pettitt AR, Allsup DJ, Bailey JR, Pratt G, Pepper C, Fegan C, Parker A, Oscier D, Allan JM, Catovsky D, Houlston RS. Common variants at 2q37.3, 8q24.21,15q21.3 and 16q24.1 influence chronic lymphocytic leukaemia risk. Nat Genet. 2010;42:132138.

Daghistani D, Toledano SR, Curless R. Monosomy 7 syndrome. Cancer Genet Cytogenet. 1990;44:263–9.

Davies HD, Leusink GL, McConnell A, Deyell M, Cassidy SB, Fick GH, Coppes MJ. Myeloid leukemia in Prader–Willi syndrome. J Pediatr. 2003;142:174–8.

Davis RE, Ngo VN, Lenz G, Tolar P, Young RM, Romesser PB, Kohlhammer H, Lamy L, Zhao H, Yang Y, Xu W, Shaffer AL, and 25 others. Chronic active B-cell-receptor signalling in diffuse large B-cell lymphoma. Nature. 2010;463:88–92.

De Moor P. A hereditary form of acute lymphoblastic leukemia. Leukemia. 1988;2(8):556. PMID:3166082.

Di Bernardo MC, Crowther-Swanepoel D, Broderick P, Webb E, Sellick G, Wild R, Sullivan K, Vijayakrishnan J, Wang Y, Pittman AM, Sunter NJ, Hall AG, Dyer MJ, Matutes E, Dearden C,

Mainou-Fowler T, Jackson GH, Summerfield G, Harris RJ, Pettitt AR, Hillmen P, Allsup DJ, Bailey JR, Pratt G, Pepper C, Fegan C, Allan JM, Catovsky D, Houlston RS. A genome-wide association study identifies six susceptibility loci for chronic lymphocytic leukemia. Nat Genet. 2008;40(10):1204–10.

Ding J, Komatsu H, Wakita A, et al. Familial essential thrombocythemia associated with a dominant-positive activating mutation of the c-MPL gene, which encodes for the receptor for thrombopoietin. Blood. 2004;103:4198–200.

Dowton SB, Beardsley D, Jamison D, Blattner S, Lie FP. Studies of a familial platelet disorder. Blood. 1985;65:557–65.

Ernst T, Chase AJ, Score J, et al. Iactivating mutations of the histone methyltransferase gene EZH2 in myeloid disorders. Nat Genet. 2011;42:722–5.

Eyster M, Saletan SL, Rabellino EM, et al. Familial essential thrombocythemia. Am J Med. 1986;89:497–502.

Feldmann J, Callebaut I, Raposo G, et al. Munc13–4 is essential for cytolytic granules fusion and is mutated in a form of familial hemophagocytic lymphohistiocytosis (FHL3). Cell. 2003;115:461–73.

Ferraris AM, Racchi O, Rapezzi D, Gaetani GF, Boffetta P. Familial Hodgkin's disease: a disease of young adulthood? Ann Hematol. 1997;74:131–4.

Fine JM, Muller JY, Rochu D, et al. Waldenstrom's macroglobulinaemia in monozygotic twins. Acta Med Scand. 1986;220:369–73.

Ford AM, Ridge SA, Cabrera ME, Mahmoud H, Steel CM, Chan LC, Greaves M. In utero rearrangements in the trithorax-related oncogene in infant leukemia. Nature. 1993;363:358–60.

Ford AM, Palmi C, Bueno C, Hong D, Cardus P, Knight D, Cazzaniga G, Enver T, Greaves M. The TEL-AML1 leukaemia fusion gene dysregulates the TGF-β pathway in early B lineage progenitor cells. J Clin Invest. 2009;119(4):826–36.

Ganly P, Walker LC, Morris CM. Familial mutations of the transcription factor RUNX1 (AML1, CBFA2) predispose to acute myeloid leukaemia. Leuk Lymphome. 2004;45(1):1–10.

Goldin LR, Pfeiffer RM, Hemminki K. Familial risk of lymphoproliferativce tumours in families of patients with chronic lymphocytic leukaemia: results from the Swedish Family-Cancer Database. Blood. 2004;104(6):1850–4.

Goldin LR, Slager SL, Caporaso NE. Familial chronic lymphocytic leukaemia. Curr Opin Haematol. 2010;17:350–5.

Goransdotter Ericson K, Fadeel B, Nilsson-Ardnor S, et al. Spectrum of perforin gene mutations in familial hemophagocytic lymphohistiocytosis. Am J Hum Genet. 2001;68:590–7.

Graham GE, Graham LM, Bridge PJ, Maclaren LD, Wolff JEA, Coppes MJ, Egeler RM. Further evidence for genetic heterogeneity in familial hemophagocytic lymphohistiocytosis (FHLH). Pediatr Res. 2000;48:227–32.

Grass S, Preuss KD, Wikowicz A, Terpos E, Ziepert M, Nikolaus D, Yang Y, Fadle N, Regitz E, Dimopoulos MA, Treon SP, Hunter ZR, Pfreundschuh M. Hyperphosphorylated paratarg-7: a new molecularly defined risk factor for monoclonal gammopathy of undetermined significance of the IgM type and Waldenstrom macroglobulinemia. Blood. 2011;117(10):2918–23.

Gunz FW, Gunz JP, Veale AMO, Chapman CJ, Houston IE. Familial leukaemia: a study of 909 families. Scand J Haematol. 1975;15:117–31.

Heim S, Mitelman F. Cancer cytogenetics. New York: Alan Liss Inc.; 1987.

Hemminki K. Re: familial multiple myeloma: a family study and review of the literature. J Natl Cancer Inst. 2002;94(6):462–3.

Hjalgrim H, Rasmussen S, Rostgaard K, Nielsen NM, Koch-Henriksen N, Munksgaard L, Storm HH, Melbye M. Familial clustering of Hodgkin lymphoma and multiple sclerosis. J Natl Cancer Inst. 2004;96(10):780–4.

Horwitz LJ, Levy RN, Rosner F. Multiple myeloma in three siblings. Arch Intern Med. 1985;145:1449–50.

Horwitz M, Goode EL, Jarvik GP. Anticipation in familial leukemia. Am J Hum Genet. 1996;59:990–8.

Horwitz M, Benson KF, Li FQ, Wolff J, Leppert MF, Hobson L, Mangelsdorf M, Yu S, Hewett D, Richards RI, Raskind WH. Genetic heterogeneity in familial acute myelogenous leukemia: evidence for a second locus at chromosome 16q21–23.2. Am J Hum Genet. 1997;61:873–81.

Houlston RS. Low penetrance susceptibility to haematological malignancy. Curr Opin Genet Dev. 2010;20:245–50.

Houlston RS, Sellick G, Yuille M, Matutes E, Catovsky D. Causation of chronic lymphocytic leukemia – insights from familial disease. Leuk Res. 2003;27:871–6.

Ishibe N, Sgambati MT, Fontaine L, et al. Clinical characteristics of familial B-CLL in the National Cancer Institute Familial Registry. Leuk Lymphoma. 2001;42:99–108.

Izraeli S. Perspective: chromosomal aneuploidy in leukemia – lessons from Down syndrome. Haematol Oncol. 2005;24(1):3–6.

Izraeli S, Rainis L, Hertzberg L, Smooha G, Birger Y. Trisomy of chromosome 21 in leukemogenesis. Blood Cell Mol Dis. 2007;39(2):156–9.

Jacobs A. Benzene and leukemia. Br J Haematol. 1989;12:119–21.

Jedlickova K, Stockton DW, Prchal JT. Possible primary familial and congenital polycythemia locus at 7q22.1–7q22.2. Blood Cell Mol Dis. 2003;31:327–31.

Judson IR, Wiltshaw E, Newland AC. Multiple myeloma in a pair of monozygotic twins: the first reported case. Br J Haematol. 1985;60:551–4.

Kalff MW, Hijmans W. Immunoglobulin analysis in families of macroglobulinaemia patients. Clin Exp Immunol. 1969;5:479–98.

Kearney L, De Castro DG, Yeung J, Procter J, Horsley SW, Eguchi-Ishimae M, Bateman CM, Anderson K, Chaplin T, Young BD, Harrison CJ, Kempski H, So CW, Ford AM, Greaves M. Specific JAK2 mutation (JAK2R683) and multiple gene deletions in Down syndrome acute lymphoblastic leukemia. Blood. 2009;113(3):646–8.

Kersey JH, Shapiro RS, Filipovich AH. Relationship of immunodeficiency to lymphoid malignancy. Pediatr Infect Dis J. 1988;7:510–2.

Kikuchi M, Tayama T, Hayakawa H, Takahashi I, Hoshino H, Ohsaka A. Familial thrombocytosis. Br J Haematol. 1995;89:900–2.

Kinlen L. Childhood leukaemia, nuclear sites, and population mixing. Br J Cancer. 2011; 104(1):12–8.

Klitz W, Aldrich CL, Fildes N, Horning SJ, Begovich AB. Localization of predisposition to Hodgkin disease in the HLA class II region. Am J Hum Genet. 1994;54:497–505.

Klusmann JH, Creutzig U, Zimmerman M, Dworzak M, Jorch N, Langebrake C, Pekrun A, Macakova-Reingardt K, Reinhardt D. Treatment and prognostic impact of transient leukemia in neonates with Down syndrome. Blood. 2007;111(6):2991–8.

Kondo T, Okabe M, et al. Familial essential thrombocythemia associated with one-base deletion in the 5′-untranslated region of the thrombopoietin gene. Blood. 1998;92:1091–6.

Kralovics R, Sokol L, Prchal JT. Absence of polycythemia in a child with aunique erythropoietin receptor mutation in a family with autosomal dominant primary polycythemia. J Clin Invest. 1998;102(1):124–9.

Kralovics R, Stockton DW, Prchal JT. Clonal hematopoiesis in familial polycythemia vera suggests the involvement of multiple mutational events in the early pathogenesis of the disease. Blood. 2003;102:3793–6.

Kurzrock R, Guterman JU, Talpaz M. The molecular genetics of Philadelphia chromosome-positive leukaemias. N Engl J Med. 1988;319:990–8.

Kwong YL, Ng MH, Ma SK. Familial acute myeloid leukemia with monosomy 7: late onset and involvement of a multipotential progenitor cell. Cancer Genet Cytogenet. 2000; 116:170–3.

Laurent EL, Talpaz M, Kantarjian H, Kurzrock R. The BCR gene and Philadelphia chromosome-positive leukaemogenesis. Cancer Res. 2001;61:2343–55.

Le Couedic JP, Mitjavila MT, Villeval JL, Feger F, Gobert S, Mayeux P, Casadevall N, Vainchenker W. Missense mutation of the erythropoietin receptor is a rare event in human erythroid malignancies. Blood. 1996;87:1502–11.

Lenz G, Davis RE, Ngo VN, Lam L, George TC, Wright GW, Dave SS, Zhao H, Xu W, Rosenwald A, Ott G, Muller-Hermelink HK, and 10 others. Oncogenic CARD11 mutations in human diffuse large B cell lymphoma. Science 2008;319(5870):1676–9.

Lynch HT, Marcus JN, Weisenburger DD, et al. Genetic and immunopatho-logical findings in a lymphoma family. Br J Cancer. 1989;59:622–6.

Lynch HT, Sanger WG, Pirruccello S, Quinn-Laquer B, Weisenburger DD. Familial multiple myeloma: a family study and review of the literature. J Natl Cancer Inst. 2001;93(19):1479–83.

Lynch HT, Weisenburger DD, Quinn-Laquer B, Watson P, Lynch JF, Sanger WG. Hereditary chronic lymphocytic leukemia: an extended family study and literature review. Am J Med Genet. 2002;115:113–7.

Lynch HT, Ferrara K, Barlogie B, et al. Familial myeloma. NEJM. 2008a;359:152–7.

Lynch HT, Ferrara KM, Weisenburger DD, Sanger WG, Lynch JF, Thomé SD. Genetic counseling for DAPK1 mutation in a chronic lymphocytic leukemia family. Cancer Genet Cytogenet. 2008b;186(2):95–102.

Ma W, Zhang X, Wang X, et al. MPL mutation profile in Jak2 mutation-negative patients with myeloproliferative disorders. Diagn Mol Pathol. 2011;20(1):34–9.

Mack TM, Cozen W, Shibata DK. Concordance for Hodgkin's Disease in identical twins suggesting genetic susceptibility to the young-adult form of the disease. N Engl J Med. 1995; 332:413–8.

McMaster ML. Familial Waldenstrom's macroglobulinemia. Semin Oncol. 2003;30:146–52.

McMaster ML, Goldin LR, Bai Y, et al. Genomewide linkage screen for Waldenstraom macroglobulinaemia susceptibility loci in high-risk families. Am J Hum Genet. 2006;79:695–701.

Menko FH, Kaspers GL, Meijer GA, Claes K, van Hagen JM, Gille JJ. A homozygous MSH6 mutation in a child with café-au-lait spots, oligodendroglioma and rectal cancer. Fam Cancer. 2004;3(2):123–7.

Miller RW. Deaths from childhood leukemia and solid tumours among twins and other sibs in the United States, 1960–67. J Natl Cancer Inst. 1971;46:203–9.

Mulligan CG. JAK2 – a new player in acute lymphoblastic leukemia. Lancet. 2008;372(9648):1448–50. Leukemia. 2007 Apr;21(4):830–3. Epub 2007 Feb 15.

Niemeyer CM, Kang MW, Shin DH, Furlan I, Erlacher M, Bunin NJ, Bunda S, Finklestein JZ, Sakamoto KM, Gorr TA, Mehta P, Schmid I, Kropshofer G, Corbacioglu S, Lang PJ, Klein C, Schlegel PG, Heinzmann A, Schneider M, Starý J, van den Heuvel-Eibrink MM, Hasle H, Locatelli F, Sakai D, Archambeault S, Chen L, Russell RC, Sybingco SS, Ohh M, Braun BS, Flotho C, Loh ML. Germline CBL mutations cause developmental abnormalities and predispose to juvenile myelomonocytic leukemia. Nat Genet. 2010;42(9):794–800.

Nowell PC, Hungerford DA. A minute chromosome in human chronic granulocytic leukemia. Science. 1960;132:1497.

Pandit B, Sarkozy A, Pennacchio LA, Carta C, Oishi K, Martinelli S, Pogna EA, Schackwitz W, Ustaszewska A, Landstrom A, Bos JM, Ommen SR, Esposito G, Lepri F, Faul C, Mundel P, López Siguero JP, Tenconi R, Selicorni A, Rossi C, Mazzanti L, Torrente I, Marino B, Digilio MC, Zampino G, Ackerman MJ, Dallapiccola B, Tartaglia M, Gelb BD. Gain-of-function RAF1 mutations cause Noonan and LEOPARD syndromes with hypertrophic cardiomyopathy. Nat Genet. 2007;39(8):1007–12.

Park S, Picard F, Dreyfus F. Erythroleukemia: a need for a new definition. Leukemia. 2002;16:1399–401.

Poley JW, Wagner A, Hoogmans MM, Menko FH, Tops C, Kros JM, Reddingius RE, Meijers-Heijboer H, Kuipers EJ, Dinjens WN, Rotterdam Initiative on Gastrointestinal Hereditary Tumors. Biallelic germline mutations of mismatch-repair genes: a possible cause for multiple pediatric malignancies. Cancer. 2007;109(11):2349–56.

Pottern LM, Linet M, Blair A, et al. Familial cancers associated with subtypes of leukemia and non-Hodgkin's lymphoma. Leuk Res. 1991;15:305–14.

Rabin KR, Whitlock JA. Malignancy in children with trisomy 21. Oncologist. 2009;14(2): 164–73.

Raval A, Tanner SM, Byrd JC. Downregulation of death associated protein kinase 1 (DAPK1) in chronic lymphatic leukemia. Cell. 2007;129(5):879–90.

Rawstron AC, Yuille MR, Fuller J, Cullen M, Kennedy B, Richards SJ, Jack AS, Matutes E, Catovsky D, Hillmen P, Houlston RS. Inherited predisposition to CLL is detectable as subclinical monoclonal B-lymphocyte expansion. Blood. 2002;100(7):2289–90.

Renier G, Ifrah N, Chevailler A, Saint-André JP, Boasson M, Hurez D. Four brothers with Waldenstrom's macroglobulinaemia. Cancer. 1989;64:1554–9.

Saarinen S, Aavikko M, Altomaki K, et al. Exome sequencing reveals germline NPAT mutation as a candidate risk factor for Hodgkin lymphoma. Blood. 2011a;118:493–6.

Saarinen S, Aavikko M, Aittomäki K, Launonen V, Lehtonen R, Franssila K, Lehtonen HJ, Kaasinen E, Broderick P, Tarkkanen J, Bain BJ, Bauduer F, Ünal A, Swerdlow AJ, Cooke R, Mäkinen MJ, Houlston R, Vahteristo P, Aaltonen LA. Exome sequencing reveals germline NPAT mutation as a candidate risk factor for Hodgkin lymphoma. Blood. 2011b;118(3):493–8.

Schlemper RJ, van der Maas APC, Eikenboom JCJ. Familial essential thrombocythemia: clinical characteristics of 11 cases in one family. Ann Hematol. 1994;68:153–8.

Scott LM, Tong W, Levine RL, Scott MA, Beer PA, Stratton MR, Futreal PA, Erber WN, McMullin MF, Harrison CN, Warren AJ, Gilliland DG, Lodish HF, Green AR. JAK2 exon 12 mutations in polycythemia vera and idiopathic erythrocytosis. N Engl J Med. 2007;356(5):459–68.

Shah S, Schrader KA, Waanders E, Timms AE, Vijai J, Miething C, Wechsler J, Yang J, Hayes J, Klein RJ, Zhang J, Wei L, Wu G, Rusch M, Nagahawatte P, Ma J, Chen SC, Song G, Cheng J, Meyers P, Bhojwani D, Jhanwar S, Maslak P, Fleisher M, Littman J, Offit L, Rau-Murthy R, Fleischut MH, Corines M, Murali R, Gao X, Manschreck C, Kitzing T, Murty VV, Raimondi SC, Kuiper RP, Simons A, Schiffman JD, Onel K, Plon SE, Wheeler DA, Ritter D, Ziegler DS, Tucker K, Sutton R, Chenevix-Trench G, Li J, Huntsman DG, Hansford S, Senz J, Walsh T, Lee M, Hahn CN, Roberts KG, King MC, Lo SM, Levine RL, Viale A, Socci ND, Nathanson KL, Scott HS, Daly M, Lipkin SM, Lowe SW, Downing JR, Altshuler D, Sandlund JT, Horwitz MS, Mullighan CG, Offit K. A recurrent germline PAX5 mutation confers susceptibility to pre-B cell acute lymphoblastic leukemia. Nat Genet. 2013;45:1226–31.

Shugart YY, Collins A. Combined segregation and linkage analysis of 59 Hodgkin's disease families indicates the role of HLA determinants. EJHG. 2000;8:460–3.

Shugart YY, Hemminki K, Vaittinen P, Kingman A, Dong C. A genetic study of Hodgkin's lymphoma: an estimate of heritability and anticipation based on the familial cancer database in Sweden. Hum Genet. 2000;106(5):553–6.

Shugart YY, Hemminki K, Vaittinen P, Kingman A. Apparent anticipation and heterogeneous transmission patterns in familial Hodgkin's and non-Hodgkin's lymphoma: report from a study based on Swedish cancer database. Leuk Lymphoma. 2001;42(3):407–15.

Skibola CF, Bracci PM, Halperin E, et al. Genetic variants at 6p21.33 are associated with susceptibility to follicular lymphoma. Nat Genet. 2009;41:873–5.

Smith ML, Cavenagh JD, Lister TA, Fitzgibbon J. Mutation of CEBPA in familial acute myeloid leukemia. N Engl J Med. 2004;351:2403–7.

Steingrimsdottir H, Einarsdottir HK, Haraldsdottir V, Ogmundsdottir HM. Familial monoclonal gammopathy: hyper-responsive B cells in unaffected family members. Eur J Haematol. 2011;86(5):396–404.

Taylor GM, Gokhale DA, Crowther D, Woll PJ, Harris M, Ryder D, Ayres M, Radford JA. Further investigation of the role of HLA-DPB1 in adult Hodgkin's disease (HD) suggests an influence on susceptibility to different HD subtypes. Br J Cancer. 1999;80(9):1405–11.

Thunberg U, Tobin G, Johnson A, Soderberg O, Padyukov L, Hultdin M, Klareskog L, Enblad G, Sundstrom C, Roos G, Rosenquist R. Polymorphism in the P2X7 receptor gene and survival in chronic lymphocytic leukemia. Lancet. 2002;360(9349):1935–9.

Tigay JH. A comparison of acute lymphoblastic leukemia in Down syndrome and non-Down syndrome children: the role of trisomy 21. J Paediatr Nurs. 2009;26(6):362–8.

Till MM, Jones LH, Penticess CR, et al. Leukaemia in children and their grand-parents: studies of immune function in six families. Br J Haematol. 1975;29:575–86.

van Dijken PJ, Woldendorp KH, van Wouwe JP. Familial thrombocytosis in infancy presenting with a leukaemoid reaction. Acta Pediatr. 1996;85:1132–4.

Van Roosbroeck K, Cox L, Tousseyn T, Lahortiga I, Gielen O, Cauwelier B, De Paepe P, Verhoef G, Marynen P, Vandenberghe P, De Wolf-Peeters C, Cools J, Wlodarska I. JAK2 rearrangements, including the novel SEC31A-JAK2 fusion, are recurrent in classical Hodgkin lymphoma. Blood. 2011;117(15):4056–64.

Wiernik PH, Wang SQ, Hu X-P, Marino P, Paietta E. Age of onset evidence for anticipation in familial non-Hodgkin's lymphoma. Br J Haematol. 2000;108:72–9.

Wiley JS, et al. A loss-of-function polymorphic mutation in the cytolytic P2X7 receptor gene and chronic lymphocytic leukemia: a molecular study. Lancet. 2002;359(9312):1114–9.

Yuille MR, Matutes E, Marossy A, Hilditch B, Catovsky D, Houlston RS. Familial chronic lymphocytic leukemia: a survey and review of published studies. Br J Haematol. 2000; 109(4):794–9.

Chapter 9
Musculoskeletal System

Bone Tumors

In general, sarcomas of bone, muscle, or connective tissue are rare, especially in children. Bone tumors comprise about 5 % of childhood cancers (3 % osteosarcomas and 2 % Ewing sarcoma), and their incidence overall is about 10 per million persons in the UK. The age-standardized rate of malignant bone tumors for white children (0–14 years of age) in the SEER Registry, 1983–1992, was 6.4 per million. Soft tissue sarcomas are slightly more common (10 per million). The rates are similar for black children in the same registry, except for Ewing sarcoma, which is nine times less common in black children (Parkin 1998).

Osteosarcoma

Osteogenic sarcoma is commoner in males than in females and shows two age peaks, one at adolescence and a second, which parallels that of chondrosarcoma, in the sixth and seventh decades. The tumor has a predilection for rapidly growing bone, and the risk is increased in Paget disease (Wu et al. 1991). Children with osteosarcoma are significantly taller at time of diagnosis than are unaffected controls (Gelberg et al. 1997). A similar but not significant difference is seen for children with Ewing sarcoma. Familial aggregations of Paget's disease are sometimes seen; several loci have been implicated, and mutations have been detected in the *TNFRSF 11A* gene in affected individuals (Hughes et al. 2000).

Familial osteosarcoma is rare, but multiple cases have been described in a number of sibships. A study of familial osteosarcoma identified 59 affected individuals from 24 families. Seven patients had Paget disease, three had a history of multiple fractures, two had bilateral retinoblastoma, and one had an osteosarcoma at another site (Hillmann et al. 2000). Sarcoma-prone families have been reported where individuals with osteosarcoma had germline mutations in *TP53* (Lynch et al. 2003), and about 3 % of children with osteosarcoma may carry germline mutations in *TP53*. They may not all have a substantial family history consistent with Li–Fraumeni syndrome (Toguchida et al. 1992; McIntyre et al. 1994).

Osteosarcoma may also occur in individuals with germline mutations of the retinoblastoma gene (relative risk up to 500 times normal), especially in the field of any irradiation (see p. 15; Mertens and Bramwell 1995). It may also occur in the multiple exostosis and multiple endostosis syndromes, Bloom syndrome (Fuchs and Pritchard 2002), and in Rothmund–Thomson disease (Cumin et al. 1996; Leonard et al. 1996). This disorder is characterized by skin atrophy, telangiectasia, hyper- and hypopigmentation, congenital skeletal abnormalities, short stature, premature aging, and a predisposition to malignancy. Truncating mutations in the causative gene, *RECQL4*, (Kitao et al. 1999; Simon et al. 2010) appear to be more strongly associated with osteosarcoma than are other types of mutations (Wang et al. 2003). However, mutations in *RECQL4* are uncommon in sporadic osteosarcoma (Nishijo et al. 2004). There has been a report of a family with familial gigantiform cementoma, where one individual developed an osteosarcoma (Rossbach et al. 2005).

There is a risk of malignant degeneration in both monostotic fibrous dysplasia (which is sporadic) and McCune–Albright syndrome, characterized by polyostotic fibrous dysplasia, cafe-au-lait skin pigmentation, and precocious puberty, in which activating mutations of Gs proteins (postzygotic mutations in the *GNAS1* gene) have been detected (see p. 275; Alman et al. 1996). Patients with polyostotic fibrous dysplasia are at higher risk of malignant degeneration than those with monostotic lesions, which is thought to reflect their greater number of lesions rather than an increased risk per lesion. Somatic mutations in GS alpha have been found in both conditions (Lumbroso et al. 2004; Pollandt et al. 2001). In genetically predisposed individuals (e.g., Li–Fraumeni syndrome), a second osteogenic sarcoma may develop in the field of radiation delivered to the initial primary cancer (Li et al. 1978). Osteogenic sarcoma occurs as part of the OSLAM syndrome, described in a single report of probable autosomal dominant inheritance of childhood osteosarcomas associated with erythroid mastocytosis and a megaloblastic marrow and limb abnormalities (Mulvihill et al. 1977).

Hereditary multiple exostoses (diaphyseal aclasis) is an autosomal dominant skeletal dysplasia with an estimated prevalence of 9 per 1,000,000 population. It is characterized by the development of numerous cartilage-capped exostoses in actively growing areas of bone (Ahn et al. 1995). The most common sites are the regions of the long bones, the pelvis, scapula, and ribs, but the skull and vertebrae are usually spared. A Madelung deformity of the forearm is common. The multiple exostoses produce bony deformities, abnormal bone growth, and mild short stature. Penetrance is almost complete radiologically but with many subclinical lesions. Growth of the exostoses is maximal during childhood and adolescence, and the diagnosis is usually made during the first decade of life. The major complication of this disorder is malignant degeneration of the exostoses. Estimates of this risk vary, but the incidence is probably less than 10 %. Patients should be alerted to the significance of a rapid change in the rate of growth and the development of pain and inflammation. Regular surveillance to detect these changes is recommended. If osteosarcomas occur, they develop at an earlier age than their sporadic counterparts, at a mean age of approximately 30 years (range 10–50 years) (Hennekam 1991). The presence of multiple exostoses in a patient with a balanced translocation t(8; 11)(q24.11; p15.5) led to the identification of one of three loci now identified, on chromosomes 8q24.1, 11p13, and 19p, in which germline mutations can cause this disorder (Ludecke et al. 1991; Wuyts et al. 1996). Germline mutations have also been identified in the *EXT1* and *EXT2* genes (Heinritz et al. 2009). Both genes encode glycosyltransferases that are involved in heparan sulfate biosynthesis. The risk for sarcoma is greater for those with *EXT1* mutations than for *EXT2* mutations. Multiple exostoses type III has been mapped to chromosome 19 (*EXT3*). Screening for sarcoma in *EXT1* mutation carriers is justified (Porter et al. 2004; Seki et al. 2001).

Multiple exostoses also occur in metachondromatosis, an autosomal dominant condition characterized by short stature, with exostoses and enchondromas occurring in the hands and long bones. The osteochondromas point towards the joint and there is a tendency for them to regress and even disappear. It is caused by mutations in the *PTPN11* gene on chromosome 12q24 (Sobreira et al. 2010).

The Langer–Giedion syndrome (trichorhinophalangeal syndrome type II) is characterized by postnatal short stature, sparse hair, unusual faces with pear-shaped nose and long philtrum, micrognathia and protruding ears, and multiple exostoses (Buhler et al. 1987). About 70 % of affected individuals have developmental delay. It is a contiguous gene syndrome on 8q24.1, involving loss of functional copies of the *TRPS1* and *EXT1* genes on chromosome 8q24 (Ludecke et al. 1995).

Exostoses–anetodermia–brachydactyly type E is probably an autosomal dominant disorder characterized by a combination of macular atrophy, multiple exostoses, and brachydactyly (Mollica et al. 1984).

A contiguous gene syndrome on chromosome 11p11, known as DEFECT 11, involves *EXT2*. In this condition, the multiple cartilaginous exostoses develop in the first few years of life, and increase in number until puberty is complete. They cause deformity and asymmetry of growth, and there is a small risk of osteosarcoma developing. This condition is usually sporadic.

Chondrosarcoma

The incidence of this tumor increases with increasing age. Chondrosarcoma is described as a complication of multiple enchondromatosis (Ollier disease; see below), inherited multiple exostoses (diaphysial achlasis; see above), Maffucci syndrome (p. 274; Hecht et al. 1997), and other conditions in which exostoses occur. The incidence of malignancy in these syndromes has been assessed as 18 % (Sun et al. 1985). Two groups have recently reported that somatic mosaic mutations in *IDH1* and *IDH2* are the predominant cause of both Ollier disease and Maffucci syndrome (Pansuriya et al. 2011; Amary et al. 2011).

Multiple enchondromatosis (Ollier disease) is usually sporadic, although several families with affected siblings have been described. Deformities, particularly of the long bones, develop because of the enchondromas, resulting in asymmetrical, bilateral limb shortening, bowing, or deformation. The enchondromas tend to grow until adolescent growth is over. Sarcomatous degeneration (chondrosarcoma) can occur in the lesions in adult life, and intracranial gliomas (Chang and Prados 1994) and ovarian juvenile granulosa cell tumors and precocious puberty have also been described in this condition (Tamimi and Bolen 1984).

Maffucci syndrome, characterized by multiple enchondromas and subcutaneous hemangiomas, is associated with a high risk of malignant transformation, a risk of 30 % for chondrosarcomas and other malignancies being reported (Albrechts and Rapini 1995; Kaplan et al. 1993). Intracranial chordoma has also been reported in this syndrome (Nakayama et al. 1994). There was a suggestion that a single germ-line mutation in parathyroid hormone-related protein (*PTHR1*), c.448CT, resulting in R105C could be an important cause of endochrondromatosis (Hopyan et al. 2002), but a subsequent study did not find any mutations in *PTHR1* in patients with enchondromatosis (Rozeman et al. 2004).

Hereditary multiple exostoses, associated with germline mutations in the *EXT2* gene, predispose to familial chondrosarcoma (Hecht et al. 1997), and loss of heterozygosity is seen in the tumor in the region of chromosome 11 where *EXT2* maps (see above).

Ewing Sarcoma

This tumor has a peak age at onset in adolescence, is rare in black races, and is not radiation induced. Its incidence is 1.7 per 1,000,000 per year. Familial cases are rare, and the tumor only rarely occurs as part of specific familial cancer syndromes. It is probably a member of a family of neoplasms that includes a skin tumors and primitive neuroectodermal tumors of bone and soft tissue. Retinoblastoma has been recorded as a first primary cancer in ten cases of Ewing sarcoma, and Ewing sarcoma has also occurred after leukemia and lymphoma (Coppes et al. 2001). An excess of inguinal hernias has been observed in children with Ewing sarcoma.

A t(11; 22)(q24; q12) translocation occurs in up to 95 % of Ewing sarcomas and also in primitive neuroectodermal tumors and in peripheral neuroepithelioma and Askin tumors. Some Ewing sarcomas without a t(11; 22) show more complex rearrangements or rearrangements involving 22q12 and other chromosomes so that, overall, 92 % of tumors have a 22q12 breakpoint and 88 % have a 11q23.3 breakpoint (Griffin et al. 1986). A der (16) t(1; 16)(q11; q11) has been observed in the later stages of tumor development (Mugneret et al. 1987). The result of the t(11; 22) is that an aberrant transcription factor protein is produced (Granwetter 1995; Lin et al. 1999). None of these genetic rearrangements are inherited.

Rhabdomyosarcoma

Soft tissue sarcomas account for up to 8 % of all childhood cancers and 2 % of childhood cancer deaths, with an incidence of about 8 per 1,000,000 per year. About half occur in children aged under 3 years, with an equal sex incidence.

Rhabdomyosarcoma accounts for two-thirds of pediatric soft tissue sarcomas (McDowell 2003) and most commonly arise in the head and neck (40 %), genitourinary tract (20 %), and extremities (20 %) (Crist and Kun 1991). On histological criteria, rhabdomyosarcoma may be classified into two main subtypes: embryonal and botryoid (two-thirds of all tumors) and alveolar (one-third).

Most rhabdomyosarcomas are sporadic, but they complicate neurofibromatosis type 1 (NF1; see p. 288, Brems et al. 2009), the Beckwith–Wiedemann syndrome (p. 221) (Lapunzina 2005), and the Li–Fraumeni syndrome (p. 271). Segregation analysis for soft tissue sarcomas in the absence of a known genetic syndrome suggests a heritability of 0.13, due to a postulated rare autosomal dominant gene (population frequency 0.00002) with a penetrance of 50 and 90 % at ages 30 and 60 years, respectively. The risk to first-degree relatives is significantly increased if the index case has two or more primaries (Burke et al. 1991).

Germline mutations in *TP53* may be detected in around 10 % of children with rhabdomyosarcoma (Diller et al. 1995), especially orbital alveolar rhabdomyosarcomas, and rhabdomyosarcoma is the second most prevalent tumor in Li–Fraumeni syndrome after breast cancer (Olivier et al. 2003). Embryonal rhabdomyosarcoma (which occurs in 6 % of tumors in Beckwith–Wiedemann syndrome) specifically shows chromosome 11p allele loss in the same region as the Beckwith–Wiedemann gene. A translocation between chromosomes 2 and 13, (2; 13)(q37; q14), has been described specifically in rhabdomyosarcoma (Meddeb et al. 1996); although it is most frequent in alveolar rhabdomyosarcoma, it has also been reported in embryonal and undifferentiated types. Embryonal rhabdomyosarcomas are the most common tumor associated with Costello syndrome (Gripp 2005), and they may also be seen in children with any of the "RASopathies" (i.e., with germline mutations in genes which are part of the Ras/mitogen activated protein kinase (MAPK) pathway), including Noonan, LEOPARD, and cardio-cutaneous-facial syndromes (Tidyman and Rauen 2009; Denayer et al. 2010). They also have been described in individuals with biallelic *PMS2* mutations (Kratz et al. 2009) and in Nijmegen breakage syndrome (Meyer and Spunt 2004) embryonal rhabdomyosarcomas are also reported in *DICER1* mutation carriers, particularly those arising from the cervix (Foulkes et al. 2011).

Other Sarcomas

Synovial sarcomas occur in adolescents and young adults, especially males, have no racial predilection, and are not noted for familial occurrence. The tumors have been shown to have X:18 chromosomal translocations t(X:18)(p11.2; q11.2), involving a breakpoint at Xp11.2, resulting in the formation of a hybrid transcript (Gilgenkrantz et al. 1989; de Leeuw et al. 1995; Carbano et al. 2002; de Leeuw et al. 1994).

A study of the family histories of children with soft tissue sarcomas showed an increased family history of the Li–Fraumeni syndrome, sarcomas, gastric cancer, and neurofibromatosis, and it was considered that one-third of cases had a genetic susceptibility (Hartley et al. 1993).

Extraskeletal myxoid chondrosarcomas have been found to show a 9:22 chromosomal translocation: t(9; 22)(q31; q12.2) causing a *NR4A3/TFG* fusion gene (Hisaoka et al. 2004).

Kaposi sarcoma (multiple idiopathic pigmented hemangiosarcoma) has rarely been described in several members of the same family, suggesting an autosomal dominant pattern of inheritance. The condition is characterized by red–purple nodules, plaques, and macules which are commonest on the extremities but can occur at any site, including internally. Edema is associated, due to tumor infiltration of lymphatics, and the lesions spread, often with metastatic dissemination, usually with fatal results, although spontaneous regression has been described. The condition is commoner in people of Italian or Jewish origin (DiGiovanna and Safai 1981). Kaposi sarcoma is usually sporadic and immunosuppressed transplant recipients; it is the most common neoplasm affecting patients with AIDS, and HIV infection is an important risk factor in its development: the KS risk of AIDS patients is 20,000-fold over that of the general population. Foster et al. (2000) found a strong association between the IL6 gene promoter polymorphism and susceptibility to Kaposi sarcoma in HIV-infected men. Homozygotes for IL6 allele G, associated with increased IL6 production, were overrepresented among patients with Kaposi sarcoma, whereas allele C homozygotes were underrepresented. A novel herpes virus, termed KS-associated herpes virus (KSHV) or human herpes virus 8 (HHV8), has been detected in Kaposi sarcoma tissues, indicating that a viral infection may be important in the etiology of this condition (Kedes et al. 1996).

Uterine leiomyomas (fibroids) occur in individuals with leiomyomatosis, where germline mutations in the fumarate hydratase (FH) gene predispose to these tumors and to type 2 papillary renal cell cancer (see p. 201).

Rhabdoid Tumors

Rhabdoid tumors are aggressive pediatric malignancies which mainly develop in infancy and early childhood. When they arise in the central nervous system, they are referred to as atypical tetratoid/rhabdoid tumors and malignant rhabdoid tumor (MRT) when they arise in other renal and extrarenal sites. Most are associated with loss of function of the *SMARCB1* gene in chromosome 22q11.2, and approximately one-third of patients with rhabdoid tumors have a germline mutation in the *SMARCB1* gene. Incomplete penetrance and gonadal mosaicism has been described in families with such mutations, and relatives of affected cases may develop rhabdoid tumors, schwannomas, or schwannomatosis (Eaton et al. 2011).

Sacrococcygeal Teratoma

After the first few years of life, most teratomas are gonadal. Familial benign cystic teratoma of the ovary has been described in three generations of a family (Brenner and Wallach 1983). Adult testicular gonadal germ cell tumors tend to be aneuploid, although infantile gonadal germ cell tumors may more often be tetraploid or diploid, which suggests that they may have a different etiology (Silver et al. 1994). In fact, most teratomas develop in the sacrococcygeal area and tend to be benign. There may be associated malformations of the sacrum, vertebrae, and gastrointestinal or urogenital tracts. Familial teratoma with an autosomal dominant mode of inheritance has been described, with variable penetrance, and some affected individuals have been described to have anterior sacral meningocoele, sacral defects, or skin dimples without teratoma (Yates et al. 1983). The Currarino triad involves the association of partial sacral agenesis with intact first sacral vertebra ("sickle-shaped sacrum"), a presacral mass, and anorectal malformation. Some cases of the Currarino syndrome may be caused by mutations in the *HLXB9* homeobox gene (Kim et al. 2007).

References

Ahn J, Lüdecke HJ, Lindow S, Horton WA, Lee B, Wagner MJ, Horsthemke B, Wells DE. Cloning of the putative tumor suppressor gene for hereditary multiple exostoses (EXT1). Nat Genet. 1995;11(2):137–43.

Albrechts AE, Rapini RP. Malignancy in Maffucci's syndrome. Dermatol Clin. 1995;13:73–8.

Alman BA, Greel DA, Wolfe HJ. Activating mutations of Gs protein in monostatic fibrous lesions of bone. J Orthop Res. 1996;14:311–5.

Amary MF, Damato S, Halai D, Eskandarpour M, Berisha F, Bonar F, McCarthy S, Fantin VR, Straley KS, Lobo S, Aston W, Green CL, Gale RE, Tirabosco R, Futreal A, Campbell P, Presneau N, Flanagan AM. Ollier disease and Maffucci syndrome are caused by somatic mosaic mutations of IDH1 and IDH2. Nat Genet. 2011;43(12):1262–5.

Bahubeshi A, Tischkowitz M, Foulkes WD. miRNA processing and human cancer: DICER1 cuts the mustard. Sci Transl Med. 2011;30;3(111):111 ps 46. doi: 10.1126/scitranslmed.3002493. Review.

Brems H, Beert E, de Ravel T, Legius E. Mechanisms in the pathogenesis of malignant tumors in neurofibromatosis type 1. Lancet Oncol. 2009;10:508–15.

Brenner SH, Wallach RC. Familial benign cystic teratoma. Int J Gynaecol Obstet. 1983;21:167–9.

Buhler EM, Buhler UK, Beutler C, et al. A final word on the tricho-rhino-phalangeal syndrome. Clin Genet. 1987;31:273–5.

Burke E, Li F, Janov AJ, et al. Cancer in relatives of survivors of childhood sarcoma. Cancer. 1991;67:1467–9.

Carbano M, Rizzo P, Powers A, et al. Molecular analyses, morphology and immuno-histochemistry together differentiate pleural synovial sarcomas from mesotheliomas: clinical implications. Anticancer Res. 2002;22(6B):3443–8.

Chang S, Prados MG. Identical twins with Ollier's disease and intracranial gliomas: case report. Neurosurgery. 1994;34:903–6.

Coppes RP, Zeilstra LJ, Kampinga HH, Konings AW. Early to late sparing of radiation damage to the parotid gland by adrenergic and muscarinic receptor agonists. Br J Cancer. 2001;85(7):1055–63.

Crist WM, Kun LE. Common solid tumours of childhood. New Engl J Med. 1991;324:461–71.

Cumin I, Cohen JY, David A, et al. Rothmund–Thomson syndrome and osteosarcoma. Med Pediatr Oncol. 1996;26:414–16.

de Leeuw B, Balemans M, Weghuis DOO, et al. Molecular cloning of the synovialsarcoma-specific molecular translocation (X:18)(p.11.2:q11.2) breakpoint. Hum Mol Genet. 1994;3:745–9.

de Leeuw B, Balemans M, Olde Weghuis D, Geurts van Kessel A. Identification of two alternative fusion genes, SYT-SSX1 and SYT-SSX2, in t(X;18)(p11.2;q11.2)-positive synovial sarcomas. Hum Mol Genet. 1995;4(6):1097–9.

Denayer E, Devriendt K, de Ravel T, et al. Tumour spectrum in children with noonan syndrome and SOS1 or RAF1 mutations. Genes Chromosomes Cancer. 2010;49:242–52.

DiGiovanna JJ, Safai S. Kaposi's sarcoma. Am J Med. 1981;71:779–83.

Diller L, Sexsmith E, Gottlieb A, et al. Germline p53 mutations are frequently detected in young children with rhabdomyosarcoma. J Clin Invest. 1995;95:1606–11.

Eaton KW, Tooke LS, Wainwright LM, Judkins AR, Biegel JA. Spectrum of SMARCB1/INI1 mutations in familial and sporadic rhabdoid tumors. Pediatr Blood Cancer. 2011;56(1):7–15.

Foster CB, Lehrnbecher T, Samuels S, Stein S, Mol F, Metcalf JA, Wyvill K, Steinberg SM, Kovacs J, Blauvelt A, Yarchoan R, Chanock SJ. An IL6 promoter polymorphism is associated with a lifetime risk of development of Kaposi sarcoma in men infected with human immunodeficiency virus. Blood. 2000;96:2562–7.

Fuchs B, Pritchard DJ. Etiology of osteosarcoma. Clin Orthop Relat Res. 2002;397:40–52.

Gelberg KH, Fitzgerald EF, Hwang S, Dubrow R. Growth and development and other risk factors for osteosarcoma in children and young adults. Int J Epidemiol. 1997;26:272–8.

Gilgenkrantz S, Mujica P, Chery M, et al. Mapping the breakpoint at 11 p11.2 in synovial sarcoma. Cytogenet Cell Genet. 1989;51:1004 [Abstract].

Granwetter L. Ewing's sarcoma and extracranial peripheral neuroectodermal tumors. Curr Opin Oncol. 1995;7:355–60.

Griffin CA, McKeon C, Israel MA, et al. Comparison of constitutional and tumour-associated 11;22 translocations: nonidentical breakpoints on chromosomes 11 and 22. Proc Natl Acad Sci USA. 1986;83:6122–6.

Gripp KW. Tumour predisposition in Costello syndrome. Am J Med Genet. 2005;137C:72–7.

Hartley AL, Birch JM, Blair V, et al. Patterns of cancer in the families of children with soft tissue sarcomas. Cancer. 1993;72:923–30.

Hecht JT, Hogue D, Wang Y, Blanton SH, Wagner M, Strong LC, Raskind W, Hansen MF, Wells D. Hereditary multiple exostoses (EXT): mutational studies of familial EXT1 cases and EXT-associated malignancies. Am J Hum Genet. 1997;60(1):80–6.

Heinritz W, Hüffmeier U, Strenge S, Miterski B, Zweier C, Leinung S, Bohring A, Mitulla B, Peters U, Froster UG. New mutations of EXT1 and EXT2 genes in German patients with multiple osteochondromas. Ann Hum Genet. 2009;73:283–91.

Hennekam RCM. Hereditary multiple exostoses. J Med Genet. 1991;28:262–6.

Hillmann A, Ozaki T, Winkelmann W. Familial occurrence of osteosarcoma. A case report and review of the literature. J Cancer Res Clin Oncol. 2000;126(9):497–502.

Hisaoka M, Ishida T, Imamura T, Hashimoto H. TFG is a novel fusion partner of NOR1 in extraskeletal myxoid chondrosarcoma. Genes Chromosomes Cancer. 2004;40:325–8.

Hopyan S, Gokgoz N, Poon R, et al. A mutant PTH/PTHrP type I receptor in enchondromatosis. Nat Genet. 2002;30:306–10.

Hughes AE, Ralston SH, Marken J, Bell C, MacPherson H, Wallace RGH, van Hul W, Whyte MP, Nakatsuka K, Hovy L, Anderson DM. Mutations in TNFRSF11A, affecting the signal peptide of RANK, cause familial expansile osteolysis. Nat Genet. 2000;24:45–8.

Kaplan RP, Wang JT, Amron DM, Kaplan L. Maffucci's syndrome: two case reports with a literature review. J Am Acad Dermatol. 1993;29:894–9.

Kedes DH, Operskalski E, Busch M, Kohn R, Flood J, Ganem D. The seroepidemiology of human herpesvirus 8 (Kaposi's sarcoma-associated herpesvirus): distribution of infection in KS risk groups and evidence for sexual transmission. Nat Med. 1996;2:918–24.

Kim I-S, Oh S, Choi S-J, Kim J-H, Park KH, Park H-K, Kim J-W, Ki C-S. Clinical and genetic analysis of HLXB9 gene in Korean patients with Currarino syndrome. J Hum Genet. 2007;52:698–701.

Kitao S, Shimamoto A, Goto M, et al. Mutations in RECQL4 cause a subset of Rothmund–Thomson syndrome. Nat Genet. 1999;22:82–4.

Kratz C, Holter S, Etzler J, et al. Rhabdomyosarcoma in patients with constitutional mismatch repair deficiency syndrome. J Med Genet. 2009;46:418–20.

Lapunzina P. Risk of tumourigenesis in overgrowth syndromes: a comprehensive review. Am J Med Genet. 2005;137C:53–71.

Leonard A, Craft AW, Moss C, Malcolm AJ. Osteogenic sarcoma in the Rothmund–Thomson syndrome. Med Pediatr Oncol. 1996;26:249–53.

Li FP, Lokich J, Lapey J, Neptune WB, Wilkins Jr EW. Familial mesothelioma after intense asbestos exposure at home. J Am Med Assoc. 1978;240:467.

Lin P, Brody RI, Hamelin AC, et al. Differential transactivation by alternative EWS-FLI1 fusion proteins correlates with clinical heterogeneity in Ewing's sarcoma. Cancer Res. 1999;59:1428–32.

Ludecke HJ, Johnson C, Wagner MJ, et al. Molecular definition of the shortest region of deletion overlap in the Langer–Gideon syndrome. Am J Hum Genet. 1991;49:1197–206.

Ludecke H-J, Wagner MJ, Nardmann J, La Pillo B, Parrish JE, Willems PJ, Haan EA, Frydman M, Hamers GJH, Wells DE, Horsthemke B. Molecular dissection of a contiguous gene syndrome: localization of the genes involved in the Langer-Giedion syndrome. Hum Mol Genet. 1995;4:31–6.

Lumbroso S, Paris F, Sultan C, European Collaborative Study. Activating Gsalpha mutations: analysis of 113 patients with signs of McCune-Albright syndrome–a European Collaborative Study. J Clin Endocrinol Metab. 2004;89:2107–13.

Lynch HT, Deters CA, Hogg D, Lynch JF, Kinarsky Y, Gatalica Z. Familial sarcoma: challenging pedigrees. Cancer. 2003;98:1947–57.

McDowell HP. Update on childhood rhabdomyosarcoma. Arch Dis Child. 2003;88:354–7.

McIntyre JF, Smith-Sorensen B, Friend SH, et al. Germline mutations of the p53 tumour suppressor gene in children with osteosarcoma. J Clin Oncol. 1994;12:925–30.

Meddeb M, Valent A, Danglot G, Nguyen VC, Duverger A, Fouquet F, Terrier-Lacombe MJ, Oberlin O, Bernheim A. MDM2 amplification in a primary alveolar rhabdomyosarcoma displaying a t(2;13)(q35;q14). Cytogenet Cell Genet. 1996;73(4):325–30.

Mertens WC, Bramwell V. Osteosarcoma and other tumors of bone. Curr Opin Oncol. 1995;7(4):349–54. Review.

Meyer WH, Spunt SL. Soft tissue sarcomas of childhood. Cancer Treat Rev. 2004;30:269–80.

Mollica F, Livolti S, Guarneri B. New syndrome: exostoses, anetodermia, and brachydactyly. Am J Med Genet. 1984;19:665–7.

Mugneret F, Aurias A, Lizard S, et al. Der(16)t(1;16) (q11;all.1) is a consistent secondary chromosome change in Ewing's sarcoma. Cytogenet Cell Genet. 1987;46:665.

Mulvihill JJ, Cralnick HR, Whang-Peng J, Leventhal BC. Multiple childhood osteosarcomas in an American family with erythroid macrocytosis and skeletal abnormalities. Cancer. 1977;40:3115–22.

Nakayama Y, Takeno Y, Tsugu H, Tomonanga M. Maffucci's syndrome associated with intracranial chordoma: case report. Neurosurgery. 1994;34:907–9.

Nishijo K, et al. Mutation analysis of the RECQL4 gene in sporadic osteosarcomas. Int J Cancer. 2004;111(3):367–72.

Olivier M, Goldgar DE, Sodha N, et al. Li Fraumeni and related syndromes: correlation between tumor type, family structure and TP53 genotype. Cancer Res. 2003;63:6643–50.

Pansuriya TC, van Eijk R, d'Adamo P, van Ruler MA, Kuijjer ML, Oosting J, Cleton-Jansen AM, van Oosterwijk JG, Verbeke SL, Meijer D, van Wezel T, Nord KH, Sangiorgi L, Toker B, Liegl-Atzwanger B, San-Julian M, Sciot R, Limaye N, Kindblom LG, Daugaard S, Godfraind C, Boon LM, Vikkula M, Kurek KC, Szuhai K, French PJ, Bovée JV. Somatic mosaic IDH1 and IDH2 mutations are associated with enchondroma and spindle cell hemangioma in Ollier disease and Maffucci syndrome. Nat Genet. 2011;43(12):1256–61.

Parkin DM. Epidemiology of cancer: global patterns and trends. Toxicol Lett. 1998;102–103:227–34. Review.

Pollandt K, Engels C, Kaiser E, Werner M, Delling G. Gsalpha gene mutations in monostotic fibrous dysplasia of bone and fibrous dysplasia-like low-grade central osteosarcoma. Virchows Arch. 2001;439(2):170–5.

Porter DE, Lonie L, Fraser M, Dobson-Stone C, Porter JR, Monaco AP, Simpson AH. Severity of disease and risk of malignant change in hereditary multiple exostoses. A genotype-phenotype study. J Bone Joint Surg Br. 2004;86:1041–6.

Rossbach HC, Letson D, Lacson A, Ruas E, Salazar P. Familial gigantiform cementoma with brittle bone disease, pathologic fractures, and osteosarcoma: a possible explanation of an ancient mystery. Pediatr Blood Cancer. 2005;44:390–6.

Rozeman LB, Sangiorgi L, Briaire-de Bruijn IH, Mainil-Varlet P, Bertoni F, Cleton-Jansen AM, Hogendoorn PC, Bovee JV. Enchondromatosis (Ollier disease, Maffucci syndrome) is not caused by the PTHR1 mutation p.R150C. Hum Mutat. 2004;24(6):466–73.

Seki H, Kubota T, Ikegawa S, Haga N, Fujioka F, Ohzeki S, Wakui K, Yoshikawa H, Takaoka K, Fukushima Y. Mutation frequencies of EXT1 and EXT2 in 43 Japanese families with hereditary multiple exostoses. Am J Med Genet. 2001;99:59–62.

Silver SA, Wiley JM, Perlman EJ. DNA ploidy analysis of pediatric germ cell tumors. Mod Pathol. 1994;7:951–6.

Simon T, Kohlhase J, Wilhelm C, Kochanek M, De Carolis B, Berthold F. Multiple malignant diseases in a patient with Rothmund-Thomson syndrome with RECQL4 mutations: case report and literature review. Am J Med Genet. 2010;152A:1575–9.

Sobreira NLM, Cirulli ET, Avramopoulos D, Wohler E, Oswald GL, Stevens EL, Ge D, Shianna KV, Smith JP, Maia JM, Gumbs CE, Pevsner J, Thomas G, Valle D, Hoover-Fong JE, Goldstein DB. Whole-genome sequencing of a single proband together with linkage analysis identifies a mendelian disease gene. PLoS Genet. 2010;6:e1000991.

Sun TC, Swee RG, Shives TC, Unni KK. Chondrosarcoma in Mafrucci's syndrome. J Bone Joint Surg. 1985;67A:1214–9.

Tamimi HK, Bolen JW. Enchondramatosis (Ollier's disease) and ovarian juvenile granulosa cell tumor. Cancer. 1984;53:1605–8.

Tidyman WE, Rauen KA. The RASopathies: developmental syndromes of Ras/MAPK pathway dysregulation. Curr Opin Genet Dev. 2009;19:230–6.

Toguchida J, Yamaguchi T, Dayton SH, et al. Prevalence and spectrum of germline mutations of the p53 gene among patients with sarcoma. N Engl J Med. 1992;326:1301–9.

Wang LL, Gannavarapu A, Kozinetz CA, et al. Association between osteosarcoma and deleterious mutations in the RECQL4 gene in Rothmund–Thomson syndrome. J Natl Cancer Inst. 2003;95:669–74.

Wu AU, Trumble TE, Ruwe PA. Familial incidence of Paget's disease and secondary osteogenic sarcoma. A report of three cases in a single family. Clin Orthop. 1991;265:306–9.

Wuyts W, Van Hul W, Wauters J, et al. Positional cloning of a gene involved in hereditary multiple exostoses. Hum Mol Genet. 1996;5:1547–57.

Yates VD, Wilroy RS, Whittington GL, Simmons JCH. Anterior sacral defects; an autosomal dominantly inherited condition. J Pediatr. 1983;102:239–42.

Chapter 10
Skin

Genetic predisposition to skin cancer is most frequently seen by dermatologists in a number of dominantly inherited conditions such as familial melanoma, the basal cell nevus syndrome, self-healing epitheliomas of Ferguson Smith, and Bazex–Dupré–Christol syndrome. There are also a number of rare skin diseases which are associated with chronic inflammation of the skin, such as epidermolysis bullosa which are associated with an increased risk of squamous cell carcinoma of the skin (SCC). These conditions will be discussed in the first part of this chapter (Tsai and Tsao 2004).

In the second part of the chapter, we will discuss inherited disorders where skin cancers occur but for which there are often more pressing medical implications, such as albinism, the chromosome breakage disorders (Bloom's syndrome (p. 226), Fanconi anemia (p. 249), ataxia telangiectasia (p. 219), xeroderma pigmentosum (p. 320)), Cowden's disease (p. 233), dermatitis herpetiformis/celiac disease, DiGeorge syndrome, familial hyperglucagonemia, Gardner's syndrome (p. 256), the basal cell nevus syndrome (Gorlin syndrome) (p. 252), hemochromatosis, multiple endocrine neoplasia type 2 (MEN2B, p. 252), neurofibromatosis type 1 (NF1, p. 288), porphyria, tuberose sclerosis (p. 307), and tylosis (p. 312).

There are some additional dermatological disorders which show some clustering in families, which may rarely be associated with skin cancer, such as lichen planus or lichen sclerosus et atrophicus, but these are not discussed here.

Specific Skin Cancers

With Julia A. Newton-Bishop

S.V. Hodgson et al., *A Practical Guide to Human Cancer Genetics*,
DOI 10.1007/978-1-4471-2375-0_10, © Springer-Verlag London 2014

Genetic Predisposition to Melanoma

Melanoma is a relatively uncommon cancer, with an incidence in most of Northern Europe of around 10 per 100,000 per annum (Parkin et al. 2001). In many countries, there is a sex difference in incidence so that in some, particularly in the UK, it has been more common in women, whereas in hot countries it is more common in men. The incidence has increased markedly this century in white people in most Western countries and in Australia and New Zealand, which have the highest rates in the world, but melanoma is fortunately rare in Asian or black skin (Eide and Weinstock 2005). The disparity in incidence between white and pigmented skins gives the first clue that genetics play a major role in determining susceptibility to a form of cancer for which the major environmental determinant is sun exposure (Jones et al. 1999).

The commonest type of melanoma is the superficial spreading type, which has the appearance of a mole progressively changing in shape, size, and color. The melanomas commonly have irregularly distributed hues of brown, grey, black, or red. These tumors are most frequent on the lower leg in women and on the trunk in males. The prognosis is determined by the Breslow thickness in millimeters, which is the thickness measured by the histopathologist from the granular layer of the skin to the deepest part of the tumor, as well as sex, age, tumor site, and other histological features such as the presence of ulceration (Balch et al. 2009). Earlier diagnosis with thinner tumors is associated with a better prognosis (Rees 2003; Barsh 1996; Elwood et al. 1990; Bahmer et al. 1990; Balch et al. 2001; Anderson and Badzioch 1991; Augustsson et al. 1990; Hayward 2003).

Epidemiological studies have established that the most potent phenotypic risk factor identified to date is the presence of numerous or clinically atypical nevi or moles (Fig. 10.1). The presence of multiple nevi, some of which are clinically

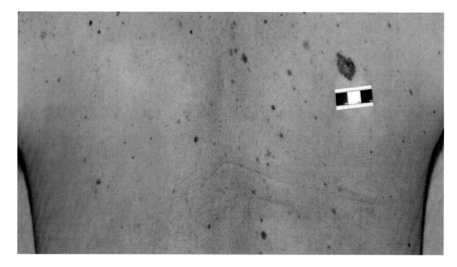

Fig. 10.1 Familial atypical mole-melanoma syndrome: a melanoma arising from a dysplastic or atypical nevus; note the irregular borders and pigmentation (Courtesy of Julia A. Newton-Bishop)

atypical, is called the atypical mole syndrome (AMS) phenotype (otherwise known as the dysplastic nevus syndrome (Tucker et al. 2002) or the familial atypical mole and multiple melanoma syndrome FAMMM (Bergman et al. 1992)). It was thought originally that this phenotype was indicative of the inheritance of high-penetrance melanoma susceptibility genes, but it is now recognized that the AMS is relatively common, for example, it was seen in 2 % of the general UK population in one study (Newton et al. 1993), and 18 % of healthy individuals had at least one clinically diagnosed atypical nevus in a Swedish study (Augustsson et al. 1991). The odds ratio for melanoma in individuals with the AMS but no family history of melanoma is in the order of 10 relative to those who have very few nevi at all (Bataille et al. 1996). The absolute risk to such people is therefore moderate. Twin studies have shown that nevi are predominantly genetically determined (Easton et al. 1991; Wachsmuth et al. 2001) and it is hypothesized that the AMS in the absence of a family history is indicative of genetic susceptibility to melanoma with some contribution from sun exposure (particularly sunny holidays). In recent times some of the associated genes have been found using genome-wide association studies (GWAS). Single nucleotide polymorphisms (SNPs) associated with nevus number and melanoma risk were in the *TERT* gene (Rafnar et al. 2009; Barrett et al. 2011), near to the locus coding for *CDKN2A* on chromosome 9 (Bishop et al. 2009) and on chromosome 22 in a gene known as *PLA2G6* (Bishop et al. 2009). *TERT* codes for telomerase, a polymerase which maintains the telomere end (or cap) which protects the chromosomes from end-to-end fusion, nucleolytic decay, and atypical recombination (Nan et al. 2011), so this observation is consistent with a previous study in which patients with more nevi had longer telomeres (Bataille et al. 2007). The biology which underpins the second two associations (on chromosome 9p and *PLA2G6*) is not yet fully understood. Finally, there is some evidence of a role for the gene coding for interferon regulatory factor 4 (*IRF4*) and nevus number and melanoma risk, but the nature of that relationship is apparently complex (Duffy et al. 2010), with age-dependent effects on nevus number. Even when all these genes are considered together, however, only about 3 % of the variation in nevus number is currently explained (unpublished Leeds in-house data) (Cannon-Albright et al. 1990; Auroy et al. 2001; van der Velden et al. 2001).

Other phenotypic risk factors relate to the presence of fair skin and hair, freckles, and a reported susceptibility to sunburn, often referred to as people's "skin type" (Gandini et al. 2005a, b). A major genetic determinant of this phenotype (and a genetic risk factor for skin cancer) is the inheritance of common polymorphisms of the melanocortin receptor 1 (*MC1R*) gene, which codes for variation in the melanocortin receptor to which MSH binds and which result in modulation of the ratio of eumelanin (black pigment) to pheomelanin (red/yellow pigment) in the skin and hair. The association was first reported by Valverde et al. (1996) but has been explored extensively by other groups working on sporadic melanoma (Raimondi et al. 2008) and familial melanoma (Demenais et al. 2010).

As genetically determined phenotypes associated with a tendency to burn in the sun have been unequivocally identified as melanoma risk factors, it is not surprising that there is also an increased risk associated with environmental factors, such as a history of severe sunburn and sunbathing (Gandini et al. 2005a, b; Chang et al. 2009).

Additional pigment genes underlying phenotypic variation in skin and melanoma susceptibility have also been explored in GWAS, and these include *SLC45A2* (Barrett et al. 2011), the *IRF4* locus, the gene coding for tyrosinase (*TYR*) (Gudbjartsson et al. 2008; Barrett et al. 2011), and the agouti signaling protein locus *ASIP* (Barrett et al. 2011; Gudbjartsson et al. 2008) which is an agonist of the MC1R and therefore functions in the same pathway as variants in *MC1R* having effects on melanin synthesis. Using what is known about the variants of *MC1R*, it is apparent that we have in all now identified susceptibility genes which "explain" 30 % of the variance in skin pigmentation in white-skinned people taking part in the GWAS (unpublished data).

GWAS have identified a number of additional melanoma susceptibility genes which are not associated with either "at-risk" phenotype (fair skin or increased nevus number) which opens up new and interesting biological pathways to better understand melanomagenesis. These include *ARNT* (Macgregor et al. 2011) two genes involved in DNA repair, *PARP1* and *ATM*, *CASP8* (caspase 8 which is an apoptosis-related gene), *CCND1*, and *MX2* (Barrett et al. 2011).

Clustering of many cases of melanoma predominantly occurs in families in which there appears to be susceptibility to melanoma alone (see below). There are very rare families demonstrating susceptibility to both cutaneous melanoma and ocular melanoma. Scandinavian families have been reported in which susceptibility to ocular and skin melanoma was linked to a gene on 9p21 (Jonsson et al. 2005) and more recently, an inherited mutation in the *BAP-1* gene on chromosome 3p was reported in an ocular melanoma patient (Harbour et al. 2010).

Low numbers of cases of melanoma have also been reported in hereditary non-polyposis colorectal cancer (Lynch syndrome, p. 256). In one recent series, 9 family members developed melanoma from 8 families in a series of 60 Lynch syndrome families (Ponti et al. 2008). There is a reported increased risk of melanoma in the Li–Fraumeni syndrome (p. 271) and inherited retinoblastoma (p. 15). In inherited retinoblastoma many of the melanomas have been reported to occur in the radiation field. There is a clear increased risk in patients with xeroderma pigmentosum in whom DNA repair defects are causal (p. 320). Inheritance of *BRCA* 2 mutations also appears to increase the risk of melanoma moderately (Liede et al. 2004).

Congenital anomalies such as neurocutaneous melanosis (Arunkumar et al. 2001; De Andrade et al. 2004) (p. 140) and giant congenital hairy nevi (p. 140) also predispose to melanoma.

Familial Melanoma

Rare families exist in which there is an increased risk of melanoma and in which the tendency to melanoma appears to be inherited as an autosomal dominant with incomplete penetrance, first recognized in the nineteenth century by Norris (1820). Within these families, the majority of melanomas are of the superficial spreading type, but there may be less common types such as nodular melanomas and lentigo maligna melanomas. Ocular melanomas may occur in some families, but this is very rare (see above). In the UK families with the most common high penetrance susceptibility gene, *CDKN2A* so far reported, there is little evidence of increased susceptibility to cancers other than melanoma. However, other groups have reported an association in particular with pancreatic carcinoma, particularly in the Netherlands and in the USA (Bergman et al. 1990; Lynch and Fusaro 1991), and other gastrointestinal cancers (see below).

In the families described with a founder mutation in the *CDKN2A* gene in the Netherlands (de Snoo et al. 2008), the increased risk of pancreatic cancer in these families was very clear in a recent study, but there was also evidence of increased risk of other cancers related to smoking such as cancers of the lip, mouth, pharynx, and respiratory system. Insufficient numbers of families from other centers have so far been studied in order to quantify the risk of nonmelanoma cancers, but it is clear that some families have an increased susceptibility to gastrointestinal cancer as well as to melanoma, which is currently being explored by the Melanoma Genetics Consortium, GenoMEL (www.genomel.org). It would seem prudent to advise family members strongly against smoking.

Some melanoma families also have the AMS, but not all. In a proportion of families, this abnormal nevus phenotype in melanoma cases may be striking. The phenotype is characterized by the presence of clinically atypical moles (by definition more than 5 mm in diameter with an irregular or blurred edge and irregularly irregular pigmentation), numerous but otherwise banal moles, and moles in unusual places such as on the buttocks, in the iris, and on the ears (Newton et al. 1993). The biological significance, even within melanoma-prone families, of this phenotype is unclear as some families with melanoma do not have abnormal nevi at all. In the UK families so far described, the members of the largest family, with nine cases of melanoma, all had normal nevi (Harland et al. 1997). Overall, it is clear that although the atypical mole syndrome is associated in some way with familial melanoma, it is a poor indicator of gene carrier status and cannot be used reliably even within these melanoma families to predict who is a gene carrier (Wachsmuth et al. 1998; Newton Bishop et al. 2000).

In deciding how atypical mole syndrome patients should be managed in terms of follow-up and risk estimation then, family history is the key. Patients with this phenotype without a personal or family history of melanoma should be taught how to self-examine their nevi and be given advice about sun protection, but long-term follow-up is not normally appropriate. Patients with a strong family history of melanoma with or without the atypical mole syndrome should retain long-term access to the pigmented lesion service. The screening of nevi in patients with the atypical mole syndrome and a family history of melanoma is specialized, and all such patients should be referred to the local Cancer Centre Pigmented Lesion Clinic, usually run by a dermatologist. In such clinics, the emphasis is on clinical and dermoscopic examination of nevi, using photography for baseline documentation. Nevi are removed only if they appear to be changing, and therefore if malignant change is suspected, they are not excised prophylactically. Additional genetic counseling may be required.

Progress has been made in understanding the genetic basis of high-risk susceptibility. Initial reports of genetic linkage in melanoma families to chromosome 1p

(Bale et al. 1989a, b) have not yet been substantiated by other groups. Strong evidence of linkage to chromosome 9p, reported by the Utah group (Cannon-Albright et al. 1992), was soon confirmed by others although genetic heterogeneity exists. The tumor suppressor gene *CDKN2A*, which codes for the cyclin-dependent kinase (CDK) inhibitor p16, lies in the identified area of 9p, and all groups working on familial melanoma have now identified germline mutations in this gene so that to date the *CDKN2A* gene remains the major identified cause of high-risk familial melanoma. Overall, germline mutations in this gene have been identified in around 40 % of families with three or more cases of melanoma but much less frequently in families with only two cases. GenoMEL estimates an overall *CDKN2A* mutation penetrance for melanoma of 0.30 (95 % confidence interval (CI)=0.12–0.62) by age 50 years and 0.67 (95 % CI=0.31–0.96) by age 80 years, with evidence of greater penetrance where gene carriers live in sunnier climates, namely, Australia (Bishop et al. 2002). The confidence intervals for these estimations remain high so that GenoMEL will continue to improve its data. It has also been demonstrated that penetrance is higher in mutation carriers who also have certain *MC1R* polymorphisms (associated with a tendency to burn in the sun) (Demenais et al. 2010). Where *CDKN2A* mutation carriers have been ascertained from populations other than family studies, then the penetrance is predictably lower: the risk of melanoma in *CDKN2A* mutation carriers was approximately 14 % (95 % CI=8–22 %) by age 50 years, 24 % (95 % CI=15–34 %) by age 70 years, and 28 % (95 % CI=18–40 %) by age 80 years in the GEM study (Begg et al. 2005; Soufir et al. 2000; Newton Bishop et al. 1994; Lal et al. 2000; Bartsch et al. 2002; Goldstein et al. 1994, 2004).

As above, in some families with germline mutations in *CDKN2A*, there is also an increased susceptibility to pancreatic carcinoma, manifest in patients over the age of 45 years (de Snoo et al. 2008). This appears to be particularly seen in families with truncating mutations such as the founder p16-Leiden mutation, but is also seen in families with the founder mutation G101W, common in Italy and France (Ghiorzo et al. 2007). Most of these G101W families in which pancreatic cancer was seen also had melanoma, but very rare mutation-positive families were reported with pancreatic cancer alone (Ghiorzo et al. 2004). In the p16-Leiden families, the incidence of pancreatic cancer was reported to be 29 times greater than population levels, and more recently a lifetime risk of 17 % was suggested. In the Italian G101W families, a 9.4-fold risk (95 % CI 0.8–5.7) was reported. The elevated risk in the p16-Leiden families is sufficiently high that MRI screening is being investigated in clinical trials as a means of early detection of pancreatic cancer.

GenoMEL has reported the predictors of *CDKN2A* mutation detection in melanoma families and shown that early age of onset, multiple primaries, multiple cases of melanoma, and the presence of pancreatic cancer are all associated with an increased probability of finding mutations (Goldstein et al. 2007), although there was no significant evidence of increased risk of pancreatic cancer risk in Australian families with *CDKN2A* mutations (Loo et al. 2003; Bishop et al. 2000; Della Torre et al. 2001; Gillanders et al. 2003; Harland et al. 2000).

There has been some suggestion of an increased risk of breast cancer in *CDKN2A* mutation-positive women (Borg et al. 2000), but this is unsubstantiated as yet and the risks of this and other cancers will be addressed by GenoMEL. Although families are reported in which both ocular and cutaneous melanomas occur (see above), there is no evidence of an increased risk of ocular melanoma in *CDKN2A* mutation carriers.

Germline mutations in *CDKN2A* have been identified in around 10–15 % of melanoma patients with multiple primaries. The prevalence of germline mutations in sporadic "population" ascertained melanoma cases however is low: in the GEM study, an identifiable mutation was identified in 1–2 %, depending on region of origin (Begg et al. 2005).

A second high-penetrance susceptibility gene was identified in 1996 when Dracopoli identified two families with the same single base pair substitution in another gene that coding for CDK4, producing a protein anomaly at the site at which p16, the *CDKN2A* product, binds (Zuo et al. 1996). Germline mutations in this gene are extremely rare. To date, only around seventeen families worldwide have been described with these mutations (Molven et al. 2005; Goldstein et al. 2007; Pjanova et al. 2007; Puntervoll et al. 2013).

However, the identification of the mutations strengthens the observation that the p16 protein is critical to melanoma carcinogenesis. Puntervoll et al. (2013) have recently reported that families with inherited *CDK4* mutations have a very similar clinical picture to those with *CDKN2A* mutations suggesting that the *CDK4* gene should be screened as well as *CDKN2A* in families who elect to proceed to gene testing.

Reported evidence of linkage to 9p in melanoma families in whom *CDKN2A* mutations could not be identified suggested that other *CDKN2A* mutations remained to be found. There was however no evidence for promoter mutations except for a mutation of the *CDKN2A*5′UTR which creates an aberrant initiation codon which has been identified in a number of families in North America, Australasia, and Europe (Liu et al. 1999). Splice site variants have been found (Harland et al. 2001, 2005) and 9p deletions (Mistry et al. 2005), but still a good proportion of melanoma families have no identifiable mutations.

CDKN2A is an unusual locus with an alternative reading frame coding for another protein p14ARF, whose role in melanoma carcinogenesis remains of great interest. In 1998 families with a susceptibility to melanoma and neural tumors were described in whom there were germline deletions at 9p (Bahuau et al. 1998) and the suggestion was that there was loss of *CDKN2A* and exon 1β, coding for p14ARF. More recently, a similar family was reported in which the deletion appeared to result in loss of exon 1β only, (Randerson-Moor et al. 2001) with no evidence of resultant impact on p16. This, the first evidence that *p14ARF* is the third high-penetrance melanoma susceptibility gene, was strengthened when a germline mutation in exon 1β, which creates an abnormal splice site, was reported in a melanoma family (Hewitt et al. 2002), and a small insertion affecting *p14ARF* was reported in a Spanish melanoma family (Rizos et al. 2001).

Overall then, the consensus is that there are 3 high-penetrance susceptibility genes effecting p16, CDK4, and p14ARF, and there is recent evidence for another at 1p22, with a probable role for *BAP-1* in families with ocular melanoma (Harbour et al. 2010). In the UK currently we have identified probable germline mutations in 53 and 68 % of three or more and four or more case families, respectively (Harland, Bishop and Newton-Bishop unpublished). This figure is lower in some other centers, particularly in areas of high incidence where lower-penetrance genes may be more evident (Goldstein et al. 2007). It is thought likely therefore that familial clustering in hot countries where people of Northern European origin live, such as Australia, has occurred as a result of inheritance of multiple lower-penetrance genes (such as those associated with pigmentation and nevus at-risk phenotypes described above) and intense sun exposure. The identification of *BAP-1* germline mutations however means that remaining families might have "boutique" mutations, or mutations peculiar to their family or a very small number of families.

Gene testing within melanoma families is taking place but the uptake is very variable internationally (de Snoo et al. 2003; Newton-Bishop et al. 2010; Kefford et al. 2002). Leachman et al. have argued the case for genetic counseling based upon a rule of threes (three or more cases in the family or three or more primaries in an individual) (Leachman et al. 2009), but the value of gene testing remains unclear to many. A positive *CDKN2A* mutation test may ultimately be of value when screening for pancreatic cancer has been shown to be effective and for families in which pancreatic cancer has occurred. There is a European screening research program called EUROPAC addressed to this issue. In the absence of pancreatic cancer, however, a positive test is unlikely to change management. As causal mutations are currently not identifiable in many families even with multiple cases of melanoma, the possibility is that there are as yet unidentified mutations, so that a negative test result is of limited utility. An online package for genetic counselors has been placed on the GenoMEL website, www.genomel.org.

The majority of the *CDKN2A* mutations identified to date appear to co-segregate with the tumor, and from what is known about the structure of the p16 protein, it is to some extent possible to predict which mutations are real and which are silent. P16 (INK4A) is a member of a family of CDK inhibitors, the other members of which are p15 (INK4B), p18 (INK4C), and p19 (INK4D). The members of the group have significant sequence homology and have a structure dictated by the presence of four or five so-called ankyrin repeats. Mutations which fall outside the ankyrin repeats were thought likely to be nonsignificant having a lower likelihood of impacting on the protein, like the common *CDKN2A* polymorphism Ala148Thr. Some splice site variants outside these repeats are however increasingly being recognized. In order to prove that identified mutations are significant, functional tests of the p16 protein have been developed. The test most widely used is a test of the ability of the mutant protein to bind to CDK4 and CDK6. But it is not a comprehensive test of function. For mutations described in large families around the world such as Arg24Pro, Met53Ile, and 23ins24, there is confidence that the mutations are real and that gene testing would produce interpretable results. For novel mutations, an abnormal functional test result would seem to be necessary before testing. GenoMEL maintains a database of these mutations (eMelanoBase) which is now part of LOVD (Leiden Open Variation Database) http://chromium.liacs.nl/LOVD2/home.php.

Giant Congenital Melanocytic Nevus

One percent of newborn infants has small congenital melanocytic nevi, but fortunately giant nevi (defined as 20 cm in diameter or larger) are very rare, estimated in one study to be one in 20,455 live births (Castilla et al. 1981). Most cases are sporadic and are thought to arise as a result of a post-zygotic mutation, possibly in the *NRAS* gene (Phadke et al. 2011). Very rare cases have been reported of more than one case in the same extended family where the mode of inheritance was postulated to be a polygenic paradominant pattern of inheritance (de Wijn et al. 2010). The risk of melanoma in congenital nevi is unclear due to its rarity, and publication bias and the published estimates of this risk for giant nevi range from 2 to 14 % (Shah 2010; Yun et al. 2012), with a significant proportion of melanomas occurring in the first 10 years of life (Shah 2010; Araim et al. 2004; Angelo et al. 2001; Makkar and Frieden 2002; Ruiz-Maldonado et al. 1992; Hoanq et al. 2002).

Imaging using MRI may identify anomalies in the CNS: both intracranial melanosis and others (Kinsler et al. 2001). Neuromelanosis may be complicated by hydrocephalus or other neurological symptoms (Kinsler et al. 2001). A very small proportion of neuromelanosis eventuates in intracranial melanoma, but the incidence is not established.

Basal Cell Carcinoma (BCC)

This epithelial tumor arises from the basal layers of the epidermis and its appendages (Fig. 10.2).

It is locally invasive, metastasis being excessively rare. It is the most common skin tumor affecting light-skinned people and appears predominantly in sun-exposed areas of the skin (head and neck predominantly although also on the trunk). It is indeed the commonest cancer overall. Arsenic is a known predisposing

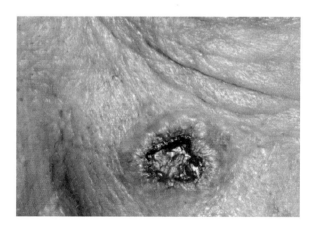

Fig. 10.2 The typical appearance of a BCC

environmental agent (Boonchai et al. 2000) but is now a rare cause. BCC may occur after radiotherapy: it was seen in the past as multiple lesions on the scalp as a sequel of the use of radiotherapy to treat scalp ringworm and now is seen more commonly as a late result of radiotherapy to treat cancer or even noncancerous conditions such as ankylosing spondylitis. The clue to the cause is the distribution so that multiple lesions in a rectangular distribution along the spine, for example, are more likely to be related to radiotherapy than genetic susceptibility. In a recent registry-based study from the Netherlands of 444,131, histologically confirmed cases between 1973 and 2008, age-adjusted incidence rates (European Standard Population) increased approximately threefold from 40 to 148 per 100,000 in males and from 34 to 141 in females. Lifetime risk of BCC was 1 in 5–6 for Dutch citizens (Flohil et al. 2011).

Most cases of BCC are sporadic but there is some evidence for clustering in families (de Zwaan and Haass 2010), and association studies have shown a similar relationship to pigment genes as for melanoma. Red-haired individuals are particularly sun sensitive, and therefore it is not surprising that variants in genes associated with red hair are associated with increased risk such as the melanocortin 1 receptor gene (*MC1R*) (Scherer et al. 2008; Han et al. 2006; Bastiaens et al. 2001a, b; Box et al. 2001a, b) and the agouti signaling protein locus (*ASIP*) (Nan et al. 2009). Polymorphisms in other pigment genes are also associated with risk such as the oculocutaneous albinism A2 gene *OCA2* (Box et al. 2001a, b) *SLC45A2* (Stacey et al. 2009a, b) and the interferon regulator gene 4, *IRF4* (Han et al. 2011). Loci not known as yet to be associated with pigmentation but which have been shown to be associated with susceptibility in GWAS include a gene coding for keratin 5, a locus near to the *CDKN2A* locus at 9p and *TERT* which codes for telomerase and therefore impacts on telomere length (Stacey et al. 2009a, b; Baird 2010). BCC and melanoma are therefore both associated with pigment genes, and it is not therefore surprising that patients not infrequently get both (Farndon et al. 1992; Gorlin 1984; Guarneri et al. 2000; Happle 2000).

Genetic disorders associated with a predisposition to basal cell carcinoma include Gorlin syndrome (the nevoid basal cell carcinoma syndrome) (p. 252) in which a characteristic facies, bony anomalies, odontogenic dental cysts, and palmar pits precede the development of multiple BCC. The number of BCC is increased in those with greater sun exposure, and radiotherapy significantly increases tumor risk both in the skin and the meninges and therefore must be avoided if at all possible. Rarer tumors include medulloblastoma and ovarian fibromas. In the UK, around 1 in 30,827 people is affected (prevalence) (Evans et al. 2010). Inherited mutations in the "patched" *PTCH1* gene at 9p 22.3 have been shown to be the cause of the nevoid basal cell carcinoma syndrome (Hahn et al. 1996; Johnson et al. 1996), loss of the second allele of *PTCH1* occurring somatically to cause BCC in gene carriers over time. Patched is a negative regulator of the hedgehog pathway which is a proproliferative signaling pathway which is now known to be important in a number of cancers as well as BCC (de Zwaan and Haass 2010). Sporadic basal cell carcinomas show chromosome 9q allele loss, and mutations in the "patched" gene which causes the basal cell nevus syndrome have been detected with high frequency in such

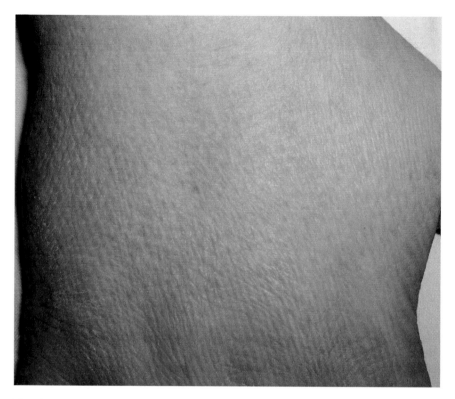

Fig. 10.3 Follicular atrophoderma (ice pick marks) in Bazex–Dupré–Christol syndrome

tumors. This supports the view that the "patched" gene is a gatekeeper for common skin cancers. Patched controls the activity of "smoothened," and recent therapeutic developments for BCC have included the exploration of smoothened inhibitors (Skvara et al. 2011) for the treatment of very advanced disease.

Increased susceptibility to BCC is also seen in xeroderma pigmentosum (p. 320), porokeratosis, albinism, Bazex–Dupré–Christol syndrome (p. 187), and the rare Rombo syndrome (p. 189) (Van Steensel et al. 2001).

Bazex Syndrome (Bazex–Dupré–Christol Syndrome)

This trait (not to be confused with the nongenetic paraneoplastic acrokeratosis also described by Bazex, in which psoriasiform changes develop on the hands, feet, and face, with abnormalities of the nails associated with internal malignancy) is characterized by follicular atrophoderma, especially on the face, hands, feet, and elbows, with the appearance of "ice pick" marks (especially on the dorsum of the hands) (Fig. 10.3) but without palmar or plantar pits and multiple milia

Fig. 10.4 Milia on the dorsa of the hands in a baby with Bazex–Dupré–Christol syndrome

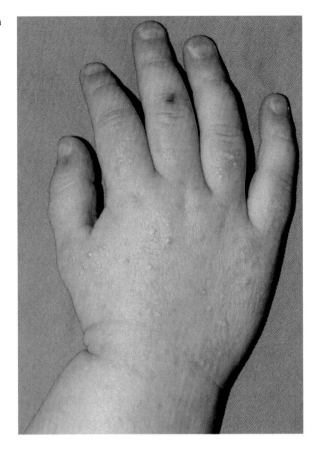

(Fig. 10.4) (Kidd et al. 1996; Vabres et al. 1995). That the disorder is fundamentally one affecting the hair follicle is illustrated by the presence of hypotrichosis in affected individuals which is obvious from infancy. As in the basal cell nevus syndrome, affected children may develop benign proliferations of the hair follicle such as trichoepitheliomas (Yung and Newton-Bishop 2005a, b) in early in life. Multiple basal cell carcinomas may develop on the face from the second decade, but there is variable expressivity which is likely to be related to the degree of sun protection given in childhood. Occasional children develop pigmented proliferative lesions described as BCC (Abuzahra et al. 2011; Parren et al. 2011), but the author's experience is that these are difficult to distinguish from "benign" proliferations described by some as trichoepitheliomas. Bazex–Dupré–Christol syndrome is inherited as an X-linked dominant trait, both males and females being affected, and is linked to DXS1192 at Xq14–q27.1 (Abuzahra et al. 2011; Parren et al. 2011).

Rombo Syndrome

Rombo syndrome is a very rare syndrome (Ashinoff et al. 1993), first described in a four-generation family, in which affected individuals developed follicular atrophy of the skin of the cheeks in childhood. In affected adults, telangiectasia and skin papules appeared, especially on the face, and the eyelashes and eyebrows were abnormal. Basal cell carcinomas occur frequently from the third decade. The clinical description bears many similarities to Bazex–Dupré–Christol syndrome described above. Parren et al. believe the two conditions to be similar but different as Rombo syndrome was reported with male-to-male transmission and is therefore thought to be an autosomal dominant trait (Parren and Frank 2011).

Squamous Cell Carcinoma (SCC)

This tumor is derived from epidermal keratinocytes. The incidence of squamous cell carcinoma shows marked geographical variation. It is most frequent in parts of the world where light-skinned people are exposed to large cumulative exposures to sunlight. Thus, it is much more frequent in southern than northern states of America, in outdoor workers, and the incidence is much higher in light-skinned than in dark-skinned peoples (Carrucci 2004). Genetic variation accounting for pigmentation of the skin and reaction to sun exposure as described above is therefore also thought to be important in determining susceptibility. Albino individuals are particularly at risk, especially if they live in the tropics. Arsenic, tar, and oil derivatives and X-rays and gamma rays also predispose to squamous cell carcinoma. In the UK, SCCs occurring as a result of exposure to these carcinogens have become significantly less common as working conditions in relevant industries have improved. Squamous cell carcinomas are more common in chronically immunosuppressed individuals, and organ transplant recipients now represent a significant proportion of patients with multiple SCC. There is some evidence that the risk is particularly high in those treated with azathioprine as a result of higher incorporation of a metabolic product of azathioprine into skin cell DNA (Kalra et al. 2011), and the move to replacing this drug with others may reduce the incidence in the future.

SCC may also arise in chronic scars, ulcers, and sinuses, but as these chronic conditions are better controlled, this is now much less frequent in the developed world. SCC are still seen however in medical conditions where scarring cannot be controlled such as hereditary skin disorders that cause blistering and ulceration (e.g., epidermolysis bullosa) and conditions associated with leukoplakia, such as dyskeratosis congenita and lichen sclerosus et atrophicus.

Squamous cell carcinoma may also occur in the ectodermal dysplasias, the Rothmund–Thomson syndrome, sclerotylosis, and hyperkeratosis lenticularis perstans. Genetic disorders predisposing to cutaneous squamous cell carcinoma may also predispose to squamous cell carcinoma in the mucous membranes, e.g., dyskeratosis congenita and ectodermal dysplasia can predispose to tongue, esophageal, and cervical carcinoma.

Epidermodysplasia Verruciformis

Epidermodysplasia verruciformis (EV) is a rare inherited skin condition in which there is defective immunity to the human papillomavirus (HPV). It usually appears to be recessively inherited, but the genetic basis for the disorder is not entirely clear and in some families the pattern of inheritance is not consistent with a recessive pattern of inheritance (Robati et al. 2009). In some chronically immunosuppressed patients such as HIV-positive patients, phenocopies may be seen (Jacobelli et al. 2011). Affected individuals develop plane (flat) viral warts in childhood on the trunk and extremities, which evolve into verrucous, polymorphic, warty lesions over time. The appearance of some of the lesions is said to resemble pityriasis versicolor or basal cell papillomas on the trunk and actinic keratoses (precancerous lesions) on exposed sites (Vohra et al. 2010). Ultimately SCC may develop within the warty plaques which may metastasize (Vohra et al. 2010; Kim et al. 2010).

Numerous HPV subtypes have been identified in affected patients, and it is reported that lesions infected with HPV 5 and 8 are more likely to transform, but rarely others are described such as HPV-22b in EV-related SCC (Kim et al. 2010).

The gene associated with recessively inherited EV was mapped to two loci, 2p21-2p24 and 17q25, and subsequently nonsense mutations in two adjacent novel genes, *EVER1* and *EVER2*, that are associated with the disease were reported at 17p25 (Ramoz et al. 2002). The EVER proteins are expressed by a number of cell types involved in immunity, e.g., dendritic cells and lymphocytes (Rezaei et al. 2011). Twenty-five percent of EV patients have no identifiable mutations in either *EVER1* or *EVER2* (Orth 2006).

Ferguson-Smith-Type Self-Healing Epithelioma (Multiple Self-Healing Squamous Epithelioma)

This is a rare, dominantly inherited disorder, which was first reported in people of Scottish descent, from Ayrshire (Shaw Dunn and Ferguson Smith 1934). It was thought that all cases are possibly descended from one individual (a founder effect), but recently the causal gene has been identified (*TGFBR1*) on chromosome 9q31-32 (Bose et al. 2006; Goudie et al. 2011a), and several different mutations were identified indicating that this is not so. Loss of function mutations in the *TGFBR1* gene has been found to underlie the disease. Interestingly missense mutations in this gene cause Marfan-related disorders with vascular involvement but no cancer susceptibility (Goudie et al. 1991, 2011a, b).

The condition is characterized by the postpubertal appearance of multiple cutaneous keratoacanthomas (Fig. 10.5), which enlarge, ulcerate, and eventually

Fig. 10.5 A keratoacanthoma on the ear of a lady with self-healing epitheliomas of Ferguson Smith

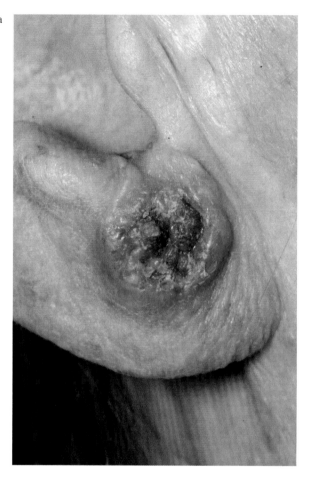

heal, sometimes with calcification, to leave pitted, irregular scars which can be very disfiguring. Most lesions occur on the head and neck, in exposed areas of skin, especially where pilosebaceous follicles are found. The lesions resemble squamous cell carcinomas, but metastasize only very rarely (to lymph nodes) and do not generally behave in an aggressive fashion. In the past, treatment for the lesions (e.g., radiotherapy) has appeared to increase the invasiveness of the tumors as has been reported in the basal cell nevus syndrome as described above (Robertson et al. 2010; Orlow 1997; Griffiths 2002; Shiflett et al. 2002; Ward et al. 2002). There is marked variation in the age at onset and number of lesions in different affected individuals. Rarely tumors are seen in extracutaneous sites in affected patients, such as anal tumors and SCC like lesions of the vulva. Management is by sun protection, which is important (without resulting in vitamin D deficiency), and the avoidance of radiotherapy was possible. The use of acitretin has been reported for advanced disease (Robertson et al. 2010), and this has been found to be helpful in controlling cutaneous lesions.

Inherited Conditions Predisposing to Dermatological Malignancy

Albinism

Oculocutaneous albinism is a group of autosomal recessively inherited disorders of melanin synthesis, whose clinical manifestations are pale skin, white hair, nystagmus, and photophobia. There is considerable genetic heterogeneity, many distinct types having been described. Actinic skin damage, squamous cell carcinoma, and basal cell carcinoma are well-recognized complications of oculocutaneous albinism; malignant melanoma is a much less common complication.

Any patient with albinism is at an increased risk of cutaneous malignancies. This susceptibility to cancer appears to be related to the lack of skin pigmentation and attests to the protective qualities of melanin. However, in patients with vitiligo or piebaldism, areas of skin where melanin (and melanocytes) is absent do not appear to be predisposed to malignancies in the same way individuals with albinism should avoid sunlight exposure and use sunscreen creams when they are exposed to it (Iannello et al. 2003; Karim et al. 2002).

Birt–Hogg–Dubé Syndrome (See p. 224)

This autosomal dominant condition is characterized by skin fibrofolliculomas, lung cysts, and a predisposition to spontaneous pneumothorax. These patients are at increased risk of developing renal neoplasms, most commonly chromophobe and oncocytic hybrid tumors. The gene responsible, *FLCL*, maps to chromosome 17 (Schmidt 2004).

Brooke–Spiegler Syndrome (Multiple Cylindromatosis)

This is an autosomal dominant condition. It is characterized by multiple benign tumors of the skin appendages. These are smooth, dome-shaped, firm, pink tumors of the head (turban tumors), including syringomas and trichoepitheliomas and sometimes spiroadenomas, which develop from early adulthood and may be very disfiguring. Basal cell epitheliomas may develop in the lesions, and radiation therapy may exacerbate this tendency (Szepietowski et al. 2001; Welch et al. 1968).

The tumors are of hairy skin and are not associated with basal or squamous cell carcinomas. The condition has been linked to chromosome 16q12–13 (Biggs et al. 1995; Fenske et al. 2000), and mutations in the *CYLD* gene have been identified as causing the condition. Genotype–phenotype correlations have not been described until recently, when in a family with mild disease (where the tumors tended to be small), the causative mutation was R758X in the *CYLD* gene (Oiso et al. 2004; Blake and Toro 2009). Loss of the cylindromatosis tumor suppressor inhibits apoptosis by activating NF-kB. It has been suggested since aspirin also inhibits the action of NF-kB, it is a logical (topical) therapeutic agent for cylindromatosis, and phase 1 clinical trials of this are currently underway (Gutierrez et al. 2002; Bernends 2003; Brummelkamp et al. 2003; Lakhani 2004).

Cheilitis Glandularis

This rare condition, which can be inherited as an autosomal dominant trait, is characterized by diffuse nodular enlargement of the lower lip, with hypertrophy of the labial mucous glands, chronic inflammation, and dilatation of the excretory ducts. There is a high risk of squamous cell carcinoma of the lower lip (Vernia 2003).

Chronic Mucocutaneous Candidiasis Syndrome

This is a rare condition characterized by chronic and recurrent *Candida* infections of the skin, nails, and oropharynx from early childhood. There may be an underlying immune defect. In over 50 % of cases, there is associated endocrine disease. Several examples of familial chronic mucocutaneous candidiasis syndrome have been recorded, some showing an autosomal recessive and some an autosomal dominant mode of transmission; some cases are not associated with endocrinopathy (Buzzi et al. 2003). Late-onset cases may be sporadic. The condition can predispose to malignancy, especially of the oropharynx. The *Candida* endocrinopathy syndrome includes hypoparathyroidism, hypothyroidism, hypoadrenocorticism, and diabetes, usually autosomal recessive in inheritance (Ahonen 1985; Coleman and Hay 1997; Buzzi et al. 2003; Myhre et al. 2004). Vertical transmission of the syndrome with hypothyroidism has been described (Kirkpatrick 1994), and a syndrome of immune deficit, mucocutaneous candidiasis, and thyroid disease has been mapped to chromosome 2p in one family. A germline mutation in the *AIRE* gene has been described in a patient with this condition and muscular atrophy (Sato et al. 2002). An immune deficit causing dominant chronic mucocutaneous candidiasis and thyroid disease maps to chromosome 2p in a single family. The autosomal recessive form of familial chronic mucocutaneous candidiasis (CANDF2) is caused by mutation in the *CARD9* gene on chromosome 9q34 (Glocker et al. 2009). Autosomal dominant candidiasis (CANDF1) maps to chromosome 2p, CANDF2 is caused by mutations in the *CARD9* gene on chromosome 9q34.3, CANDF3 (restricted to nails of the hands and feet) maps to chromosome 11, CANDF4 is caused by mutations in the *CLEC7A* gene on chromosome 12p13.2-p12.3, CANDF5 by mutations in the *IL17RA* gene on chromosome 22q11, and *CANDF6* by mutations in the *IL17F* gene on chromosome 6p12.

Familial chronic nail candidiasis has been described with ICAM-1 deficiency with autosomal recessive inheritance (Zuccurello et al. 2002).

Congenital Generalized Fibromatosis

This is a very rare, probably autosomal recessive, condition characterized by the development of multiple rubbery, firm and fibroblastic tumors of the skin, striated muscle, bones, and viscera from infancy. Multiple subcutaneous nodules proliferate early in life, but tend to regress spontaneously. The visceral involvement may be fatal. Some X-ray features resemble those of Ollier disease (Sty et al. 1996). Autosomal dominant families have been described with the infantile form of this condition (Zand et al. 2004).

Dyskeratosis Congenita

This is classically an X-linked condition although other inheritance patterns have been described in some families, suggesting genetic heterogeneity, characterized by reticulated hyperpigmentation of the skin, with depigmented spots, nail dystrophy (in 98 % of patients, sometimes apparent at birth), and leukoplakia of the mucous membranes (87 %) with atrophy of the lingual papillae in affected males. Signs of the condition usually develop in the first decade of life, but may not occur until puberty. There may be enamel dystrophy of the teeth. The skin changes are progressive, with development of poikiloderma, telangiectasia, and atrophy. Hypertrophic squamous epithelium occurs in mucous epithelia. Bullous skin eruptions and hyperkeratosis, especially of the palms and soles, may occur, and atrophy of the skin of the palms may lead to loss of dermatoglyphics. Blepharitis, ectropion, and nasolacrimal obstruction may occur, and there are dental caries. Subnormal intelligence is sometimes a feature (42 % of cases). Leukoplakia develops, particularly of the oral mucosa, and also in the rectum and genitourinary tract (Davidson and Connor 1988; Fogarty et al. 2003). There is thought to be an immune dysfunction, with reduced cellular immunity and T cell function, leading to opportunistic infections. Complications include pancytopenia (due to bone marrow failure) and squamous and basal cell carcinomas of the skin and mucous membranes, often developing in areas of leukoplakia, after the age of 20 years. Squamous cell carcinoma of the mouth, rectum, cervix, vagina, esophagus, and skin may occur, and there may be multiple primaries. An increased incidence of solid tumors (which can be multiple) has been claimed, with a total incidence of malignancy of 12 % (Kawaguchi et al. 1990). Female carriers are generally normal. Excessive spontaneous chromatid breaks have been reported in some cases of this condition, and an increased X-irradiation-induced chromatid breakage has been demonstrated in fibroblasts. Hematopoietic stem cell transplantation has been tried as therapy in affected patients (Nobili et al. 2002).

Linkage to markers at Xq28(D9S52) was demonstrated, and mutation in the gene encoding dyskerin *(DKC1) KKC1* gene is responsible for the condition. Dyskeratin is a protein necessary for the function of telomerase, so the disorder is caused by a defect in the maintenance of telomeres with reduced apoptosis (Kirwan and Dokal 2008). Late-onset cases, or of aplastic anemia, may also be due to mutations in *TERC* (Arngrimsson et al. 1993). Disease anticipation has been shown to be associated with progressive telomere shortening (Montanaro et al. 2003; Shay and Wright 2004; Vuilamy et al. 2004).

Ectodermal Dysplasias

These conditions comprise a heterogeneous group of congenital diffuse disorders of the epidermis and appendages (Pinheiro and Freire-Maia 1994). Three forms of autosomal dominant ectodermal dysplasia are described, and each of these may predispose to squamous cell carcinoma of the skin and nail beds. The hidrotic type, Clouston syndrome, is characterized by thickened, deformed hypoplastic nails, thin sparse hair, and thick dyskeratotic skin of the palms and soles. Areas of hyperpigmentation occur, especially in skin overlying joints (Escobar et al. 1983). A biochemical defect of keratin may be present, and ultrastructural abnormalities of the hair may be demonstrated. Hypohidrotic ectodermal dysplasia is rare, with hypodontia, hypotrichosis, and variable hypohidrosis. The Rapp–Hodgkin syndrome comprises anhydrotic ectodermal dysplasia and cleft lip and palate. The hair in this condition is short and wiry, the teeth small and conical, and the nails abnormal (Cirillo Silengo et al. 1982). Anhydrotic ectodermal dysplasia is an X-linked recessive condition; the cancer risk is not specifically increased in affected males.

The molecular basis of some of these are being identified – for instance, the X-linked form has been shown to be due to germline mutations in the gene encoding NEMO/1KK gamma, and an autosomal dominant form to germline I Kappa B alpha mutations (Courtois et al. 2003; Lane et al. 2003).

Epidermolysis Bullosa

This is a heterogeneous group of inherited disorders characterized by extreme skin fragility and recurrent blisters. Classification is based upon the level at which blistering occurs. Superficial blistering occurs in epidermolysis bullosa simplex, with breakdown occurring in the basal cells. This type is often inherited as an autosomal dominant trait and is clinically mild, without scarring, and mucous membranes are spared. Nails may be mildly involved. The autosomal dominant Dowling–Meera form of epidermolysis bullosa simplex can be severe in infancy; the histology of this type is characteristic and can be detected in fetal skin biopsies. In junctional epidermolysis bullosa, the split occurs in the lamina lucida, causing extensive blistering on the skin and mucosal surfaces. Severe scarring may occur. There are several clinical types of junctional epidermolysis bullosa, all inherited as autosomal recessive traits. Germline mutations in several keratin genes have been found to underlie the different forms of epidermolysis bullosa, the type of mutation correlating with phenotype (Jonkman et al. 2003; Porter and Lane 2003; Uitto et al. 2002; Lin and Carter 1989; Korge and Kreig 1996).

In dystrophic epidermolysis bullosa, blistering occurs in the dermis. Dominant and recessive forms are described, but the severe forms are usually recessively inherited. Bullae develop, particularly on the extremities, leading to severe mitten-like scarring and deformity (mutilans). Gastrointestinal involvement is common, leading to esophageal strictures, erosions, and webs, and life-threatening hemorrhage may occur. Chronic anemia and hypoalbuminemia occur. Dental enamel is defective, and there may be laryngeal involvement.

In epidermolysis bullosa, squamous cell carcinoma may develop in the scars, but this tendency is much more marked in the dystrophic type. These carcinomas may occur at multiple sites, mainly on the limbs (Mallipeddi 2002; Tomita et al. 2003). They arise in young individuals (75 % develop in the 20–40-year age group) and are characteristically well or moderately well differentiated, but aggressive in behavior and metastasize readily (Goldberg et al. 1988). The carcinomas may develop on mucosal surfaces, including esophagus, stomach, bronchus, bladder, and tongue (Tidman 1990). Basal cell carcinomas may also develop in epidermolysis bullosa scars.

Simplex forms of epidermolysis bullosa are caused by mutations in the genes for the basal epidermal keratins *K5* and *K14* (Coulombe et al. 1991), and *K1* and *K10* mutations occur in epidermolytic ichthyosis. Dystrophic epidermolysis bullosa results from mutations in the anchoring fibril collagen gene *COL7A*, whereas the junctional form is due to mutations in *laminin 5* (Eady and Dunnill 1994). Families with autosomal dominant epidermolysis bullosa simplex have shown linkage to the *K14* gene and others to the *K5* gene. Mutations in the *K14* gene have been demonstrated in affected individuals (Bonifas et al. 1991), and a mutation in type VII collagen has been demonstrated in a family with dystrophic epidermolysis bullosa (Bale and DiGiovanna 1997). The genes in which mutations cause epidermolysis bullosa generally encode proteins in or around the hemidesmosome, the sited anchorage of the basal cell to the cell membrane, and the severity of disease determined by the functional position of the affected protein (Fuchs 1996). These genes include *KRT5, KRT14, PLEC1, DST, ITGB4, ITGA6, COL17A1, LAMA3, LAMB3, LAMC2,* and *COL7A1.* Germline mutations in two adjacent genes (*EVER1* and *EVER2*) have been detected in individuals with this condition (Ramoz et al. 2002; Tate et al. 2004; Majewski and Jablonska 2004).

KID Syndrome

This rare condition is characterized by keratitis, ichthyosis, and deafness. It usually occurs as a sporadic condition, but instances of vertical transmission have been described, indicating autosomal dominant inheritance. There are hyperkeratotic plaques on the skin and reticulated keratosis of the face, with keratoderma. Ichthyosis develops soon after birth, especially over extensor aspects of the skin. Sensorineural deafness is present from birth, and loss of visual acuity develops due to corneal vascularization and opacification. Hair is sparse and the nails may be dystrophic. Recurrent *Candida* infection of the skin occurs in 50 % of cases, although no consistent immunological defect has been demonstrated. Cutaneous infections and abscesses may develop, and multiple squamous cell carcinomas ensue.

Germline mutations in the *GJB2* gene encoding connexin 26 cause this syndrome (Yotsumoto et al. 2003; Janecke et al. 2005).

Multiple Cylindromatosis

This is an autosomal dominant condition. It is characterized by multiple, smooth, dome-shaped, firm, pink tumors of the head (turban tumors), including syringomas and trichoepitheliomas, and these may be very disfiguring. Basal cell epitheliomas may develop in the lesions, and radiation therapy may exacerbate this tendency.

The tumors are of hairy skin and are not associated with basal or squamous cell carcinomas. The condition has been linked to D16S411 and D16S416 on chromosome 16q12–13.

Flegel Disease (Hyperkeratosis Lenticularis Perstans)

This is an autosomal dominant condition characterized by punctate keratoses affecting the extensor surfaces of the legs and the dorsa of the feet, with palmar and plantar scaly papules and pits. Keratinosomes may be deficient. There is a risk of squamous and basal cell carcinomas (Li et al. 1997; Miljkovic 2004).

Juvenile Hyaline Fibromatosis

This is an autosomal recessive condition characterized by multiple subcutaneous scalp. The tumors may be disfiguring, and there is associated gingival hyperplasia. Joint contractures and osteolytic bony lesions often occur. Excision of the tumors may be followed by recurrence (Fayad et al. 1987; Katagiri et al. 1996). The gene for this condition maps to 4q21, and mutations in *CMG2* (capillary morphogenesis gene-2) appear to cause both juvenile hyaline fibrosis and infantile systemic hyalinosis (Rahman et al. 2002; Paller et al. 2003).

Klippel–Trenaunay Syndrome

This is usually a sporadic condition, characterized by the triad of capillary or cavernous hemangiomas, hemihypertrophy, and varicosities. Additional dermatological features include abnormal pigmentation, papillomas, and varicose ulcers. Arteriovenous aneurysms and lymphatic abnormalities are common (Viljeon 1988).

A de novo translocation t(8;14) (q22.3;q13) has been found in abnormal tissue in this condition (Wang et al. 2001). At least one gene (*RASA1*) in which germline mutations cause this syndrome has been identified (Eerola et al. 2003; Tian 2003), although the latter finding has been recently thrown into doubt (Barker et al. 2006).

Lichen Planus

This fairly common dermatological condition may predispose to cutaneous malignancy. Familial cases have been described, and in these cases the disease affects younger individuals and is a more widespread eruption (also spreading to involve nails and mucous membranes) than in isolated cases (Sandhu et al. 2003). There may be genetic heterogeneity in etiology in lichen planus, with idiopathic cases of cutaneous lichen planus showing some HLA associations (La Nasa et al. 1995; Sandhu et al. 2003).

Porokeratosis of Mibelli

This is a rare, autosomal dominant defect of skin keratinization. Centrifugally spreading patches are surrounded by horny ridges, and there is central atrophy. Onset is usually in childhood, and lesions may occur anywhere on the skin, enlarge slowly, and are usually asymptomatic. Squamous cell carcinoma, Bowen's disease, and basal cell carcinoma may develop in the keratoatrophodermic lesions, particularly on the extremities. X-ray treatment may increase the tendency to develop carcinoma. There are other rare forms of porokeratosis: disseminated superficial actinic porokeratosis and porokeratosis plantaris, palmaris, et disseminata, which are also inherited as autosomal dominant conditions predisposing to skin cancer but which occur more in adults and are more likely to be symptomatic. Sporadic cases also occur, and malignancy may be more common in sporadic cases. Males are more often affected than females (Gotz et al. 1999; Goerttler and Jung 1975).

Proteus Syndrome

This is a very rare condition (named after the Greek god Proteus) and is usually sporadic. Possible transmission of the condition from father to son has been described once (Goodship et al. 1991), but there is considerable debate about this in view of diagnostic pitfalls (Turner 1999). Somatic mosaicism was postulated to explain some cases (Reardon et al. 1996), and this hypothesis has been supported by the identification of somatic mosaic activating mutations in *AKT1* in most if not all cases of well-characterized Proteus syndrome (Lindhurst et al. 2011). Congenital lipomas occur, sometimes with hemangiomatous or lymphangiomatous elements, and progress and are associated with partial or complete hemihypertrophy, asymmetry, and disfiguration. Accelerated growth is seen in the first few years of life. Exostoses of the skull cause macrocephaly and skull asymmetry with frontal bossing. Localized deformities develop, especially of the hands and feet, and hemihypertrophy (segmental to total) is common. Dermatological features include pigmented nevi, diffuse areas of hyperpigmented and depigmented areas of skin, and linear verrucous epidermal nevi, and massive cerebroid gyriform hyperplasia with rugosity of the soles of the feet is a characteristic feature. Bony and adipose overgrowth may lead to bizarre macrodactyly. Subcutaneous hamartomatous tumors, pigmented areas of skin, bony abnormalities, and lung cysts have been described (Nishimura and Koslowski 1990). Intelligence is usually normal. There is a theoretical risk of malignancy in this overgrowth syndrome, and a testicular mesothelioma at the age of 4 years has been described in a severe case (Barker et al. 2001).

Mutations in *PTEN* have been detected in a subset of cases. The second *PTEN* allele has been shown to be inactivated in the abnormal tissue (Zhou et al. 2000, 2001; Smith et al. 2002).

Sclerotylosis (Scleroatrophic and Keratotic Dermatosis of Limbs; Scleroatrophic Syndrome of Huriez)

This rare autosomal dominant condition is characterized by scleroatrophy of the skin of the hands and feet, hypoplastic nails, and palmoplantar keratoderma. Skin cancer (squamous cell carcinoma) and bowel cancer are said to be common in this condition, and squamous cell carcinomas of the tongue and tonsil also occur. Aggressive squamous cell carcinomas develop on the skin with early onset (third to fourth decade) in about 15 % cases. Linkage has been established with the MN blood group on chromosome 4q28–3. In the scleroatrophic syndrome of Huriez, the histopathologic findings of an almost complete absence of epidermal Langerhans cells in affected skin may explain the susceptibility to squamous cell carcinoma in these lesions (Delaporte et al. 1995; Hamm et al. 1996; Downs and Kennedy 1998; Guerriero et al. 2000; Lee et al. 2000).

Steatocystoma Multiplex

In this condition, multiple, small, rubbery, elevated, cystic lesions develop, usually in adolescence. The lesions may become infected and this leads to scarring. Autosomal dominant inheritance is the rule. Keratin 17 (*K17*) mutations can cause this condition and PC type 2 (Corden and McLean 1996; Smith et al. 1997).

Syringomas

A rare condition with multiple facial syringomas, sometimes with neonatal teeth and oligodontia, has been identified as an autosomal dominant condition (Morrison and Young 1996; Metze et al. 2001).

Trichoepithelioma

This is an autosomal dominant inherited tendency to multiple, small, flesh-colored, translucent tumors from childhood, mainly on the face. There is a risk of basal cell carcinoma developing in the lesions. The condition has been mapped to chromosome 9p21, close to D9S126 (Harada et al. 1996; Clarke et al. 2002). The condition is caused by mutations in the *CYLD* gene, thus allelic with Brooke–Spiegler syndrome (Saggar et al. 2008). Brooke–Spiegler (p. 192) syndrome is an autosomal dominant syndrome characterized by multiple cylindromas and trichoepitheliomas.

Tylosis

Tylosis, or focal epidermolytic palmoplantar keratoderma occurring after infancy, is associated with early-onset squamous cell carcinoma of the esophagus in three families. The tylosis is characterized by abnormal thickening of the palmoplantar skin. Neonatal onset of palmoplantar keratosis is a different disorder and not associated with esophageal cancer. The genetic locus for the tylosis esophageal cancer (*TOC*) gene has been localized to 17q25 (Langan et al. 2004) and the responsible gene has recently been identified (see section on Esophageal Cancer).

Lichen Sclerosis Et Atrophicus

This dermatological disorder is much more common in females than in males (10:1), has a predilection for the vulva, particularly in postmenopausal women, and is the most commonly encountered vulvar dystrophy. Extragenital lesions are most common on the trunk, arms, neck, and face. The lesions are greyish, polygonal, flat papules, which may coalesce into plaques which atrophy. The vulvar lesions predispose to carcinoma of the vulva, with a reported incidence of up to 10 % of affected adult women. The lesions show elevated p53 levels and 17p loss of heterozygosity (LOH). Several cases of familial lichen sclerosis with more than one affected generation have been described, including premenopausal women and children, but these are very rare (Shirer and Ray 1987; Carlson et al. 1998).

Mast Cell Disease

This includes a wide spectrum of clinical entities, with urticaria pigmentosa with or without systemic lesions, and may rarely be associated with malignant mast cell leukemia. Symmetrical hyperpigmented macules or papules may develop from infancy, most commonly on the trunk; they urticate on mild trauma. Vesiculation, erythema, and telangiectasia may develop. Pruritus is common and may be accompanied by flushing, tachycardia, and malaise. Familial instances with autosomal dominant trait inheritance have been described (Shaw 1968). A somatic point mutation in *KIT* may be detected in peripheral blood mononuclear cells in patients with mastocytosis with an associated hematological disorder (Nagata et al. 1995; Fritsch-Polanz et al. 2001; Ferger et al. 2002; Chang et al. 2001). *TET2* mutations have been found in the bone marrow of affected cases (Tefferi et al. 2009).

Multiple Cutaneous Leiomyomas

This is an autosomal dominant condition in which many small smooth muscle tumors develop in the skin. These tumors appear as single or multiple small, firm, painful dermal nodules, fixed to the skin, especially noted on the limbs, trunk, and face, and develop more often in the third decade of life, although they can occur in childhood. Uterine myomas may be associated; 54 % of affected females in one family described in the literature had uterine myomas. These may rarely develop into leiomyosarcomas (Berendes et al. 1971), and there is also an increased risk of type II papillary renal cancer or renal cancer with collecting duct morphology. Affected individuals have reduced fumarate hydratase (FH) activity in lymphoblastoid cells. In the majority of cases, the condition is due to germline heterozygous mutations in the *FH* gene, a component of the tricarboxylic acid cycle (Martinez-Mir et al. 2003; Tomlinson et al. 2002). Homozygotes (or compound heterozygotes for FH mutations) cause the fumarase metabolic deficiency syndrome characterized by developmental delay and death in the first decade (Tomlinson et al. 2002; Alam et al. 2003). However, not all mutation carrier parents of children with FH deficiency have a predisposition to leiomyomata.

Screening affected individuals should include regular abdominal imaging for renal abnormalities (MRI scans are preferred as tumours can be isoechogenic) (Garman et al. 2003; Wei et al. 2006) which should be initiated early, because cases of renal cancer have been described in individuals as young as 11y with germline FH mutations (Alrashdi et al. 2010) (see p. 140).

Multiple Lipomatosis: Familial

This rare autosomal dominant condition is characterized by the development of multiple, encapsulated, subcutaneous, non-tender, smooth lipomas on the forearms, trunk, thighs, and arms. The lipomas are often symmetric, usually begin in early adulthood, and grow to a certain size and then stabilize; regression is rare, as is malignant degeneration. The distribution of the lipomas may follow that of the peripheral nerves (Leffell and Braverman 1986). In one family the condition was linked to an *RB1* gene mutation with low-penetrance retinoblastoma susceptibility (Genuardi et al. 2001). Germline mutations in the *HMGA2* gene may be responsible for dominant familial multiple lipomatosis, and that somatic mutations in this gene may be responsible for encephalocutaneous lipomatosis (Prontera et al. 2009).

Multiple Lipomatosis: Symmetric

This is a separate condition, predominantly occurring in adult males, and autosomal inheritance has been suggested. The primary defect is thought to be in adrenergic-stimulated lipolysis. Clinically, lipomatous masses develop in a symmetric distribution at the back of the neck and shoulders, the breast areas, abdomen, and pubic regions. There may be atrophy of uninvolved fat. Visceral lipomatosis can be life-threatening. Autonomic and peripheral neuropathy is associated, and alcoholism is thought to precipitate its development in many cases. The condition is probably heterogeneous and may not be genetic, but may be confused with multiple lipomatosis. Autosomal dominant inheritance of multiple familial lipomatosis with polyneuropathy has been described (Wilson and Boland 1994; Stoll et al. 1996; Nisoli et al. 2002), and mutations in the mitochondrial genome, possibly resulting in faulty noradrenergic modulation of proliferation and differentiation of brown fat cells (Gamez et al. 1998; Nisoli et al. 2002; Enzi et al. 2002).

NAME Syndrome: Carney Complex

Carney complex is an autosomal dominant multiple endocrine neoplasia and lentiginosis syndrome characterized by spotty skin pigmentation; cardiac, skin, and breast myxomas; and a variety of endocrine tumors. The skin features include common and blue nevi and psammomatous melanotic schwannomas. Endocrine overactivity occurs. Pituitary tumors, adrenal cortical rest tumors, pheochromocytoma, Leydig cell tumors, large cell calcifying Sertoli cell tumor of the testis, schwannomas, and myxoid breast fibroadenomas and ductal adenomas have all been described in this condition (Carney 1995). The most common manifestation is an ACTH-independent Cushing's syndrome due to primary pigmented nodular adrenocortical disease (PPNAD).

The condition is genetically heterogeneous. Mutations in the gene encoding the protein kinase A type 1-alpha regulatory subunit (*PRKAR1A*) on chromosome 17q have been identified in about three quarters of affected individuals (Kirschner et al. 2000a, b; Veugelers et al. 2004); other families show linkage to chromosome 2p16 (Stratakis et al. 1996), and chromosome 2 abnormalities have been described in the tumors (Matyakhina et al. 2003) (see p. 228).

This syndrome is distinct from the Carney triad, an association between stromal gastric sarcoma, pulmonary chondroma, and extra-adrenal paraganglioma (Carney 1999).

Pachyonychia Congenita

This rare autosomal dominant condition is characterized by thickened nails (which are very difficult to cut), with yellow discoloration, follicular keratosis in 59 %, plantar keratosis in 72 %, and leukokeratosis in 57 % of cases. The nail abnormalities may be seen soon after birth, and paronychial inflammation occurs. Subcutaneous hamartomatous cysts, bullae, ichthyosis, and hyperkeratosis may develop. Blistering may occur over pressure areas, and there may be deafness, hair and dental abnormalities, hyperhidrosis, and corneal opacification. Oral leukoplakia is seen. Malignant changes may occur in the oral lesions, in cysts, or at sites of chronic plantar ulcerations, so that areas of chronic ulceration or bullous formation should be observed for the possible development of malignancy (Su et al. 1990). Steatocystoma multiplex is considered to be the same condition. Germline mutations in the K17 gene may underlie certain types of this condition (Smith et al. 1997); others may be due to missense mutations in keratin 17 (Smith et al. 1997; Feinstein et al. 1988; Hodes and Norins 1977; Stieglitz and Centerwall 1983).

Pachyonychia congenita (PC) types 1 and 2 are described. These are similar but type 1 gets oral leukokeratoses, whereas type 2 has premature dentition and multiple sebaceous cysts. Mutations in the keratin 17 (K17) gene can cause PC type 2 or steatocystoma multiplex PC types 1 and 2 with hypertrophic nail dystrophy, focal keratoderma, and sebaceous cysts (Corello et al. 1998). PC type 1 is due to K6a and K16 mutations (Swenssen 1999).

Palmar Keratoses

It has been claimed that palmar and plantar keratoses are more common in individuals with bladder and lung cancer, occurring in 70–90 % of cases and in only 36 % of controls, but it is difficult to assess the significance of this finding since it is based on only a few studies (Cuzick et al. 1984). Keratin gene or connexin abnormalities may underlie this group of conditions (Bale and DiGiovanna 1997; Kelsell et al. 2000; Kimyai-Asadi et al. 2002; Radi et al. 2005).

There are many subtypes, including palmoplantar keratoderma, the Clarke–Howel–Evans syndrome (see Esophageal Cancer) (Malde, Meleda, Smith 2003). Mutations of the KRT1 and KRT9 genes may cause the epidermolytic form of PPK. Both epidermolytic and nonepidermolytic forms of palmoplantar keratoderma have been observed with various mutations in the KRT1 gene (Chiu et al. 2007).

Pilomatrixoma (Benign Calcifying Epithelioma of Malherbe)

Pilomatrixomas appear in young adults, most commonly on the arms, face, and neck, as asymptomatic, firm, lobular, bluish nodules, which may be painful and occasionally inflamed. They are usually sporadic but have rarely been found to occur in families. They occur in both sexes, possibly with autosomal dominant inheritance. Multiple calcifying epitheliomas have been reported in association with myotonic dystrophy (Harper 1972; Hubbard and Whittaker 2004) and with Rubinstein–Taybi syndrome (Masuno et al. 1998). Activating mutations in CTNNB1 are detected in a high proportion of tumors (Chan et al. 1999).

References

Abuzahra F, Parren L, Frank J. Multiple familial and pigmented basal cell carcinomas in early childhood – Bazex-Dupré-Christol syndrome. J Eur Acad Dermatol Venereol JEADV. 2011;26(1):117–21. doi:10.1111/j.1468-3083.2011.04048.x. Epub 2011 Mar 24.

Ahonen P. Autoimmune polyendocrinopathy-candidosis-ectodermal dystrophy (APECED): autosomal recessive inheritance. Clin Genet. 1985;27:535–42.

Alam NA, Rowan AJ, Wortham N, et al. Genetic and functional analyses of FH mutations in multiple cutaneous and uterine leiomatosis, hereditary leiomyomatosis and renal cancer, and fumarate hydratase deficiency. Hum Mol Genet. 2003;12:1–12.

Alrashdi I, Levine S, Paterson J, Saxena R, Patel SR, Depani S, Hargrave DR, Pritchard-Jones K, Hodgson SV. Hereditary leiomyomatosis and renal cell carcinoma: very early diagnosis of renal cancer in a paediatric patient. Fam Cancer. 2010;9(2):239–43.

Anderson DE, Badzioch MD. Hereditary cutaneous malignant melanoma: a 20-year family update. Anticancer Res. 1991;11:433–8.

Angelo C, Groeso MG, Stella P, et al. Becker's nevus syndrome. Cutis. 2001;68:123–4.

Araim M, Nosaka K, Koshiara K, et al. Neurocutaneous melanosis associated with Dandy Walker malformation and a meningohydroencephalocele. J Neurosurg Spine. 2004;100:501–5.

Arngrimsson R, Dokal I, Luzzato L, Connor JM. Dyskeratosis congenita. Three additional families show linkage to a locus in Xq28. J Med Genet. 1993;30:618–9.

Arunkumar MJ, Ranjan A, Jacob M, Rajshekhar V. Neurocutaneous melanosis: a case of primary intracranial melanoma with metastasis. Clin Oncol. 2001;13:52–4.

Ashinoff R, Jacobson M, Belsito DV. Rombo syndrome: a second case report and review. J Am Acad Dermatol. 1993;28:1011–4.

Augustsson A, Stierner U, Rosdahl I, Suurkula M. Common and dysplastic nevi as risk factors for cutaneous malignant melanoma in a Swedish population. Acta Derm Venereol. 1990;71:518–24.

Augustsson A, Stierner U, Suurkula M, et al. Prevalence of common and dysplastic nevi in a Swedish population. Br J Dermatol. 1991;124:152–6.

Auroy S, Avril MF, Chompret A, et al. Sporadic multiple primary melanoma cases: CDKN2A germline mutations with a founder effect. Genes Chromosomes Cancer. 2001;32(3):195–202.

Bahmer FA, Fritsch P, Kreusch J, et al. Terminology in surface microscopy. J Am Acad Dermatol. 1990;23(6):1159–62.

Bahuau M, Vidaud D, Jenkins RB, et al. Germ-line deletion involving the INK4 locus in familial proneness to melanoma and nervous system tumors. Cancer Res. 1998;58:2298–303.

Baird DM. Variation at the TERT locus and predisposition for cancer. Expert Rev Mol Med. 2010;12:e16.

Balch CM, Soong SJ, Gershenwald JE, et al. Prognostic factors analysis of 17,600 melanoma patients: validation of the American joint committee on cancer melanoma staging system. J Clin Oncol. 2001;19(16):3622–34.

Balch CM, Gershenwald JE, Soong SJ, et al. Final version of 2009 AJCC melanoma staging and classification. J Clin Oncol. 2009;27:6199–206.

Bale SJ, DiGiovanna JJ. Genetic approaches to understanding the keratinopathies. Adv Dermatol. 1997;12:99–113.

Bale SJ, Dracopoli NC, Tucker MA, et al. Mapping the gene for hereditary cutaneous malignant melanoma-dysplastic nevus to chromosome 1p. N Engl J Med. 1989a;320:1367–72.

Bale SJ, Dracopoli NC, Tucker MA, et al. Mapping the gene for hereditary cutaneous malignant melanoma dysplastic nevus syndrome to chromosome 1p. N Engl J Med. 1989b;320:1367–72.

Barker K, Zhou X-P, Araki T, et al. PTEN mutations are uncommon in Proteus syndrome. J Med Genet. 2001;38:480–1.

Barker KT, Foulkes WD, Schwartz CE, Labadie C, Monsell F, Houlston RS, Harper J. Is the E133K allele of VG5Q associated with Klippel-Trenaunay and other overgrowth syndromes? J Med Genet. 2006;43:613–4.

Barrett JH, Iles MM, Harland M, Taylor JC, Aitken JF, Andresen PA, Akslen LA, Armstrong BK, Avril MF, Azizi E, Bakker B, Bergman W, Bianchi-Scarrà G, Bressac-de Paillerets B, Calista D, Cannon-Albright LA, Corda E, Cust AE, Dębniak T, Duffy D, Dunning AM, Easton DF, Friedman E, Galan P, Ghiorzo P, Giles GG, Hansson J, Hocevar M, Höiom V, Hopper JL, Ingvar C, Janssen B, Jenkins MA, Jönsson G, Kefford RF, Landi G, Landi MT, Lang J, Lubiński J, Mackie R, Malvehy J, Martin NG, Molven A, Montgomery GW, van Nieuwpoort FA, Novakovic S, Olsson H, Pastorino L, Puig S, Puig-Butille JA, Randerson-Moor J, Snowden H, Tuominen R, Van Belle P, van der Stoep N, Whiteman DC, Zelenika D, Han J, Fang S, Lee JE, Wei Q, Lathrop GM, Gillanders EM, Brown KM, Goldstein AM, Kanetsky PA, Mann GJ, Macgregor S, Elder DE, Amos CI, Hayward NK, Gruis NA, Demenais F, Bishop JA, Bishop DT, GenoMEL Consortium. Genome-wide association study identifies three new melanoma susceptibility loci. Nat Genet. 2011;43(11):1108–13.

Barsh GS. The genetics of pigmentation: from fancy genes to complex traits. Trend Genet. 1996;12:299–305.

Bartsch DK, Sina-Frey M, Lang S, Wild A, Gerdes B, Barth P, Kress R, Grutzmann R, Colombo-Benkmann M, Ziegler A, Hahn SA, Rothmund M, Rieder H, et al. CDKN2A germline mutations in familial pancreatic cancer. Ann Surg. 2002;236(6):730–7.

Bastiaens MT, ter Huurne JA, Kielich C, et al. Melanocortin-1 receptor gene variants determine the risk of nonmelanoma skin cancer independently of fair skin and red hair. Am J Hum Genet. 2001a;68:884–94.

Bastiaens M, ter Huurne J, Gruis N, Bergman W, Westendorp R, Vermeer BJ, Bouwes Bavinck JN. The melanocortin-1-receptor gene is the major freckle gene. Hum Mol Genet. 2001b;10(16):1701–8.

Bataille V, Newton Bishop JA, Sasieni P, Swerdlow AJ, Pinney E, Griffiths K, et al. Risk of cutaneous melanoma in relation to the numbers, types and sites of nevi: a case–control study. Br J Cancer. 1996;73(12):1605–11.

Bataille V, Kato BS, Falchi M, et al. Nevus size and number are associated with telomere length and represent potential markers of a decreased senescence in vivo. Cancer Epidemiol Biomark Prev. 2007;16:1499–502.

Begg CB, Orlow I, Hummer AJ, et al. Lifetime risk of melanoma in CDKN2A mutation carriers in a population-based sample. J Natl Cancer Inst. 2005;97:1507–15.

Berendes U, Kuhner A, Schnyder UW. Segmentary and disseminated lesions in multiple hereditary cutaneous leiomyoma. Humangenetik. 1971;13:81–2.

Bergman W, Watson P, de Jong J, Lynch HT, Fusaro RM. Systemic cancer and the FAMMM syndrome. Br J Cancer. 1990;61:932–6.

Bergman W, Gruis NA, Frants RR. The Dutch FAMMM family material: clinical and genetic data. Cytogenet Cell Genet. 1992;59:161–4.

Bernends R. Cancer: cues for migration. Nature. 2003;425:247–8.

Biggs PJ, Wooster R, Ford D, et al. Familial cylindromatosis (turban tumor syndrome) gene localized to chromosome 16q12–13: evidence for its role as a tumor suppressor gene. Nat Genet. 1995;11:441–3.

Bishop D, Goldstein A, Demenais F. Geographical variation in CNKN2A penetrance for melanoma. Am J Hum Genetics. 2000;67:16.

Bishop DT, Demenais F, Goldstein AM, et al. Geographical variation in the penetrance of CDKN2A mutations for melanoma. J Natl Cancer Inst. 2002;94(12):894–903.

Bishop DT, Demenais F, Iles MM, et al. Genome-wide association study identifies three loci associated with melanoma risk. Nat Genet. 2009;41:920–5.

Blake PW, Toro JR. Update of cylindromatosis gene (CYLD) mutations in Brooke-Spiegler syndrome: novel insights into the role of deubiquitination in cell signaling. Hum Mutat. 2009;30:1025–36.

Bonifas JM, Rothman AL, Epstein Jr EH. Epidermolysis bullosa simplex: evidence in two families for keratin gene abnormalities. Science. 1991;2254(5035):1202–5.

Boonchai W, Walsh M, Cummings M, et al. Expression of p53 in arsenic-related and sporadic basal cell carcinoma. Arch Dermatol. 2000;136:195–8.

Borg A, Sandberg T, Nilsson K, et al. High frequency of multiple melanomas and breast and pancreas carcinomas in CDKN2A mutation-positive melanoma families. J Natl Cancer Inst. 2000;92(15):1260–6.

Bose S, Morgan LJ, Booth DR, Goudie DR, Ferguson-Smith MA, Richards FM. The elusive multiple self-healing squamous epithelioma (MSSE) gene: further mapping, analysis of candidates, and loss of heterozygosity. Oncogene. 2006;25:806–12.

Box NF, Duffy DL, Irving RE, et al. Melanocortin-1 receptor genotype is a risk factor for basal and squamous cell carcinoma. J Invest Dermatol. 2001a;116:224–9.

Box NF, Duffy DL, Chen W, Stark M, Martin NG, Sturm RA, Hayward NK. MC1R genotype modifies risk of melanoma in families segregating CDKN2A mutations. Am J Hum Genet. 2001b;69(4):765–73.

Brummelkamp TR, Nijman SMB, Dirac AMG, Bernards R. Loss of the cylindromatosis tumor suppressor inhibits apoptosis by activating NF-kB. Nature. 2003;424:797–801.

Buzzi F, Badolato R, Mazza C, et al. Autoimmune polyendocrinopathy C-ED syndrome; time to review diagnostic criteria. J Clin Endo Metab. 2003;88:3146–8.

Cannon-Albright LA, Goldgar DE, Wright EC, et al. Evidence against the reported linkage of the cutaneous melanoma-dysplastic nevus syndrome locus to chromo-some 1p36. Am J Hum Genet. 1990;46:912–8.

Cannon-Albright LA, Goldgar DE, Meyer LJ, et al. Assignment of a locus for familial melanoma, MLM, to chromosome 9p13-p22. Science. 1992;258:1148–52.

Carlson JA, Ambros R, Malfetano J, et al. Vulvar lichen sclerosis and squamous cell carcinoma: a cohort, case control, and investigational study with historical perspective; implications for chronic inflammation and sclerosis in the development of neoplasia. Hum Pathol. 1998;29:932–48.

Carney JA. Carney complex; the complex of myxomas, spotty pigmentation. Endocrine overactivity and schwannomas. Semin Dermatol. 1995;14:90–8.

Carney JA. Gastric stromal sarcoma, pulmonary chondroma and extra-adrenal paraganglioma (Carney Triad): natural history, adrenocortical component and possible familial occurrence. Mayo Clin Proc. 1999;74:543–52.

Carrucci JA. Squamous cell carcinoma in organ transplant recipients; approach to management. Skin Ther Lett. 2004;9:5–7.

Castilla EE, da Graca Dutra M, Orioli-Parreiras IM. Epidemiology of congenital pigmented nevi: I. Incidence rates and relative frequencies. Br J Dermatol. 1981;104:307–15.

Chan EF, Gat U, McNoff JM, Fuchs E. A common human skin tumor is caused by activating mutation in beta catenin. Nat Genet. 1999;21:410–3.

Chang H, Tunq RC, Schlesinger T, et al. Familial cutaneous mastocytosis. Pediatr Dermatol. 2001;18(4):271–6.

Chang YM, Barrett JH, Bishop DT, et al. Sun exposure and melanoma risk at different latitudes: a pooled analysis of 5700 cases and 7216 controls. Int J Epidemiol. 2009;38: 814–30.

Chiu H-C, Jee S-H, Sheen Y-S, Chu C-Y, Lin P-J, Liaw S-H. Mutation of keratin 9 (R163W) in a family with epidermolytic palmoplantar keratoderma and knuckle pads. (Letter). J Dermatol Sci. 2007;45:63–5.

Cirillo Silengo M, Dan GF, Bianco MC, et al. Distinctive hair changes (pili torti) in Rapp Hodgkin ectodermal dysplasia syndrome. Clin Genet. 1982;21:297–300.

Clarke J, Loffreda M, Helm KF. Multiple familial trichoepitheliomas: a folliculosebaceous-apocrine genodermatosis. Am J Dermatopathol. 2002;24:402–5.

Coleman R, Hay RJ. Chronic mucocutaneous candidiasis associated with hypothyroidism: a distinct syndrome? Br J Dermatol. 1997;136:24–9.

Corden LD, McLean WH. Human keratin diseases: hereditary fragility of specific epithelial tissues. Exp Dermatol. 1996;5(6):297–307.

Corello SP, Smith FJ, Sittevis-Smith JH, et al. Keratin mutations cause either steatocystoma multiplex or pachyonychia congenital type 2. Br J Dermatol. 1998;39:475–80.

Coulombe PA, Hutton ME, Letai A, et al. Point mutations in human keratin 14 genes of epidermolysis bullosa simplex patients: genetic and functional analyses. Cell. 1991;66:1301–11.

Courtois G, Smahi A, Reichenbach J, et al. A hypermorphic I kappa B alpha mutation is associated with autosomal dominant anhidrotic ectodermal dysplasia and T cell immunodeficiency. J Clin Invest. 2003;112:1108–15.

Cuzick J, Harris R, Mortimer PS. Palmar keratoses and cancers of the bladder and lung. Lancet. 1984;323:530–3.

Davidson HR, Connor JM. Dyskeratosis congenita. J Med Genet. 1988;25:843–6.

De Andrade DO, Dravet C, Rayboud C, et al. An unusual case of neurocutaneous melanosis. Epileptic Disord. 2004;6:145–52.

de Snoo FA, Bergman W, Gruis NA. Familial melanoma: a complex disorder leading to controversy on DNA testing. Fam Cancer. 2003;2(2):109–16.

de Snoo FA, Bishop DT, Bergman W, et al. Increased risk of cancer other than melanoma in CDKN2A founder mutation (p16-Leiden)-positive melanoma families. Clin Cancer Res. 2008;14:7151–7.

de Wijn RS, Zaal LH, Hennekam RC, et al. Familial clustering of giant congenital melanocytic nevi. J Plast Reconstr Aesthet Surg JPRAS. 2010;63:906–13.

de Zwaan SE, Haass NK. Genetics of basal cell carcinoma. Australas J Dermatol. 2010;51:81–92; quiz 93–4.

Delaporte E, N'guyen-Mailfer C, Janin A, et al. Keratoderma with scleroatrophy of the extremities or sclerotylosis (Huriez syndrome): a reappraisal. Br J Dermatol. 1995;133:409–16.

Della Torre G, Pasini B, Frigerio S, et al. CDKN2A and CDK4 mutation analysis in Italian melanoma-prone families: functional characterization of a novel CDKN2A germ line mutation. Br J Cancer. 2001;85(6):836–44.

Demenais F, Mohamdi H, Chaudru V, et al. Association of MC1R variants and host phenotypes with melanoma risk in CDKN2A mutation carriers: a GenoMEL study. J Natl Cancer Inst. 2010;102:1568–83.

Downs AM, Kennedy CT. Scleroatrophic syndrome of Huriez in an infant. Pediatr Dermatol. 1998;15:207–9.

Duffy DL, Iles MM, Glass D, et al. IRF4 variants have age-specific effects on nevus count and predispose to melanoma. Am J Hum Genet. 2010;87:6–16.

Eady RA, Dunnill MG. Epidermolysis bullosa: hereditary skin fragility diseases as paradigms in cell biology. Arch Dermatol Res. 1994;287(1):2–9.

Easton D, Cox G, Macdonald A, et al. Genetic susceptibility to nevi- a twin study. Br J Cancer. 1991;64:1164–7.

Eerola I, Boon LM, Mulliken JB, Burrows PE, Dompmartin A, Watanabe S, Vanwijck R, Vikkula M. Capillary malformation-arteriovenous malformation, a new clinical and genetic disorder caused by RASA1 mutations. Am J Hum Genet. 2003;73:1240–9.

Eide MJ, Weinstock MA. Association of UV index, latitude, and melanoma incidence in nonwhite populations–US Surveillance, Epidemiology, and End Results (SEER) Program, 1992 to 2001. Arch Dermatol. 2005;141:477–81.

Elwood JM, Whitehead SM, Davison J, Stewart M, Galt M. Malignant melanoma in England: risks associated with nevi, freckles, social class, hair colour, and sunburn. Int J Epidemiol. 1990;19(4):801–10.

Enzi G, Busetto L, Ceschin E, Coin A, Digito M, Pigozzo S. Multiple symmetric lipomatosis: clinical aspects and outcome in a long-term longitudinal study. Int J Obes. 2002;26:253–61.

Escobar V, Goldblatt LI, Bixler D, et al. Clouston syndrome: an ultrastructural study. Clin Genet. 1983;24:140–6.

Evans DG, Howard E, Giblin C, et al. Birth incidence and prevalence of tumor-prone syndromes: estimates from a UK family genetic register service. Am J Med Genet A. 2010;152A:327–32.

Farndon PA, Del Mastro RG, Evans DGR, et al. Location of gene for Gorlin syndrome. Lancet. 1992;339:581–2.

Fayad MN, Yacoub A, Salman S, et al. Juvenile hyaline fibromatosis: two new patients and review of the literature. Am J Med Genet. 1987;26:123–31.

Feinstein A, Friedman J, Schewach-Millet M. Pachonychia congenita. J Am Acad Dermatol. 1988;19:705–11.

Fenske C, Banergee P, Holden C, Carter N. Brook–Spiegler syndrome locus assigned to 16q 12–13. J Invest Dermatol. 2000;114:1057–8.

Ferger F, Ribadean DA, Leriche L, et al. Kit and c-kit mutations in mastocytosis: a short overview with special reference to novel molecular and diagnostic concepts. Int Arch Allergy Immunol. 2002;127:110–4.

Flohil SC, de Vries E, Neumann HA, et al. Incidence, prevalence and future trends of primary basal cell carcinoma in the Netherlands. Acta Derm-Venereol. 2011;91:24–30.

Fogarty PF, Yamaguchi H, Wiestner A, et al. Late presentation of dyskeratosis congenita as apparently acquired aplastic anemia due to mutations in telomerase RNA. Lancet. 2003;362:1628–30.

Fritsch-Polanz R, Jordan JH, Eeli XA, et al. Mutation analysis of C-Kit in patients with myelodysplastic syndrome without mastocytosis and cases of systemic mastocytosis. Br J Haematol. 2001;13:357–64.

Fuchs E. The cytoskeleton and disease: genetic disorders of intermediate filaments. Ann Rev Genet. 1996;30:197–231.

Gamez J, Playan A, Andreu AL, et al. Familial multiple symmetric lipomatosis associated with the A8344G mutation of mitochondrial DNA. Neurology. 1998;51:258–60.

Gandini S, Sera F, Cattaruzza MS, et al. Meta-analysis of risk factors for cutaneous melanoma: II. Sun exposure. Eur J Cancer. 2005a;41:45–60.

Gandini S, Sera F, Cattaruzza MS, et al. Meta-analysis of risk factors for cutaneous melanoma: III. Family history, actinic damage and phenotypic factors. Eur J Cancer. 2005b;41:2040–59.

Garman ME, Blumberg MA, Ernst R, Rainer SS. Familial leiomyomatosis: a review and discussion of pathogenesis. Dermatology. 2003;207:210–3.

Genuardi M, Klutz M, Devriendt K, et al. Multiple lipomas linked to an RBI gene mutation in a large pedigree with low penetrance retinoblastoma. Eur J Hum Genet. 2001;9(9):690–4.

Ghiorzo P, Pastorino L, Bonelli L, et al. INK4/ARF germline alterations in pancreatic cancer patients. Ann Oncol. 2004;15(1):70–8.

Ghiorzo P, Gargiulo S, Nasti S, et al. Predicting the risk of pancreatic cancer: on CDKN2A mutations in the melanoma-pancreatic cancer syndrome in Italy. J Clin Oncol. 2007;25:5336–7; author reply 5337–8.

Gillanders E, Hank Juo SH, Holland EA, et al. Localization of a novel melanoma susceptibility locus to 1p22. Am J Hum Genet. 2003;73(2):301–13.

Glocker E-O, Hennigs A, Nabavi M, Schaffer AA, Woellner C, Salzer U, Pfeifer D, Veelken H, Warnatz K, Tahami F, Jamal S, Manguiat A, Rezaei N, Amirzargar AA, Plebani A, Hannesschlager N, Gross O, Ruland J, Grimbacher B. A homozygous CARD9 mutation in a family with susceptibility to fungal infections. New Eng J Med. 2009;361:1727–35.

Goerttler EA, Jung EG. Porokeratosis of Mibelli and skin carcinoma: a critical review. Humangenetik. 1975;26:291–6.

Goldberg GI, Eisen AZ, Bauer EA. Tissue stress and tumor promotion. Arch Dermatol. 1988;124:737–41.

Goldstein AM, Dracopoli NC, Engelstein M, Fraser MC, Clark Jr WH, Tucker MA. Linkage of cutaneous malignant melanoma dysplastic nevi to chromosome 9p, and evidence for genetic heterogeneity. Am J Hum Genet. 1994;54:489–96.

Goldstein AM, Struewing JP, Fraser MC, Smith MW, Tucker MA. Prospective risk of cancer in CDKN2A germline mutation carriers. J Med Genet. 2004;41:421–4.

Goldstein AM, Chan M, Harland M, Hayward NK, Demenais F, Bishop DT, Azizi E, Bergman W, Bianchi-Scarra G, Bruno W, Calista D, Albright LA, Chaudru V, Chompret A, Cuellar F, Elder DE, Ghiorzo P, Gillanders EM, Gruis NA, Hansson J, Hogg D, Holland EA, Kanetsky PA, Kefford RF, Landi MT, Lang J, Leachman SA, MacKie RM, Magnusson V,

Mann GJ, Bishop JN, Palmer JM, Puig S, Puig-Butille JA, Stark M, Tsao H, Tucker MA, Whitaker L, Yakobson E, Lund Melanoma Study Group, Melanoma Genetics Consortium (GenoMEL). Features associated with germline CDKN2A mutations: a GenoMEL study of melanoma-prone families from three continents. J Med Genet. 2007;44(2):99–106. Epub 2006 Aug.

Goodship J, Redfearn A, Milligan D, et al. Transmission of proteus syndrome from father to son? J Med Genet. 1991;28:781–6.

Gorlin RJ. Proteus syndrome. J Clin Dysmorphol. 1984;2:8–9.

Gotz A, Kopera D, Wach F, et al. Porokeratosis Mibelli; case report and literature review. Hantarz. 1999;50:435–8.

Goudie DR, Yuille MAR, Affara NA, Ferguson-Smith MA. Localisation of the gene for multiple self healing squamous epithelioma (Ferguson–Smith type) to the long arm of chromosome 9. Cytogenet Cell Genet. 1991;58:1939.

Goudie DR, D'Alessandro M, Merriman B, et al. Multiple self-healing squamous epithelioma is caused by a disease-specific spectrum of mutations in TGFBR1. Nat Genet. 2011a;43:365–9.

Goudie DR, D'Alessandro M, Merriman B, et al. Multiple self-healing squamous epithelioma is caused by a disease-specific spectrum of mutations in TGFBR1. Nat Genet. 2011b;43:365–71.

Griffiths GM. Albinism & immunity: what's the link? Curr Mol Med. 2002;2:479–83.

Guarneri B, Borgia F, Cannaro SP, et al. Multiple familial BCCs and a case of seg-mental manifestations. Dermatology. 2000;200:299–302.

Gudbjartsson DF, Sulem P, Stacey SN, et al. ASIP and TYR pigmentation variants associate with cutaneous melanoma and basal cell carcinoma. Nat Genet. 2008;40:886–91.

Guerriero C, Albanesi C, Girolomoni G, De Simone C, Capizzi R, Amerio P, Tulli A. Huriez syndrome: case report with a detailed analysis of skin dendritic cells. Br J Dermatol. 2000;143:1091–6.

Gutierrez PP, Eggenmena T, Holler D, et al. Phenotype diversity in familial cylindromatosis: a frameshift mutation in the tumor expressor gene CYLD underlies different tumors of skin. J Invest Dermatol. 2002;119:527–31.

Hahn H, Wicking C, Zaphiropoulous PG, et al. Mutations of the human homolog of Drosophila patched in the nevoid basal cell carcinoma syndrome. Cell. 1996;85:841–51.

Hamm J, Traupe H, Brocker EB, et al. The scleroatrophic syndrome of Huriez: a cancer-prone genodermatosis. Br J Dermatol. 1996;134:512–8.

Han J, Kraft P, Colditz GA, et al. Melanocortin 1 receptor variants and skin cancer risk. Int J Cancer. 2006;119:1976–84.

Han J, Qureshi AA, Nan H, et al. A germline variant in the interferon regulatory factor 4 gene as a novel skin cancer risk locus. Cancer Res. 2011;71:1533–9.

Happle R. Nonsyndromic type of hereditary multiple basal cell carcinoma. Am J Med Genet. 2000;95:161–3.

Harada H, Hashimoto K, Ko MSH. The gene for multiple familial trichoepithelioma maps to chromosome 9p21. J Invest Dermatol. 1996;107:41–3.

Harbour JW, Onken MD, Roberson ED, et al. Frequent mutation of BAP1 in metastasizing uveal melanomas. Science. 2010;330:1410–3.

Harland M, Meloni R, Gruis N, et al. Germline mutations of the CDKN2 gene in UK melanoma families. Hum Mol Genet. 1997;6:2061–7.

Harland M, Holland EA, Ghiorzo P, et al. Mutation screening of the CDKN2A promoter in melanoma families. Genes Chromosomes Cancer. 2000;28(1):45–57.

Harland M, Mistry S, Bishop DT, Bishop JA. A deep intronic mutation in CDKN2A is associated with disease in a subset of melanoma pedigrees. Hum Mol Genet. 2001;10(23):2679–86.

Harland M, Taylor CF, Bass S, et al. Intronic sequence variants of the CDKN2A gene in melanoma pedigrees. Genes Chromosomes Cancer. 2005;43:128–36.

Harper PS. Calcifying epithelioma of Malherbe. Association with myotonic muscular dystrophy. Arch Dermatol. 1972;106:41–4.

Hayward NK. Genetics of melanoma predisposition. Oncogene. 2003;22:3053–62.

Hewitt C, Lee Wu C, Evans G, et al. Germline mutation of ARF in a melanoma kindred. Hum Mol Genet. 2002;11(11):1273–9.

Hoanq MP, Sinkre P, Albores-Savedras J. Rhabdomyosarcoma arising in a congenital melanocytic naevus. Am J Dermatopathol. 2002;24:26–9.

Hodes ME, Norins AL. Pachyonychia congenita and steatocystoma multiplex. Clin Genet. 1977;11:359–64.

Hubbard VG, Whittaker SJ. Multiple familial pilomatrixomas: an unusual case. J Cutan Pathol. 2004;31:281–3.

Iannello S, Fabbri G, Bosco P, et al. A clinical variant of familial Hermansky–Pudlak syndrome. Medscape Gen Med. 2003;5:3.

Jacobelli S, Laude H, Carlotti A, et al. Epidermodysplasia verruciformis in human immunodeficiency virus-infected patients: a marker of human papillomavirus-related disorders not affected by antiretroviral therapy. Arch Dermatol. 2011;147:590–6.

Janecke AR, Hennies HC, Gunther B, et al. GJB2 mutations in keratitis-ichthyosis-deafness syndrome including its fatal form. Am J Med Genet. 2005;133:128–31.

Johnson RL, Rothman AL, Xie J, et al. Human homolog of patched, a candidate gene for the basal cell nevus syndrome. Science. 1996;272:1668–71.

Jones W, Harman C, Ng A, Shaw J. The incidence of malignant melanoma in Auckland, New Zealand: highest rates in the world. World J Surg. 1999;23:732–5.

Jonkman MF, Rulo HF, Duipmans JC. From gene to disease: epidermolysis bullosa due to mutations in or around the hemidesmosome. Ned Tijschr Geneeskd. 2003;147:1108–13.

Jonsson G, Bendahl PO, Sandberg T, et al. Mapping of a novel ocular and cutaneous malignant melanoma susceptibility locus to chromosome 9q21.32. J Natl Cancer Inst. 2005;97: 1377–82.

Kalra S, Zhang Y, Knatko EV, et al. Oral azathioprine leads to higher incorporation of 6-thioguanine in DNA of skin than liver: the protective role of the Keap1/Nrf2/ARE pathway. Cancer Prev Res. 2011;4:1665–74.

Karim MA, Suzuki K, Fukai K, et al. Apparent genotype–phenotype correlation in childhood, adolescent and adult Chegiac; Higashi syndrome. Am J Med Genet. 2002;108:16–22.

Katagiri K, Takasaki S, Fujiwara S, et al. Purification and structural analysis of extracellular matrix of a skin tumor from a patient with juvenile hyaline fibromatosis. J Dermatol Sci. 1996;13:37–8.

Kawaguchi K, Sakamaki H, Onozawa Y, et al. Dyskeratosis congenita (Zinsser–Cole– Engman syndrome). Virchows Arch A Pathol Anat Histopathol. 1990;417:247–53.

Kefford R, Bishop JN, Tucker M, et al. Genetic testing for melanoma. Lancet Oncol. 2002;3(11):653–4.

Kelsell DP, Wilgoss AL, Richard G, et al. Connexin mutations associated with palmoplantar keratoderma and profound deafness in a single family. Eur J Hum Genet. 2000;8:141–4.

Kidd A, Carson L, Gregory DW, de Silva D, Holmes J, Dean JC, Haites N. A Scottish family with Bazex-Dupré-Christol syndrome: follicular atrophoderma, congenital hypotrichosis, and basal cell carcinoma. J Med Genet. 1996;33:493–7.

Kim T, Park JC, Roh MR, et al. Development of aggressive squamous cell carcinoma in epidermodysplasia verruciformis associated with human papillomavirus type 22b. Dermatology. 2010;220:326–8.

Kimyai-Asadi A, Ketcher LB, Ji LMH. The molecular basis of hereditary palmarplantar keratodermas. J Am Acad Dermatol. 2002;47(3):327–43.

Kinsler VA, Aylett SE, Coley SC, et al. Central nervous system imaging and congenital melanocytic nevi. Arch Dis Child. 2001;84:152–5.

Kirkpatrick CH. Chronic mucocutaneous candidiasis. J Am Acad Dermatol. 1994;31:S14–7.

Kirschner LS, Carney JA, Pack SD, et al. Mutations in the gene encoding the protein kinase A type 1-alpha regulatory subunit in patients with Carney complex. Nat Genet. 2000a;26:89–92.

Kirschner LS, Sandrini F, Monbo J, Lin JP, Carney JA, Stratakis CA. Genetic heterogeneity and spectrum of mutations of the PRKAR1A gene in patients with the Carney complex. Hum Mol Genet. 2000b;9:3037–46.

Kirwan M, Dokal I. Dyskeratosis congenita: a genetic disorder of many faces. Clin Genet. 2008;73:103–12.

Korge BP, Krieg T. The molecular basis for inherited bullous disease. J Mol Med. 1996;74:59–70.

La Nasa G, Cottoni E, Mulgaria M, et al. HLA antigen distribution in different clinical subgroups demonstrates genetic heterogeneity in lichen planus. Br J Dermatol. 1995;132:897–900.

Lakhani SR. Putting the brakes on cylindromatosis? N Engl J Med. 2004;350:187–8.

Lal G, Liu L, Hogg D, Lassam NJ, Redston MS, Gallinger S. Patients with both pancreatic adenocarcinoma and melanoma may harbor germline CDKN2A mutations. Genes Chromosomes Cancer. 2000;27:358–61.

Lane JE, Bowman PH, Cohen DJ. Epidermodysplasia verruciformis. South Med J. 2003;96:613–5.

Langan JE, Cole CG, Huckle EJ, Bryne S, McRonald FE, Rowbottom L, Ellis A, Shaw JM, Leigh IM, Kelsell DP, Dunham I, Field JK, Risk JM. Novel microsatellite markers and single nucleotide polymorphisms refine the tylosis with esophageal cancer t(TOC) minimal region on 17q25 to 42.5 kb: sequencing does not identify the causative gene. Hum Genet. 2004;114:534–40.

Leachman SA, Carucci J, Kohlmann W, et al. Selection criteria for genetic assessment of patients with familial melanoma. J Am Acad Dermatol. 2009;61:677 e1-14.

Lee Y-A, Stevens HP, Delaporte E, Wahn U, Reis A. A gene for an autosomal dominant scleroatrophic syndrome predisposing to skin cancer (Huriez syndrome) maps to chromosome 4q23. (Letter). Am J Hum Genet. 2000;66:326–30.

Leffell DJ, Braverman JM. Familial multiple lipomatosis. J Am Acad Dermatol. 1986;15:275–9.

Li TH, Hsu CK, Chiu HC, Chang CH. Multiple asymptomatic hyperkeratotic papules on the lower part of the legs. Hyperkeratosis lenticularis perstans (HLP) (Flegel disease). Arch Dermatol. 1997;133(7):910–1, 913–4.

Liede A, Karlan BY, Narod SA. Cancer risks for male carriers of germline mutations in BRCA1 or BRCA2: a review of the literature. J Clin Oncol. 2004;22:735–42.

Lin AN, Carter DM. Epidermolysis bullosa: when the skin falls apart. J Pediatr. 1989;114:349–56.

Lindhurst MJ, Sapp JC, Teer JK, Johnston JJ, Finn EM, Peters K, Turner J, Cannons JL, Bick D, Blakemore L, Blumhorst C, Brockmann K, Calder P, Cherman N, Deardorff MA, Everman DB, Golas G, Greenstein RM, Kato BM, Keppler-Noreuil KM, Kuznetsov SA, Miyamoto RT, Newman K, Ng D, O'Brien K, Rothenberg S, Schwartzentruber DJ, Singhal V, Tirabosco R, Upton J, Wientroub S, Zackai EH, Hoag K, Whitewood-Neal T, Robey PG, Schwartzberg PL, Darling TN, Tosi LL, Mullikin JC, Biesecker LG. A mosaic activating mutation in AKT1 associated with the Proteus syndrome. N Engl J Med. 2011;365(7):611–9.

Liu L, Dilworth D, Gao L, Monzon J, Summers A, Lassam N, et al. Mutation of the CDKN2A 5'UTR creates an aberrant initiation codon and predisposes to melanoma. Nat Genet. 1999;21:1–5.

Loo JC, Liu L, Hao A, et al. Germline splicing mutations of CDKN2A predispose to melanoma. Oncogene. 2003;22(41):6387–94.

Lynch HT, Fusaro RM. Pancreatic cancer and the familial atypical multiple mole melanoma (FAMMM) syndrome. Pancreas. 1991;6(2):127–31.

Macgregor S, Montgomery GW, Liu JZ, Zhao ZZ, Henders AK, Stark M, Schmid H, Holland EA, Duffy DL, Zhang M, Painter JN, Nyholt DR, Maskiell JA, Jetann J, Ferguson M, Cust AE, Jenkins MA, Whiteman DC, Olsson H, Puig S, Bianchi-Scarrà G, Hansson J, Demenais F, Landi MT, Dębniak T, Mackie R, Azizi E, Bressac-de Paillerets B, Goldstein AM, Kanetsky PA, Gruis NA, Elder DE, Newton-Bishop JA, Bishop DT, Iles MM, Helsing P, Amos CI, Wei Q, Wang LE, Lee JE, Qureshi AA, Kefford RF, Giles GG, Armstrong BK, Aitken JF, Han J, Hopper JL, Trent JM, Brown KM, Martin NG, Mann GJ, Hayward NK. Genome-wide association study identifies a new melanoma susceptibility locus at 1q21.3. Nat Genet. 2011;43(11):1114–8. doi:10.1038/ng.958.

Majewski S, Jablonska S. Why epidermodysplasia verruciformis is a very rare disease and has raised such interest. Int J Dermatol. 2004;43:309–11.

Makkar HS, Frieden IJ. Congenital melanogtic nevi: an update for the pedi-atrician. Curr Opin Pediatr. 2002;14:397–403.

Mallipeddi R. Epidermolysis and cancer. Clin Exp Dermatol. 2002;27:616–23.

Martinez-Mir A, Glaser B, Chuang GS, et al. Germline fumarate hydratase mutations in families with multiple cutaneous and uterine leiomyomata. J Invest Dermatol. 2003;121:741–4.

Masuno M, Imaizumir K, Ishi T, et al. Pilomatrixoma in Rubinstein–Taybi syndrome. Am J Med Genet. 1998;77:81–2.

Matyakhina L, Pack S, Kirschner LS, et al. Chromosome 2(2p16) abnormalities in Carney complex tumors. J Med Genet. 2003;40:268–77.

Metze D, Wigbes B, Hildebrand A. Familial syringomas: a rare clinical variant. Hantarzt. 2001;52:1045–8.

Miljkovic J. An unusual generalized form of hyperkeratosis lenticularis perstans (Flegel's disease). Wien Klin Wochenschr. 2004;116 Suppl 2:78–80.

Mistry SH, Taylor C, Randerson-Moor JA, et al. Prevalence of 9p21 deletions in UK melanoma families. Genes Chromosomes Cancer. 2005;44:292–300.

Molven A, Grimstvedt MB, Steine SJ, et al. A large Norwegian family with inherited malignant melanoma, multiple atypical nevi, and CDK4 mutation. Genes Chromosomes Cancer. 2005;44:10–8.

Montanaro L, Tazzan PL, Dereuzini M. Enhanced telomere shortening in transformed lymphoblasts from patients with X-linked dyskeratosis. J Clin Pathol. 2003;56:583–6.

Morrison PJ, Young ID. Syringomas, natal teeth and oligodontia: a new ectodermal dysplasia. Clin Dysmorphol. 1996;5:63–6.

Myhre AG, Stray-Pedersen A, Spangen S, Eide E, Veimo D, Knappskog PM, Abrahamsen TG, Husebye ES. Chronic mucocutaneous candidiasis and primary hypothyroidism in two families. Eur J Pediatr. 2004;163(10):604–11.

Nagata H, Worobec AS, Oh CK, et al. Identification of a point mutation in the catalytic domain of the protooncogene c-kit in peripheral blood mononuclear cells of patients who have mastocytosis with an associated hematologic disorder. Proc Natl Acad Sci USA. 1995; 92:10560–4.

Nan H, Kraft P, Hunter DJ, et al. Genetic variants in pigmentation genes, pigmentary phenotypes, and risk of skin cancer in Caucasians. Int J Cancer. 2009;125:909–17.

Nan H, Qureshi AA, Prescott J, et al. Genetic variants in telomere-maintaining genes and skin cancer risk. Hum Genet. 2011;129:247–53.

Newton Bishop JA, Bataille V, Pinney E, Bishop DT. Family studies in melanoma: identification of the atypical mole syndrome (AMS) phenotype. Melanoma Res. 1994;4(4):199–206.

Newton Bishop J, Harland M, Wachsmuth R, et al. Genotype/phenotype and penetrance studies in melanoma families with germline CDKN2A mutations. J Invest Dermatol. 2000; 114:28–33.

Newton JA, Bataille V, Griffiths K, et al. How common is the atypical mole syndrome phenotype in apparently sporadic melanoma? J Am Acad Dermatol. 1993;29:989–96.

Newton-Bishop JA, Chang YM, Iles MM, et al. Melanocytic nevi, nevus genes, and melanoma risk in a large case–control study in the United Kingdom. Cancer Epidemiol Biomark Prev. 2010;19:2043–54.

Nishimura G, Koslowski K. Proteus syndrome. (Report of three cases.). Australas Radiol. 1990;34:47–52.

Nisoli E, Regianini L, Briscini L, et al. Multiple symmetric lipomatosis may be the consequence of defective noradrenergic modulation of proliferation and differentiation of brown fat cells. J Pathol. 2002;198:378–87.

Nobili B, Rossi G, De Stefano P, Zecca M, Giorgiani G, Perrotta S, Canazzio A, Locatelli F. Successful umbilical cord blood transplantation in a child with dyskeratosis congenita after a fludarabine-based reduced-intensity conditioning regimen. Br J Haematol. 2002; 119:573–4.

Norris W. A case of fungoid disease. Edinb Med Surg J. 1820;16:562–5.

Oiso N, Mizuno N, Fukai K, et al. Mild phenotype of familial cylindromatosis associated with an R758X nonsense mutation in the CYLD tumor suppressor gene. Br J Dermatol. 2004;151:1084–6.

Orlow S. Albinism: an update. Semin Cutan Med Surg. 1997;16:24–9.

Orth G. Genetics of epidermodysplasia verruciformis: insights into host defense against papillomaviruses. Semin Immunol. 2006;18:362–74.

Paller AS, Norton K, Teevi A, et al. Mutations in the capillary morphogenesis gene-2 result in the allelic disorder Juvenile hyaline fibromatosis and infantile systemic hyalinosis. Am J Hum Genet. 2003;73:957–66.

Parkin DM, Bray F, Ferlay J, et al. Estimating the world cancer burden: Globocan 2000. Int J Cancer J Int Du Cancer. 2001;94:153–6.

Parren LJ, Frank J. Hereditary tumor syndromes featuring basal cell carcinomas. Br J Dermatol. 2011;165:30–4.

Parren LJ, Abuzahra F, Wagenvoort T, Koene F, Van Steensel MA, Steijlen PM, Van Geel M, Frank J. Linkage refinement of Bazex-Dupré-Christol syndrome to an 11·4-Mb interval on chromosome Xq25-27.1. Br J Dermatol. 2011;165(1):201–3. doi:10.1111/j.1365-2133.2011.10219.x.

Phadke PA, Rakheja D, Le LP, et al. Proliferative nodules arising within congenital melanocytic nevi: a histologic, immunohistochemical, and molecular analyses of 43 cases. Am J Surg Pathol. 2011;35:656–69.

Pinheiro M, Freire-Maia N. Ectodermal dysplasias: a clinical classification and a causal review. Am J Med Genet. 1994;53:153–62.

Pjanova D, Engele L, Randerson-Moor JA, et al. CDKN2A and CDK4 variants in Latvian melanoma patients: analysis of a clinic-based population. Melanoma Res. 2007; 17:185–91.

Ponti G, Losi L, Pellacani G, et al. Malignant melanoma in patients with hereditary nonpolyposis colorectal cancer. Br J Dermatol. 2008;159:162–8.

Porter RM, Lane EB. Phenotypes, genotypes and their contribution to under-standing keratin function. Trend Genet. 2003;19:278–85.

Prontera P, Stangoni G, Manes I, Mencarelli A, Donti E. Encephalocraniocutaneous lipomatosis (ECCL) in a patient with history of familial multiple lipomatosis (FML). (Letter). Am J Med Genet. 2009;149A:543–5.

Puntervoll HE, Yang XR, Vetti HH, Bachmann IM, Avril MF, Benfodda M, Catricalà C, Dalle S, Duval-Modeste AB, Ghiorzo P, Grammatico P, Harland M, Hayward NK, Hu HH, Jouary T, Martin-Denavit T, Ozola A, Palmer JM, Pastorino L, Pjanova D, Soufir N, Steine SJ, Stratigos AJ, Thomas L, Tinat J, Tsao H, Veinalde R, Tucker MA, Bressac-de Paillerets B, Newton-Bishop JA, Goldstein AM, Akslen LA, Molven A. Melanoma prone families with CDK4 germline mutation: phenotypic profile and associations with MC1R variants. J Med Genet. 2013;50(4):264–70. doi:10.1136/jmedgenet-2012-101455. Epub 2013 Feb 5.

Radi O, Parma P, Imbeaud S, Nasca MR, Uccellatore F, Maraschio P, Tiepolo L, Micali G, Camerino G. XX sex reversal, palmoplantar keratoderma, and predisposition to squamous cell carcinoma: genetic analysis in one family. Am J Med Genet. 2005;138:241–6.

Rafnar T, Sulem P, Stacey SN, et al. Sequence variants at the TERT-CLPTM1L locus associate with many cancer types. Nat Genet. 2009;41:221–7.

Rahman N, Dunstan M, Tearc MD, et al. The gene for juvenile hyaline fibromatosis maps to chromosome 4q21. Am J Hum Genet. 2002;71:975–80.

Raimondi S, Sera F, Gandini S, et al. MC1R variants, melanoma and red hair color phenotype: a meta-analysis. Int J Cancer. 2008;122:2753–60.

Ramoz N, Rueda LA, Bouadjar B, et al. Mutations in two adjacent novel genes are associated with epidermodysplasia verruciformis. Nat Genet. 2002;32:579–81.

Randerson-Moor JA, Harland M, Williams S, Cuthbert-Heavens D, Sheridan E, Aveyard J, et al. A germline deletion of p14(ARF) but not CDKN2A in a melanoma-neural system tumor syndrome family. Hum Mol Genet. 2001;10:55–62.

Reardon W, Harding B, Winter R, Baraitser M. Hemihypertrophy, hemimegalencephaly and polydactyly. Am J Med Genet. 1996;66:144–9.

Rees JL. Genetics of hair and skin colour. Ann Rev Genet. 2003;37:67–90.

Rezaei N, Hedayat M, Aghamohammadi A, et al. Primary immunodeficiency diseases associated with increased susceptibility to viral infections and malignancies. J Allergy Clin Immunol. 2011;127:1329–41 e2; quiz 1342–3.

Rizos H, Puig S, Badenas C, et al. A melanoma-associated germline mutation in exon 1beta inactivates p14ARF. Oncogene. 2001;20(39):5543–7.

Robati RM, Marefat A, Saeedi M, et al. Four familial cases of epidermodysplasia verruciformis: mother and three sons. Dermatol Online J. 2009;15:8.

Robertson SJ, Bashir SJ, Pichert G, et al. Severe exacerbation of multiple self-healing squamous epithelioma (Ferguson-Smith disease) with radiotherapy, which was successfully treated with acitretin. Clin Exp Dermatol. 2010;35:e100–2.

Ruiz-Maldonado R, Tamayo L, Laterza AM, Duran C. Giant pigmented nevi: clinical, histopathologic, and therapeutic considerations. J Pediatr. 1992;120:906–11.

Saggar S, Chernoff KA, Lodha S, Horev L, Kohl S, Honjo RS, Brandt HRC, Hartmann K, Celebi JT. CYLD mutations in familial skin appendage tumors. J Med Genet. 2008;45:298–302.

Sandhu K, Handa S, Kanwar AJ. Familial lichen planus. Pediatr Dermatol. 2003;20(2):186.

Sato K, Nakajima K, Imamura H, Deguchi T, Horinouchi S, Yamazaki K, Yamada E, Kanaji Y, Takano K. A novel missense mutation of AIRE gene in a patient with autoimmune polyendocrinopathy, candidiasis and ectodermal dystrophy (APECED), accompanied with progressive muscular atrophy: case report and review of the literature in Japan. Endocr J. 2002;49(6):625–33.

Scherer D, Bermejo JL, Rudnai P, et al. MC1R variants associated susceptibility to basal cell carcinoma of skin: interaction with host factors and XRCC3 polymorphism. Int J Cancer. 2008;122:1787–93.

Schmidt LS. Birt–Hogg–Dube syndrome, a genodermatosis that increases risk for renal carcinoma. Curr Mol Med. 2004;4:877–85.

Shah KN. The risk of melanoma and neurocutaneous melanosis associated with congenital melanocytic nevi. Semin Cutan Med Surg. 2010;29:159–64.

Shaw JM. Genetic aspects of urticaria pigmentosa. Arch Dermatol. 1968;97:137–8.

Shaw Dunn J, Ferguson Smith J. Self healing squamous epithelia of the skin. Br J Dermatol. 1934;46:519–22.

Shay JW, Wright WE. Telomeres in dyskeratosis congenita. Nat Genet. 2004;36:437–8.

Shiflett SL, Kaplan J, Ward DM. Chediak–higashi syndrome: a rare disorder of lysosomes and L related organelles. Pigment Cell Res. 2002;5:451–67.

Shirer JA, Ray MC. Familial occurrence of lichen sclerosis et atrophicus: case reports of a mother and daughter. Arch Dermatol. 1987;123:485–8.

Skvara H, Kalthoff F, Meingassner JG, et al. Topical treatment of Basal cell carcinomas in nevoid Basal cell carcinoma syndrome with a smoothened inhibitor. J Investig Dermatol. 2011;131:1735–44.

Smith F. The molecular genetics of keratin disorders. Am J Clin Dermatol. 2003;4:347–64.

Smith FJ, Corden LD, Rugg EL, et al. Missense mutations in keratin 17 cause either pachyonychia congenita type 2 or a phenotype resembling steatocystoma multiplex. J Invest Dermatol. 1997;108:220–3.

Smith JM, Kirk EPE, Theodosopoulos G, et al. Germline mutation of the tumor suppressor PTEN in Proteus syndrome. J Med Genet. 2002;39:937–40.

Soufir N, Bressac-de Paillerets B, Desjardins L, et al. Individuals with presumably hereditary uveal melanoma do not harbour germline mutations in the coding regions of either the P16INK4A, P14ARF or cdk4 genes. Br J Cancer. 2000;82(4):818–22.

Stacey SN, Sulem P, Masson G, et al. New common variants affecting susceptibility to basal cell carcinoma. Nat Genet. 2009a;41:909–14.

Stacey SN, Sulem P, Masson G, Gudjonsson SA, Thorleifsson G, Jakobsdottir M, Sigurdsson A, Gudjartsson DF, Sigurgeirsson B, Benediktsdottir KR, Thorisdottir K, Ragnarsson R, and 52 others. New common variants affecting susceptibility to basal cell carcinoma. Nat Genet. 2009b;41:909–14.

Stieglitz JB, Centerwall WR. Pachyonychia congenita (Jadassohn–Lewandowsky syndrome) a seventeen member four generation pedigree with unusual respiratory and dental involvement. Am J Med Genet. 1983;14:21–8.

Stoll C, Alembik Y, Truttman M. Multiple familial lipomatosis with polyneuropathy, an inherited dominant condition. Ann Genet. 1996;39:193–6.

Stratakis CA, et al. Carney complex, a familial multiple neoplasia and lentiginosis syndrome: analysis of 11 kindreds and linkage to the short arm of chromosome 2. J Clin Invest. 1996;97:699–705.

Sty JR, Ruiz ME, Carmody TJ. Congenital generalized fibromatosis. Extraosseus accumulation of bone seeking radiopharmaceutical. Clin Nucl Med. 1996;21:413–4.

Su WPD, Chun SI, Hammond DE, et al. Pachyonychia congenita: a clinical study of 12 cases and review of the literature. Pediatr Dermatol. 1990;7:33–8.

Swenssen O. Pachyonychia congenita. Keratin gene mutations with pleiotropic effect. Hantarzt. 1999;50:483–90.

Szepietowski JC, Wasik F, Szybejko-Machaj G, et al. Brook–Spiegler syndrome. J Eur Acad Dermatol Venereol. 2001;15:346–9.

Tate G, Suzuki T, Kishimoto K, et al. Novel mutations of EVER1/TMC6 gene in a Japanese patient with Epidermodysplasia verruciformis. J Hum Genet. 2004;49:223–5.

Tefferi A, Levine RL, Lim K-H, Abdel-Wahab O, Lasho TL, Patel J, Finke CM, Mullally A, Li C-Y, Pardanani A, Gilliland DG. Frequent TET2 mutations in systemic mastocytosis: clinical, KITD816V and FIP1L1-PDGFRA correlates. Leukemia. 2009;23:900–4.

Tian XL. Identification of an angiogenic factor that when mutated causes susceptibility to klippel Trenaunay syndrome. Nature. 2003;427:640–5.

Tidman MJ. Skin malignancy in epidermolysis bullosa. In: Priestly GC, Tidman MJ, Weiss JB, Eady RAJ, editors. Epidermolysis bullosa. Crowthorne: Dystrophic Epidermolysis Bullosa Research Association; 1990. p. 156–60.

Tomita Y, Sato-Matsumura KC, Sawamura D, Matsumura T, Shimizu H. Simultaneous occurrence of three squamous cell carcinomas in a recessive dystrophic epidermolysis bullosa patient. Acta Derm Venereol. 2003;83:225–6.

Tomlinson IP, Alam NA, Rowan AJ, et al. Germline mutations in FH predispose to dominantly inherited uterine fibroids, skin leiomyomata and papillary renal cell cancer. Nat Genet. 2002;30:406–10.

Tsai KY, Tsao H. The genetics of skin cancer. Am J Med Genet. 2004;131C:82–92.

Tucker MA, Fraser MC, Goldstein AM, et al. A natural history of melanomas and dysplastic nevi: an atlas of lesions in melanoma-prone families. Cancer. 2002;94:3192–209.

Turner ML. Birt–Hogg–Dube syndrome: a novel marker of kidney neoplasia. Arch Dermatol. 1999;135(10):1195–202.

Uitto J, Pulkkinent L, Ringpfeil F. Progress in molecular genetics of heritable skin diseases: the paradigms of epidermolysis bullosa and pseudoxanthoma elasticum. J Invest Dermotol Symp Proc. 2002;7(1):6–16. pseudoxanthoma elasticum.

Vabres P, Lancombe D, Rabinowitz LG, et al. The gene for Bazex–Dupre–Christol syndrome maps to chromosome Xq. J Invest Dermatol. 1995;105:87–9.

Valverde P, Healy E, Sikkink S, et al. The Asp84Glu variant of the melanocortin 1 receptor (MC1R) is associated with melanoma. Hum Mol Genet. 1996;5(10):1663–6.

van der Velden PA, Sandkuijl LA, Bergman W, Pavel S, van Mourik L, Frants RR, Gruis NA. Melanocortin-1 receptor variant R151C modifies melanoma risk in Dutch families with melanoma. Am J Hum Genet. 2001;69(4):774–9.

Van Steensel MA, Jaspers NG, Steijlen PM. A case of Rombo syndrome. Br J Dermatol. 2001;144:1215–8.

Vernia S. Cheilitis glandularis: a rare entity. Br J Dermatol. 2003;148:362.

Veugelers M, Wilke D, Burton K, et al. Comparative PRKAR1A genotype-phenotype analyses in humans with Carney complex and prkar1a haploinsufficient mice. Proc Natl Acad Sci. 2004;101:14222–7.

Viljeon DL. Klippel–Trenaunay–Weber syndrome (angio-osteohypertrophy syndrome). J Med Genet. 1988;25:250–2.

Vohra S, Sharma NL, Shanker V, et al. Autosomal dominant epidermodysplasia verruciformis: a clinicotherapeutic experience in two cases. Indian J Dermatol Venereol Leprol. 2010;76:557–61.

Vuilamy T, Marrone A, Szydlo R, et al. Telomerase is a ribonucleoprotein complex required for synthesis of DNA repeats at the ends of telomeres. The RNA component of this is mutated in dyskeratosis congenita. Nat Genet. 2004;36:447–9.

Wachsmuth RC, Harland M, Bishop JA. The atypical-mole syndrome and predisposition to melanoma. N Engl J Med. 1998;339:348–9.

Wachsmuth RCG, Rupert M, Barrett JH, Saunders CL, Randerson-Moor JA, Eldridge A, et al. Heritability and gene-environment interactions for melanocytic nevus density examined in a UK adolescent twin study. J Invest Dermatol. 2001;117(2):348–52.

Wang Q, Timur AA, Szafranski P, Sadgephour A, Jurecic V, Cowell J, Baldini A, Driscoll DJ. Identification and molecular characterization of de novo translocation t(8;14) (q22.3;q13) associated with a vascular and tissue overgrowth syndrome. Cytogenet Cell Genet. 2001;95(3–4):183–8.

Ward DM, Shiflett SL, Kaplan J. Chediak–Higashi syndrome: a clinical and molecular view of a rare lysosomal storage disease. Curr Mol Med. 2002;2:469–77.

Wei M-H, Toure O, Glenn GM, Pithukpakorn M, Neckers L, Stolle C, Choyke P, Grubb R, Middelton L, Turner ML, Walther MM, Merino MJ, Zbar B, Linehan WM, Toro JR. Novel mutations in FH and expansion of the spectrum of phenotypes expressed in families with hereditary leiomyomatosis and renal cell cancer. J Med Genet. 2006;43:18–27.

Welch JP, Wells RS, Kerr CB. Ancell-Spiegler cylindromas (turban tumors) and Brook-Fordyce trichoepitheliomas: evidence for a single genetic entity. J Med Genet. 1968;5:29–35.

Wilson D, Boland J. Sporadic multiple lipomatosis: a case report and review of the literature. West Va Med J. 1994;90:145–6.

Yotsumoto S, Hashignchi T, Chen X. Novel mutations in GJBZ encoding connexin 26 in Japanese patients with keratitis–ichthyosis–deafness syndrome. Br J Dermatol. 2003;148:649–53.

Yun SJ, Kwon OS, Han JH, Kweon SS, Lee MW, Lee DY, Kim MB, Kim YC, Yoon TY, Chung KY, Kim IH, Kim KH, Suh KS, Lee SJ, Seo YJ, Kim KH, Park HJ, Roh MR, Ahn KJ, Yoon TJ, Kim MH, Li KS, Park JS, Shin BS, Ko JY, Ahn HH, Kim HJ, Park SD, Jang SJ, Won YH. Clinical characteristics and risk of melanoma development from giant congenital melanocytic naevi in Korea: a nationwide retrospective study. Br J Dermatol. 2012;166(1):115–23. doi:10.1111/j.1365-2133.2011.10636.x.

Yung A, Newton-Bishop JA. A case of Bazex-Dupre-Christol syndrome associated with multiple genital trichoepitheliomas. Br J Dermatol. 2005a;153:682–4.

Yung A, Newton-Bishop JA. A case of Bazex-Dupre-Christol syndrome associated with multiple genital trichoepitheliomas. (Letter). Br J Dermatol. 2005b;153:664–99.

Zand DJ, Huff D, Everman D, Russell K, Saitta S, McDonald-McGinn D, Zackai EH. Autosomal dominant inheritance of infantile myofibromatosis. Am J Med Genet. 2004;126A:261–6.

Zhou XP, Marsh DJ, Hampel H, Mulliken JB, Gimm O, Eng C. Germline and germline mosaic mutations associated with a Proteus-like syndrome of hemihypertrophy, lower limb asymmetry, arteriovenous malformations and lipomatosis. Hum Mol Genet. 2000;9:765–8.

Zhou XP, Hampel H, Thiele H, et al. Association of germline mutation in the PTEN tumor suppressor gene and a subset of Proteus sand Proteus-like syndromes. Lancet. 2001;358:210–1.

Zuccurello D, Salpietro DC, Gangemi S, et al. Familial chronic nail candidiasis with ICAM-1 deficiency: a new form of chronic mucocutaneous candidiasis. J Med Genet. 2002;39:671–5.

Zuo L, Weger J, Yang Q, et al. Germline mutations in the p16^{INK4a} binding domain of CDK4 in familial melanoma. Nat Genet. 1996;12:97–9.

Chapter 11
Inherited Cancer-Predisposing Syndomes

Ataxia Telangiectasia (OMIM 208900)

This autosomal recessive disorder, with a birth incidence of about 1 in 300,000, is characterized by the development of cerebellar ataxia in the first decade, along with choreoathetosis, dysarthria, and abnormalities of ocular movements. Mental retardation is not usually a feature. The neurological features are progressive, leading to confinement to a wheelchair in the second decade of life. Oculocutaneous telangiectasia develops in childhood (often after ataxia is apparent) and then spreads to involve other exposed cutaneous areas. Vitiligo, café-au-lait spots, and macular hyperpigmentation may occur. The development of acanthosis nigricans is associated with the development of neoplasia. An immune deficiency occurs, with disordered B cell and T helper cell function, thymic hypoplasia, reduced levels of IgA (70 %) and IgE (80 %), and reduced T cells. Frequent bacterial (pulmonary or sinus) infections occur secondary to immunodeficiency. The serum alpha-fetoprotein is consistently elevated. There is an inconsistently increased incidence of spontaneous structural chromosomal aberrations (30–50-fold) (chromatid gaps, breaks and interchanges, and telomere fusions) in cultured white cells and fibroblasts, and this is markedly increased by exposure to X-radiation and radiomimetic agents. Peripheral blood lymphocytes may show abnormal clones of cells with a stable cytogenetic rearrangement, usually involving chromosome 14, particularly involving the T cell receptor genes on 14q11, 7q14, and 7q35. Clones of cells with these translocations may develop into T cell promyelocytic leukemia. Other translocations involve the immunoglobulin genes in B lymphocytes. In vivo sensitivity to X-rays is also observed. Recombination is increased by a factor of 30–200 (Tomanin et al. 1989; Peterson et al. 1992; Viniou et al. 2001; Sun et al. 2002).

There is a 30–40 % risk of malignancy developing, most frequently Hodgkin and non-Hodgkin lymphoma (60 %) and lymphoblastic T cell leukemia (27 %) (Johnson 1989). The lymphoreticular neoplasms develop before the age of 16 years, and epithelial carcinomas (including medulloblastomas; gastric, basal cell, hepatocellular, parotid, laryngeal, skin, and breast carcinomas; uterine leiomyomas; and ovarian

S.V. Hodgson et al., *A Practical Guide to Human Cancer Genetics*,
DOI 10.1007/978-1-4471-2375-0_11, © Springer-Verlag London 2014

dysgerminoma) may develop in patients surviving longer (Spector et al. 1982). Severe reactions have been described to standard doses of radiotherapy in this condition.

The *ATM* gene was cloned in 1995 (Savitsky et al. 1995). Its product, ATM, has a central role in orchestrating the response to double-strand breaks. It is a serine/threonine kinase that mediates checkpoint regulation and homologous repair by phosphorylating a number of proteins; without it, cells display aberrant cell-cycle progression and increased chromosomal breakage, especially when exposed to ionizing radiation. McConville et al. (1996) and others have reported families with a milder clinical and cellular phenotype due to certain ataxia-telangiectasia mutations (Sariozzi et al. 2002; Chessa 2003) causing reduced ATM function. The *ATM* carrier frequency is estimated to be about 1 %, and early studies showed that these heterozygotes have an increased risk of cancer, particularly breast cancer (Morrell et al. 1990). This was supported by studies conducted after the gene was identified (Athma et al. 1996; Thomson et al. 2005). These epidemiological studies were confirmed directly when Renwick et al. identified 12 deleterious mutations in 443 affected cases compared to 2 out of 521 controls resulting in an estimated relative risk of 2.37 (Renwick et al. 2006). One limitation of the study however was that the significance of 35 of 37 missense mutations identified could not be determined. To try to solve this problem, Tavtigian et al. used an in silico approach to test the hypothesis that missense mutations in evolutionary conserved residues would be more common among breast cancer patients than in controls. Suggestive of a dominant-negative model, they found that missense mutations ranked highly deleterious were associated with an even greater risk of breast cancer than truncation or splice site mutations, demonstrating that not all variants have equal risk predisposition (Tavtigian et al. 2009; Thorensten et al. 2003), but this remains controversial.

Ataxia-Telangiectasia-Like Disorder (ATLD) (OMIM 604391)

A small proportion of "AT" cases have mutations in the *MRE11* gene rather than *ATM*, causing a disorder known as ATLD. The lymphocytes of such patients show increased levels of translocations involving immune system genes, and chromosomal radiosensitivity is seen, but B lymphocytes may not be affected and the cancer risk is less (Stewart et al. 1999; Duker 2002; De la Torre et al. 2003). *MRE11* is part of the MRN (MRE11–RAD50–NBN) complex. MRN appears to be the primary sensor of DNA damage, signaling ATM to sites of double-strand breaks to initiate the DNA damage response (Lavin 2007). It also has important downstream functions that include tethering and processing the two broken ends of the DNA strand to generate 3′ overhangs for either non-homologous end-joining or homologous repair. Its role in maintaining genome integrity is underscored by chromosome instability and cell-cycle checkpoint defects common to all patients with recessive loss of any one of these components. Heterozygous mutations in *NBN* and *RAD50* (Heikkinen et al. 2006) have been associated with an increased risk for breast cancer (mainly in countries where founder mutations in these genes have been identified). Rare germline mutations in *MRE11* have also been proposed to be breast cancer alleles – in one study of eight tumors showing concomitant reduction/loss of all three MRN-complex proteins, mutation analysis revealed two germline mutations in *MRE11*: a missense mutation Arg202Gly and a truncating mutation Arg633X (Bartkova et al. 2008). This study remains to be verified in large case-control studies. One likely truncating mutation in *MRE11A* was identified in 360 women with ovarian carcinoma (Walsh et al. 2011).

Bannayan–Riley–Ruvalcaba Syndrome (Bannayan–Zonana Syndrome, Ruvalcaba–Riley–Smith Syndrome)

Bannayan–Riley–Ruvalcaba syndrome (BRRS, MIM 153480), a rare autosomal dominant congenital disorder, is characterized by macrocephaly, lipomatosis, hemangiomatosis, and speckled penis (Gorlin et al. 1992). Other features include Hashimoto thyroiditis, gastrointestinal (GI) hamartomatous polyposis most likely not associated with GI malignancy, hypotonia, and variable mental retardation and psychomotor delay. While a lipid storage myopathy is still considered a component to BRRS, its original etiology, long-chain acyl-coA dehydrogenase (LCHAD) deficiency, has been questioned.

Germline *PTEN* mutations were originally found in two classic BRRS families (Marsh et al. 1997), and thus, a subset of BRRS is allelic to Cowden syndrome (see p. 233) (Marsh et al. 1999). Subsequently, 60 % of a series of BRRS probands were found to have germline *PTEN* mutations (Marsh et al. 1999). Of those that were mutation negative after PCR-based mutational analysis of exons 1–9 and flanking intronic regions, 10 % have been found to carry large deletions including or encompassing *PTEN* (Zhou et al. 2003a, b). Genotype–phenotype association analysis reveals that BRRS carrying germline *PTEN* mutations were at increased risk of neoplasia, especially malignant breast disease, and lipomatosis compared to those without *PTEN* mutations (Marsh et al. 1999).

Traditionally, medical management of BRRS has been symptomatic. However, given the genotype–phenotype association and that a subset of BRRS is allelic to Cowden syndrome, individuals with BRRS, especially those found to have germline *PTEN* mutations, should undergo similar surveillance and management to individuals with Cowden syndrome (p. 233). Because thyroid cancers can occur even in the teens in BRRS, it would be prudent to begin annual comprehensive physical examinations, paying particular attention to the neck, in the early teens.

Beckwith–Wiedemann Syndrome (EMG Syndrome and IGF2 Overgrowth Disorder) (OMIM 130650)

This syndrome, with an estimated incidence of 1 in 14,000, is characterized by major (pre- and/or postnatal overgrowth, anterior abdominal wall defects (diastasis recti, umbilical hernia, or exomphalos), and macroglossia) and minor features (earlobe grooves or helical rim pits, facial nevus flammeus, visceromegaly (liver, kidney, spleen), neonatal hypoglycemia, hemihypertrophy, renal anomalies, cryptorchidism, and, infrequently, cardiac defects). In addition embryonal tumors occur in ~8 % of patients (though the risk depends on the underlying specific genetic/epigenetic abnormality) (Wiedemann et al. 1983; Hatada et al. 1996; Koufos et al. 1989).

There are no consensus clinical diagnostic criteria for Beckwith–Wiedemann syndrome (BWS). Strict diagnostic criteria were suggested by Elliott and Maher (1994) that required the presence of (1) three major features or (2) two major features plus three minor features (from ear creases or pits, hypoglycemia, nephromegaly, or hemihypertrophy), but less strict diagnostic criteria have also been proposed, for example, at least two from (a) positive family history; (b) macrosomia (height and weight >97 percentile); (c) anterior linear earlobe creases/posterior helical ear pits; (d) macroglossia; (e) exomphalos/umbilical hernia; (f) visceromegaly involving one or more intra-abdominal organs including liver, spleen, kidneys, adrenal glands, and pancreas; (g) embryonal tumor (e.g., Wilms tumor, hepatoblastoma, rhabdomyosarcoma) in childhood; (h) hemihypertrophy; (i) adrenocortical cytomegaly; (j) renal abnormalities including structural abnormalities, nephromegaly, and nephrocalcinosis; and (k) cleft palate (rare) and one from (a) polyhydramnios, (b) neonatal hypoglycemia, (c) facial nevus flammeus, (d) hemangioma, (e) characteristic facies including midfacial hypoplasia and infraorbital creases, (f) cardiomegaly/structural cardiac anomalies/rarely cardiomyopathy, and (g) diastasis recti and advanced bone age (http://www.geneclinics.org). However, molecular genetic testing can diagnose most cases (Cooper et al. 2005).

The characteristic craniofacial dysmorphological features of Beckwith–Wiedemann syndrome (BWS) are most apparent before the age of 3 years, and after the age of 5 years, there are often only minor dysmorphisms. The differential diagnosis of BWS includes Perlman syndrome, Simpson–Golabi–Behmel syndrome, and other overgrowth disorders, such as Weaver or Sotos syndrome.

The genetics of BWS are complex (Choufani et al. 2010; Lim and Maher 2010). Most cases are sporadic but ~15 % of cases are familial. The inheritance pattern of familial cases is dependent on the nature of the genetic cause (see later), but in most cases it will be autosomal dominant trait with parent-of-origin effects such that the penetrance is more complete when the mother is the transmitting parent, and examples of transmitting males with affected children are rare. As there is wide variation in expression of the disease and the features of BWS tend to become less apparent with age, it is likely that some familial cases of BWS are misdiagnosed clinically as sporadic cases because minor manifestations in relatives are overlooked. Though characterization of the molecular pathology in an individual case may indicate whether the disorder is likely to be sporadic or familial, careful examination of close relatives (particularly the mother) should be performed.

An association between twinning and BWS has been recognized. Thus a greater than expected number of twins have been described among BWS children, and these are usually female monozygotic twins that are discordant for BWS (Bliek et al. 2009).

The parent-of-origin effects on the penetrance and expression of familial BWS suggested a genomic imprinting disorder, and molecular tests (see below) have confirmed that BWS results from abnormal function/expression of imprinted genes (in particular the paternally expressed growth factor *IGF2* and the maternally expressed growth suppressor *CDKN1C*) contained within a cluster of imprinted genes at chromosome 11p15.5. Interestingly, the frequency of BWS and some other genomic imprinting disorders appears to be increased in children conceived by assisted reproductive technologies (both ICSI and in vitro fertilization) (DeBaun et al. 2003; Maher et al. 2003; Lim et al. 2009). Though the relative risk of having a child with BWS is increased after BWS (probably up to tenfold), the absolute risk appears to be small (less than 1 in 1,000).

BWS may result from chromosomal rearrangements (duplications or translocations/inversions of distal chromosome 11p), uniparental disomy of 11p15.5, mutations, or epimutations directly involving the two 11p15.5 imprinting control regions (IC1 and IC2). In addition germline mutations in *CDKN1C* or inactivation of *NLRP2* in the mother can cause familial BWS (Cooper et al. 2005; Choufani et al. 2010; Lim and Maher 2010).

Chromosome 11p15.5 was first implicated in BWS by the finding of paternally derived duplications of 11p15.5 in BWS patients. Subsequently maternally inherited balanced rearrangements of 11p15 were also demonstrated to be associated with BWS. It is estimated that up to 3 % of BWS patients have a cytogenetically visible chromosome duplication or rearrangement. Chromosome 11 paternal uniparental disomy is found in approximately 20 % of sporadic cases of BWS. Typically uniparental disomy in BWS is mosaic paternal isodisomy, and although the disomic region always includes the imprinted gene cluster at 11p15.5, involvement of more centromeric regions of 11p and of 11q is variable. A few patients diagnosed with BWS have been demonstrated to have whole genome paternal uniparental disomy, and these cases appear to have an increased risk of neoplasia (e.g., pheochromocytoma, hepatoblastoma) (Romanelli et al. 2011).

Epigenetic errors at two putative imprinting control regions within 11p15.5 (IC1 and IC2) have also been implicated in BWS. Thus, 5 % of BWS patients have an imprinting defect at the distal imprinting center (IC1) such that the maternal *IGF2* and *H19* alleles display a paternal epigenotype (hypermethylation and silencing of *H19* and biallelic *IGF2* expression). In up to 50 % of cases, there is loss of paternal methylation at IC2 (KvDMR1) that is associated with silencing of *CDKN1C* expression and variable loss of imprinting (biallelic expression) of *IGF2*. Cases associated with assisted reproductive technologies and those that occur in twins are very likely to have loss of paternal methylation at IC2 (KvDMR1). In general the risk of recurrence after a child with an imprinting center epimutations is very low if an *in cis* duplication or deletion has been excluded. However in rare cases, an epimutation may result as an *in trans* effect of maternal homozygosity for a *NALP2* mutation (Meyer et al. 2009).

Germline inactivating *CDKN1C* mutations occur in about half of familial cases and 5 % of sporadic cases (Lam et al. 1999). *CDKN1C* is expressed from the maternal allele (though there is a small level of paternal allele expression), and so a paternally transmitted mutation has minimal effect of the children who inherit the mutation. In contrast a maternally inherited *CDKN1C* mutation will cause BWS (Maher and Reik 2000).

Genotype–phenotype correlations have been described for hemihypertrophy and exomphalos. Most cases with hemihypertrophy have mosaic uniparental disomy. There is a high incidence of exomphalos in patients with *CDKN1C* mutations and IC2 imprinting center defects, but exomphalos is infrequent in patients with uniparental disomy or IC1 imprinting center defects. In addition to patients with classical BWS, Morison et al. (1996) reported that some patients with overgrowth and nephromegaly or Wilms tumor may have biallelic *IGF2* expression, and they coined the term "IGF2 overgrowth disorder" to describe these patients (Gicquel et al. 2003).

Patients with BWS have an increased risk of neoplasia. Wiedemann (1983) reviewed 388 children with BWS and found 29 children (7.5 %) with 32 tumors. Most tumors (26/29) were intra-abdominal (including 14 Wilms tumor, 5 adrenal carcinomas, and 2 hepatoblastomas). Most tumors occur before the age of 5 years. A clinical association between hemihypertrophy and neoplasia in BWS was noted, and among patients with BWS, the risk of Wilms tumor is highest in those with uniparental disomy and IC1 imprinting center defect, and the risk of Wilms tumor appears minimal in those with IC2 imprinting center defects and *CDKN1C* mutations (Engel et al. 2000; Weksberg et al. 2003; DeBaun et al. 2002; Cooper et al. 2005). Thus, in one study the risk of embryonal tumors was 9 % at age of 5 years in all cases but 24 % in those with uniparental disomy (Cooper et al. 2005). As the risk of Wilms tumor appears to be very low in children with IC2 imprinting defects and *CDKN1C* mutations, there is no indication for Wilms tumor surveillance (e.g., 3-monthly renal ultrasonography) in such cases. However, hepatoblastoma can occur in children with IC2 defects, and though the absolute risk of hepatoblastoma is low and the utility of screening for hepatoblastoma alone is unproven, some parents may request surveillance by serum alpha-fetoprotein measurements.

Birt–Hogg–Dubé Syndrome (OMIM135150)

Following the description of familial renal oncocytoma (Weirich et al. 1998), it was reported that some familial renal oncocytoma kindreds contained affected individuals with rare hamartomatous tumors of the hair follicle known as fibrofolliculoma (Toro et al. 1999). Fibrofolliculomas are a characteristic feature of the dominantly inherited multisystem familial cancer syndrome Birt–Hogg–Dubé syndrome (Birt et al. 1977). Benign whitish-grey papular skin tumors develop on the face and upper body in the third decade, and histological examination reveals fibrofolliculomas or trichodiscomas (Birt et al. 1977; Rongioletti et al. 1989). Additional features include lipomas and cystic lung lesions and pneumothorax. In some reports, colonic polyposis is described (the combination of skin fibrofolliculomas and colorectal polyps described by Hornstein and Knickenberg (1975) is now considered to be BHD syndrome), and an increased risk of colorectal cancer has been reported in some studies but not in others (Zbar et al. 2002; Nahorski et al. 2010). Lifetime risk of renal cell carcinoma in BHD is about 30 % with a mean age of diagnosis of ~50 years (Menko et al. 2009). A variety of histopathological subtypes of RCC have been described in Birt–Hogg–Dubé syndrome; a hybrid oncocytoma/chromophobe is characteristic, but other types including chromophobe and clear cell (conventional) RCC may occur (Pavlovich et al. 2002; Menko et al. 2009). Germline BHD gene (*FLCN*) mutations may be detected in ~5 % of patients with features of non-syndromic inherited RCC and also in kindreds with familial pneumothorax (Woodward et al. 2008; Graham et al. 2005).

The suggested diagnostic criteria for BHD syndrome require the presence of one major (at least 5 fibrofolliculomas–trichodiscomas, at least one histologically confirmed, of adult onset or a pathogenic germline mutation) or two minor criteria (multiple lung cysts (bilateral basal lung cysts with no other apparent cause, with or without spontaneous primary pneumothorax) or renal cancer: early-onset (<50 years) and/or multifocal/bilateral renal cancer and/or renal cancer of mixed chromophobe/oncocytic histology) or a first-degree relative with BHD syndrome.

The *BHD* gene maps to 17p11.2 and encodes a 64-kDa protein (Nickerson et al. 2002). A frameshift mutation hotspot in a mononucleotide tract (C_8) in exon 11 accounts for ~50 % of mutations and most mutations are protein truncating (see http://www.lovd.nl/flcn). Molecular genetic diagnostic testing diagnosis should consist of sequence analysis and analysis (e.g., MLPA) for exonic deletions and amplifications. Two naturally occurring animal models of Birt–Hogg–Dubé syndrome, in the German shepherd dog and rat, have been described (Jonasdottir et al. 2000; Okimoto et al. 2004). The folliculin protein may negatively regulate AMPK and mTOR-related pathways, though the effects on mTOR may be context dependent and folliculin function has not yet been fully elucidated (Menko et al. 2009).

Surveillance for renal tumors is recommended by annual MRI scan of the kidney starting at the age of 20 years. As in von Hippel–Lindau disease, renal tumors <3 cm can be monitored and nephron-sparing surgery performed when they reach 3 cm. In view of the risk of pneumothorax, caution should be exercised for circumstances which might precipitate pneumothorax, such as general anesthesia. Individuals with BHD syndrome who develop pneumothorax will have lung cysts (usually basal), and so a lung CT scan may predict risk of pneumothorax. Fibrofolliculomas are benign and do not need treatment other than for cosmetic reasons. The role of colonoscopy in BHD syndrome is uncertain, but in families in which colorectal cancer has occurred, 3-yearly colonoscopy from age 45 years is indicated.

Blackfan–Diamond Syndrome (OMIM 105650)

This rare disorder (>1 in 250,000 births) is characterized by congenital hypoplastic anemia with normal leucocyte and platelet counts. Approximately 10–25 % are familial with the majority sporadic. Approximately 30–40 % have other congenital anomalies such as upper limb and craniofacial anomalies. There is an increased risk of leukemia (Alter 1987). Gustavsson et al. (1997) estimated that 10–20 % of cases followed a recessive or dominant inheritance pattern, and they mapped a gene to chromosome 19q13 for both recessive and dominant forms. Subsequently Draptchinskaia et al. (1999) demonstrated germline mutations in the *RPS19* gene in Blackfan–Diamond anemia (DBA, MIM105650). Overall about 25 % of DBA patients have *RPS19* mutations, but multiple loci have now been identified (Gazda et al. 2001; Boria et al. 2010). Interestingly, there are at least ten forms of DBA, all of which are due to germline mutations in genes responsible for ribosome synthesis. DBA is a consequence of defective ribosome biogenesis and defective protein translation (Boria et al. 2010). While germline mutations in *RPL5* seemed to confer increased risk of thumb, but not craniofacial anomalies, none of those with *RPL11* mutations had such anomalies (Gazda et al. 2008).

Bloom Syndrome (OMIM 210900)

This rare autosomal recessive condition is much more common in Ashkenazi Jews than in other ethnic groups. It is characterized by low birth weight, growth deficiency, and a sunlight-sensitive erythematous and telangiectatic rash, especially on the face from the first year of life. Sun exposure accentuates these changes, and may induce bullae, with bleeding and crusting on the face (especially the lips and eyelids). The nose is prominent in a long thin face, and there is clinodactyly. Spotty hypopigmentation and hyperpigmentation may be seen on the skin, and also "twin spots," which may be due to somatic recombination (Bloom 1966). Adult height is usually less than 150 cm. Intelligence is normal. There is a severe immune defect with reduced gammaglobulin (IgA and IgM) levels, leading to a high incidence of chronic severe infections of the respiratory and GI tract. About 20 % of patients with Bloom syndrome develop neoplasms, half of these before the age of 20 years, and tumors may be multiple. Neoplasms are predominantly lymphatic and non-lymphatic leukemia, lymphoma, and carcinomas of the mouth, stomach, esophagus, colon, cervix, and larynx. Early cervical screening should be offered to affected women. Screening for other cancers may be problematic, although regular oral examinations by a dental surgeon and colonoscopy are also probably worthwhile. Myeloid leukemia and myelodysplastic syndrome have been reported, often with monosomy for chromosome 7 (Ellis and German 1996; Aktas et al. 2000; Poppe et al. 2001). Wilms tumor has been described in four children with Bloom syndrome, and one of these four children had a sib who developed a hepatocellular carcinoma at age of 15 years (Cairney et al. 1987; Jain et al. 2001).

Few patients survive into adulthood, but in those that do, colorectal cancer has been reported. In one case, this occurred in the context of ulcerative colitis (Wang et al. 1999), whereas in other case, an attenuated familial adenomatous polyposis (FAP) phenotype was observed (Lowy et al. 2001). Interestingly, a mucinous (i.e., hereditary non-polyposis colorectal cancer-like) transverse colon cancer, with normal p53 expression, has been reported in a 16-year-old with Bloom syndrome. These observation led investigators to study the gene, *BLM*, identified by Ellis et al.

(1995) in individuals from the population with colorectal cancer. One mutation, *BLM: 2281del6ins7* is seen in approximately 1 in 110 Ashkenazi Jews, so this population was studied in detail. Overall, 1 in 54 Jews with colorectal cancer carried this allele, whereas the allele was seen in 1 in 118 controls (odds ratio, 2.76; 95 % CI, 1.4–5.5) (Gruber et al. 2002). This finding was supported by data showing that mice heterozygous for *Blm* developed twice the number of intestinal tumors when crossed with mice carrying a mutation of the *Apc* tumor suppressor gene (Goss et al. 2002). Somatic mutations in length repeats within *BLM* are also quite frequent in sporadic colorectal cancer (Calin et al. 1998) and, interestingly, tend to be associated with mucinous colorectal cancers (Calin et al. 2000). Knocking out *BLM* in karyotypically stable colorectal cancer cell lines results in increased sister chromatid exchange and homologous recombination (but without gross chromosomal rearrangements) (Traverso et al. 2003). Finally, in a murine model, chromosomal instability and tumor predisposition seem to correlate inversely with BLM protein levels (McDaniel et al. 2003). Taken together, these findings suggest that homozygous individuals are at considerably increased risk for colorectal cancer and that heterozygosity for *BLM* can be added to the I1307K *APC* allele as a genetic risk factor for colorectal cancer in the Jewish population, I1307K, however, is at least 6 times as prevalent as BLM^{Ash}, and thus the clinical significance of the latter allele is very limited. Another possible founder mutation has been reported in Japan: *BLM: 631delCAA* (Kaneko et al. 2004), and studies of this allele in colorectal cancer in Japan would be of interest.

At the nuclear level, an elevated frequency of chromosomal breaks is observed, with an increase in sister chromatid exchanges, and an abnormal profile of DNA replication intermediates is reported in this condition (Lonn et al. 1990). The exact mechanism by which BLM maintains replication fidelity is debated. In a mouse model of Bloom syndrome, viable mice were prone to cancers at many sites, and cell lines showed elevated levels of mitotic recombination (and therefore loss of heterozygosity) (Luo et al. 2000). These data were supported by results in human cancer cells, as discussed above (Traverso et al. 2003).

There is a registry for cases of Bloom syndrome to help affected individuals and their families and to assist in the assessment of the natural history of the disease. The registry can be contacted at http://med.cornell.edu/bsr/. According to this website, as of 2009, there were 265 persons with Bloom syndrome registered.

Blue Rubber Bleb Nevus Syndrome (OMIM112200)

This may occur as an autosomal dominant trait, but is usually sporadic and of unknown etiology. Multiple vascular nipple-like lesions occur, especially on the trunk and upper arms and mucous membranes, and intestinal, hepatic, and pulmonary angiomas may develop (Dobru et al. 2004). Bleeding from these lesions can lead to anemia (Fukhro et al. 2002). Central nervous system (CNS) hemangioma and cerebellar medulloblastoma may also occur (Satya-Murti et al. 1986; Kim

2000). It has been suggested that this syndrome is a variant of familial (autosomal dominant) venous malformations which has been mapped to chromosome 9p by linkage studies in two large kindreds (Gallione et al. 1995), and germline mutations in the endothelial cell-specific receptor tyrosine kinase gene *TIE2* (*TEK*) have been detected in some families; somatic mutations in the same gene can be demonstrated in sporadic cases (Nobuhara et al. 2006; Limaye et al. 2009).

Carney–Stratakis Syndrome (Carney Dyad; Dyad of Paragangliomas and Stromal Tumors) (OMIM606864)

Carney–Stratakis syndrome (CSS) or Carney dyad should not be confused with the more classic Carney triad, the latter of which comprises paragangliomas (PGL), gastrointestinal stromal tumors (GIST), and pulmonary chondromas. In contrast to Carney triad which occurs sporadically, CSS is an autosomal dominant condition characterized by PGL or pheochromocytoma and GIST (Stratakis and Carney 2009). Recently, germline heterozygous mutations in *SDHB*, *SDHC*, or *SDHD*, encoding three of the four subunits of succinate dehydrogenase (mitochondrial complex II), were found in individuals and families with CSS (McWhinney et al. 2007; Pasini et al. 2008). In this initial series, 8 of 11 CSS individuals harbored *SDH* mutations. At this time, it is difficult to determine whether individuals with PGL and GIST but who are *SDH* mutation negative actually have Carney triad but have yet to develop the third component (Alrashdi et al. 2010). Because of the rarity of CSS and the short time from discovery of its genetic basis, one must assume that medical management and surveillance are similar to that recommended for those with PGL/pheochromocytoma syndromes caused by germline mutations in *SDHA-D* genes (see page 42).

Carney Complex (NAME Syndrome, LAMB Syndrome, Carney Syndrome) (OMIM 160980)

Carney complex (CNC) is a rare autosomal dominant heritable multiple neoplasia syndrome characterized by cardiac, endocrine, cutaneous, and neural tumors and a variety of mucocutaneous pigmented lesions. CNC is linked to at least two different loci. Germline mutations in *PRKAR1A*, on 17q22–q24, have been shown to cause a subset of CNC (Kirschner et al. 2000a, b). The gene on 2p15–p16, which may account for 20 % of all CNC families, has yet to be identified. Some believe that a third minor locus might also be involved.

This rare condition is characterized by cardiac, breast, and cutaneous myxomas, pigmented skin lesions, and micronodular pigmented adrenal hyperplasia (Koopman and Happle 1991). The tumors are commonly multicentric or bilateral, and the mean age at diagnosis of the first manifestation is 18 years. Most patients have two or more manifestations of the condition. Pituitary adenomas and testicular tumors (Sertoli or Leydig cell in about 50 % of affected males) are associated, and the hormones secreted by these tumors cause characteristic phenotypic effects (Carney et al. 1986). Skin lesions include lentigines, blue nevi, dermal fibromas, and myxoid neurofibromas. The pigmentation is spotty, particularly on the face (in 70 % of cases), hands, and feet, and is similar to that seen in Peutz–Jeghers syndrome (PJS), although in the latter the lesions are seen more in the buccal region and palate, and the visceral lesions appear to be quite distinct in these two syndromes (Carney et al. 1985; Lodish and Stratakis 2011). Further, inner canthal pigmentation is virtually only seen in CNC. Eyelid myxomas are found in 16 % of affected patients. The tumors are usually benign, but liposarcomas and other malignant tumors may develop. The cardiac tumors are life threatening via embolism or by direct mass effect. Recently pancreatic cancer has been found in 9 of 354 cases of Carney complex (1 adenocarcinoma, 2 acinar cell carcinomas, and 3 intraductal mucinous neoplasms where histology was available), and loss of heterozygosity for *PRKAR1A* was suggested, with lack of expression of the protein in 5/6 tumors studies (Gaujoux et al. 2011).

CNC was found to be linked to 17q22–q24 and 2p15–p16. Germline loss-of-function mutations in *PRKR1A*, encoding the type 1A subunit of the protein kinase A receptor on 17q22–q24, have been found in a subset of CNC (Kirschner et al. 2000a, b). Nonsense-mediated decay of mutant transcript appears to be the mechanism leading to loss of function (Kirschner et al. 2000a). Over 380 CNC patients with >20 years of follow-up in a bi-institutional series were analyzed for genotype–phenotype associations (Bertherat et al. 2009). There were 80 different germline *PRKR1A* mutations. Mutations in this gene were more commonly found in individuals with a combination of myxomas (affecting multiple organs), psammomatous melanotic schwannomas (PMS), thyroid tumors, and large cell calcifying Sertoli cell tumor (LCCSCT) than in individuals with CNC without this combination of clinical features. The "hot spot" mutation, c.491_492delTG, was more commonly associated with lentigines, cardiac myxoma, and thyroid tumors than all other *PRKAR1A* mutations combined (Bertherat et al. 2009). Individuals with isolated PPNAD tended to carry either the c.709-7 to c.709-2delATTTTT or c.1 A>G, and these are the only two mutations that have incomplete penetrance. In general, splice site mutations tended to occur with milder disease. Nonetheless, penetrance of *PRKAR1A* mutation is >95 % by age 50 years. Germline *PDE11A* variation seems to modify germline *PRKAR1A* mutations, conferring 4–5-fold increased prevalences of PPNAD and LCCSCT compared to those without *PDE11A* variants (Libe et al. 2011).

As with other inherited tumor syndromes, mutation analysis by bidirectional Sanger sequencing should begin with a clinically affected individual. Once a family-specific mutation in *PRKR1A* is found, then predictive testing may be offered. Clinical and biochemical screening for CNC and medical surveillance for affected patients remain the gold standard for the care of patients with CNC. In brief, for postpubertal pediatric and for adult patients of both sexes with established CNC, the following annual studies are recommended: echocardiogram, measurement of urinary free cortisol levels (which may be supplemented by diurnal cortisol or the overnight 1 mg dexamethasone testing), and serum IGF1 levels (Stratakis et al. 1999). Male patients should also have testicular ultrasonography at the initial evaluation; microscopic LCCSCT (large cell calcifying Sertoli cell tumor) may be followed by annual ultrasound thereafter (Stratakis et al. 2001). Thyroid ultrasonography should be obtained at the initial evaluation, and may be repeated, as needed (Stratakis et al. 2001). Transabdominal ultrasonography in female patients is recommended during the first evaluation but need not be repeated, unless there is a detectable abnormality, because of the relatively low risk of ovarian malignancy (Stratakis et al. 2001). Because cardiac myxoma is responsible for a significant amount of morbidity and mortality, pediatric patients with CNC should have echocardiography during their first 6 months of life and annually thereafter; biannual echocardiographic evaluation may be necessary for patients with history of an excised myxoma.

Cockayne Syndrome (OMIM 216400)

This is a very rare autosomal recessive disorder characterized by growth failure leading to extremely short stature, evident within the first few years after birth (described as "cachectic dwarfism"), lack of subcutaneous fat, cutaneous photosensitivity, deafness, progressive optic atrophy, neurological deterioration with a leukodystrophy, and mental retardation. There is brain dysmyelination with calcium deposits. There is a typical "salt and pepper" retinitis and/or cataracts. These features develop from late infancy, but there is considerable variability of the phenotype, even within families (Mahmoud et al. 2002). Characteristic facial features include large ears, sunken eyes, and limbs that are relatively long. There is type II hyperlipoproteinemia. Knee contractures may occur, causing a "horse-riding stance," and delayed neural development and neurological degeneration cause mental retardation. Mean age at death is 12.5 years, but varies a great deal. There appears to be a deficiency of DNA repair after exposure to UV light and deficiency in cellular repair of oxidative DNA damage. Death usually occurs before the age of 20 years, and malignancy is not reported to be specifically increased in this condition. The disease is genetically heterogeneous, and genes for complementation groups CS-A and CS-B have been identified (Stefanini et al. 1996). Cockayne syndrome type A is caused by biallelic mutations in the gene encoding the group 8 excision repair cross-complementing protein (ERCC8; www.omim.org/entry/609412) on chromosome 5q11. Cockayne syndrome type B (CSB; www.omim.org/entry/133540) is caused by mutation in the *ERCC6* gene (www.omim.org/entry/609413) on chromosome 10q11. Bertola et al. (2006) analyzed the *ERCC8* gene in Brazilian families with typical CSA and identified homozygosity or compound heterozygosity for *ERCC8* mutations in them, with no clear genotype/

phenotype correlation. The CS-B gene product is involved in transcription-coupled and/or global genome nucleotide excision repair of DNA damage induced by UV light and other oxidative DNA damage (Mahmoud et al. 2002; Osterod et al. 2002; Tuo et al. 2003). Notably, in contrast to human Cockayne syndrome, homozygous knockout mice for the murine orthologue of the human CSA gene ($Csa_3/_3$) develop skin tumors after chronic exposure to UV light (van der Horst et al. 2002). The reason why humans with Cockayne syndrome do not develop skin cancer is not known. Interestingly, other cases of Cockayne syndrome with features overlapping with those of xeroderma pigmentosum (XP) are due to mutations in the *XPB*, *XPD*, or *XPG* genes (Rapin et al. 2000). *XPG* and *CSB* mutations may also be responsible for the cerebro-oculo-facio-skeletal (COFS) syndrome (Graham et al. 2001). COFS is another autosomal recessive neurodegenerative disorder with growth failure, joint contractures, cataracts, microcornea, and optic atrophy.

Celiac Disease

Patients with celiac disease have an increased risk of esophageal cancer, cancer of the mouth and pharynx, small bowel carcinoma, and lymphoma. Although non-Hodgkin lymphoma is the main cause of cancer death in celiac disease (Corrao et al. 2001), in a series of small bowel cancers, 13 % of adenocarcinoma cases and 39 % of lymphomas occurred in patients with celiac disease providing evidence that celiac disease confers susceptibility to adenocarcinoma of the small bowel as well as lymphoma (Howdle et al. 2003). Small bowel adenocarcinomas associated with celiac disease have a high frequency of microsatellite instability (MSI) and somatic inactivation of *MLH1* or *MSH2* (Potter et al. 2004). Although the absolute risk of malignancy in celiac disease is small, those cases complicated by malignancy often appear to have been poorly controlled, and treatment reduces the risk of malignancy (Houlston and Ford 1996; Ferguson and Kingstone 1996).

Celiac disease itself shows familial aggregation and a strong human leucocyte antigen (HLA) association. Familial clustering appears to reflect multifactorial inheritance with major genetic risk factors (HLA-DQ2 and HLA-DQ8) and environmental factors. It appears that genes within the HLA class II DQ region are necessary but not sufficient for celiac disease to develop. About 95 % of all patients have a DQ2 allele with DQ2 homozygotes being at highest risk. Of the remaining 5 %, most are DQ8 positive. It is estimated that HLA class II genes account for 50 % of genetic susceptibility to celiac disease, and non-HLA-associated genes are also implicated (Treem 2004). Hovhannisyan et al. (2008) showed that the HLA-DQ8 beta-57 polymorphism promotes the recruitment of T cell receptors bearing a negative signature charge in the complementary determining region 3-beta (CDR3-beta) during the response against native gluten peptides presented by HLA-DQ8 in celiac disease. These T cells showed a cross-reactive and stronger response to deamidated gluten peptides.

Common Variable Immunodeficiency (CVID) (OMIM 607594)

This comprises a heterogeneous group of disorders characterized by hypogamma-globulinemia, humoral immunodeficiency, and susceptibility to infection. Some patients may also have defects in some aspects of cell-mediated immunity. Many cases are acquired, but genetic factors have been implicated in some cases, and autosomal recessive inheritance is proposed. There is an increased incidence of lymphoid malignancy in patients with common variable immunodeficiency (Kersey et al. 1988). In three families with a variant of CVID, a dominantly inherited combination of cold urticaria and antibody deficiency, with susceptibility to infection and autoimmunity, referred to as PLAID (PLCγ2-associated antibody deficiency and immune dysregulation), researchers identified deletions in *PLCG2*. This led to gain in phospholipase C gamma 2 function and subsequent abnormal regulation of numerous leucocyte subsets (Ombrello et al. 2012). Cancers have not been reported in these families.

Constitutional Mismatch Repair Deficiency (CMMRD), also known as Autosomal Recessive Childhood Cancer Predisposition Syndrome (OMIM 276300)

It has become appreciated that biallelic mutations in *MLH1*, *MSH2*, *MSH6*, and most commonly, *PMS2* can be responsible for an autosomal recessive condition characterized by mainly childhood and adolescent malignancies, particularly hematological (lymphomas and leukemias) and brain tumors, including medulloblastomas, glioblastomas, and oligodendrogliomata, other cancers (GI or uterine cancer), and dermatological features of NF (café-au-lait patches) (De Vos et al. 2004; Menko et al. 2004; reviewed in Wimmer and Etzler 2008). This has in the past been described as a variant of Turcot syndrome (p. 311) (De Rosa et al. 2000; Bougeard et al. 2003), and it is interesting to speculate what proportion of Turcot syndrome is attributable to mutations in APC and the MMR genes, particularly as both autosomal dominant and recessive forms of Turcot syndrome have been described.

Costello Syndrome (OMIM 218040)

This rare multisystem condition is also known as fasciocutaneous syndrome and is usually sporadic, possibly representing new mutations. The facial features are similar to Noonan syndrome, with increasingly coarse features with age, and nasal papillomata. There is excess skin on the hands. Developmental delay after postnatal failure to thrive and short stature are usual. There is an increased risk of cancer, possibly up to 17 %, particularly rhabdomyosarcomas, neuroblastomas, and transitional carcinomas of the bladder, and screening by 3–6-monthly abdominal ultrasound and 6–12-monthly urinary catecholamine estimations until 5 years of age and annual urinalysis thereafter recommended until 10 years of age (DeBaun 2002; Gripp et al. 2002, 2006).

The diagnosis is based on clinical findings, with confirmation of the diagnosis requiring identification of a germline heterozygous gain-of-function missense mutations in the *HRAS* proto-oncogene (Aoki et al. 2005; Gripp and Lin 2012). The mutation frequency is 90 %, with virtually all mutations involving exon 2 (first coding exon) of *HRAS*. Therefore, if the diagnosis is suspected but no *HRAS* mutation is found, then other differential diagnoses should be considered. Top differential diagnoses include other syndromes involving the RAS/MAPK pathway (so-called RASopathies) including type 1 neurofibromatosis (see p. 288), Noonan syndrome (see p. 297), cranio-cardio-facial syndrome, and Legius syndrome (Gripp and Lin 2012).

Cowden Syndrome (Multiple Hamartoma Syndrome) (OMIM 158350)

Cowden syndrome (CS) is an autosomal dominantly inherited multiple hamartoma syndrome characterized by an increased risk of breast, thyroid, and endometrial cancer. Germline mutations in *PTEN*, encoding a lipid and protein phosphatase on 10q23.3, are associated with a subset (25–80 %) of CS (Eng et al. 2003; Zhou et al. 2003a, b; Eng and Peacocke 1998; Zbuk and Eng 2007; Tan et al. 2011).

Clinical diagnosis is often a challenge, because of the protean manifestations of CS, many of which can occur in isolation in the general population. For this reason, the true incidence is not known. After identification of *PTEN* as the *CS* gene, a molecular-based study revealed the incidence to be at least 1 in 200,000 (Nelen et al. 1997, 1999), although this is likely still to be an underestimate. Because CS is underdiagnosed, the proportion of apparently sporadic cases and familial cases (two or more affected individuals) is not precisely known. As a broad estimate, perhaps 40–65 % of CS cases are familial (Marsh et al. 1998; Marsh et al. 1999; Eng, unpublished observations, 2011).

The lack of uniform diagnostic criteria for CS prior to 1995 led to the formation of the International Cowden Consortium (C. Eng, Coordinator and Chair, engc@ccf.org), which represented a group of centers mainly in North America and Europe interested in systematically studying this syndrome to localize the susceptibility gene. The consortium arrived at a set of consensus operational diagnostic criteria based on published data and expert opinion (Nelen et al. 1996; Eng and Parsons 1998). These criteria have been revised annually in the context of new molecular-based data and are reflected in the practice guidelines of the US-based National Comprehensive Cancer Network Genetics/High-Risk Panel (NCCN 1999; Eng 2000a, b; Hobert and Eng 2009) (www.nccn.org for 2005 and 2006 revisions which remain the best sets of criteria) as follows:

1. Pathognomic criteria:

   (a) Mucocutaneous lesions:

   - Trichilemmomas, facial
   - Acral keratoses
   - Papillomatous papules
   - Mucosal lesions (e.g., scrotal tongue)
   - Lhermitte–Duclos disease (LDD)

2. Major criteria:

   (a) Breast carcinoma, invasive
   (b) Thyroid carcinoma, epithelial, especially follicular thyroid carcinoma and follicular variant of papillary thyroid carcinoma
   (c) Macrocephaly (megalencephaly) (>97th percentile)
   (d) Endometrial carcinoma

3. Minor criteria:

   (a) Other anatomic thyroid lesions, e.g., adenoma, multinodular goiter, Hashimoto's thyroiditis
   (b) Developmental delay
   (c) GI hamartomas (GI polyposis of any histology)
   (d) Fibrocystic disease of the breast
   (e) Lipomas
   (f) Fibromas
   (g) Genitourinary tumors (e.g., renal cell carcinoma, uterine fibroids) or malformation (e.g., bicornuate uterus, duplicated collecting ducts)

Operational Diagnosis in an Individual:

1. Mucocutaneous lesions alone if:

   (a) There are 6 or more facial papules, of which 3 or more are trichilemmomas
   (b) There are cutaneous facial papules and oral mucosal papillomatosis
   (c) There are oral mucosal papillomatosis and acral keratoses
   (d) There are palmoplantar keratoses, 6 or more

2. 2 Major criteria, but one must include macrocephaly or LDD
3. 1 Major and 3 minor criteria
4. 4 Minor criteria

Operational Diagnosis in a Family Where One Individual Is Diagnostic for Cowden Syndrome (by Clinical Criteria or by Gene Status):

1. Pathognomonic criterion/criteria
2. Any one major criterion with or without minor criteria
3. Two minor criteria

While the original intent of the International Cowden Consortium operational diagnostic criteria and the NCCN criteria were for the gene hunt (former) and for early clinical practice (both sets of criteria), the criteria would result in a dichotomous response, namely, meets criteria or does not meet criteria. Necessarily, these related two sets of operational criteria were based on retrospective data from exaggerated cases (full criteria mainly by pathognomic and major criteria) and familial cases. Recently, multiple logistic regression analysis of comprehensive *PTEN* mutation data from a >10-year prospective accrual of probands by a minimum of relaxed Consortium operational criteria from multiple centers, including the community, has resulted in a continuous score, the *PTEN* Cleveland Clinic Score (www.lerner.ccf.org/gmi/ccscore/), based on key phenotypic features (Tan et al. 2011). Because the key phenotypic features present in children and adults are quite different, two sets of criteria are utilized depending on age groups. A *PTEN* CC score of >10 in adults, relating to a prior probability of >3 % of finding a pathogenic *PTEN* mutation, was selected as the clinical threshold for considering *PTEN* testing/referral to genetic specialists (Tan et al. 2011).

More than 90 % of individuals affected with CS are believed to manifest a CS phenotype by the age of 20 years (Nelen et al. 1996; Eng 2000b). By the end of the third decade (i.e., 29 years), 99 % of affected individuals are believed to have developed at least the mucocutaneous signs of the syndrome, although any of a number of component features can manifest as well. The most commonly reported manifestations are mucocutaneous lesions; thyroid abnormalities; fibrocystic disease and carcinoma of the breast; multiple, early-onset uterine leiomyoma; and macrocephaly (specifically, megencephaly) (Starink et al. 1986; Hanssen and Fryns 1995; Mallory 1995; Longy and Lacombe 1996; Eng 2000b; Ngeow et al. 2011).

The two most well-documented component malignancies are carcinomas of the breast and epithelial thyroid gland (Starink et al. 1986; Zbuk and Eng 2007; Hobert and Eng 2009). Historically, lifetime risks for female breast cancer are estimated to range from 25 to 50 % (Starink et al. 1986; Longy and Lacombe 1996) in contrast to 11 % in the general population. The age at diagnosis ranges between 14 and 65 years, with a mean around 40–45 years (Starink et al. 1986; Longy and Lacombe 1996). The histopathology of CS breast cancer is adenocarcinoma of the breast, both ductal and lobular (Schrager et al. 1997). Male breast cancer may be a minor component of the syndrome (Marsh et al. 1998; Fackenthal et al. 2001). In a recent prospectively accrued series of *PTEN* pathogenic mutation-positive CS and CSL cases, lifetime risk for female (invasive) breast cancer was calculated to be 85 % with age- and sex-adjusted standardized incidence rates (SIR) of >25 (Table 11.1) (Tan et al. 2012). This is much higher than pre-gene estimates and should be duly considered during risk management. Interestingly, this series did not note an elevated *PTEN*-related male breast cancer risk. The lifetime risk for differentiated thyroid cancer can be as high as 10 % in males and females with CS. A recent prospective series has revealed that individuals with germline pathogenic *PTEN* mutations have a 35 % lifetime risk of epithelial thyroid carcinoma (1) with SIR of 50–72 (Ngeow et al. 2011; Tan et al. 2012). In this large series, follicular thyroid

Table 11.1 Lifetime risks of *PTEN*-related malignancies and age-related penetrance

Malignancy	Lifetime risk (%)	Penetrance by age 50 years (%)	Comments
Breast cancer	85	40	Females at risk only
Thyroid cancer		25	
Endometrial cancer	28	20	Females only
Colorectal cancer	10	1	
Renal cell cancer	34	10	
Melanoma	6	5	

carcinoma (FTC) was overrepresented among adults with *PTEN* mutations. While papillary thyroid carcinomas (PTC) were also observed, one-third of these were the follicular variant (FvPTC). All six children (<18 years of age) who were found to have pathogenic *PTEN* mutations had thyroid cancer, but interestingly all were PTC (Ngeow et al. 2011). With this new series, it is now obvious that the age at diagnosis of thyroid cancers is truly earlier (mean age 37.5 years) than that in the general population, and even children can develop PTC. Interestingly, *PTEN* frameshift mutations were found in 31 % of those with thyroid cancer and only 17 % of those who did not (Ngeow et al. 2011).

Endometrial carcinoma was also considered to be a putative component cancer of CS in previous genotype–phenotype and case studies (Marsh et al. 1998; DeVivo et al. 2000; Eng 2000b). In a prospective series of pathogenic *PTEN* mutation-positive CS and CSL cases accrued from academic and community-based healthcare facilities, the SIR of endometrial cancer was >40, with lifetime risk of 28.2 % (Table 11.1) (Tan et al. 2012). For the first time, elevated lifetime risks of renal carcinomas (34 %) and melanoma (6 %) were noted in *PTEN* mutation-positive individuals.

Prior to 2010, exponents believed that hamartomatous polyps were component of CS but that colorectal carcinomas were not part of the disease spectrum. However, in a recent prospective study of a series of individuals carrying pathogenic *PTEN* mutations, >90 % of those who received colonoscopies were found to have polyps (Heald et al. 2010). Surprisingly, polyps of all histologies and an elevated SIR (10–100) for colorectal cancers were noted, with the earliest age at diagnosis of cancer being 35 years and the oldest 50 years (Tan et al. 2012). The lifetime risk of *PTEN-related* colorectal cancer is almost 10 % (Tan et al. 2012). All but one person with colorectal cancer had pre-/coexisting colonic polyposis.

The most common nonmalignant component lesions include trichilemmomas (hamartoma of the infundibulum of the hair follicle) and papillomatous papules (90–100 %), thyroid adenomas and goiter (67 %), breast fibroadenomas and fibro-cystic disease (75 %), macrocephaly (>80 %), and genitourinary abnormalities (40 %) including uterine fibroids and malformations (Mester et al. 2011; Ngeow et al. 2011). A rather striking nonmalignant hamartoma is LDD or dysplastic gangliocytoma of the cerebellum (Eng et al. 1994), which usually manifests later in life, initially with subtle degrees of dysmetria on intent, progressing to frank ataxia. A small series of incident LDD cases revealed that many adult-onset LDD carried germline *PTEN* mutations (Zhou et al. 2003a).

CS was mapped to 10q22–q23 (Nelen et al. 1996). Germline mutations in *PTEN* have been found in 85 % of CS probands diagnosed by the strict International Cowden Consortium criteria, when accrued by select academic centers (Marsh et al. 1998; Zhou et al. 2003b). In contrast, a large series accrued from the community revealed that ~25 % of probands meeting the strict International Cowden Consortium criteria were found to carry pathogenic *PTEN* mutations (Tan et al. 2011). These mutations result in loss of function, and the majority occur in exons 5, 7, and 8, which encode the phosphatase domain, although mutations can occur throughout the gene including the promoter (Zhou et al. 2003b). Germline mutations in *PTEN* have also been found in approximately 60 % of individuals with BRRS accrued from select academic tertiary referral centers (see section on Bannayan–Riley–Ruvalcaba syndrome, (BRRS) p. 221) (Marsh et al. 1997; 1999). Thus CS and BRRS are allelic. Compared to *PTEN* mutations in CS, mutations in BRRS tend to occur in the 3′ half of the gene (Eng et al. 2003). There is a genotype–phenotype association in CS (Marsh et al. 1998): families found to have germline *PTEN* mutations have an increased risk of malignancy, in particular, breast cancer. The presence of both CS and BRRS features in a single family, of glycogenic acanthosis of the esophagus, or of LDD, increases the prior probability of finding a *PTEN* mutation (Marsh et al. 1999; McGarrity et al. 2003; Zhou et al. 2003b).

Germline *PTEN* mutations have also been described in up to 20 % of Proteus syndrome and up to 50 % of Proteus-like syndrome cases (Zhou et al. 2000, 2001; Smith et al. 2002). Germline mutations in *PTEN* have been described in single patients with megencephaly and VATER association and with megencephaly and autism (Dasouki et al. 2001; Reardon et al. 2001). Multiple studies of individuals with autism or autism with macrocephaly have now confirmed that *PTEN* mutations occur in ~10 % of those with autism spectrum disorder and macrocephaly (Butler et al. 2005; Herman et al. 2007; Varga et al. 2009).

It was puzzling that the *PTEN* mutation frequency in classic CS in the general population was 25 %, yet the original linkage studies suggested no genetic heterogeneity. Recently, a new gene named *KLLN* (encoding KILLIN) was discovered immediately upstream of *PTEN*, with *KLLN* and *PTEN* sharing a single bidirectional promoter. Germline epimutation (promoter methylation) of *KLLN* was shown to be associated with approximately one-third of CS and CS-like individuals who lacked germline *PTEN* mutations (Bennett et al. 2010). Interestingly, individuals with germline *KLLN* epimutation had a higher frequency of breast and renal cancers than those with germline pathogenic *PTEN* mutation (Bennett et al. 2010). The age-/sex-adjusted SIR for epithelial thyroid carcinoma for *KLLN* epimutation was found to be 45, but in contrast to *PTEN* mutation, classic PTC was overrepresented in those with *KLLN* epimutation (Ngeow et al. 2011). Finally, approximately 10 % of individuals with CS without germline *PTEN* mutations were shown to carry germline missense variants in *SDHB* or *SDHD* (Ni et al. 2008, 2012). Individuals carrying these *SDH* variants had a higher frequency of breast and thyroid cancers. Interestingly, individuals with germline *PTEN* mutations who also carry *SDHx* variants had a higher risk of breast cancer than those with germline *PTEN* mutations alone (Ni et al. 2012). Again, unlike CS with *PTEN* mutations, the thyroid cancers found in cases with *SDH* mutations were mainly classic PTC (Ngeow et al. 2011). Recently, germline *AKT1* and *PIK3CA* mutations have been demonstrated in some cases of Cowden syndrome (Orloff et al. 2013).

All individuals with or suspected of having CS or any PTEN-related disorder should be referred to cancer genetic professionals. *PTEN* mutation analysis is a useful molecular diagnostic test and, in families with a known *PTEN* mutation, is a good predictive test. With the recent independent validation of germline *SDHx* variants in CS/CSL individuals (Ni et al. 2012), *SDHx* testing should also be seriously considered. Once the *KLLN* epimutation data are validated in independent series, *KLLN* should be considered in the armamentarium of CS testing.

Until now, surveillance recommendations are based on expert opinion, governed by the component neoplasia, breast carcinoma, epithelial thyroid carcinoma and adenocarcinoma of the endometrium, and now colonic polyps and cancer (Eng 2000b; Pilarski and Eng 2004; Heald et al. 2007; Hobert and Eng 2009) (www.nccn. org). Because of a recent prospective series of CS/CSL individuals, we suggest consideration of new potential surveillance recommendations based on the prospective risk data as outlined in Table 11.2 (Tan et al. 2012), although the cancer risk estimates are subject to ascertainment bias and may be overestimated in some series. For example, clinicians should consider thyroid examination and baseline ultrasound at diagnosis of CS or upon finding a mutation defining CS, even in children (Ngeow et al. 2011). Females should begin annual clinical breast examination and breast self-examination around the age of 25 years. Annual breast imaging (mammography, breast MRI) should begin at 30 years. Because of accumulating data on *PTEN*-related colonic polyposis and cancer, colonoscopic surveillance could begin by 35–40 years or 5 years younger than the youngest age at diagnosis of colon cancer in the family (Heald et al. 2010; Levi et al. 2011) (Table 11.2). The optimal interval for colonoscopies is currently unknown, but could be modified by polyp load. In the past, the recommendation was for the endometrium to be screened clinically beginning at the age of 35–40 years or 5 years younger than the earliest age of endometrial cancer diagnosis in the family: annual blind repeal biopsies prior to menopause and transabdominal ultrasound after menopause. The NCCN in its recent (2009 onwards) revisions has removed endometrial screening because no formal evaluation studies have been completed. However, in view of the new prospective data which have yielded a much higher lifetime risk of endometrial cancer than previously believed, endometrial surveillance could be reconsidered (Table 11.2) (Tan et al. 2012). Clinicians who look after CS patients should be mindful to note any other seemingly non-component neoplasias, which might be overrepresented in a particular family as well.

With the elucidation of the PTEN-AKT-mTOR signaling pathway, targeted therapeutics hold great promise. mTOR inhibitors are being used in clinical trials for Cowden syndrome patients, specifically *PTEN* hamartoma tumor syndrome, and efficacy has been demonstrated in a related phakomatosis, tuberous sclerosis complex, and in the somatic setting in malignancies where upregulation of mTOR signaling is evident.

Table 11.2 Recommendations for diagnostic workup and cancer surveillance in patients with *PTEN* mutations

	Pediatric (<18 years)	Adult male	Adult female
Baseline workup	Targeted history and physical examination	Targeted history and physical examination	Targeted history and physical examination
	Baseline thyroid ultrasound	Baseline thyroid ultrasound	Baseline thyroid ultrasound
	Dermatological examination	Dermatological examination	Dermatological examination
	Formal neurological and psychological testing		
Cancer surveillance			
From diagnosis	Annual thyroid ultrasound and skin examination	Annual thyroid ultrasound and skin examination	Annual thyroid ultrasound and skin examination
From age 30[a]	As per adult recommendations		Annual mammogram (for consideration of breast MRI instead of mammography if dense breasts)
			Annual endometrial sampling or transvaginal ultrasound (or from 5 years before age of earliest endometrial cancer in family)
From age 40[a]	As per adult recommendations	Biannual colonoscopy[b]	Biennial colonoscopy[b]
		Biannual renal ultrasound/MRI	Biennial renal ultrasound/MRI
Prophylactic surgery	Nil	Nil	Individual discussion of prophylactic mastectomy or hysterectomy

[a]Surveillance may begin 5 years before the earliest onset of a specific cancer in the family, but not later than the recommended age cutoff

[b]The presence of multiple nonmalignant polyps in patients with *PTEN* mutations may complicate noninvasive methods of colon evaluation. More frequent colonoscopy should be considered for patients with a heavy polyp burden

Denys–Drash Syndrome (OMIM 194080)

This rare disorder is characterized by male pseudohermaphroditism, Wilms tumor, and a characteristic glomerulonephropathy causing progressive renal failure. Not all patients have the complete triad, and nephropathy plus Wilms tumor or urogenital abnormalities are sufficient to make the diagnosis. Wilms tumor in Denys–Drash syndrome presents early (mean age 18 months) and is usually bilateral (Jadresic et al. 1991). Gonadoblastoma may also occur. The nephropathy is characterized by focal or diffuse glomerulosclerosis and typically presents with proteinuria, progressing to nephrotic syndrome and hypertension, and then reaching end-stage renal failure by 3 years of age (Coppes et al. 1993). Males (XY karyotype) with Denys–Drash syndrome usually have ambiguous genitalia or phenotypically normal female external genitalia (male pseudohermaphroditism). In addition, the internal genitalia are frequently dysplastic or inappropriate (Mueller 1994).

The risk of Wilms tumor in children with truncating *WT1* mutations or missense mutations in the zinc finger domains (as is typical for Denys–Drash syndrome) is estimated to be >50 %, and screening with 3–4 monthly renal ultrasonography is recommended (Scott et al. 2006). Indeed the risk of Wilms tumor in Denys–Drash syndrome is high enough for bilateral prophylactic nephrectomy to be suggested for children with incomplete Denys–Drash syndrome (e.g., pseudohermaphroditism, hypogonadism, and renal failure) (Hu et al. 2004). Molecular genetic analysis of patients with this syndrome has demonstrated de novo germline *WT1* mutations in most cases (Royer-Pokora et al. 2004). The majority of mutations affect the zinc finger domains and are thought to have a dominant negative effect on genital development (Little et al. 1993). Denys–Drash syndrome is allelic with Frasier syndrome.

Down Syndrome (OMIM 190685)

The risk of acute leukemia in Down syndrome (DS) (trisomy 21) is 20–30 times that of the general population. This increased risk relates both to acute lymphoblastic and acute myeloid leukemia (AML). The cumulative risk of leukemia in DS is 2.1 % by age of 5 years and 2.7 % by age of 30 years. The most common type is acute nonlymphocytic leukemia subtype M7-megakaryocytic leukemia, a type very rare in individuals with normal karyotypes. Acute megakaryoblastic leukemia (AMKL) is particularly prevalent, with an estimated 500-fold increased risk compared to the general population, and a transient form of AMKL, transient myeloproliferative disorder (TMD), is seen in about 10 % of newborn cases with DS, which usually resolves, but about 20 % will develop AMKL within the first 4 years of life (Hasle et al. 2000; Klusmann et al. 2007; Rabin and Whitlock 2009). Leukemia comprises about 60 % of all malignancies and 90 % of all childhood malignancies in DS. The standard incidence rate (SIR) for leukemia in DS is 56 at 4 years and 10 at 5–29 years of age. This risk is particularly pronounced for AML, usually early onset, 49 % developing below 1 year of age (Hasle 2001). AML-M after myelodysplastic syndrome is characteristic, as is trisomy 8 with reduced granulocyte lineage. Leukemic clones in DS are nearly always megaloblastic with *GATA1* (zinc finger transcription factor required for erythroid and megakaryocytic development) mutations conferring a clonal advantage (Groet et al. 2003). Leukemic blasts in DS-AMKL harbor mutations in *GATA1*, which encodes a hematopoietic transcription factor. Most mutations cluster in exon 2 resulting in a truncated mutant protein, GATA1s, lacking the amino-terminal transcriptional activating domain. These mutations are also demonstrable at birth, thus representing an early intrauterine event, and a persistent subclone of TL cells may develop into AMKL as a result of additional mutations (Hitzler and Zipursky 2004).

There is an increased frequency of *JAK2R683* mutations in acute lymphoblastic leukemia in Down syndrome. The overall occurrence of solid tumors (especially breast cancer) in DS is reduced, except for retinoblastoma and germ cell tumors (Look 2003).

Familial Adenomatous Polyposis (OMIM175100)

This is the most common of the hereditary polyposis syndromes, with a prevalence of about 1 in 8,000. It is inherited as an autosomal dominant trait with high penetrance but variable age at onset, and the mutation rate is high (15–20 % of cases are considered to be new mutations, although this may be an overestimate, and some single generation cases may be due to biallelic germline mutations in *MUTYH*) (Sieber et al. 2003a, b). Some sporadic cases (about 15 %) are mosaic for the *APC* mutation. Polyps usually develop in the teens, and penetrance is almost complete by age of 40 years in classical cases (Fig. 11.1). Progression to malignancy is inevitable, and colorectal carcinoma develops in untreated cases by the fourth to fifth decade, or even in childhood, 20–30 years earlier than in nonfamilial colon cancer. Histologically, single crypt adenomas are a characteristic feature. Polyps also occur elsewhere in the GI tract. Gastric polyps in FAP are of two types: benign hyperplastic fundic gland polyps occur in most patients, and adenomas may also occur, usually in the pyloric region of the stomach, but at a much lower frequency. Gastric cancer may develop, even in young patients. Adenomatous duodenal polyps occur in most patients with FAP (over 80 %), are most numerous around the ampulla of Vater, and are associated with a significant risk of malignant transformation. The severity of duodenal polyposis is assessed using the Spigelman scale. Duodenal cancer is now the leading cause of death in this condition if colorectal cancer is prevented and occurs in about 5 % of cases (Spigelman et al. 1995; Brosens et al. 2005; Groves et al. 2002). Carcinoma of the gallbladder and bile ducts may also occur.

Extra-intestinal lesions develop in most patients with FAP and may be apparent before the bowel lesions. Epidermoid cysts may occur in two-thirds of patients, and although they can develop anywhere on the body, they are most noticeable on the scalp. These are very rare in normal children before puberty. Osteomas of the mandible may be detected in more than 90 % of patients using orthopantomograms and are uncommon in the general population (4 %). A third of patients may have impacted teeth, and dentigerous cysts and supernumerary and unerupted teeth may occur. Exostoses may develop in the skull, digits, and long bones, and cortical thickening is described.

The most common extraintestinal manifestation of FAP is multiple areas of retinal pigmentation, called congenital hypertrophy of the retinal pigment

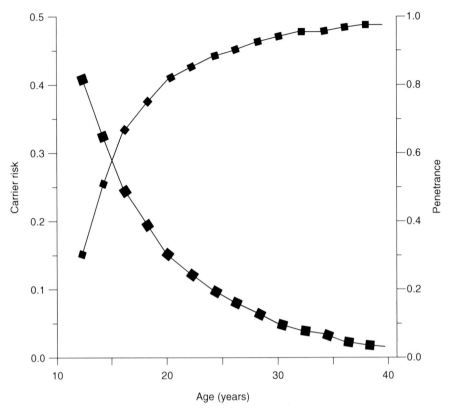

Fig. 11.1 Age-related carrier risk (*larger squares*) for relatives at 50 % prior risk of FAP, that is an affected parent, and a negative bowel examination at that age. The age-related risk was derived from the age-related penetrance data (*smaller squares*) (Adapted from Burn et al. 1991, with permission from J. Burn)

epithelium (CHRPE). These are found in about three-quarters of affected individuals. These are discrete, darkly pigmented, rounded lesions, 50–200 mm in diameter, and may have depigmentation around them (Fig. 11.2). Smaller, solitary, unilateral lesions may be seen in normal people, but it is rare for normal individuals to have more than three lesions. In FAP four or more CHRPEs are often present, characteristically large, oval, pigmented lesions with surrounding halo (type A lesions) which are specific for FAP; CHRPEs in controls are usually small dots (type B) (Olschwang et al. 1993). The larger lesions are probably congenital and appear to be choristomas of myelinated axons; the small lesions may show enlarged retinal pigment epithelial cells with increased pigment (Parker et al. 1990). There are interfamilial differences in predisposition to CHRPE in FAP, related to the position of the mutation in the *APC* gene, mutations distal to exon 9 being more prone to be associated with such lesions (Bunyan et al. 1995). However, there are exceptions to this (Pack et al. 1996), and there is intrafamilial variability in numbers of CHRPEs (Hodgson et al. 1994). Nevertheless, it has

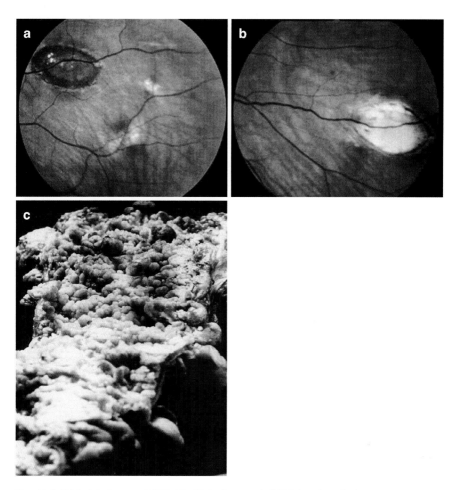

Fig. 11.2 FAP: (**a**) pigmented CHRPE, (**b**) depigmented CHRPE, and (**c**) florid colonic polyposis (Reproduced with permission from Cambridge University Press)

been estimated that in families in which CHRPEs appear to be a feature of the disease, the finding of fewer than three lesions in an individual at 50 % risk reduces the carrier risk, whereas the presence of more than three lesions conveys a very high probability that the individual is affected (Burn et al. 1991).

Frequency of Complications in FAP:

- Congenital hypertrophy of the retinal pigment epithelium (70–80 %)
- Thyroid cancer (2–3 %)
- Epidermoid cysts (50 %)
- Brain tumor (1 %)
- Osteoma (50–90 %)
- Hepatoblastoma (1 %)

- Desmoid tumor (10–15 %)
- Supernumerary teeth (11–27 %)
- Adrenal gland adenomas (7–13 %)

(Adapted from Vasen et al. 2009)

Desmoid disease is common in FAP, occurring in about 10–15 % of cases. It is nearly twice as common in females as in males and occurs at an earlier age in females (Brosens et al. 2005). Desmoids are more common in some families than in others, and this is related to the position of the germline APC mutation (mutations beyond codon 1444 being more likely to cause the disease). Histologically, they are composed of very vascular, fibrous tissue and may be diffuse or encapsulated. They occur predominantly in the small bowel mesentery, peritoneum, or abdominal wall, although they occasionally develop at extra-abdominal sites and often develop after a surgical procedure or pregnancy; 10 % resolve; 50 % may remain stable for prolonged periods; 30 % fluctuate; and 10 % grow rapidly. Desmoid tumors do not metastasize but do infiltrate locally and can cause major morbidity and death, being one of the most common causes of death in FAP. They tend to recur after surgery, so treatment with nonsteroidal anti-inflammatory drugs (sulindac), antiestrogens, or, in resistant cases, cytotoxic chemotherapy or radiotherapy with computerized tomography monitoring is preferable.

Extraintestinal cancers associated with FAP include papillary carcinoma of the thyroid, brain tumors (medulloblastoma, astrocytoma), and hepatoblastoma. Papillary carcinoma of the thyroid, characteristically the cribriform variant, appears to occur at increased frequency in young women (under 35 years of age) with FAP and in individuals with specific mutations in the APC gene, particularly at codon 1061 (Fenton et al. 2001). Brain tumors (especially astrocytomas) are rare overall, but the relative risk is high in individuals with FAP: 23 to age of 29 years for all brain tumors (7 for all ages) and 99 to age of 29 years for cerebellar medulloblastomas. Some cases of Turcot syndrome are a variant of FAP (see p. 311). A number of cases of hepatoblastoma have been described in children with FAP, and although the absolute risk is small, the relative risk is high (<500), and screening might be considered in high-risk families, although not usually performed (Hirschman et al. 2005).

Classically, the diagnosis of FAP is made clinically by the finding of more than 100 adenomatous polyps in the colon and rectum, with histological evidence of single crypt adenomas. However, there is a milder form of the disease, attenuated FAP (AFAP), characterized by the presence of fewer adenomas and later onset of disease, which is seen in about 8 % of cases. The differential diagnosis is from other causes of intestinal polyposis, most importantly MUTYH-associated polyposis (p. 287) and other causes of inherited bowel cancer, such as Lynch syndrome and individuals with germline mutations in *POLD1* and *POLE* (Palles et al. 2013). Individuals with AFAP usually have fewer than 100 adenomas, and such a phenotype may be caused by mutations in the first 4 exons of the *APC* gene (Olschwang et al. 1993; Knudsen et al. 2010) or by biallelic mutations in *MUTYH*. Biallelic germline *MUTYH* mutations have been assessed as causing 30 % of cases of >15 and <100 and 8 % classical polyposis with no APC mutation (Sieber et al. 2003a, b).

The FAP gene (*APC*) was localized to chromosome 5q21 following the report of a mentally retarded man who had Gardner syndrome and a constitutional deletion of chromosome 5q (Herera et al. 1986). Characterization of the mutation in the *APC* gene in an affected individual in the family (possible in >90 % cases) allows predictive testing to be made available to at-risk relatives. The gene is large and has 15 exons, of which exon 15 is the largest. Most mutations in FAP patients are frameshift (2/3) or nonsense (1/3) mutations which result in the production of a truncated protein (Nagase and Nakamura 1993). Many different mutations have been described, but there are common ones, at codons 1061, 1450, and 1309 in exon 15. The *APC* gene product functions as a tumor suppressor with subcellular location and interaction with catenins. It contains a number of coiled-coil heptad repeats at the 5' end that promote oligomerization; the central part of the gene contains beta-catenin-binding domains, involved in cell–cell interaction, and Armadillo repeats, and the 3' end contains tubulin-binding domains, with properties of binding to microtubules (Ilyas and Tomlinson 1997; Fodde et al. 2001).

Phenotype–genotype correlations are apparent (Stormorken et al. 2007), with the common mutations (1309 and 1061) being associated with a severe phenotype (Nugent et al. 1994), mutations before exon 9 usually being associated with a lack of CHRPE, and mutations in the first 6 exons being associated with a more variable and often milder phenotype, including "attenuated FAP" (Foulkes 1995). *APC* mutations found in "attenuated FAP" most commonly occur in exon 4, but many individuals with this "attenuated" form do not appear to have *APC* mutations; some may have MUTYH-associated polyposis. The observation that very short variant proteins may result in a less severe phenotype tends to support the "dominant negative" theory, but large deletions of the gene may be found in individuals with a severe phenotype, so that other factors including the loss of the mild APC mutant allele (Spirio et al. 1998) or the effects of other polymorphic alleles such at the *NAT1* and *NAT2* genes (Crabtree et al. 2004) may also be involved in the pathogenesis of the disease process.

Usually there is reasonable consistency with regard to severity of adenomatous disease in different individuals with FAP within a single family, but some exceptions to this have been reported, with very variable age at onset of polyps in different cases, some presenting decades later than their affected relatives (Evans et al. 1993).

The frequency of extracolonic features in FAP is associated with mutations in specific regions of the *APC* gene (Fig. 11.3).

The phenotypic effects of a germline *APC* mutation may be affected by FAP modifier genes which include *MOM* in mice and genes encoding DNA methyltransferase and COX-2 (Fearon 1997; Crabtree et al. 2002, 2003).

A polymorphism in the APC gene was detected in an individual with a family history of colorectal cancer but not polyposis. Subsequent analysis suggested that this germline T–A mutation, predicted to result in a change from isoleucine to lysine position 1307 of the protein, predisposed to the development of somatic mutations of the *APC* gene and that gene carriers were therefore predisposed to colorectal cancer without florid polyposis, with a twofold increase in risk of bowel cancer in mutation carriers (Rozen et al. 2002). The mechanism for this at a molecular level appears to be that the polymorphism which converts an AAATAAAA sequence to (A)8 predisposes to the development of somatic mutations in the *APC* gene. This mutation is almost entirely restricted to the Ashkenazim (about 6 % of the Ashkenazi population probably carry this variant) (Laken et al. 1997), and there has been much debate about whether population screening for this mutation should be advocated in Ashkenazim, with colonoscopic

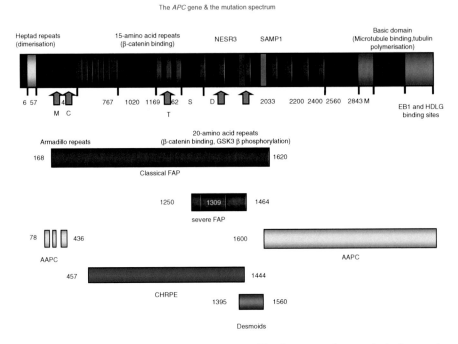

Fig. 11.3 The APC gene and the mutation spectrum The frequency of extracolonic features in FAP is associated with mutations in specific regions of the APC gene (With permission from Ian Tomlinson) *AAPC* attenuated FAP, T thyroid cancer

surveillance for gene carriers. Currently the increase in risk is not thought to be sufficient for such a measure to be appropriate. Other germline variants such as E1317Q may be associated with an attenuated phenotype (Lamlum et al. 2000), but the evidence for this is less clear (Hahnloser et al. 2003), and recent data suggest that there is no increased colorectal neoplasia risk in carriers of this variant (Theodoratou et al. 2008).

Management

Surveillance of the colorectum in patients at risk of FAP should begin before the age of 20 years; the risk of developing colorectal cancer before this age is very low, but some affected individuals do develop severe polyposis before the age of 10 years, so endoscopic surveillance should be commenced between 11 and 15 years, earlier if symptoms related to colonic problems occur beforehand (Vasen et al. 2008). Flexible sigmoidoscopy is probably sufficient before the age of 20 years as the polyps almost invariably develop in the distal colon initially, but colonoscopy should be performed annually from 20 years until florid polyposis develops.

Patients with FAP should be offered total colectomy with ileorectal anastomosis or proctocolectomy with restorative ileoanal anastomosis once colonic polyps have developed (Church 2006). The risk of colorectal cancer is significant once polyps have begun to develop, irrespective of polyp density (Phillips and Spigelman 1996). After surgery conserving the rectal stump, subsequent management should include lifelong surveillance of the rectal stump by yearly sigmoidoscopy as there is a 3.5 % risk of colorectal cancer in it after 5 years, rising to 10 % at 10 years. Proctocolectomy removes this risk and may be done after 50 years of age. In addition, since upper GI cancer is reported to occur in 5 % of patients, with an estimated prevalence of duo-denal dysplasia of up to 90 %, initial surveillance by means of upper GI endoscopy with a side-viewing endoscope to allow detailed examination of the papilla, or a forward-viewing endoscope in early Spigelman stage cases, recommended to start at about 25 years of age, to give a baseline for subsequent follow-up (Arvanitis et al. 1990; Debinski et al. 1995; Theodoratu et al. 2008) (Fig. 11.4). If adenomas are detected, they should be biopsied; larger adenomas may be removed and further surveillance continued with 1–5-yearly duodenoscopy, depending on the Spigelman severity score (Dunlop 2002; Vasen et al. 2008). Duodenal cancer in FAP patients below 30 years of age is extremely rare, and the overall risk of duodenal cancer is small (5 %), but with a Spigelman stage lll–lV, the risk of cancer is 7–36 %.

Palpation of the thyroid gland and possibly ultrasound in young women with FAP have been suggested, but the rarity of death from thyroid cancer in this disease makes this of questionable benefit unless there is a family history of thyroid cancer, and this is not usually performed.

Relatives of affected individuals should be ascertained with the help of a genetic register, and those at risk of inheriting the disease should be offered screening and genetic testing if possible. Screening of at-risk relatives is commenced between the ages of 11 and 13 years by annual sigmoidoscopy because the rectum is involved by adenomas at an early stage, and polyps rarely develop before 11 years of age. However, if symptoms arise, it may be necessary to arrange endoscopy earlier because there are case reports of colonic polyps developing in young children (Distante et al. 1996). Where the APC mutation has been characterized, predictive testing may be offered to children in the family, and once a child has been found to carry the APC mutation in the family, it is appropriate to consider colonoscopy in their early teens to establish the extent of polyposis. In an at-risk child where a pre-dictive genetic test is not available, if polyps are found, these are biopsied (to confirm they are adenomatous and to exclude malignancy) and colonoscopy is arranged. Although small numbers of polyps can be managed by endoscopic resection, because of the inevitability of florid polyposis developing and the risk of malignant change, definitive surgery (see above) is usually arranged at this stage. In the absence of posi-tive findings, sigmoidoscopy is continued annually, with colonoscopies with dye spray after 20 years of age, to exclude more proximal polyposis. This is continued to at least the age of 40 years, by which time the risk to an individual with an affected parent has fallen below 1 % (see Fig. 11.1). However, since very variable age at onset has been described in some families, it is advisable to continue screening well beyond this age (Evans et al. 1993). Endoscopic surveillance should also be offered to indi-viduals with attenuated polyposis and their close relatives (Heiskanen et al. 2000), with colonoscopic surveillance 2-yearly from age 18–20 years, and upper GI surveil-lance as for classical FAP (Debinsky et al. 1995; Vasen et al. 2008). If colectomy is necessary, ileorectal anastomosis should be offered; since the risk of duodenal cancer is also present, upper GI surveillance should also be recommended as above.

Spigelman Score of Duodenal Polyposis

criterion	1 point	2 points	3 points
Polyp number	1–4	5–20	>20
Polyp size (mm)	1–4	5–10	>10
Histology Dysplasia	Tubular Mild	Tubulovill. Moderate	Villous Severe

Fig. 11.4 Spigelman score of duodenal polyposis

Predictive testing based on mutation analysis may be available, and individuals who have not inherited the mutation can be discharged from follow-up. A more cautious approach to management is indicated where the predictive test was based upon linkage analysis, surveillance being indicated until the estimated chance that the individual is affected is calculated as below 0.1 % on Bayesian risk analysis combining clinical and molecular data. Prenatal diagnosis is available by mutation or linkage analysis in informative families, although the uptake rate is low. The acceptability of such testing in a disorder such as FAP is a very personal matter, and the decision about whether to opt for such testing should be one made by the family after nondirective genetic counseling. Many parents wish their children to be tested for FAP at a very young age, but there are arguments for delaying such testing until clinical screening would normally be instituted, since, until this time, clinical management would not be affected (Hyer and Fell 2001).

The effectiveness of intervention strategies, such as the administration of aspirin, are being evaluated (Mathers et al. 2003), but are not sufficient to obviate the need for colectomy in affected individuals once polyps have developed. In FAP, the CAPP1 study showed that aspirin had a modest effect on polyp progression and significantly reduced the size of the largest polyps in 200 FAP patients, but no effect on polyp number (Burn et al. 2011). There has been some evidence that the administration of oral sulindac (a nonsteroidal anti-inflammatory drug) or cyclo-oxygenase-2 (COX-2) inhibitors in general may cause regression of duodenal adenomas (Phillips et al. 2002). Carcinoma of the rectal stump may occur (in about 10 % of cases) after surgical removal of the colon and ileorectal anastomosis, and COX-2 inhibitors may also be effective in reducing polyp recurrence in the colorectum (Steinbach et al. 2000), but these have been shown to increase cardiovascular morbidity in the VICTOR and APPROVE research studies and are therefore not recommended – but there is a delayed effect on colorectal cancer incidence, as seen in the CAPP2 study. Fish oils have long been thought to be protective against GI cancers, and a special formulation of eicosapentaenoic acid (EPA) was able to reduce polyp number and size (West et al. 2010).

Fanconi Anemia (OMIM 227650)

Fanconi anemia (FA) is an autosomal recessive chromosomal instability disorder which is characterized by congenital abnormalities, defective hemopoiesis and a high risk of developing AML and certain solid tumors. The birth incidence of FA is around 3 per million. Affected individuals can have mild growth retardation (63 %), and median height of FA individuals lies around the 5th centile. Other clinical features include areas of skin hyper- and hypopigmentation (64 %), skeletal defects (75 %) including radial limb defects (absent thumb with or without radial aplasia), abnormalities of ribs and hips, scoliosis, and cardiac (13 %) and renal (34 %) malformations. Other associated anomalies include microphthalmia (38 %) and developmental delay (16 %). The phenotypic abnormalities are variable and there is marked variability between affected individuals in the same sibship. Importantly, up to one-third of FA cases do not have any obvious congenital abnormalities and are only diagnosed when another sibling is affected or when they develop a hematological problem. However, most FA cases do have some subtle clinical features, such as dermatological manifestations.

The pancytopenia usually develops between the ages of 5 and 9 years (median age 7 years), and symptoms due to this develop progressively. The cumulative incidence of any hematological abnormality in FA is up to 90 %, and the cumulative incidence of leukemia is around 10 % by age of 25 years. The crude risk (irrespective of age) for MDS is around 5 % and for leukemia is 5–10 % (Alter et al. 2003). FA patients that survive into early adulthood are around 50 times more likely to develop solid tumors compared to the general population, and in one study 29 % developed a solid tumor by the age of 48 years (Rosenberg et al. 2003). In particular, there is a high risk of hepatic tumors (which may be related to androgen use) but also squamous cell carcinomas of the esophagus, oropharynx, and vulva (Alter 2003; Rosenberg et al. 2003).

The hallmark feature of FA cells is chromosomal hypersensitivity to DNA cross-linking agents such as mitomycin C (MMC) or diepoxybutane (DEB), and the resulting increase in chromosome breakage provides the basis for a diagnostic test (Auerbach 1993). The characteristic chromosomal findings are excess tri- and quadriradial and complex interchanges. The basic defect appears to be a deficiency of the repair of DNA strand cross-links. The relationship between the DNA repair defects and chromosomal aberrations found in this condition and the susceptibility to cancer is not fully understood; an increased mutation rate or incidence of tumor-promoting translocations may be a factor.

There is some evidence that heterozygotes for FA have an increased risk of certain cancers, especially leukemia and gastric and colonic cancers, with a relative risk of 3 reported, but this did not reach statistical significance (Swift et al. 1980; reviewed in Tischkowitz and Hodgson 2003). A separate study of 125 relatives of FA patients failed to reproduce these observations (Potter et al. 1983), and a more recent study of 36 UK families also found no excess of cancers in relatives of FA cases (OR 0.97, $P=0.62$) (Tischkowitz et al. 2008). Chromosome breakage testing in FA heterozygotes is complicated by overlap with the normal range (Pearson et al. 2001). Prenatal diagnosis has been achieved by demonstrating increased spontaneous and induced chromosome breakage in fetal cells (cultured amniocytes or chorionic villus cells) (Auerbach et al. 1985).

Sixteen FA genes have been identified since 1992 (see Fig. 11.5). *FANCA* mutations account for almost two-thirds of cases, *FANCC* and *G* for 25 %, and *FANCE* and *FANCF* for a further 8 %. There are only a handful of FA cases that have not yet been genetically diagnosed. Diagnosis by direct mutation detection is available. Molecular studies have established that a common pathway exists, both between the FA proteins and other proteins involved in DNA damage repair, such as *NBS1*, *ATM*, *BRCA1*, and *BRCA2* (reviewed in Venkitaraman 2004).

FANCD1 has been shown to be *BRCA2* (Howlett et al. 2002). FA cases due to biallelic *BRCA2* mutations are rare but seem to be associated with an increased risk of medulloblastoma or Wilms tumor that may precede development of aplastic anemia (Hirsch et al. 2004; Offit et al. 2003) or an earlier onset of leukemia (Wagner et al. 2004). A family history of breast or ovarian cancer might provide clues in these cases. At present it is not known whether such cases should have intensive screening for solid tumors or whether they would benefit from more aggressive treatment with earlier stem cell transplants. The finding that FA can be caused by biallelic *BRCA2* mutations should be taken into account when counseling *BRCA2* mutation carriers, although interestingly no homozygosity for some frequent mutations, such as 6174delT, has been identified.

Perhaps not surprisingly, *PALB2* (partner and localizer of *BRCA2*) has also been found to be a FA gene (*FANCN*, arrow on figure), and like *BRCA2/FANCD1*, children with biallelic *PALB2/FANCN* mutations tend to have more serious cancer-related phenotypes, with early-onset Wilms Tumor, acute myeloid leukemia, and medulloblastomas predominant (Reid et al. 2007; Xia et al. 2007; Tischkowitz and Xia 2010). The *BRCA1* partner, *BRIP1* (also known as *BACH1*), is also a FA gene – *FANCJ* (Levran et al. 2005; Levitus et al. 2005). Notably, children with FA type J tend to develop solid tumors, rather than the leukemia seen with *FANCD1/BRCA2* and *FANCN/PALB2*.

Continuing the DNA damage repair/cancer/FA theme, a handful of children with FA or FA-like disorders have been found to carry biallelic mutations in *XRCC2* (Shamseldin et al. 2012) or *RAD51C* (Vaz et al. 2010). In contrast to the genes mentioned above, cancer has yet been noted in these children. Interestingly, while

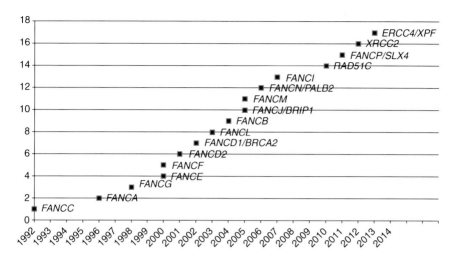

Fig. 11.5 Tempo of discovery of 16 FA genes (Figure courtesy of Marc Tischkowitz MD, PhD)

some data have suggested that monoallelic *XRCC2* mutations seem to moderately increase the risk for breast cancer (Park et al. 2012), monoallelic *RAD51C* mutations predispose to ovarian cancer only (Meindl et al. 2010; Loveday et al. 2011).

Until recently it was thought that biallelic *BRCA1* mutations were embryonic lethal, but such a case has now been described in an individual who had short stature, microcephaly, developmental delay and was diagnosed with ovarian carcinoma at age 28 (Domchek et al. 2013). She was found to have one allele with a *BRCA1* c.2457delC (p.Asp821Ilefs*25) truncating mutation, and a hypomorphic c.5207T>C missense mutation (p.Val1736Ala) on the other allele. This possibly unique combination of clinical features resemble FA, but are likely distinct from it. Unfortunately DEB testing was not carried out and cannot be done as the patient has died.

At diagnosis patients should have a full hematological assessment that should include examination of the bone marrow; HLA typing in anticipation of possible bone marrow transplantation should be performed. Other investigations at presentation should include audiometry, ultrasound of the renal tract, an endocrine assessment, especially if there is evidence of growth failure, and an ophthalmology assessment. Referral to hand surgeons and plastic surgeons may be indicated to consider correction of radial ray defects with a view to improving function and appearance. It is important that siblings are also tested as they may not have any congenital abnormalities.

If there is no hemopoietic defect at time of diagnosis, hematological monitoring may only be required once per year, but as the patient becomes older and develops hematological complications, hematologists play an increasingly central role. Many patients who develop bone marrow failure initially respond to treatment with androgens and hemopoietic growth factors. Eventually most patients become refractory to these therapies, and the definitive treatment currently available for bone marrow failure is hemopoietic stem cell transplantation.

Frasier Syndrome (OMIM 136680)

This disorder is caused by mutations in the *WT1* gene and so is allelic with Denys–Drash syndrome. It is characterized by male pseudohermaphroditism, streak gonads, and steroid-resistant nephritic syndrome and renal failure from focal and segmental glomerulosclerosis, but although gonadoblastoma is frequent, the risk of Wilms tumor is much less, and the glomerulopathy progresses more slowly than in Denys–Drash syndrome. The risk of Wilms tumor has been estimated at 5–10 % risk, and affected children should also be offered surveillance by 3–4-monthly renal ultrasonography (Scott et al. 2006). The *WT1* intron 9 splicing mutations that cause Frasier syndrome alter the balance of WT1 isoforms (Klamt et al. 1998) and cause Frasier syndrome if the karyotype is 46,XY and isolated nephrotic syndrome if the karyotype is 46,XX (Chernin et al. 2010).

Gorlin Syndrome (Nevoid Basal Cell Carcinoma Syndrome) (OMIM 109400)

This is an autosomal dominant condition with a minimal prevalence of 1 in 70,000 of the population. The main features of this syndrome are multiple basal cell carcinomas (BCC) of the skin (most common in sun-exposed areas) and palmar and plantar pits (occurring in 65 % of cases) (see Fig. 11.6a). The basal cell skin lesions arise as pink or brown papules from the age of puberty onwards. Only 15 % manifest before puberty, and 10 % or more of patients have no skin lesions at the age of 30 years. They mainly affect the thorax, neck, and face. UV light increases the incidence of the BCC; they are more common in white-skinned patients, and therapeutic radiation is often associated with progression of BCC that is present within the radiation field. Only a small proportion of carcinomas become locally invasive, but they can cause severe destruction, particularly around the eyes and orifices. Metastasis is very rare. There are many associated non-dermatological features, including hypertelorism with a broad nasal bridge and frontal and parietal bossing and a prominent chin. Odontogenic keratocysts of the jaw are common (see Fig. 11.6b). These are multiple, usually bilateral, recurrent, and slow growing and occur in 85 % of mutation carriers by the age of 40 years. Squamous cell carcinomas have been reported within keratocysts in patients with Gorlin syndrome who have been treated by radiotherapy for facial BCC (Moos and Rennie 1987). Variable skeletal abnormalities are associated, including "bridging" of the sella with calcification of the falx cerebri (see Fig. 11.6c); bifid (usually third, fourth, or fifth), absent, or rudimentary ribs fusion defects of the cervical spine; polydactyly or syndactyly, short fourth metacarpals, flame-shaped lucencies of the metacarpals and/or phalanges, and Sprengel deformity. Ocular abnormalities have been reported, including exotropia, chalazia and coloboma, and congenital blindness. All except the skeletal features increase with age, but there is considerable variability of expression of these features in different affected people

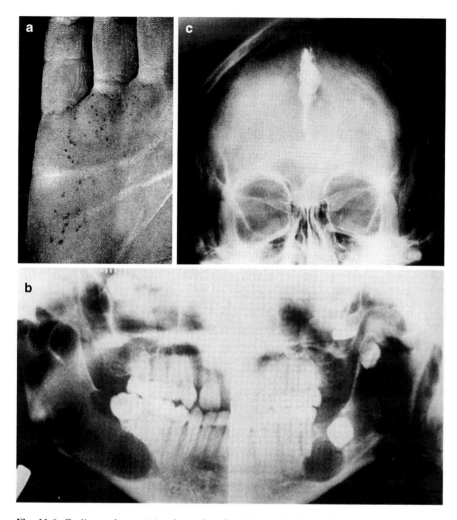

Fig. 11.6 Gorlin syndrome: (**a**) palmar pits, (**b**) odontogenic keratocyles and (**c**) calcified falx cerebri (courtesy of Robert Gorlin). Reproduced with permission from Cambridge University Press

(Gorlin 1987, 1995). The condition is inherited as an autosomal dominant trait with almost complete penetrance but highly variable expression. Diagnostic features are described in Table 11.3.

A variety of other, less common, abnormalities have been noted in affected people, including milia, epidermoid cysts, chalazia and comedones of the skin, cleft lip and palate, pectus carinatum, and hypogonadotropic hypogonadism in males. Hamartomatous upper GI polyposis has also been reported (Schwartz 1978). There is a definite increase in incidence of non-dermatological malignancies, including squamous cell carcinoma and fibrosarcoma in the jaw cysts, and nasopharyngeal carcinomas. Mental retardation has been reported in about 3 % of cases, but its true

Table 11.3 Diagnostic criteria for Gorlin syndrome (Evans et al. 1993)

Major criteria
More than two BCCs or one BCC under 20 years at diagnosis
Histologically proven odontogenic keratocysts of the jaw
Three or more cutaneous palmar or plantar pits
Bifid, fused, or markedly splayed ribs
First-degree relative with Gorlin syndrome
Minor criteria
Height-adjusted macrocephaly
One of the following orofacial characteristics: cleft lip or palate, frontal bossing, coarse face, moderate or severe hypertelorism
One of the following skeletal abnormalities: Sprengel, pectus excavatum (marked), severe syndactyly
One of the following radiological features: bridging of the sella turcica, hemi-/fused/elongated vertebral bodies, modeling defects and flame-shaped lucencies of the hands and feet
Ovarian fibroma, medulloblastoma
The diagnosis requires the presence of two major or one major and one minor features

Reproduced from X with permission from X – author to insert credit line at proof stage

incidence is unclear. Detailed CT and MRI have revealed a high incidence of asymmetric or dilated ventricles in 24 %, and one in ten individuals has dysgenesis or agenesis of the corpus callosum (Kimonis et al. 2004). Childhood medulloblastoma may occur in the first 2 years of life, and meningioma and craniopharyngioma have been described. Bilateral ovarian fibromas (which can be hormonally active) are common in affected women, and there is a risk of ovarian fibrosarcoma or other malignancy developing in these lesions (Ismail and Walker 1990).

Seminoma has been reported in males. Cardiac fibromas may occur from early childhood; these may remain static or possibly regress or enlarge with age. Other tumors that have been described in association with Gorlin syndrome include renal fibroma, melanoma, neurofibroma, leiomyoma, and rhabdomyoma/sarcoma. Mesenteric lymphatic or chylous cysts may occur.

Surveillance of affected people should consist of yearly dermatological examinations and 6-monthly evaluation of the jaw cysts by means of an oropantogram, since odontogenic cysts can erode locally and be very destructive, and early enucleation of these cysts can prevent this. Infants should be kept under surveillance for signs of medulloblastoma, and some have recommended 6-monthly MRI until the age of 7 years (after which the risk declines significantly) (Kimonis et al. 2004). Cranial ultrasound may also be a useful investigation because care should be taken to restrict exposure to radiation to a minimum in view of the extreme radiation sensitivity in this condition. Pelvic ultrasound scanning may detect ovarian tumors, but in view of the low incidence of this complication, regular scanning is generally not advised.

Genetic counseling should be facilitated by molecular genetic analysis. Affected children may show few features. However, if at the age of 5 years an at-risk child has no abnormality on X-ray of spine or skull and has no osteomas or dermatological lesions, the risk of the child being a gene carrier is very small (Farndon et al. 1992).

Gorlin syndrome is caused by mutations in the human homologue (*PTCH*) of the *Drosophila* segment polarity gene *patched* which maps to chromosome 9q (Hahn et al. 1996; Johnson et al. 1996). There is no evidence of locus heterogeneity in Gorlin syndrome, and most reported mutations are predicted to cause protein truncation. No genotype–phenotype relationships have been identified (Wicking et al. 1997). *PTCH* encodes a transmembrane glycoprotein that acts as an antagonist in the Hedgehog signaling pathway. *PTCH* inhibits smoothened (SMO), which in turn activates transcription factors in the *Wnt* and decapentaplegic pathways. It appears likely that some manifestations of Gorlin syndrome (e.g., symmetrical developmental defects, such as macrocephaly) result from haploinsufficiency but that basal cell carcinomas and other tumors require inactivation of both alleles in a two-step mechanism of tumorigenesis (Levanat et al. 1996). Interestingly, too much activity in the Hedgehog pathway leads to Gorlin syndrome with the associated cancer risk, whereas underactivity causes holoprosencephaly (Roessler et al. 1997; Odent et al. 1999).

Hemihypertrophy/Hemihyperplasia

Isolated hemihypertrophy/hemihyperplasia (IH) refers to asymmetric regional body overgrowth secondary to abnormal cell proliferation in individuals without any other underlying diagnosis. IH should be distinguished from hemiatrophy and from asymmetrical overgrowth that can be associated with Beckwith–Wiedemann syndrome (BWS), proteus syndrome, neurofibromatosis type 1, mosaic trisomy 8, and disorders associated with vascular malformations such as Klippel–Trenaunay syndrome. IH may be associated with a significant risk of learning disability, genitourinary abnormalities, and neoplasia (Viljeon et al. 1984). The most frequently associated neoplasm is Wilms tumor, but there are also reported associations with adrenal cortical tumors and hepatoblastoma (Viljeon et al. 1984). Estimates of the tumor risks associated with IH are variable (e.g., risk of Wilms tumor 1 to 3 % (Viljeon et al. 1984; Dempsey-Robertson et al. 2012)) and may be influenced by ascertainment bias. In a prospective study of 168 children for 10 years, the tumor incidence was ~6 % (6 Wilms and 2 adrenal cortical carcinomas out of the total of 10 tumors) (Hoyme et al. 1998).

There is overlap between the molecular abnormalities described in BWS (e.g., paternal uniparental disomy for chromosome 11p15.5, imprinting center 1 epimutations) and those detectable in a subset of patients with IH (Grundy et al. 1991). However, it has been suggested that the results of such testing cannot reliably distinguish between those children who will and will not develop an embryonal tumor and that tumor surveillance (abdominal ultrasound every 3 months until 7 years and serum alpha-fetoprotein measurement every 3 months until 4 years) should be offered to all children with IH (Clericuzio and Martin 2009). In contrast, Scott et al. (2006) recommended that abdominal ultrasound screening should only be offered to children with hemihypertrophy with paternal uniparental disomy 11p15 or isolated *H19* hypermethylation.

Hereditary Non-polyposis Colorectal Cancer, Lynch Syndrome (OMIM 120435)

This condition is commonly abbreviated as HNPCC and now preferably termed Lynch syndrome.

Background: History and Epidemiology

Lynch et al. (1985) delineated two disorders characterized by an autosomal dominantly inherited predisposition to colon cancer without florid polyposis. These disorders, "Lynch syndromes I and II" (the latter reserved for families with extracolonic cancers), are not distinct entities (Lynch et al. 1993). Paradoxically, in some "HNPCC" pedigrees, colorectal cancer is absent and led to the reintroduction of the term "Lynch syndrome" to describe this condition (Umar et al. 2004a). The condition is due to inherited changes in the DNA mismatch repair (MMR) genes, most commonly *MLH1*, *MSH2*, and *MSH6* and less frequently *PMS2*. Early studies suggested that in most affected individuals, there is a high risk of colon cancer, up to 80 % lifetime risk, somewhat lower in females (40 %) than in males (Dunlop et al. 1997), with an early age at diagnosis of colon cancer (40–50 years compared with 60–70 years in the general population), a preponderance of right-sided tumors (60–70 % versus 15 %), and susceptibility to multiple primary cancers (25 % versus 5 %) and metachronous cancers (23 %) (Lynch and de la Chapelle 1999), and about 5 % of colorectal cancers occur before 30 years of age (Vasen et al. 2001).

In individuals with Lynch syndrome, there is a predisposition to a variety of extracolonic cancers, most commonly endometrial but also ovarian, gastric, pancreatic, hepatobiliary tract, urothelial, and small intestine (Watson and Lynch 2001). Estimates of the cumulative lifetime risks of the various cancer types in gene mutation carriers are 28–78 % for colorectal cancer in males (24–52 % in females), 27–72 % for endometrial cancer in women, 19 % for gastric cancer, 18 % for biliary tract cancer, 1–12 % for urinary tract cancer and 3–13 % for ovarian cancer in women, and with a 1–4 % risk of brain tumors and 4–7 % risk of small bowel tumors, representing a significantly increased relative risk for these tumor types (reviewed in Vasen et al. 2007). The estimated cumulative risks of colorectal cancer by age 70 years in individuals with Lynch syndrome have been reported as 41 % (95 % confidence intervals [CI], 25–70 %) for *MLH1* mutation carriers, 48 % (95 % CI, 30–77 %) for *MSH2*, and 12 % (95 % CI, 8–22 %) for *MSH6*. For endometrial cancer, corresponding risks were 54 % (95 % CI, 20–80 %), 21 % (95 % CI, 8–77 %), and 16 % (95 % CI, 8–32 %). For ovarian cancer, they were 20 % (95 % CI, 1–65 %), 24 % (95 % CI, 3–52 %), and 1 % (95 % CI, 0–3 %). The estimated cumulative risks by age 40 years did not exceed 2 % (95 % CI, 0–7 %) for endometrial cancer or 1 % (95 % CI, 0–3 %) for ovarian cancer. The estimated lifetime risks for other tumor types did not exceed 3 % with any of the gene mutations (Bonadona et al. 2011; Aarnio et al. 1995, 1999; Barrow et al. 2013). These risks are lower than those published previously.

The estimated relative risks for extracolonic cancer vary with different germline mutations: those for small intestinal cancer are 291 for *MLH1* mutation carriers and 102 for *MSH2* mutation carriers; for gastric cancer 4 and 19, respectively; for ovarian cancer 6 and 8, respectively; and for urinary tract cancer 75 in *MSH2* mutation carriers only (Vasen et al. 2001). Overall, *MSH2* mutations appear to confer a higher risk of cancer than *MLH1* mutations, mainly due to an increased risk of urinary tract and endometrial cancers in *MSH2* mutation carriers. *MSH6* mutations are associated with less of a risk of colorectal cancer but an increased risk of endometrial and, to a lesser extent, urothelial cancer (Wijnen et al. 1999; Vasen et al. 2001).

Clinical Features and Pathology

Florid polyposis does not occur in Lynch syndrome, but colonic adenomas (particularly right sided) have been reported to be more common than in controls: 30 % of Lynch syndrome patients have at least one colonic adenoma, and 20 % have multiple lesions, compared with 11 and 4 % in age- and sex-matched controls (Lanspa et al. 1990; Gaglia et al. 1995). Other studies have, however, suggested that the prevalence of adenomas is not greatly increased, but they develop more rapidly through the adenoma–carcinoma sequence in this disease (Jass 1995). If multiple adenomas do occur, it is very rare to find more than 50, which differentiates Lynch syndrome from FAP, in which characteristically there are more than 100 polyps. A subgroup of patients with Lynch syndrome develop flat adenomas (slightly elevated lesions with adenomatous changes confined to the colonic crypts) (Lynch et al. 1990a, b, c), although it is not clear that this subset can be distinguished by molecular means.

The MMR defect results in instability of microsatellite DNA in the tumors, causing microsatellite instability (MSI) in over 90 % tumors in Lynch syndrome compared with 15 % in sporadic tumors.

The pathology of colorectal cancers in Lynch syndrome is notable for a slight overrepresentation of mucinous carcinomas, mainly well differentiated and rarely of the signet-ring cell type, with a medullary pattern in about 9 % of cases. Lymphocytic infiltration and tumor budding with de-differentiation are more common in Lynch syndrome than in sporadic cancers, and in Lynch syndrome, there are characteristically more *APC*, *CTNNB1*, and *KRAS* mutations than in sporadic cancers, whereas DNA methylation and *BRAF* mutations are rare (Jass 2004). Interestingly, a higher level of antibody reactivity against such frameshift peptides (FSPs) can be demonstrated in patients with microsatellite unstable Lynch syndrome and healthy MMR mutation carriers than in controls, indicating that these FSPs are recognized by the patients' T cells. This may account for the observed high levels of inflammatory response with lymphocyte infiltration in tumors in individuals with Lynch syndrome.

The dermatological features of Muir–Torre syndrome (Smyrk et al. 2001) with sebaceous adenomas and carcinomas may occur occasionally in individuals with Lynch syndrome, but genotype–phenotype correlations are not evident, beyond the observation that *MSH2* mutations are more likely to cause this than *MLH1* (Lucci-Cordisco et al. 2003).

Turcot syndrome is defined as the co-occurrence of colorectal polyps and brain tumors (see p. 311). This can be caused by germline mutations in the *APC* gene or germline mutations in one of the MMR genes. Some children have been described with adenomatous colonic polyps, primary brain tumors, leukemia, and café-au-lait skin patches, with an autosomal recessive inheritance pattern, and the condition has been shown to be due to homozygosity or compound heterozygosity for mutations in the MMR genes *MLH1*, *MSH2*, *MSH6* or *PMS2* (Ricciardone et al. 1999; Whiteside et al. 2002; Menko et al. 2004, reviewed in Bandipalliam 2005) (see p. 232).

There is evidence that colorectal cancers exhibiting MSI have a better survival than those that do not (Bubb et al. 1996; Gryfe et al. 2000), and this may also be true for those with Lynch syndrome (Sankila et al. 1996; Watson et al. 1998), although this has been disputed (Farrington et al. 2002; Clark et al. 2004).

Diagnostic Features

For practical purposes, and for research, criteria for the diagnosis of Lynch syndrome known as the Amsterdam criteria were drawn up in 1991 (see Table 11.4).

Table 11.4 The original Amsterdam criteria: AC1

1. At least three relatives (all related to each other) affected by colorectal cancer, one a first-degree relative of the other two
2. At least two successive generations affected
3. Colorectal cancer diagnosed before 50 years of age in one relative
4. Familial adenomatous polyposis excluded

Vasen et al. (1991); Reproduced with permission from Dr. H. Vasen

Table 11.5 The revised Amsterdam criteria: AC2

1. At least three relatives (all related to each other) affected by a Lynch syndrome-related cancer,[a] one a first-degree relative of the other two
2. At least two successive generations affected
3. Lynch syndrome-related cancer diagnosed before 50 years of age in one relative
4. Familial adenomatous polyposis excluded

Vasen et al. (1999); Reproduced with permission from Dr. H. Vasen
[a]The only cancers permitted are colorectal carcinoma, endometrial adenocarcinoma, small intestinal adenocarcinoma, transitional cell carcinoma of the renal pelvis, and transitional cell carcinoma of the ureter

Table 11.6 The revised Bethesda guidelines

Tumors from individuals should be tested for MSI in the following situations
1. Colorectal cancer diagnosed in a patient who is less than 50 years of age
2. Presence of synchronous, metachronous colorectal, or other Lynch syndrome-associated, tumors, regardless of age
3. Colorectal cancer with the MSI-H histology (such as tumor-infiltrating lymphocytes, Crohn's-like lymphocytic reaction, mucinous/signet-ring differentiation, or medullary growth pattern) diagnosed in a patient who is less than 60 years of age
4. Colorectal cancer diagnosed in one or more first-degree relatives with a Lynch syndrome-related tumor, with one of the cancers being diagnosed under age 50 years
5. Col orectal cancer diagnosed in two or more first- or second-degree relatives with Lynch syndrome-related tumors, regardless of age

Adapted from Umar et al. (2004a, b)

Subsequently, because of the increased relative risk for the related tumors referred to above, the occurrence of an endometrial or upper GI carcinoma in a young individual in such a family was included to indicate affected status with regard to Lynch syndrome (Amsterdam 2 (AC2) criteria; Vasen et al. 1999; Aarnio et al. 1995, 1999) (see Table 11.5).

The seven-point Bethesda guidelines were introduced to increase the sensitivity of diagnosis, identifying 94 % of patients with a pathogenic mutation, but with low specificity (25 %) (Rodriguez-Bigas et al. 1997). These guidelines were introduced initially to indicate who might benefit from MSI analysis, not to replace the Amsterdam criteria, which was originally designed to identify families most likely to carry mutations in the causative genes. On the basis of further research into the sensitivity and specificity of the original guidelines, they have recently been changed, simplified, and in some ways made broader (Umar et al. 2004a). These guidelines differ from the original in that fulfilling the Amsterdam criteria is no longer included, the presence of colonic adenomas alone is not sufficient for inclusion, and the age at diagnosis for inclusion has been (Table 11.6).

A logistic model that takes into account various clinical parameters of the family has been proposed to estimate the probability of a mutation being present in *MLH1* or *MSH2* (Wijnen et al. 1998). One study showed that in a high-risk clinical setting, virtually all *MLH1* and *MSH2* mutation carriers can be identified by applying only the first 3 of the original 7 Bethesda guidelines; on the other hand, the specificity is substantially reduced (Syngal et al. 2000). However, *MSH6* mutation carriers tend to be diagnosed with cancer at a later age than individuals with inherited mutations in *MLH1* and *MSH2* (median 66 years at diagnosis) and are more often rectal in site (Klarsov et al. 2011); they are less likely to be diagnosed using the above criteria. Studies in the population have indicated that identifying all mutation carriers using family history alone is not possible (Aaltonen et al. 1998). Other models (such as the so-called "Amsterdam-Plus" model) have tried to improve on previous models by including additional information such as the number of family members with one or more adenoma or double primary cancers (Lipton et al. 2004). Further improvements incorporating molecular markers found in the cancers may soon be possible, and there is an argument for looking for microsatellite instability (MSI) or immunohistochemical staining for the MMR proteins in all colorectal cancers in individuals affected below a certain cutoff age, such as 60 years. A series of recommendations have been established for the process of evaluation of at-risk patients; see below (Wijnen et al. 1997; Vasen et al. 1989, 1995).

Recommendations for the process of molecular evaluation of patients identified as being at risk, based on meeting the Bethesda guidelines (adapted from Umar et al. 2004a) modified recently, suggest doing immunohistochemical staining (IHC) first, using four antibodies in patients with family histories conforming to criteria for Lynch syndrome, but doing MSI analysis first in families with a less strong family history (Vasen et al. 2007). This is because MSI is very sensitive (almost 100 %), but although less sensitive, immunohistochemistry (IHC) can indicate the gene to test for germline mutations. False positives with IHC may occur and are probably due to the antibody detecting a truncated form of the protein. MSH6 staining is usually absent in cases due to a *MSH2* mutation (although the reverse is not observed) and is not always abnormal in tumors arising in *MSH6* mutation carriers (Berends et al. 2002). Tumors in individuals with Lynch syndrome characteristically demonstrate MSI, but this may also occur in 15 % of all colorectal cancers. Testing the tumor for MSI using a panel of microsatellites (BAT 25, BAT 26, and three others) helps to identify tumors from individuals with an increased likelihood of having Lynch syndrome (Boland et al. 1998), but as more microsatellites are used, the number of MSI-high tumors increases, and the test becomes less specific for Lynch Syndrome (Laiho et al. 2002; Reyes et al. 2002). The yield of mutations (positive predictive value) in families meeting the Amsterdam criteria is about 50 % and sensitivity 40 %, while the yield in families meeting the Bethesda criteria is 10–20 % and the sensitivity is about 90 %.

MLH1 methylation is common (86 %) in MSI-high tumors from non-Lynch syndrome subjects (de la Chapelle 2004), so lack of such methylation makes Lynch syndrome more likely. *BRAF* mutations are rarely seen in Lynch syndrome-related cancers, and their presence in a colorectal cancer occurring in a hereditary colorectal cancer family makes a MMR gene mutation unlikely (Wang et al. 2003a, b). Taken together, these observations suggest that pathological analysis of colorectal cancers can considerably simplify germline mutation analysis in hereditary colorectal cancer families:

1. The optimal approach to evaluation is MSI or immunohistochemical analysis of tumors, followed by germline MMR gene testing in patients with MSI-H tumors or tumors with a loss of expression of one of the MMR genes.
2. After the mutation is identified, at-risk relatives can be referred for genetic counseling and predictive testing.
3. An alternative approach, if tissue testing is not feasible, is to proceed directly to germline analysis of the MMR genes, but this is not currently cost-effective, but may become more attractive if MMR gene mutations are offered as part of cancer panel gene testing.
4. If no MMR gene mutation is found in a proband with an MSI-H tumor and/ or a clinical history of Lynch syndrome, the genetic test result is non-informative.

The patients and the at-risk individuals should be counseled as for Lynch syndrome, and high-risk surveillance should be undertaken.

Molecular Genetics

The most common genes in which germline mutations may cause this disease are *MSH2* on chromosome 2p16, *MLH1* on chromosome 3p21 which account for approximately 90 % of cases of Lynch syndrome, *MSH6* on 2p15, and much less commonly, *PMS2* on chromosome 7p22, which can be a rare cause of childhood brain cancer, when biallelic mutations are present (De Vos et al. 2004, see pages 9, 226 and 304 for more details). Mutations in *MSH3* are very rarely reported in patients with colorectal cancer (Nicoliades et al. 1994; Akiyama et al. 1997; de la Chapelle 2004). Interpretation of reported mutations in *PMS2* is complicated by the presence of pseudogenes (Hayward et al. 2004). Up to one-half of individuals diagnosed with colorectal cancer before the age of 35 years may have a germline mutation in one of these genes (Liu et al. 1995), but only a minority of patients with colorectal cancer diagnosed between the ages of 35 and 45 years without a family history of colorectal cancer have such mutations. The overall contribution of Lynch syndrome to colorectal cancer is probably 2–3 % (de la Chapelle 2004), but only extensive, multimodal mutation analysis can find more than 75 % of all mutations. Alu-mediated exonic deletions are particularly common in *MSH2*.

All these genes are involved in the same pathway for repair of mismatches in DNA, and MSI may be demonstrated as DNA replication errors detectable in tumor relative to genomic DNA (Parsons et al. 1993; Liu et al. 1995; Shia et al. 2005). Frameshift mutations of the transforming growth factor (TGF) type II receptor gene (TGFBR2) and other growth-/apoptosis-related genes such as *BAX* are common and are due to the runs of mono- or dinucleotide repeats present in these target genes. Analysis of a series of families with Lynch syndrome suggests that perhaps half of the cases are due to mutations in the *MSH2* gene, 30–40 % to mutations in the *MLH1* gene, less than 10 % are attributable to mutations in *MSH6*, and only a handful are due to mutations in other genes. When multiple analysis techniques are used, most families that fulfill the Amsterdam Criteria are found to have germline Lynch syndrome mutations (DiFiore et al. 2004; Wagner et al. 2003). Founder mutations in the genes causing Lynch syndrome are known; for instance, there is an *MLH1* deletion of exon 16 in the Finns (Nystrom-Lahti et al. 1995), and a founder mutation in *MSH2*, known as p.Ala636Pro, probably accounts for a third of all Lynch syndrome cases in the Ashkenazi Jewish population (Foulkes et al. 2002). Attenuated forms of FAP may rarely masquerade as Lynch syndrome, usually due to unusual mutations in the *APC* gene (Spirio et al. 1993). Other genes that may be involved in colorectal cancer predisposition, with single reports of germline mutations reported in cases, include *AXIN2* and TGFBR2. Subsequent data have suggested that the latter mutation is most likely to be a neutral polymorphism (Lu et al. 1998; de la Chapelle 2004).

A small minority of cases of Lynch syndrome can be caused by constitutional *MLH1* epimutations, with soma-wide allele-specific promoter methylation and transcription silencing of this gene. These epimutations are reversible, resulting in non-Mendelian inheritance of the phenotype. These were initially identified in cases with early-onset colorectal cancer showing loss of staining for MLH1 and MSI in the tumor, but with no identified germline mutation in the *MLH1* gene. Deletion of the unmethylated *MLH1* gene was demonstrated in the tumor (Hitchins and Ward 2009). In many cases the somatic methylation was mosaic, and the case sporadic, but some familial cases have been described, with apparent variability in the degree of somatic methylation of the *MLH1* gene. The risk of a Lynch syndrome phenotype in the first-degree relatives of such cases is less than 50 %, as the methylation defect appears to be unstable, leading to non-Mendelian inheritance patterns, but it is recommended that first-degree relatives of cases should be screened as for Lynch syndrome.

Constitutional epimutations in *MSH2* have been detected in some cases of Lynch syndrome with loss of staining for MSH2 and MSH6, and MSI, in tumor samples, but with no detectable germline mutation in *MSH2*. In these cases a germline deletional mutation has been detected in the final exons of the upstream gene *EPCAM* (*TACSTD2*). This deletion disrupts the transcription termination signal from *EPCAM*, resulting in read-through into *MSH2*. This results in methylation of the *MSH2* gene particularly in epithelial tissues where EPCAM expression is upregulated, causing a mosaic somatic methylation pattern (Kovacs et al. 2009). The risk of endometrial cancer in *EPCAM* deletion carriers appears to be significantly lower than in carriers of *MSH2* mutations, although the risk of colorectal cancer is comparable (Lightenberg et al. 2013).

Heterozygous cells repair DNA normally in Lynch syndrome (or at levels that generally do not have clinical consequences), but in cells where the second allele has been inactivated, for instance, by deletion, in the colonic epithelium, a mutator phenotype is generated and MSI is seen. Genes with microsatellite sequences in their coding regions (such as *TGFBR2*) are prone to somatic mutation, which is thought to promote the carcinogenic progression (de la Chapelle 2004). It has been suggested that the DNA MMR defect in Lynch syndrome generates increased numbers of novel and potentially immunogenic mutations, which result in an increased immunologic response to tumors in affected individuals. MSI can be demonstrated in hyperplastic endometrium in women without Lynch syndrome, but not in normal endometrium, and is also detectable in about 20 % of endometrial cancers (Baldinu et al. 2002). Similar findings have been described in individuals with Lynch syndrome with colorectal cancer and also even before the diagnosis of cancer.

Extracolonic Cancer in Lynch Syndrome (See also Endometrial Cancer, p. 102)

Endometrial cancer is the fifth most common cancer in women in the UK, accounting for 7 % of invasive cancers in women, occurring in 1 in 100 women by 75 years of age. The commonest histological type (90 %) is adenocarcinoma (see p. 102).

Women with Lynch syndrome have a very high lifetime risk of endometrial cancer. Tumors characteristically demonstrate MSI+(due to impaired repair of mismatch DNA errors), and complex atypical endometrial hyperplasia appears to be the premalignant endometrial lesion (Lohse et al. 2002; Sutter et al. 2004). Carriers of *MSH6* mutations have the highest endometrial cancer risk (Wijnen et al. 1999), and the risk is higher in *MSH2* than *MLH1* mutation carriers (Vasen et al. 2001; Huang et al. 2004). Women with Lynch syndrome have a lifetime risk of endometrial cancer of up to 60 %, with the highest incidence between 40 and 60 years of age, average 49.3 years. The characteristics of endometrial cancer in Lynch syndrome, which appear to be different from sporadic cancers, include more poorly differentiated histology (83 % versus 27 % in sporadic cancers) with Crohn's-like lymphoid reaction (100 % versus 27 %), lymphangio-invasive growth (67 % versus 0 %), and tumor invasion by lymphocytes (100 % versus 36 %) (Van den Bos et al. 2004).

The risk of ovarian cancer in women with Lynch syndrome is about 8% (see p. 107), highest in *MLH1* and *MSH2* mutation carriers. There is an increased risk of pancreatic cancer in Lynch syndrome, RR of 8, with cumulative risk of 4 % by the age of 70 years (Kastrinos et al. 2009). It is still unclear whether the risk of breast cancer is increased in individuals with Lynch syndrome. An increased risk of breast cancer has been reported recently, and the tumors have been shown to be deficient in the relevant MMR protein, especially in *MLH1* mutation carriers (Engel et al. 2012; Barrow et al. 2009; Jensen et al. 2009), although other studies have failed to demonstrate an increased risk (Watson et al. 2008). More recent studies have again suggested that there is an increased risk for breast cancer in MMR mutation carriers (Win et al. 2012). Engel et al. (2012) reported a significantly increased risk of prostate cancer in Lynch syndrome (SIR 2.5 (1.4–4)), highest in *MSH2* mutation carriers, and similar small increases in risk were reported in two other studies (Grindedal et al. 2009; Barrow et al. 2012) (see p. 116). Immunohistochemistry showed loss of the relevant MMR gene protein in most tumors tested. There is an increased risk of urothelial cancer in Lynch syndrome (see p. 141). The risk of gastric cancer is also increased, with a lower age at diagnosis than in the general population; the risk appears to be higher in countries where the background risk of gastric cancer is high (p. 51).

Screening

First-degree relatives of individuals affected by Lynch syndrome should be offered screening for colorectal cancer and possibly for other cancers seen in their family. Since colorectal adenomas are assumed to be the premalignant lesions (for colorectal cancer), and the majority of lesions are right sided, colonoscopy is the screening method of choice (Hodgson et al. 1995; Vasen et al. 2007, 2013). Asymptomatic at-risk relatives (with an affected first-degree relative with Lynch syndrome) should be offered annual colonoscopy from the age of 25 (Umar et al. 2004b). Interval cancers have been detected in individuals screened at 2-yearly intervals, so annual examinations are probably optimal but often not very practical, and therefore a "compromise" has been made by starting 18-monthly colonoscopies from 20 to 25 years of age, since fewer than 1 % of patients with Lynch syndrome develop colorectal cancer before the age of 20 years. The adenoma–carcinoma progression rate appears to be very much increased in Lynch syndrome above that in the general population (Jass 1995). If adenomas are found, they are removed, and colonoscopy should be repeated annually. There is good evidence that such screening does reduce cancer morbidity and mortality in screened individuals (Jarvinen et al. 1995; Renkonen-Sinisalo et al. 2000) and lead to the detection of CRC at an earlier stage, with a reduction of the risk of CRC by 63 %, and reduced colorectal cancer mortality (Vasen et al. 2007, 2013).

When colorectal cancer is detected in an affected individual, many centers advocate subtotal or even total colectomy because of the significant risk of a second colorectal cancer, but the evidence for and against such management options is still lacking, and there is currently a European trial to evaluate this (Olschwang et al. 2005). Prophylactic hysterectomy and subtotal colectomy may be considered in certain cases of Lynch syndrome (Celentano et al. 2011). Lifetime surveillance for rectal cancer should be continued after such surgery. The risk of rectal cancer has been assessed at 12 % over a 12-year follow-up period (Jarvinen et al. 2000). Such surgery could also be offered to MMR gene mutation carriers who have been found to have recurrent or dysplastic adenomas. Carrier women found to have colon cancer require careful preoperative assessment for ovarian and uterine cancer. Even if there is no evidence of current malignancy, prophylactic hysterectomy and bilateral oophorectomy at the time of colon surgery should be considered when there is a strong family history of these neoplasms. In view of the substantial risk of a second CRC after partial colectomy, the option of subtotal colectomy should be considered when undertaking surgery for a first colorectal cancer.

Aspirin significantly reduces the incidence of cancer in Lynch syndrome, so treatment with regular small doses may be advisable, but the pros and cons of such treatment should be carefully discussed in view of the side effects of such treatment.

It has been claimed that individuals with Lynch syndrome may have a survival benefit from treatment with adjuvant chemotherapy (Elsaleh et al. 2001), although the evidence for this is conflicting; current evidence suggests that tumors demonstrating MMR deficiency are resistant to chemotherapeutic agents including 5-FU, methylating agents, and antimetabolites (Bignami et al. 2003; Clark et al. 2004).

Because of the increased risk of gynecological cancers (ovarian and endometrial) in females with Lynch syndrome (possibly up to a half of total cancer risk), women with this disease and those at high risk of inheriting it should probably be followed up with annual bimanual pelvic examination and transvaginal ultrasound scan for ovarian and uterine cancers from 30 years of age. Transvaginal ultrasound with Doppler examination may delineate ovarian lesions, and a serum CA125 is also suggested annually (Jacobs and Lancaster 1996), but the efficacy of such surveillance is still unproven. Regular endometrial aspiration and biopsy (pipette or hysteroscopic biopsy) is more sensitive than ultrasound for the detection of premalignant lesions such as atypical endometrial hyperplasia and endometrial cancer (Wood and Duffy

2003), but since endometrial cancer has a relatively good prognosis, and the efficacy of surveillance is as yet unknown, screening would be best performed in the setting of a prospective study (Vasen et al. 1996, 2013) (see section on "Endometrial cancer"). Hysterectomy and bilateral oophorectomy largely prevent the development of endometrial and ovarian cancer and may be considered in women with Lynch syndrome after childbearing age, especially if colorectal cancer surgery is scheduled.

A high incidence of other Lynch syndrome-associated cancers in particular families may be an indication for screening for the specific cancer within that kindred showing an increased frequency of these extracolonic cancers. Thus, dermatological surveillance may be offered in Muir–Torre families. The estimated risk of urothelial cancer in Lynch syndrome varies from 5 to 20 %, highest in *MSH2* mutation carriers. These usually present with painless hematuria, and the prognosis is relatively good. Surveillance for urological malignancy could be offered by abdominal ultrasound and cytological examination of an early-morning urine sample for red blood cells and cytology, and tumor-specific markers, from 30 to 35 years of age, although this is controversial and not of proven efficacy (Myrhoj et al. 2008).

Most gastric cancers in Lynch syndrome are of the intestinal type, so regular upper GI endoscopy may lead to early detection of precursor lesions and early cancer. Precursor lesions have been ascertained in MMR gene mutation carriers: *H. pylori* infection was observed in 26 %, atrophy in 14 %, and intestinal metaplasia also in 14 % (Renkonen-Sinisalo et al. 2000). Gastroscopies annually, with eradication of *Helicobacter pylori* infection, when present, could therefore be considered from the age of 35 years in individuals with a strong family history of gastric cancer (Park et al. 2000) or those in areas with a high background risk of gastric cancer such as Japan, although the efficacy of such screening has not yet been established. (For more discussion see p. 61, Renkonen-Sinisalo et al. 2002; ten Kate et al. 2007; Vasen et al. 2007).

Because some studies have found a slight increase in the risk of prostate cancer in men with Lynch syndrome, screening by PSA analysis could be considered, but as no evidence exists for the benefits of screening for prostate cancer in MMR gene mutation carriers at the present time, this should only be considered as part of a research study (http://impact-study.co.uk).

Screening for pancreatic cancer has not been shown to be of benefit, so any surveillance should only be performed as part of a research study.

Genetic Counseling in Lynch Syndrome

Now that it is possible to delineate the mutation responsible for this disease in some families, it is possible to carry out predictive testing for the condition in families in which the pathogenic mutation has been detected in an affected individual. Such testing should only be offered with a full counseling protocol. Discussions should include providing information about the chances of developing cancer at a given age, and about the possible emotional effects of receiving a positive or a negative result, and the potential implications with regard to insurance and employment (Aktan-Collan et al. 2000). Before using such molecular tests, it is important to be confident of the pathogenicity of the mutation by, for example, the demonstration that it segregates with the disease or has been shown to be pathogenic in other families, and that the nature of the mutation is likely to cause disruption of function.

The ascertainment and counseling of at-risk family members are of great importance and should be encouraged; there is often poor communication between different parts of a family. Genetic registers of families with this disease facilitate the follow-up of affected and at-risk individuals and the ascertainment of other individuals within a family who may benefit from screening (see screening for "Colorectal cancer", p. 69).

Hyperparathyroidism–Jaw Tumor Syndrome (CDC73-Related Disorders) (OMIM 145001)

Hyperparathyroidism–jaw tumor syndrome (HPT-JT) is an autosomal dominant disorder characterized by parathyroid adenoma or carcinoma, ossifying fibroma of the mandible and/or maxilla, and renal cysts, adenomas, and carcinomas. Germline mutations in *HRPT2*, currently known as *CDC73*, encoding parafibromin, are associated with HPT-JT (Carpten et al. 2002; Newey et al. 2010). Typically, HPT-JT patients present with solitary parathyroid adenomas or carcinomas. Rarely, they present with double neoplasias. Parathyroid carcinomas are extremely rare and are not components of any other heritable syndrome. So its presence should raise the genetic differential diagnosis of HPT-JT. Approximately 80 % of HPT-JT patients present with hyperparathyroidism (HPT). Parathyroid carcinoma, manifesting as primary hyperparathyroidism, occurs in approximately 10–15 % of affected individuals. A unique pathologic feature of parathyroid lesions in HPT-JT is the high frequency of cystic changes. About 30 % of patients also develop fibro-osseous lesions, primarily in the mandible and/or maxilla. Kidney lesions have been reported including bilateral cysts, renal adenoma, hamartomas, and papillary or chromophobe RCC. It is important to be aware that in some families, only parathyroid lesions are present (FIHP). Thus, HPT-JT (>50–80 % of patients), parathyroid carcinoma (20 % of all apparently sporadic cases), and familial isolated hyperparathyroidism (FIHP; 15 %) associated with germline mutations in *CDC73* are under the umbrella term *CDC73*-related disorders (Newey et al. 2010).

Germline mutations in *CDC73*, located on 1q25–q31, cause HPT-JT (Teh et al. 1996; Carpten et al. 2002). *CDC73* has 17 exons spanning 18.5 kb of genomic distance. HPT-JT-associated mutations are truncating, mainly (>80 %) frameshift and nonsense, with the majority occurring in exon 1 (Carpten et al. 2002; Newey et al. 2010). Recently, a germline large deletion in *CDC73* was reported (Cascon et al. 2011) Because this gene was recently identified, it remains unknown whether a genotype–phenotype association exists. The penetrance for HPT is 80 %, which mainly will develop by the late teens. The *CDC73* transcript is 2.7 kb and is predicted to encode a 531-amino acid protein. While the gene is ubiquitously expressed, its function remained unknown for some time. Subsequently, parafibromin was shown to bind RNA Pol II as part of the PAF1 transcriptional regulatory complex (Yart et al. 2005) and importantly was found to mediate histone H3 K9 methylation which silences cyclin D1 expression (Yang et al. 2010).

Individuals and families who have or are suspected of having HPT-JT should be offered clinical cancer genetic consultation, which includes genetic counseling. When HPT-JT is suspected in a family or individual, DNA-based testing may be offered to establish the diagnosis and for medical management. Because *CDC73* has been identified, molecular-based differentiation of the various complex syndromes associated with hereditary primary HPT has become possible. Clinical surveillance and prophylactic maneuvers in HPT-JT are based on expert opinion. Annual blood-based biochemical tests for ionized calcium and intact parathyroid hormone levels beginning by or slightly after age 10 have been advocated. Following the example of multiple endocrine neoplasia type 1 (MEN 1), some believe that surgical intervention should occur once serum levels confirm the presence of HPT. Parathyroid disease in HPT-JT is typically asynchronous adenomas although the potential for malignancy needs to be seriously considered (Howell et al. 2003; Shattuck et al. 2003). While some groups advocate removal only of the enlarged parathyroid gland with continued regular monitoring, the alternative approach would be complete parathyroidectomy with fresh parathyroid autotransplantation to the forearm (or sternocleidomastoid) (Marx et al. 2002; Chen et al. 2003). Because of the unclear frequencies of jaw manifestations and renal neoplasias, it is unknown if surveillance for these component features would prove useful. The more aggressive among HPT-JT exponents would suggest orthopentography of the jaw every 3 years as well as abdominal ultrasound or CT scan with and without contrast at least every 5 years after syndrome diagnosis to screen for polycystic disease, Wilms tumor or carcinoma, and renal hamartomas (Chen et al. 2003; Newey et al. 2010).

Juvenile Polyposis Syndrome (JPS) (OMIM 174900)

Solitary juvenile intestinal polyps are relatively common in the pediatric population, occurring in approximately 1–5 %. A clinical diagnosis of juvenile polyposis syndrome (JPS) is made when multiple (>5) juvenile colonic polyps occur in any one individual (Waite and Eng 2003) or any number of juvenile polyps in an individual with a family history of juvenile polyposis. Despite its name, the age at diagnosis is bimodal, in childhood and in the mid-50s. JPS is an autosomal dominant hamartoma polyposis syndrome, often clinically diagnosed when other inherited hamartoma polyposis syndromes, such as PJS (see p. 299), Gorlin syndrome (see p. 252), BRRS (see p. 221), and hereditary mixed polyposis syndrome, have been excluded. The prevalence of JPS is believed to be 1 in 100 000. The number of polyps varies between individuals, even in the same family, but can be anywhere from 5 to 200. They are most often found in the lower bowel (98 %) but can also develop in the stomach (15 %) and small intestine (7 %). Patients can become symptomatic from their polyps, with hematochezia, melena, rectal prolapse, intussusception, or abdominal pain. There is an increased lifetime risk for malignancy of 10–60 % for GI (colorectal, gastric, and duodenal) and possibly pancreatic cancer (Jass et al. 1988).

Histopathology plays a critical role in the diagnosis of JPS. The typical JPS polyp is unilobulated and pedunculated, spherical in shape with a smooth outer surface. In contrast to other hamartomatous polyps, these lack a smooth muscle core but instead show an internal dense inflammatory response, with predominant mesenchymal stroma that entraps normal epithelial cells, often forming dilated cysts. Less typical (20 %) are JPS polyps that are multilobulated, with each lobe separated by well-defined clefts (Jass et al. 1988).

As well as the colonic polyps, gastric polyposis may occur, often with quite large polyps, carrying the risk of GI bleeding and gastric cancer; gastric involvement is more common in individuals with *SMAD4* mutations than in those with *BMPR1A* mutations. Congenital anomalies have been reported in 11–20 % of individuals with JPS, more often in the sporadic cases (Coburn et al. 1995). These can involve the GI tract (including malrotation of the gut), heart, CNS, and genitourinary system. Clubbing of the fingertips is common, as is macrocephaly and congenital cardiac anomalies. JPS is associated with mutations in one of at least two genes. Germline mutations in *SMADH4* and *BMPR1A* have been found in approximately 40 % of JPS probands (Howe et al. 1998, 2001; Zhou et al. 2001). Germline mutations in *SMADH4* account for 15–25 % of JPS, while mutations in *BMPR1A* account for another 15–25 %. Both *SMADH4* and *BMPR1A* belong to the TGF beta superfamily. BMPR1A is phosphorylated by, and dimerises with, a specific type II BMP receptor. In turn, this activated complex signals through the intracellular SMAD1 or related SMAD5 and SMAD8 proteins, increasing their affinity for SMAD4, and gaining access to the nucleus for the transcriptional regulation of downstream target genes (Massague 2000; Eng 2001; Waite and Eng 2003). The prominent role of the BMP pathway in cardiac development and in the development of the GI tract might explain the association of some JPS with congenital cardiac anomalies and malrotation of the gut (Waite and Eng 2003). Further investigation might reveal cardiac anomalies predominating in those with *BMPR1A* mutations compared to those with *SMADH4* mutations. To date, the only genotype–phenotype correlation observed is the marked prevalence of giant gastric polyps in individuals with *SMADH4* mutations as compared to families with germline *BMPR1A* alterations (Friedl et al. 2002; Aretz et al. 2007). It is likely that there is at least one other JPS gene that has not been identified yet. While other members of the TGF–SMAD superfamily would be ideal candidates, no germline mutations in the genes encoding *SMAD1*, *SMAD2*, *SMAD3*, and *SMAD5* have been identified to date (Bevan et al. 1999), although a few cases of JPS have been ascribed to *ENG* mutations, with hereditary hemorrhagic telangiectasia (HHT). Features of HHT such as telangiectasia, epistaxis, and arteriovenous malformations can sometimes be seen in JPS, where the germline mutation is in *SMAD4* (reviewed in Gammon et al. 2009). While there were early reports of germline *PTEN* mutations in "JPS," these were not confirmed as the individuals labeled as "JPS" either had features suggestive of Cowden syndrome or were too young for the manifestations of Cowden syndrome to be apparent. Indeed, when a single hospital series of individuals given the diagnosis of JPS were analyzed for the presence of *PTEN* mutations, only one was found to harbor such a mutation, and he was subsequently found to have pathognomonic cutaneous features of CS (Kurose et al. 1999). A second study of 55 individuals in whom JPS has been diagnosed included only one with a germline *PTEN* mutation and Cowden syndrome (Waite and Eng 2003) or *PTEN* hamartoma tumor syndrome (PHTS). Clinical cancer genetic consultation, which includes genetic counseling, should be offered to all probands and families with JPS or suspected to have JPS. As with most inherited cancer syndromes with known susceptibility genes, the known affected individual should be tested for mutations in *SMADH4* and *BMPR1A*. Once the family-specific mutation is known, all first-degree relatives can be offered genetic testing in the setting of clinical cancer genetic consultation including genetic counseling. In such families, a mutation-negative result in a family member offered predictive testing is a true negative. An individual believed to have JPS and found to have a germline *PTEN* mutation should be informed he/she has PHTS or Cowden syndrome and medically managed as in CS (see p. 233).

Infantile JP is a rare subtype of JPS which presents before the age of two. It presents with rectal bleeding, intussusception, and diarrhea and may be fatal. It is usually sporadic, due to de novo mutations, such as contiguous deletions involving *BMPR1A* and *PTEN*.

Clinical Surveillance

Individuals with germline *SMADH4* or *BMPR1A mutations* should undergo upper and lower endoscopy from about 15 years of age to determine whether they have polyps at that time, whether these require further medical attention and to decide upon the interval of further endoscopies. In asymptomatic at-risk individuals, screening endoscopies should begin from 15 years age. Symptomatic individuals should have upper and lower endoscopies at the time of symptomatology. If no polyps are noted, then the screening interval may be every 2–3 years of age so long as the individuals remain asymptomatic. Suggested screening for individuals with juvenile polyposis is 18-monthly colonoscopies from the mid-teens and upper GI endoscopy from 25 years (Cairns et al. 2010), but because no large trials of such surveillance have been done, the evidence supporting this recommendation is limited.

When polyps are found, they should be removed, followed by an endoscopy at 1 year. When the tract is polyp-free, then screening intervals of 2–3 years can occur. If a JPS individual presents with nonmetastatic colorectal cancer, subtotal or total colectomy should be advocated at the time of surgery. Probands or families with the clinical diagnosis of JPS but are mutation negative at both *BMPR1A* and *SMADH4* should be managed as if they had mutation-proven JPS. Because large deletions and promoter mutations have not been systematically looked for in these 2 genes, it is possible that current "mutation-negative" JPS patients might harbor deletions and promoter mutations.

Klinefelter Syndrome

In men, the incidence of cancer of the breast is about 1 % of the frequency in females. It has been estimated that about 3.8 % of males with breast cancer have Klinefelter syndrome, giving an extrapolated risk of breast cancer in males with the 47XXY karyotype of about 7 %. This is almost equivalent to the population risk of the disease in females to age 70 years. Studies vary in the extent of risk increase estimated: a relative risk of 5–49 in men has been estimated (Hasle et al. 1995; Swerdlow et al. 2005). There is an increased risk of breast cancer in males carrying mutations in *BRCA2*, but little data are available on the breast cancer risk in individuals with Klinefelter syndrome who carry such mutations.

Extragonadal malignant germ cell tumors (teratomas, usually mediastinal, diagnosed before the age of 30 years) are significantly more prevalent in Klinefelter syndrome (relative risk 67), and any individual with early sexual development or testicular growth should be screened by measurement of germ cell tumor markers, including alpha-fetoprotein and human chorionic gonadotropin-B (Nichols 1992; Derenoncourt et al. 1995; Hasle et al. 1995; Ganslandt et al. 2000; Yong et al. 2000). Testicular tumors may be more common (perhaps secondary to cryptorchidism), and an association with AML and lymphoma has been proposed (Attard-Montalto et al. 1994), but this has not been substantiated (Machatschek et al. 2004) and may be due to the fact that cytogenetic studies are often performed in individuals with hematological malignancies (Hasle et al. 1995; Keung et al. 2002). A large study of the cancer risks in Klinefelter syndrome by the UK Clinical Cytogenetics Group found an increase in risk for breast (RR 5.2–49.2) and lung (RR 1–1.9) cancers and Hodgkin lymphoma (RR0.8-3.9) and a reduction in risk of prostate (RR 0.02–0.7) cancer (Swerdlow et al. 2005).

The overall risk of cancer in Klinefelter syndrome is not substantially increased (RR 0.7–1.1), any increase being seen mainly in the age group 15–30 years of age, so that no routine cancer surveillance is recommended.

Kostmann Syndrome (Kostmann Infantile Agranulocytosis, SCN3,) (OMIM #610738)

This is a rare autosomal recessive disorder characterized by granulocytopenia and monocytosis in infancy. There is an increased risk of myelodysplastic syndrome and/or AML in the severe congenital neutropenia syndromes, such that in follow-up study (mean 6 years), malignant transformation occurred in 10 % (Freedman et al. 2000). Neutropenia may respond to treatment with recombinant human granulocyte colony-stimulating factor. Recurrent homozygous mutations in the gene encoding HAX1, a mitochondrial protein implicated in preventing apoptosis in myeloid cells, have been identified in children with Kostmann syndrome (Klein et al. 2007). Other autosomal recessive severe congenital neutropenias

(SCN) are mainly caused by mutations in *ELA2*, encoding ELANE, the neutrophil elastase gene. This variety of SCN is sometimes referred to as SCN1 (OMIM #202700). Mutations in *GFI1*, *WAS*, *CSF3R*, or *G6PC3* are also seen, but are much less common (Xia et al. 2009). More than a third of all cases of SCN remain unexplained.

Li–Fraumeni Syndrome (OMIM #151623)

Clinical Features

Li–Fraumeni syndrome (LFS) is a rare autosomal dominant disorder characterized by sarcoma, breast cancer, brain tumor, leukemia/lymphoma, and adrenocortical carcinoma (ACC) (Li and Fraumeni 1969; Li et al. 1988). Germline mutations in the *TP53* tumor suppressor gene on 17p13.1 have been found in approximately 70 % of LFS (Malkin et al. 1990; Srivastava et al. 1990; Varley et al. 1997). Deleterious *TP53* mutations leading to LFS occur in between 1 in 5,000 and 1 in 20,000 births.

The major component malignancies in LFS include sarcomas, breast cancer, brain tumors, ACC, and acute leukemia (Li and Fraumeni 1969; Garber et al. 1991; Li et al. 1991). Other associated cancers may include Wilms tumor; cancers of the colon, stomach, lung, and pancreas; as well as melanoma and gonadal germ cell tumors (Garber et al. 1991; Varley et al. 1997; Birch et al. 2001), although some of these are isolated observations in a single family, and so, their exact frequencies in mutation-positive individuals are unknown. The operational diagnostic criteria for LFS, the so-called classic criteria, are as follows (Li and Fraumeni 1969):

- An individual (index case) with a sarcoma diagnosed before age of 45 years
- A first-degree relative with any cancer before age of 45 years
- A third family member who is a first- or second-degree relative with either a sarcoma diagnosed at any age or any cancer diagnosed before age of 45 years

There are several sets of operational criteria for the diagnosis of LFS-like (LFL) families, such as the Eeles criteria (Eeles 1995) and the Manchester criteria (Varley 2003). The most recent set of criteria are the Chompret criteria, which have been recently modified (Tinat et al. 2009):

- Proband with tumor belonging to LFS tumor spectrum (e.g., soft tissue sarcoma, osteosarcoma, brain tumor, premenopausal breast cancer, adrenocortical carcinoma, leukemia, lung bronchoalveolar cancer) before age 46 years and at least one first- or second-degree relative with LFS tumor (except breast cancer if proband has breast cancer) before age 56 years or with multiple tumors
- Proband with multiple tumors (except multiple breast tumors), two of which belong to LFS tumor spectrum and first of which occurred before age 46 years

- Patient with adrenocortical carcinoma or choroid plexus tumor, irrespective of family history

At least one of these three separate parts need to be fulfilled for the Chompret criteria to be fulfilled.

Genetics

Germline *TP53* mutations cause LFS. In contrast to other cancer syndromes, missense mutations are the most common variety in LFS (Varley 2003; Ribeiro et al. 2001). Earlier studies had found that the mutation frequency in families meeting the standard clinical criteria for LFS is 70–80 % in most clinical laboratories (Varley et al. 1997; Friedl et al. 1999; Frebourg et al. 1995; Varley 2003). In families meeting the LFL criteria, the frequency is lower – 8 % using the Eeles criteria and 22–40 % using the Manchester criteria (Eng et al. 1997; Varley et al. 1997; Varley 2003; Birch et al. 1990, 1994). In a recent study, the classic criteria had high specificity (91 %) but low sensitivity (40 %), whereas the relaxed LFL criteria of Eeles were very sensitive (97 %) but not specific (16 %). The Chompret criteria offer the best compromise – 95 % sensitivity and 52 % specificity (Gonzalez et al. 2009).

The French LFS working group studied 474 French families suggestive of LFS, of which 232 fulfilled the Chompret criteria. Overall, they identified a germline mutation in 82 families (17 %). The percentage of positive results was much higher in those that met Chompret criteria (29 %) than in those that did not (6 %) (Bougeard et al. 2008). A more recent study added important details – among 525 patients sent to one US laboratory for testing, 17 % were positive for a germline *TP53* mutation. Notably, all positive cases had at least one family member with a sarcoma or breast, brain or adrenocortical carcinoma (ACC). All eight persons tested who had a choroid plexus tumor were positive for *TP53* mutations (Gonzalez et al. 2009). In contrast, others have found that about 50 % of children with choroid plexus carcinomas carry germline *TP53* mutations, and positive cases meet the classic criteria and had a very poor outcome. No cases that failed to meet the criteria carried germline mutations, and most had better outcomes. None of six children with a choroid plexus papilloma had a mutation (Tabori et al. 2010). As for ACC, 14 of 21 with a childhood ACC had a germline mutation, regardless of family history of cancer (Gonzalez et al. 2009).

Based on a segregation analysis of relatives of children with childhood sarcomas, the risk of cancer in LFS was estimated to be 50 % by age 30 years and 90 % by age 60 years. Molecular data have broadly confirmed these findings – the penetrance of *TP53* mutations for cancer is greater than 90 % for women (~75 % for men, the difference is mainly accounted for by high incidence of breast cancer diagnoses in women with LFS) (Chompret et al. 2000). Before age 10 years, the most commonly seen cancers are soft tissue sarcomas, brain tumors, and ACC. For those 11–20 years, osteosarcomas predominate, and for those above 20 years of age, breast cancer and brain tumors are the most common manifestations, and all other epithelial tumors listed above tend to occur in those over age 20 years.

Genotype–phenotype correlations have been observed in some studies but not in others. For example, in one, families with missense mutations in the DNA-binding domain trended towards an overall higher cancer incidence, particularly of those of the breast and CNS, with an earlier age at onset, when compared to families with protein truncating or inactivating mutations or families with no mutation at all (Birch et al. 1998). Further, a systematic database study of all LFS families revealed that the mean age of breast cancer diagnosis in $TP53$ mutation-positive families was 34.6 years in contrast to 42.5 years in mutation-negative families ($P=0.0035$) (Olivier et al. 2003). In mutation-positive families, brain tumors were overrepresented in those families with missense mutations in the DNA-binding loop that contacts the minor groove of DNA. Development of ACCs was associated with missense mutations in the loops opposing the protein–DNA contact surface ($P=0.0003$) (Olivier et al. 2003). In contrast, a study of 56 $TP53$ mutation-positive individuals from 107 kindreds ascertained through cases of childhood soft tissue sarcoma reported no difference in phenotype between patients with missense mutations compared to those with truncating mutations (Hwang et al. 2003). Differences in patient accrual, study design, and mutation site classification may have contributed to these disparate findings, and thus more studies or a pooled analysis are needed to clarify this issue.

The frequency of germline $TP53$ mutations in patients with multiple primary cancers unselected for family history and in those with apparently sporadic LFS component tumors has been extensively studied. While early studies suggested that only 1 % of early-onset breast cancer cases will harbor a germline $TP53$ mutation (Sidransky et al. 1992; Lalloo et al. 2003), the frequencies may be higher in cases of sporadic osteosarcomas, 2–3 % (McIntyre et al. 1994), 9 % for rhabdomyosarcomas (Diller et al. 1995), and 2–10 % for brain tumors (Felix et al. 1995). Perhaps the most striking association occurs in cases of childhood ACC. In a series of 14 ACC patients unselected for family history, 11 (82 %) carried a germline $TP53$ mutation (Gonzalez et al. 2009), and this is one reason why the Chompret criteria allow for ACC in the absence of family history (although it is fair to say that germline TP53 mutations are very rare in those diagnosed over 20 years old). Interestingly of 36 cases of childhood ACC in southern Brazil, 35 carried an identical R337H (p. Arg337His) mutation. There is a single common origin for all carriers of the Brazilian R337H mutation (Pinto et al. 2004). The cancer family history in mutation-positive cases was not striking (there was no evidence for LFS in the 30 mutation-positive kindred), suggesting a low-penetrance and possibly tissue-specific effect of this particular mutation (Figueiredo et al. 2006). More recent data, however, have shown that other cancers can occur in R337H carriers (Gomes et al. 2012; Seidinger et al. 2011). Another recent development is the finding that most

LFS-related breast cancers are ER-positive, HER2-positive tumors (Wilson et al. 2010; Masciari et al. 2012). This may help in determining when to offer *TP53* testing to young women with breast cancer who do not meet classic or Chompret criteria, when generally the yield is low (Tinat et al. 2009).

Genetic and Medical Management

The management of LFS is not straightforward. Many are reluctant to offer predictive testing for minors in families with a known pathogenic *TP53* mutation in view of the difficulties in screening for such a wide spectrum of cancers in childhood without proven benefit from screening. However, it may be useful to view *TP53* mutation analysis as a molecular diagnostic test for LFS, especially in the setting of LFL. While breast cancer screening by MRI can be instituted, little effective surveillance is widely available for many of the other component tumors. On the other hand, most clinical cancer geneticists will acknowledge that a predictive test that is negative in the setting of a known family-specific germline *TP53* mutation can be useful. Such an informative negative test will relieve that particular family member from LFS-directed clinical surveillance as his/her cancer risk would be no different from that of the general population. Recently, a prospective study applying an intensive screening protocol originating at the Hospital for Sick Children, Toronto (see Table. 11.7), has provided some hope that aggressive screening can be of benefit, particularly in detecting small, operable brain tumors and in finding intra-abdominal tumors at a readable stage (Villani et al. 2011). Further large-scale studies with longer follow-up are required before this, or similar screening protocols can be accepted for wide-scale use (Table. 11.7).

Maffucci Syndrome (OMIM 166000)

Maffucci syndrome (OMIM 166000) is a sporadic condition, in which osteochondromatosis (mostly enchondromas) and hemangiomas occur (in the related Ollier syndrome only cartilaginous tumors occur). Cavernous or capillary hemangiomas, phlebectasia, and lymphangiomas may develop and can be disfiguring. The dyschondroplasia may result in shortening of bones, fractures, and deformities from enchondromas. Many mesenchymal neoplasias may occur, possibly in 15–30 % of cases (Harris 1990; Albrechts and Rapini 1995). Chondrosarcoma is the most common malignancy to develop in this condition (75 %), but fibrosarcoma, angiosarcoma, osteosarcoma, ovarian granulosa cell tumors or teratomas, acute myeloid leukemia, and gliomas have been reported (Sun et al. 1985; Schwartz et al. 1987; Christian and Ballon 1990; Chang and Prados 1994). Multiple primary tumors may develop (Loewinger et al. 1977; Amary et al. 2011).

Maffucci syndrome was long suspected to result from constitutional mosaicism, and most cases are now known to be caused by mosaicism for specific

Table 11.7 Surveillance strategy for individuals with germline TP53 mutations

Children
Adrenocortical carcinoma
Ultrasound of abdomen and pelvis every 3–4 months
Complete urinalysis every 3–4 months
Blood tests every 4 months: β-human chorionic gonadotropin, alpha-fetoprotein, 17-OH-progesterone, testosterone, dehydroepiandrosterone sulfate, androstenedione
Brain tumour
Annual brain MRI
Soft tissue and bone sarcoma
Annual rapid total body MRI
Leukaemia or lymphoma
Blood test every 4 months: complete blood count erythrocyte sedimentation rate, lactate dehydrogenase
Adults
Breast cancer
Monthly breast self-examination starting at age 18 years
Clinical breast examination twice a year, starting at age 20–25 years, or 5–10 years before the earliest known breast cancer in the family
Annual mammography and breast MRI screening starting at age 20–25 years, or at earliest age of onset in the family
Consider risk-reducing bilateral mastectomy
Brain tumour
Annual brain MRI
Soft tissue and bone sarcoma
Annual rapid total body MRI
Ultrasound of abdomen and pelvis every 6 months
Colon cancer
Colonoscopy every 2 years, beginning at age 40 years, or 10 years before earliest known colon cancer in the family
Melanoma
Annual dermatological examination
Leukaemia or lymphoma
Complete blood count every 4 months
Erythrocyte sedimentation rate, lactate dehydrogenase every 4 months

Adapted with permission from Villani et al. (2011)

missense mutations in isocitrate dehydrogenase 1 (*IDH1*) or in *IDH2* (most commonly p.Arg132Cys substitution in *IDH1*) (Amary et al. 2011; Pansuriya et al. 2011).

McCune–Albright Syndrome (OMIM 174800)

McCune–Albright syndrome (MAS) is a nonheritable disorder classically characterized by the triad of polyostotic fibrous dysplasia (POFD), café-au-lait spots, and sexual precocity. Somatic gain-of-function mutations in the *GNAS1* locus on

20q13.2-q13.3 have been described in affected tissues. Since these mutations arise post-zygotically, affected individuals are considered somatic mosaics.

POFD is characterized by fibrous tissue proliferation with destruction of bone, leading to pathological fractures and pseudoarthroses. The diagnosis of McCune–Albright syndrome is usually clinically obvious and is confirmed by excess circulating levels of one or more hormones (thyroid hormone, cortisol, growth hormone, or estrogen) in the absence of the respective stimulating hormones. Fibrous dysplasia is usually diagnosed by its characteristic ground-glass (but occasionally sclerotic) appearance on X-ray, although it can be confused with osteofibrous dysplasia or hyperparathyroidism–jaw tumor syndrome (Hammami et al. 1997; Weinstein et al. 2002). Deafness and blindness may result from pressure within the cranial foramina. In addition, café-au-lait patches, with irregular borders, and multiple endocrinopathies occur. The most frequent endocrine disturbances are precocious puberty, especially in females, but thyroid dysfunction, hyperparathyroidism, acromegaly, Cushing syndrome, or hyperprolactinemia may occur. Osteosarcomatous transformation in areas of fibrous dysplasia has been described as a complication of this condition (Taconis 1988). Recently, four patients with severe McCune–Albright syndrome (two of whom had perioral freckling reminiscent of Peutz–Jeghers syndrome and three of whom had a detectable *GNAS1* mutation in peripheral blood) were found to harbor multiple hamartomatous gastrointestinal polyps in the stomach and/or duodenum. The authors suggested that gastrointestinal polyps may be frequent in patients with McCune–Albright syndrome (Zacharin et al. 2011).

It had been suggested that this disorder might be caused by somatic mutations in an autosomal dominant lethal gene, which would only be compatible with survival if present in mosaic form (Happle 1989). Subsequently, mutations in the *GNAS1* gene that encodes a subunit of the stimulatory G protein GS alpha were identified (Weinstein et al. 1991). It has been postulated that somatic mutations of this type occur early in embryogenesis and result in a mosaic population of cells, which would explain the sporadic occurrence and variable abnormalities in this syndrome (Marie et al. 1997). Subsequent to the initial description of somatic mosaic *GNAS1* mutations in this syndrome, alternative exons with multiple transcripts and imprinting were described (Weinstein et al. 2002; Rickard and Wilson 2003). Loss of exon 1A imprinting causes pseudohypoparathyroidism type Ib (Weinstein et al. 2002). *GNAS1* is biallelically expressed in most human tissues, but shows exclusive or preferential expression from the maternal allele in some tissues, including pituitary, thyroid, and ovary (Weinstein et al. 2002). In pituitary tumors that harbor an activating *GNAS1* mutation, the mutation almost always occurs on the maternal allele (Weinstein et al. 2002). Therefore the clinical manifestations observed in each McCune–Albright syndrome patient might be affected by which parental allele harbors the *GNAS1* gene mutation.

Since McCune–Albright syndrome and POFD result from somatic mosaic mutations, and not germline mutations, in *GNAS1*, these syndromes are virtually never inherited. Patients with fibrous dysplasia should not be treated with radiation, as it is ineffective and may increase the risk for malignant transformation. It would be prudent for all POFD patients to be screened for endocrine manifestations of McCune–Albright syndrome.

Mosaic Variegated Aneuploidy Syndrome 1 (OMIM #257300)

The term mosaic variegated aneuploidy (MVA) was first used by Warburton and colleagues to describe a rare clinical entity associated with specific cytogenetic findings in cell lines (Warburton et al. 1991). The clinical picture is severe microcephaly, growth deficiency, mild physical abnormalities, and mental retardation. Many other features have been reported. Malignancies have also been found, with myelodysplasia, rhabdomyosarcoma, leukemia, and Wilms tumor reported. Cytogenetically, the main features are aneuploidy for different chromosomes occurring mosaically; the proportion of cells showing aneuploidy varies considerably, but often more than a quarter of all cells show aneuploidy. Based on these findings, it was postulated that the underlying molecular defect was homozygosity for an autosomal recessive gene mutation that predisposed to mitotic instability. Other cases of affected children whose parents were consanguineous supported this conjecture (Tolmie et al. 1988; Papi et al. 1989). It has been noted that in MVA 3 of 14 reported cases developed a malignancy (Jacquemont et al. 2002). The finding of homozygous mutations in *BUB1B* (Hanks et al. 2004) confirmed the earlier prediction and are of particular interest because of the associated cancer predisposition. Surprisingly, an adult male with multiple gastrointestinal tumors, including carcinoma of the ampulla of Vater, stomach, and colon, was found to be homozygous for a *BUB1B* mutation that created a de novo splice site (Rio Frio et al. 2010). It is likely that the attenuated phenotype observed was attributable to "leaky" splicing and a sufficient amount of functional normal BUBR1 protein being present.

BUB1B encodes BUBR1, a protein that is essential for mitosis. BUBR1 regulates the mitotic spindle. Somatic mutations in *BUB1B* are rare in most cancers studied thus far, but have been identified (Cahill et al. 1998), and genes that regulate mitosis are likely to have an important role in cancer (Lengauer et al. 1997). The question of whether cancers can arise solely from chromosomal instability has been debated (Rajagopalan et al. 2003; Sieber et al. 2003a, b). The recent findings in mosaic variegated aneuploidy and in clonal mosaicism (from genome sequencing studies) (Jacobs et al. 2012) support the notion that aneuploidy is a sufficient cause of carcinogenesis and perhaps suggest a bigger role for aneuploidy in cancer predisposition. Screening for cancer in patients with MVA is challenging, particularly in view of its rarity and very variable penetrance, and no studies of surveillance in individuals with this condition have been reported. In view of the identification of mutations in another gene in a variation of MVA, the original syndrome has been termed by some MVA1 (see below).

Mosaic Variegated Aneuploidy Syndrome 2 (OMIM #614114)

A variant of MVA, currently referred to as MVA2 (MVA syndrome type 2), is caused by biallelic mutations in the gene encoding the centrosome protein CEP57, but no individuals with biallelic mutations in this gene have been reported to have been diagnosed with cancer (Snape et al. 2011), although so far, only 4 such cases have been reported overall.

Multiple Endocrine Neoplasia Type 1 (OMIM 131100) and the *CDKN*-opathies

Multiple Endocrine Neoplasia Type 1 and CDKN-opathies also known as Wermer syndrome, is an autosomal dominant inherited cancer syndrome occurring in 1–2/100,000 live births and characterized by the classic triad of pituitary tumors, parathyroid neoplasia, and pancreatic endocrine neoplasia (Falchetti et al. 2010). Germline mutations in *MEN1*, encoding MENIN, on 11q13, are associated with MEN 1 (Larsson et al. 1988; Larsson and Friedman 1994; Chandrasekharappa et al. 1997; Thakker 2000).

Clinical Features

The major endocrine features of MEN 1 are parathyroid tumors, typically hyperplasia (and not single adenomas), enteropancreatic endocrine tumors, and pituitary tumors, typically pituitary prolactinomas. As defined by the consensus diagnostic criteria, a diagnosis of MEN 1 is made in a person with 2 of the 3 major endocrine tumors. Familial MEN 1 is defined as at least one MEN 1 case plus at least one first-degree relative with 1 of these 3 tumors (Brandi et al. 1987; Falchetti et al. 2010). Primary HPT is the most common manifestation and, usually, the first sign of MEN 1, occurring in 80–100 % of all such patients (Falchetti et al. 2010). These tumors are typically multiglandular and often hyperplastic. The mean age at onset of MEN 1-related HPT is 30 years earlier in patients with MEN 1 than in the general population (20–25 years versus 50 years). Parathyroid carcinoma is not known to be associated with MEN 1, unlike in HPT-JT, the latter caused by mutations in the *HRPT2/CDC73* gene (see section on HPT-JT/CDC73-related disorders).

Pancreatic islet cell tumors, now referred to as neuroendocrine carcinomas of the pancreas, usually gastrinomas (manifesting as Zollinger–Ellison syndrome) and insulinomas, and less commonly VIPomas (vasoactive intestinal peptide), glucagonomas, and somatostatinomas, are the second most common endocrine manifestations, occurring in up to 30–80 % of patients by age of 40 years (Falchetti et al. 2010). These are usually multifocal and can arise in the pancreas or more commonly, as small (0.5 cm) foci throughout the duodenum. Gastrinomas represent over half of the pancreatic islet cell tumors in MEN 1 and are the major cause of morbidity and mortality in these patients (Skogseid et al. 1994; Norton et al. 1999; Brandi et al. 2001). Most result in peptic ulcer disease (Zollinger–Ellison syndrome), and half are malignant at the time of diagnosis Weber et al. 1995; Norton et al. 1999). Nonfunctional tumors of the enteropancreas, some of which produce pancreatic polypeptide, are seen in 20 % of patients. Approximately 15–50 % of individuals with MEN 1 develop a pituitary tumor. Two-thirds are microadenomas (≤ 1.0 cm in diameter) and the majority are prolactin-secreting (Corbetta et al. 1997). Other manifestations include carcinoids of the foregut (typically bronchial or thymic, with the former more common in females and the latter in males), skin tumors including lipomas (30 %), facial angiomas (85 %), and collagenomas (70 %) (Skogseid et al. 1994) and adrenal cortical lesions, including cortical adenomas, diffuse or nodular hyperplasia, or rarely carcinoma (Falchetti et al. 2010). These adrenal lesions do not show loss of heterozygosity for the *MEN1* locus and might represent a secondary phenomenon (Skogseid et al. 1992; Burgess et al. 1996). Thyroid adenomas, pheochromocytoma (PC) (usually unilateral), collagenoma, facial angiofibroma, spinal ependymoma, leiomyoma, and melanoma have also been reported, but their frequency is not known (Falchetti et al. 2010).

Genetics

Germline loss-of-function mutations in *MEN1*, on 11q13 and encoding MENIN, have been found in 80–90 % of MEN 1 probands belonging to families and approximately 65 % of nonfamilial probands (Larsson et al. 1988; Larsson and Friedman 1994; Chandrasekharappa et al. 1997; Falchetti et al. 2010). Exonic and whole gene deletions are found in another 1–4 % (Falchetti et al. 2010). Loss of the wild- type allele in many familial and sporadic MEN 1-associated tumors, as well as the fact that most mutations result in protein truncation, suggests that *MEN1* is a tumor suppressor gene.

Over 1,400 *MEN1* mutations have been reported to date, and like most tumor suppressor gene-associated loss-of-function mutations, they are nonsense, frameshift, and missense and are scattered throughout the gene. Despite almost 15 years of investigation from the time of gene discovery, no genotype–phenotype associations are evident (Giraud et al. 1998; Wautot et al. 2002; Falchetti et al. 2010).

The protean role of MENIN is becoming clearer, and its localization to the nucleus and its interactions with proteins, chief of which is JUN-D, initially suggested that it may play a role in transcriptional regulation (Agarwal et al. 1999, 2003; Kim et al. 2003). While other MENIN partners such as NF-kappa-B, SMAD3, and REL-A have been described in vitro, it remains unclear whether these relationships hold in vivo. Subsequently, MENIN was shown to regulate H3 K4 methylation and expression of p18 and p27, a relationship which was corroborated by a knockout mouse model (Karnik et al. 2005; Scacheri et al. 2006). We now know that MENIN can bind DNA sequences throughout the genome, and the relationship of MENIN and epigenetic control is complex. It is interesting to know that wild-type, but not mutant, MENIN physically interacts with p53 and that overexpression of MENIN leads to gamma-irradiation-induced apoptosis, p21 expression, and proliferation inhibition (Bazzi et al. 2008). These observations do explain, at least partially, how MENIN can regulate proliferation and apoptosis in the endocrine cell through physical interactions with p53 (Bazzi et al. 2008). It is also possible that it plays a role in other regulatory pathways that lead to the control of cell growth and/ or genomic integrity, but this remains to be seen.

Genetic and Medical Management

Individuals or families with MEN 1 or suspected of having MEN 1 should be referred for clinical cancer genetic consultation, which includes genetic counseling. The frequency of MEN 1 among patients with apparently sporadic component tumors varies but can be high for some tumor types. For instance, approximately one-third of patients with Zollinger–Ellison syndrome will have a clinical diagnosis of MEN 1 (Bardram and Stage 1985; Roy et al. 2001). Only 2–3 % of patients presenting with primary HPT have MEN 1 (Uchino et al. 2000), although familial isolated hyperparathyroidism (FIHP) is allelic (Pannett et al. 2003). In fact, 15 % of FIHP patients have been found to carry germline mutations in *CDC73* (see HPT-JT section). Other genetic differential diagnoses to consider in primary hyperparathyroidism include MEN 2 (see next section) and familial benign hypercalcemia caused by *CASR* mutations (Falchetti et al. 2010). Thus, germline *MEN1* mutation analysis can be a useful molecular diagnostic in the setting of apparently sporadic presentations of MEN1-component neoplasias. Finding a *MEN1* mutation is diagnostic of MEN1. Mutation analysis for *MEN1* and other genes, such as *HRPT2/CDC73*, can help differentiate MEN1 from HPT-JT in the setting of HPT presentation. HPT-JT also carries a risk for parathyroid carcinoma.

Among patients with pituitary tumors, the prevalence of MEN 1 is 2.5–5 % (Scheithauer et al. 1987; Corbetta et al. 1997), but is as high as 14 % in patients with prolactinoma (Corbetta et al. 1997). These results underscore the importance of carefully taking a thorough medical and family history in patients with a diagnosis of a MEN 1-associated endocrine tumor, even seemingly in isolation. Familial isolated pituitary somatotropinomas are rarely, if ever, due to germline *MEN1* mutations. Instead, 15 % of such familial isolated somatotropinomas are due to germline mutations in *AIP* encoding aryl hydrocarbon receptor-interacting protein (Vierimaa et al. 2006; Falchetti et al. 2010). Although germline *CDKN1B/p27* mutations have been reported to be associated with a MEN 1-like syndrome which includes pituitary tumors (Pellegata et al. 2006), a more recent systematic study did not reveal any *CDKN1B/p27* mutations (Agarwal et al. 2009). Involvement of genes in the CDKN/cyclin pathway is certainly in alignment given what we know of MENIN function (see above), but we suspect that the phenotypic spectrum of *CDKN1B* germline mutation is still evolving.

Approximately 25 % of Zollinger–Ellison syndrome is due to germline *MEN1* mutations (Falchetti et al. 2010). Thus, all such presentations should be referred to cancer genetic consultation for consideration of *MEN1* testing in the setting of genetic counseling. There are at least two reports of Zollinger–Ellison syndrome associated with germline mutations in the *CDKN1B/p27* gene (Agarwal et al. 2009).

The precise strategy for clinical surveillance of individuals with or at risk for MEN 1 remains controversial and based, for the most part, on expert opinion. The most aggressive surveillance protocols originate from Sweden, while the more

Table 11.8 Sample surveillance program for patients with MEN 1 and asymptomatic MEN 1[a]

For individuals known to have clinical MEN 1 or mutation in *MEN1*
From age of 5 years
1–2-yearly clinical examination and biochemical measurement of total serum calcium (corrected for albumin) and/or ionized calcium, fasting intact parathyroid hormone, prolactin
Every 2–5 years from age of 15–20 years
Upper abdominal CT or MRI scan
MRI scan of the pituitary with gadolinium contrast
MRI scan of the mediastinum in males
For individuals at 50 % risk of having clinical MEN 1 whose genetic status is unknown
From age 5 years, annually
Serum prolactin
From age 10 years, annually
Fasting total calcium (corrected for albumin) and/or ionized serum calcium
Fasting serum intact PTH
From age 20 years, annually
Fasting serum gastrin concentration if individual has symptoms of Zollinger–Ellison syndrome (reflux or diarrhea)

[a]Mutation carriers (From Dreijerink and Lips 2005; Brandi et al. 2001; Falchetti et al. 2010)

conservative is from the USA and UK. As an illustration, a sample surveillance protocol is shown in Table 11.8 (Dreijerink and Lips 2005).

While surveillance, early diagnosis, and/or prevention form the mainstay of MEN 1 management, somatostatin analogues have been used to treat symptoms. Trials of anti-VEGF inhibitors and similar therapies are also being developed. Epigenetic modulation, given the role of MENIN, may be quite successful in the future.

Multiple Endocrine Neoplasia Type 2
MEN 2 – OMIM 171400

MEN 2, also known as Sipple syndrome, is an autosomal dominant inherited cancer syndrome occurring in 1 in 300,000 live births and comprises three subtypes depending on the combination of clinical features (Schimke 1984; Zbuk and Eng 2007; Eng 2010). MEN 2A, the most common clinical subtype, is characterized by medullary thyroid carcinoma (MTC), pheochromocytoma (PC), and hyperparathyroidism (HPT). MEN 2B, the least common subtype, is similar to MEN 2A except that component neoplasias occur earlier than that in MEN 2A, clinically apparent HPT is rarely, if ever, seen, and other features such as marfanoid habitus, ganglioneuromatosis of the mucosa, and medullated corneal nerve fibers are present (Gorlin et al. 1968). Familial MTC (FMTC) is characterized by MTC only in any given family (Farndon et al. 1986). Germline mutations in the *RET* proto-oncogene, on 10q11.2, have been found in 95 % of all MEN 2 probands (Eng et al. 1996a, b; Kloos et al. 2009).

Multiple Endocrine Neoplasia Type 2A

MTC is the most frequent complication of MEN 2A and occurs in more than 95 % of clinically affected patients. PC develops in about 50 % of patients, but there are interfamilial variations in predisposition, and the variations in frequency of PC have been correlated with specific *RET* mutations (Eng et al. 1996a, b; Zbuk and Eng 2007; Frank-Raue et al. 2011) (see below). Similarly, the incidence of HPT, which occurs in 15–30 % of patients, is also correlated with allelic variation (Eng et al. 1996a, b; Schuffenecker et al. 1998; Zbuk and Eng 2007). MTC is almost always the first manifestation of MEN 2A. Clinical epidemiologic studies suggested that about 25 % of all MTC presentations are MEN 2 and are characterized by C cell hyperplasia. MTC arise from these parafollicular C cells, which derive from the neural crest, and secrete calcitonin. Other hormones may also be secreted by this tumor, including adrenocorticotropic hormone (ACTH), melanocyte-stimulating hormone (MSH), prolactin, serotonin, VIP, somatostatin, prostaglandins, and gastrin, so the symptomatology may be complex. About one-third of patients with MTC develop diarrhea, which resolves on removal of the thyroid gland. MEN 2A-related MTCs often present clinically between 20 and 40 years of age, and up to a quarter present with cervical lymphadenopathy. They may metastasize to liver, lungs, and bone. Over 90 % of MEN 2A-related PC are bilateral and multifocal, and occur, on average, about 8 years after MTC, with a mean age at diagnosis of 37 years (Howe et al. 1993), and are bilateral in approximately 50 % of affected patients. In the recent past, many believed that PC rarely precedes MTC, but population-based registries of PC have shown that germline *RET* mutations can be found in individuals with PC only (Neumann et al. 2002). However, extra-adrenal or malignant PC is infrequent in MEN 2. Up to 50 % of patients with PC are asymptomatic, and a rise in urinary catecholamines and vanillylmandelic acid (VMA) may be a late feature. Hypertension may develop, but paroxysmal hypertension, especially related to postural changes, is more typical of PC. An increase in the adrenaline–noradrenaline ratio in the urine may be noted earlier, as would serum chromogranin-A levels. Although clinical penetrance for MEN 2A is incomplete (approximately 45 % at age of 50 years and 60–75 % at age of 70 years), hyperplasia of thyroid C cells, which is the precursor of MTC, has a much earlier age at onset. C cell hyperplasia may be detected in asymptomatic mutation carriers by such biochemical screening tests and increases the apparent penetrance of MEN 2A to 93 % at age of 31 years (Easton et al. 1989).

Multiple Endocrine Neoplasia Type 2B

MEN 2B is similar to MEN 2A except that the mean age of tumor development in the former is an average 10 years earlier than the latter (Schimke 1984; Eng et al.

2001). Interestingly, clinically apparent HPT is rarely, if ever, observed in individuals with MEN 2B (Zbuk and Eng 2007; Kloos et al. 2009). Instead, they have characteristic stigmata including multiple mucosal neuromas and intestinal ganglioneuromatosis. There is a thin, asthenic marfanoid build, with some muscle wasting and possibly weakness. Joint laxity, kyphoscoliosis, pectus excavatum, pes cavus, and genu valgum are common. The face is elongated, the eyebrows are large and prominent, and the lips are enlarged and nodular, secondary to the neuromata – "blubbery" (Gorlin et al. 1968; Schimke 1984) (see Fig. 11.4). There may be multiple mucosal neuromas, which can be plexiform, and are visible on the eyelids, conjunctivae, and corneas. Enlarged corneal nerves (medullated corneal nerve fibers) may be seen. Cutaneous neuromas may also occur, and rarely, there may be café-au-lait patches and facial lentigines. The skin features may thus resemble those of NF 1, from which MEN 2B must be distinguished. Bowel malfunction, usually presenting with constipation or even obstruction, may result from ganglioneuromatosis of the gut (Carney et al. 1976). This must be distinguished from Hirschsprung's disease (see below) and Cowden syndrome, where ganglioneuromatous polyps are common (Zbuk and Eng 2007; Heald et al. 2010).

MTC and PC develop in virtually all patients with MEN 2B. The tumors are bilateral and multicentric, and metastasize locally and distantly, often before the disease is recognized. MEN 2B-related MTC develop at a younger age (mean age at diagnosis, 20 years, often at very young ages) than MEN 2A and has been observed to be metastatic even before the age of 4 years (Wells et al. 1978; Eng et al. 2001; Kloos et al. 2009). While it is widely believed that the prognosis for MEN 2B-related MTC is worse than that in MEN 2A, well-controlled studies suggest that this is largely due to lead time bias.

Familial Medullary Thyroid Carcinoma

This is a relatively infrequent clinical subtype of MEN 2, believed to represent 5–10 % of all MEN 2 cases. FMTC is characterized by familial later-onset MTC without evidence of PC or HPT (Farndon et al. 1986). Given our current knowledge of the genetics of MEN 2, it is believed that FMTC and MEN 2A are artificially divided subtypes and may be on a continuum but representing phenotypes resulting from different penetrance (Zbuk and Eng 2007).

Molecular Genetics of MEN 2

The *MEN 2* locus was mapped to 10q11.2 and, subsequently, germline gain-of-function mutations in the *RET* proto-oncogene were found in probands with MEN 2A, MEN 2B, and FMTC (Gardner et al. 1993; Mulligan et al. 1993; Eng et al. 1994, 1995a, b; Bolino et al. 1995; Santoro et al. 1995; Zbuk and Eng 2007; Kloos et al. 2009).

Before the identification of *RET* as the MEN 2 susceptibility gene, the clinical penetrance of MEN 2A was said to be 70 % by the age of 70 years (Ponder et al. 1988). However, when molecular diagnosis became possible, the penetrance of MEN 2A when biochemical tests were used was found to be 100 % by the age of 70 years (Easton et al. 1989). Similarly, although early epidemiologic studies suggested that approximately 25 % of all MTC cases were due to MEN 2, when *RET* was identified, individuals with MTC tested without family history details or clinical details had a germline mutation frequency of approximately 25 % (Decker et al. 1995). Other studies have found frequencies ranging from 5 to 10 % (Eng et al. 1995; Wohlik et al. 1996; Schuffenecker et al. 1997; Wiench et al. 2001; Kloos et al. 2009). A population-based series of apparently sporadic PC, defined as no family history and no syndromic features, found a 5 % frequency of germline *RET* mutations (Neumann et al. 2002). Germline *RET* mutations have been identified in >95 % of all MEN 2, with 98 % of MEN 2A probands, 97 % in MEN 2B, and 85 % in FMTC (Eng et al. 1996a, b; Gimm et al. 1997; Smith et al. 1997; Kloos et al. 2009).

The characteristic mutational spectrum found in MEN 2A includes missense mutations in one of cysteine codons 609, 611, 618, 620 (exon 10), or 634 (exon 11) (Eng et al. 1996a, b; Kloos et al. 2009; Moline and Eng 2011). Approximately 85 % of MEN 2A individuals carry a codon 634 mutation (Eng et al. 1996a, b; Kloos et al. 2009; Moline and Eng 2011). Genotype–phenotype analyses reveal that codon 634 mutations are associated with the presence of PC and HPT (Eng et al. 1996a, b; Zbuk and Eng 2007; Kloos et al. 2009), and the C634R mutation is most often associated with the development of HPT (Mulligan et al. 1994; Eng et al. 1996a, b; Schuffenecker et al. 1998; Kloos et al. 2009). Rare "one-off" missense mutations seen in MEN 2A include those involving codons 630 and 790 (Eng et al. 1996a, b; Eng 1999), although the codons 790 and 791 mutations may be polymorphisms (Erlic et al. 2010). FMTC-associated mutations occur at the same cysteine codons as those in MEN 2A, although mutations at codons 609–620 are more frequent in FMTC than MEN 2A. The C634R mutation is associated with HPT, so FMTC families have C634Y and other 634 mutations (Eng et al. 1996a, b; Zbuk and Eng 2007; Kloos et al. 2009). Germline mutations found almost exclusively in FMTC include E768day (exon 13), V804L, and V804M (exon 14), although one family segregating V804L has been described with older-onset unilateral PC in 2 members (Eng et al. 1996a, b; Nilsson et al. 1999; Kloos et al. 2009). Germline M918T and A883F mutations occur in 95 and 2 %, respectively, of MEN 2B patients (Eng et al. 1996a, b; Gimm et al. 1997; Smith et al. 1997) and never in MEN 2A or FMTC. Interestingly, at least four MEN 2B patients appear to carry a V804M mutation in the presence of a RET variant of unknown significance (Miyauchi et al. 1999; Kloos et al. 2009).

Variable penetrance is apparent: *RET* codons 918, 883, and 634 mutations have the highest penetrance, predisposing to MEN 2B and MEN 2A with MTC, PC, and HPT involvement (Eng et al. 1996a, b; Eng 2000b; Kloos et al. 2009). Mutations at codons 609–620 have a broad range of penetrance and expressivity, with 50 % penetrance by the age of 36 years for MTC, 68 years for pheochromocytoma, and 82 years for HPT (Frank-Raue et al. 2011), and penetrance for MTC by 50 years ranged from 60 % for codon 611 mutations to 86 % for codon 620 mutations.

Molecular-Based Medical Management in MEN 2

RET testing in MEN 2 is considered the paradigm for the practice of clinical cancer genetics. Since *RET* mutations have been identified in >95 % of individuals with MEN 2, RET gene testing as a molecular diagnostic and predictive test is standard practice (Eng et al. 1996a, b, 2001; Kloos et al. 2009). In addition, all cases of MTC, irrespective of syndromic features or family history, should be offered *RET* gene testing in the setting of clinical cancer genetic consultation if possible.

In a MEN 2 family without a known mutation, *RET* testing should begin with an affected individual. Once a family-specific mutation is found, all at-risk family members should be offered testing before the age of 5 years in MEN 2A/ FMTC and before the age of 2 years, preferably within the first year, in MEN 2B (Kloos et al. 2009). For those individuals found to have a mutation, a prophylactic total thyroidectomy is recommended for all MEN 2 subtypes. This should be completed before the age of 5–6 years for MEN 2A/FMTC and before the age of 2 years, some believe 6 months, for MEN 2B (Wells et al. 1994; Kloos et al. 2009). The precise timing of prophylactic surgery remains controversial for FMTC, and in cases with codon 609, 768, and 804 mutations, which seem to have a lower penetrance and perhaps later onset of MTC (Eng et al. 1996a, b; Shannon et al. 1999; Frank-Raue et al. 2011), current ATA Guidelines suggest that prophylactic thyroidectomy can wait beyond age 5 if basal/stimulated calcitonins and neck ultrasounds are normal (Kloos et al. 2009). Clinical surveillance following thyroidectomy is dictated by what is found during the surgery. If the patient is found to have invasive MTC at the time of surgery, screening should include calcium-stimulated calcitonin testing every 3–6 months for the first 2 years, every 6 months from 3 to 5 years after surgery, and then annually. If only a small focus of MTC is found at the time of surgery, follow-up screening should involve annual basal (unstimulated) calcitonin for 5–10 years. If no cancer is present in the thyroid at the time of prophylactic surgery, no follow-up screening is indicated, even if C cell hyperplasia is present. All individuals who have undergone thyroidectomy need thyroid hormone replacement therapy and monitoring.

MEN 2-related PC almost always occurs after MTC. All mutation-positive individuals should undergo annual screening for PC beginning at 6 years. This usually consists of 24-h urine studies for VMA, metanephrines, and catecholamines. Some centers also advocate annual serum measurements for catecholamine levels and chromogranin-A. Abdominal ultrasound or CT/MRI scans for routine surveillance remains controversial.

In MEN 2, HPT is usually later onset and has age-related penetrance (Schuffenecker et al. 1998; Frank-Raue et al. 2011). Clinical surveillance in MEN 2A includes annual measurement of serum ionized calcium and intact parathyroid hormone levels beginning at the time of MEN 2 diagnosis. Once HPT is detected, removal of all four parathyroid glands is necessary. At that time or at the time of thyroidectomy, whichever occurs first, all glands and the thymus are removed. Half of the parathyroid gland should be pulverized and autografted into an easily accessible muscle of the arm or neck to control the body's calcium levels and can be easily removed should HPT recur (Wells et al. 1994; Kloos et al. 2009). Since clinically evident HPT is rare in MEN 2B, parathyroid screening is not generally recommended for this subtype.

Management of *RET* mutation-negative MEN 2 families remains a conundrum. If there are sufficient clinically affected members in such families, linkage analysis using 10q11 markers within and around RET could be performed. In the event that the family is not large enough or informative for linkage, then management should follow that in the pre-*RET* testing era, and at-risk individuals should undergo annual screening for MTC (stimulated calcitonin screening), PC, and HPT from the age of 6–35 years. Prophylactic thyroidectomy is usually not routinely offered to this subgroup.

Muir–Torre Syndrome (OMIM 158320)

Muir–Torre syndrome is a rare autosomal dominant condition, first described in 1967 in an individual who had multiple benign sebaceous adenomas and keratoacanthoma of the skin and multiple internal malignancies (large bowel, duodenum, and larynx) (Muir et al. 1967). The skin stigmata of this condition include sebaceous hyperplasia, adenoma, and carcinoma, with keratoacanthoma and basal cell cancer (BCC). The internal neoplasias include tumors of the colon, stomach and esophagus, breast, uterus, ovaries, bladder, and larynx and squamous cell carcinomas of the mucous membranes (Grignon et al. 1987). The syndrome is defined by dermatologists as a combination of at least one sebaceous gland tumor and a minimum of one internal malignancy (Cohen et al. 1991). The condition usually becomes manifest from the fifth decade of life, and multiple skin lesions develop.

It has become apparent that the main hereditary cause of Muir–Torre syndrome is mutations in the MMR genes *MSH2*, *MLH1* and *MSH6*. The presence of identical mutations in families with HNPCC/Lynch syndrome and Muir–Torre syndrome confirms that this syndrome is nearly always a variant of Lynch syndrome (Sieber et al. 2003a, b; Aretz et al. 2013; Bartkova et al. 2008; Kolodner et al. 1994) (but see note below on MUTYH-associated polyposis). The implication of this conclusion is that individuals with sebaceous carcinoma and a mutation in a MMR gene should be considered to be at an elevated lifetime risk of all the cancers that are known to occur in Lynch syndrome. In a large, single-institution study, 27 of 41 patients with Muir–Torre syndrome had mutations in *MLH1* or *MSH2* (Mangold et al. 2004). Interestingly, 25 of the 27 mutations were in *MSH2*, confirming multiple earlier observations that found far more mutations in *MSH2* than in *MLH1* (Lucci-Cordisco et al. 2003). Because the ascertainment criteria in the recent study of Mangold et al. were a sebaceous gland neoplasm and at least one internal neoplasm in the same patient (regardless of site of cancer or family history), it is not surprising that not all individuals with germline MMR gene mutations fell within the Bethesda guidelines for gene testing. Probably all sebaceous neoplasms occurring in the context of Muir–Torre syndrome are associated with MSI (Kruse et al. 2003), or loss of expression of MSH2 (or rarely MLH1 and MSH6) (Fiorentino et al. 2004), so all patients with sebaceous neoplasms should be offered either or both of these tests. If either test suggests a MMR gene mutation, analysis should be carried out, even in the absence of an internal malignancy or a positive family history. The situation may be particularly challenging on the rare occasion when a child is diagnosed with a sebaceous neoplasm (which are usually periocular) (Omura et al. 2002); as in the absence of family history, testing of a minor may be warranted. From a laboratory standpoint, the spectrum of mutations in *MSH2* is similar to that seen in non-Muir–Torre-associated Lynch syndrome, no genotype–phenotype associations within *MSH2* are seen (Mangold et al. 2004), and a search for genomic deletions is indicated if sequenced-based analysis is negative (Barana et al. 2004).

Screening for cancer in relatives of individuals with this disorder is obviously important and should be similar to that outlined for Lynch syndrome, with extracolonic surveillance, particularly of the skin. It is interesting to note that in many families with Muir–Torre syndrome, only one person is affected by a sebaceous cancer, suggesting that other modifying factors may be present. In one Quebec family, which was later identified to carry a germline deletion in *MLH1*, the one person who developed sebaceous carcinoma only did so after receiving a heart transplant and subsequent immunosuppression (Paraf et al. 1995). The generality of this finding has been confirmed in a more recent study (Harwood et al. 2003).

When exposed to N-nitrosomethylbenzylamine, mice heterozygous for the gene encoding the fragile histidine triad gene, Fhit, developed a syndrome akin to human Muir–Torre syndrome (Fong et al. 2000). In human sebaceous carcinomas, FHIT protein was absent only from those tumors that were microsatellite stable, suggesting an alternative pathway to skin tumors in this syndrome (Holbach et al. 2002). No germline mutations in *FHIT* have been identified in Muir–Torre (or any other human cancer) syndrome. On the other hand, there have been reports of sebaceous carcinomas in MUTYH-associated polyposis (see below) and thus not all Muir-Torre syndrome is due to MMR gene mutations (Vogt et al. 2009).

MUTYH-Associated Polyposis (MAP) (OMIM 608456)

Biallelic mutations in the *MUTYH* gene have been shown to be responsible for an autosomal recessive form of adenomatous polyposis. The *MUTYH* gene is involved in repair of oxidative DNA damage, and adenomas from affected patients show characteristic DNA repair errors. The number of colonic polyps in this condition tends to be between 15 and 200, significantly fewer than in classical FAP, although approximately 8 % of cases of polyposis with no detectable germline APC mutation, particularly cases with relatively few (100–500) polyps, have been found to carry biallelic mutations in the *MUTYH* gene (Sampson and Jones 2009). The disorder accounts for approximately 30 % of cases of attenuated polyposis, with 15–100 colonic adenomas; biallelic *MUTYH* mutations have been reported in 26–29 % of patients with 10–100 polyps and 7–29 % of patients with 100–1,000 polyps. Biallelic mutations have occasionally been reported in patients with fewer than 10 adenomas (Aretz et al. 2006; Brand et al. 2012; Al-Tassan et al. 2002; Sampson et al. 2003; Sieber et al. 2003a, b) and have been reported when a single colorectal cancer is the sole phenotype (Lubbe et al. 2009). Duodenal adenomas are found in 17–25 % of individuals with MAP; the lifetime risk of duodenal cancer is about 4 %. Osteomas and CHRPE have also been reported in MAP patients (Sieber et al. 2003a, b; Bartkova et al. 2008; Aretz et al. 2013). An extended spectrum of tumor manifestations of biallelic mutations in *MUTYH* have been described (Vogt et al. 2009).

Management of patients with *MUTYH*-associated polyposis should be along the lines of FAP management, with upper GI surveillance, since affected individuals do have a risk of upper GI neoplasia. Screening should be initiated from the same age as recommended in AFAP (between 18 and 20 years). Because patients may develop only a few adenomas and CRC is often localized in the proximal colon, colonoscopy at 2-yearly intervals is preferable to sigmoidoscopy (Vasen et al. 2008).

Upper gastrointestinal endoscopy is advised, starting from 25 to 30 years of age, frequency depending on severity (Vasen et al. 2008). While this subject remains controversial, on balance, it seems that heterozygotes face little or no increased risk of GI polyps and colorectal cancer and do not require surveillance, but it is important to be certain that close relatives of affected individuals are offered genetic testing at least for the two common *MUTYH* mutations.

N Syndrome (OMIM 310465)

This rare, X-linked recessive disorder was described in a single family (two affected brothers) and was characterized by mental retardation, chromosome breakage, and a predisposition to T cell leukemia. It is suggested to be caused by a mutation of DNA polymerase alpha (Floy et al. 1990).

NAME Syndrome

See Carney Complex (above).

Neurofibromatosis Type 1 (NF1) (Von Recklinghausen Disease, Peripheral NF) (OMIM 162200)

NF1 is the most common form of NF, with a prevalence of about 1 per 3,000 persons. Inheritance is autosomal dominant with variable expression, but approximately 50 % of cases represent new mutations. Characteristic clinical features are listed in Table 11.9. Conventional diagnostic criteria require two or more of the following features: (1) six or more café-au-lait lesions (more than 5 mm greatest diameter in children and more than 15 mm greatest diameter in adults); (2) two or more neurofibromas or one plexiform neurofibroma; (3) axillary or inguinal

Table 11.9 Clinical features of NF1

Neurofibromas
Café-au-lait spots
Axillary freckling
Lisch nodules
Intellectual impairment
Epilepsy
Macrocephaly
Short stature
Kyphoscoliosis
Pseudoarthrosis
Renal artery stenosis
NS Neoplasia: Optic glioma, astrocytoma and glioma, neurilemomas, neurofibrosarcoma or malignant schwannomas
Endocrine Neoplasia: Phaeochromocytoma, carcinoid
Other Neoplasia: Wilms' tumor, Rhabdomyosarcoma, Leukemia, Neuroblastoma

freckling; (4) two or more Lisch nodules; (5) optic glioma; (6) characteristic osseous lesion (sphenoid dysplasia or cortical thinning of long bone, with or without pseudoarthrosis); and (7) a first-degree relative (parent, sibling, or child) with NF1 according to the above criteria.

The approximate frequencies of disabling nonneoplastic complications of NF1 were estimated by Huson et al. (1989) to be 33 % for intellectual handicap (3 % moderate–severe retardation, 30 % minimal retardation or learning difficulties), 5 % for scoliosis requiring surgery, 4 % for epilepsy, 2 % for severe pseudoarthrosis, and 2 % for renal artery stenosis. Café-au-lait spots occur in more than 99 % of patients with NF1 but are not specific and may fade in older patients (de Raed et al 2003).

The diagnosis of NF1 among at-risk relatives can usually be made early: Huson et al. (1989) found that all gene carriers have developed six or more café-au-lait spots by the age of 5 years, and 90 % of affected subjects have Lisch nodules by this age. Lisch nodules were reported to be present in 93–100 % of adults (aged over 20 years) with NF1 (Huson et al. 1989; Lubs et al. 1991; De Raed et al. 2003). Unlike café-au-lait spots and neurofibromas, multiple Lisch nodules are specific for NF1 and have only been reported rarely in NF2. In addition, Lisch nodules frequently develop before neurofibromas (Lubs et al. 1991), which, in the absence of molecular genetic testing, is very useful in the differentiation between minimally affected and unaffected individuals. In children with possible NF1 and no Lisch nodules, the ophthalmological assessment should be repeated periodically. Slit-lamp examination allows Lisch nodules to be distinguished from common iris nevi.

Individuals with NF1 are at increased risk of a variety of neoplastic lesions, including optic glioma, neurofibrosarcoma, brain gliomas, pheochromocytoma, and leukemia. Estimates of the increased risk of neoplasia are variable because of differences in the methods of ascertainment, and some older studies have not distinguished between NF1 and NF2. Sorensen et al. (1986) reported that the common perception of NF as a severe disorder with greatly increased risk of cancer is incorrect. Although probands in a hospital-based study had a fourfold increase in the incidence of malignant neoplasms or benign CNS tumors, the relative risk among affected relatives was only 1.5 (0.9 in males, 1.9 in females). There was a significant excess of glioma, and although the relative risk of pheochromocytoma was greatly increased (because it is rare in the general population), the absolute risk was small. In a population-based study, Huson et al. (1989) estimated the overall risk of malignant or CNS tumors to be approximately 5 % (0.7 % for optic glioma, 0.7–1.5 % for other CNS tumors, 1.5 % for rhabdomyosarcoma, and 1.5 % for peripheral nerve malignancy). Endocrine tumors (pheochromocytomas, pancreatic apudomas) may occur in 3.1 %, and spinal and visceral neurofibromas each occur in about 2.1 % of patients. Stiller et al. (1994) reported a relative risk of chronic myelomonocytic leukemia of 221 in NF1, whereas the relative risks for acute lymphoblastic leukemia (ALL) and non-Hodgkin lymphoma were 5.4 and 10, respectively. There is a small increase in the risk of breast cancer in women with NF1, and targeted early breast cancer screening has recently been suggested for these women (Evans 2012).

Specific Tumor Types in NF1

Neurofibromas are benign tumors that usually involve the skin, although they can be subcutaneous or, rarely, visceral. Solitary neurofibromas may occur in an individual without a germline *NF1* mutation. The number of cutaneous neurofibromas increases with advancing age but shows wide variation (Huson et al. 1989) (Fig. 11.7). Two types of neurofibroma are distinguished: the common discrete variety in which the lesion arises from a single site along a peripheral nerve and has well-defined margins. Cutaneous neurofibromas are usually present in adults with NF1 and are most common on the trunk. About 20 % have head and neck lesions, and more than 100 neurofibromas are found in most older patients. Though cutaneous neurofibromas usually do not become apparent until puberty but can continue to increase in size and number throughout adulthood.

Plexiform neurofibromas are peripheral nerve tumors that extend along the nerve and can involve multiple nerve branches. Plexiform neurofibromas are often associated with local soft tissue overgrowth and, when the cranial nerves are involved, cause marked disfigurement. Plexiform neurofibromas appear as large, soft, subcutaneous swellings with ill-defined margins and may be present in about 25 % of NF1 patients (usually on the trunk), but facial involvement is rare (Huson et al. 1988). The principal complication of neurofibromas is cosmetic disfigurement, but there is also the risk of malignant change (malignant peripheral nerve sheath tumor, MPNST) (Evans et al. 2002; De Raedt et al. 2003). Malignant change is usually signaled by pain and rapid increase in size, and all patients should be alerted to the significance of these events. Plexiform neurofibroma is locally aggressive and may grow along the nerve of origin to involve the spinal cord or brain. The risk of malignant change was estimated to be 2–4 % (Huson et al. 1988), but a

Fig. 11.7 Neurofibromatosis type 1. Dermal neurofibromata (Reproduced from the third edition, with permission from Cambridge University Press; Courtesy of Susan Huson)

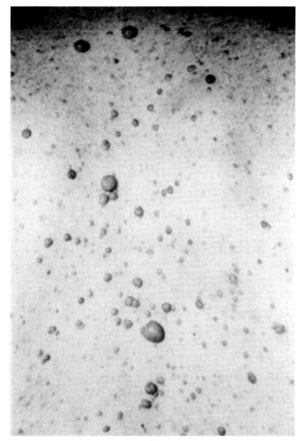

population-based longitudinal study reported a lifetime risk of 8–13 % (median age at diagnosis 26 years) (Evans et al. 2002).

Optic glioma is the most frequently reported CNS lesion in NF1, and about a third of children with optic glioma have NF1. Estimates of the incidence of optic glioma in NF1 patients vary: Huson et al. (1988) found in a population-based study that less than 2 % of patients with NF1 had a symptomatic glioma, but Lewis et al. (1984) observed a frequency of up to 15 % with routine cranial magnetic resonance imaging. Symptomatic optic gliomas usually present before 6 years of age. Histologically, optic gliomas are pilocytic astrocytomas, and these are generally nonprogressive tumors and are usually treated conservatively.

Other CNS gliomas reported in NF1 include brain stem gliomas, pilocytic astrocytomas of the hypothalamus and third ventricle, and, infrequently, diffuse gliomas of the cerebral hemispheres, cerebellum, or spinal cord. Although brain stem glioma may produce aqueduct stenosis and hydrocephalus, NF1 patients are also at risk for nonneoplastic lesions, such as dural ectasia and aqueduct stenosis without mass lesions.

NF1 is a well-recognized, but infrequent, cause of pheochromocytoma. The most frequent age at diagnosis of phaeochromocytoma in NF1 patients is in the fifth decade (Walther et al. 1999b). Onset before the age of 20 years is uncommon, and this tumor is virtually unknown in childhood (Knudson and Strong 1972).

The other endocrine tumor that has been associated with NF1 is duodenal carcinoid. Typically, this is somatostatinoma with distinctive histological appearance (psammoma bodies) and somatostatin immunoreactivity (Griffiths et al. 1987; Swinburn et al. 1988). A variety of embryonal tumors have been reported in children with NF1, including rhabdomyosarcoma, Wilms tumor, and neuroblastoma (McKeen et al. 1978; Hartley et al. 1988). In addition, children with NF1 are predisposed to myeloid malignancies (200–500 times the normal risk), particularly juvenile myelomonocytic leukemia (Bader and Miller 1978; Clark and Hutter 1982).

The *NF1* gene maps to chromosome 17 and was identified in 1990 (Wallace et al. 1990; Viskochil et al. 1990). The *NF1* gene product (neurofibromin) is a negative regulator of Ras GTPase proteins, and the *NF1* gene appears to function as a classical tumor suppressor gene such that *NF1* wild-type allele loss has been detected in both malignant neurofibroma. *NF1* is a large gene (61 exons contained within 300 kb of DNA) and has a high mutation rate. De novo mutations usually arise in the paternal germline though microdeletions may be most often of maternal origin. Comprehensive mutation analysis can identify *NF1* mutations in >90 % of patients satisfying NIH diagnostic criteria (Boyd et al. 2009). Mutation analysis of the *NF1* gene is helpful in individuals who do not fulfill clinical diagnostic criteria or if prenatal or preimplantation diagnosis is being considered. Though in general the precise nature of an *NF1* mutation does not correlate with clinical phenotype, up to 5 % of cases have a complete *NF1* gene deletion which is associated with increased numbers of neurofibromas, more severe intellectual impairment, facial dysmorphisms, and increased risk of MPNST. Germline mutations in *SPRED1* cause Legius syndrome which is characterized by similar cutaneous findings to NF1 (multiple cafe-au-lait macules and axillary freckling) but not Lisch nodules or neurofibromas.

Patients with NF1 should be kept under surveillance, with annual clinical examination (every 2 years in children), but routine biochemical or radiological screening is probably not indicated in a service setting (Huson et al. 1988). The affectation status for most at-risk relatives can be reliably established on clinical criteria because penetrance is close to 100 % for offspring of unequivocal cases (Riccardi and Lewis 1988). Although presymptomatic diagnoses of *NF1* by mutation analysis or linked DNA markers should be possible for most cases, it is not usually undertaken unless clinical diagnostic criteria are equivocal. Although detection of a *NF1* mutation might allow prenatal diagnosis, a limitation of molecular genetic testing is that the severity of the disorder usually cannot be predicted as NF1 characteristically has very wide variations in expression. Parents of apparently sporadic cases should undergo careful assessment for subclinical signs of NF1 (e.g., detailed skin examination with Wood's light and ophthalmological testing for Lisch nodules). Mosaic NF1 may be segmental, generalized (when disease is usually mild) or gonadal. Segmental mosaics present with localized cutaneous involvement (CALs/neurofibromas).

Neurofibromatosis Type 2 (NF2) (Central Neurofibromatosis and Bilateral Acoustic Neuroma Neurofibromatosis) (OMIM 607379)

NF2 is an autosomal dominantly inherited disorder estimated to have an incidence of about 1 in 33,000 persons per year and a prevalence of 1 in 55,000 (Evans et al. 2010). More than 50 % of cases have no family history of *NF2* and result from de novo mutations. It has been estimated that about a third of patients are mosaic, and the *NF2* mutation cannot be detected in blood (only in tumor tissue). NF2 accounts for 7 % of the patients with vestibular schwannomas (Evans et al. 2005). The hallmark of NF2 is bilateral vestibular schwannomas (acoustic neuromas), but there is also a predisposition to other CNS tumors, such as meningioma, astrocytoma, ependymoma, and schwannomas of the dorsal spinal roots. NF1 and NF2 are distinct disorders, with the *NF1* and *NF2* genes mapping to chromosomes 17 and 22, respectively.

The clinical features of NF2 as reported by Evans et al. (1992, 1997; Eng et al. 2003; MacCollin et al. 2003) in a large UK study are shown in Table 11.10. Although peripheral neurofibromas may occur in NF2, they are rarely numerous, and Lisch nodules (iris hamartomas), axillary or groin freckling, and multiple (six or more) café-au-lait spots are not features of NF2. However, café-au-lait patches do occur in excess: Kanter et al. (1980) found that 61 % of NF2 patients had at least one café-au-lait spot or neurofibroma but that none had more than five, and Evans et al. (1992) found only one out of 97 patients had six café-au-lait patches. Glial tumors are less common than meningioma or schwannomas, and astrocytomas and ependymomas are usually low grade, affecting the lower brain stem or upper spinal cord. A mononeuropathy that occurs particularly in children and a generalized peripheral neuropathy that occurs in adults are increasingly recognized features of NF2 in some cases (Evans et al. 1992; Lloyd and Evans 2013).

The Manchester diagnostic criteria are widely used (see Table 11.11), but all clinical diagnostic criteria have a low sensitivity for diagnosing mosaic individuals without bilateral vestibular schwannomas and a family history.

Table 11.10 Clinical features of NF2

Clinical features	Frequency (%)
Vestibular schwannoma	85
Meningioma	45
Spinal tumors	26
Skin tumors	68
Café-au-lait patch	43
Cataracts	38
Ependymoma	3
Astrocytoma	4
Optic sheath meningioma	4

Adapted from Evans et al. (1992)

Table 11.11 Diagnostic criteria for NF2

Bilateral vestibular schwannomas
Or
Family history of NF2 plus (a) unilateral vestibular schwannoma or (b) any two of meningioma, glioma, neurofibroma, schwannoma, and posterior subcapsular lenticular opacities
Or
Unilateral vestibular schwannoma plus any two of meningioma, schwannoma, glioma, neurofibroma, or posterior subcapsular opacities
Or
Multiple meningioma plus (a) unilateral vestibular schwannomas or (b) two or more of schwannoma, glioma, neurofibroma, or cataract

The age of onset of NF2 is variable. Symptoms of vestibular schwannomas (usually hearing loss, which may be unilateral, sometimes vestibular disturbance or tinnitus) typically begin in the second or third decade (mean age of 23 years), but NF2 can present in the first or seventh decade (Kanter et al. 1980; Martuza and Eldridge 1988; Evans et al. 1992). Penetrance is more than 95 % at the age of 50 years, and the mean age at diagnosis is 28 years. The first manifestation of NF2 in some cases may be a congenital cataract. Some studies have suggested that there is an earlier age at onset in familial cases with maternal transmission (Kanter et al. 1980; Evans et al. 1992); however, there is no evidence of imprinting of the *NF2* gene, and this observation may result from a tendency for severely affected men not to have children.

The proportion of NF2 patients reported to have other non-acoustic CNS tumors is variable. Kanter et al. (1980) estimated it at 18 % and Evans et al. (1992) at 45 %, but studies of single families have shown a higher incidence. Higher frequencies may reflect more complete ascertainment through diagnosis of asymptomatic tumors and also interfamilial variations in predisposition to other non-acoustic CNS tumors. Meningiomas in NF2 are frequently multiple and may be intracranial or spinal.

NF2 has been subdivided into two forms, according to a mild phenotype (Gardner type) with late onset (above 25 years) and a more severe form (Wishart) with early onset and multiple meningiomas and spinal tumors. However, many cases do not fit neatly into either category (Baser et al. 2002b).

Individuals in the following categories should be evaluated for evidence of NF2 (Martuza and Eldridge 1988): (1) acoustic neuroma at age less than 30 years, (2) child with meningeal or Schwann cell tumor, (3) multiple CNS tumors with no diagnosed cause, and (4) adolescent or adult with one or more neurofibromas but no family history of NF1, no Lisch nodules, and only a few café-au-lait spots. A careful skin examination, ophthalmological assessment, and audiometry with brain stem auditory-evoked response should be performed initially, and an MRI brain scan (to detect acoustic neuroma and other intracranial tumors) should be arranged for those individuals with any abnormalities suggestive of NF2. Skin neurofibromas occur infrequently in NF2, but skin tumors should be carefully sought. The most common types of skin tumors are (1) discrete subcutaneous swellings appearing to arise from peripheral nerves and (2) well-circumscribed, slightly raised lesions with a roughened appearance and prominent hairs (Evans et al. 1992).

Relatives of affected people should be investigated for stigmata of NF2. Congenital cataracts should be sought by detailed ophthalmoscopy, and annual clinical examination (for evidence of cutaneous stigmata) should be performed during childhood. From the age of 10 years, annual audiometry and brain stem auditory-evoked potential should be performed (Evans et al. 1992). Skin and eye examinations are also indicated. A gadolinium-enhanced MRI scan is a sensitive investigation and, if available, performed annually from age 10. In many cases, surveillance will be continued until the age of 40 years, but the decision about when to discontinue screening will depend on the individual family. Although early diagnosis and surgery will prevent progressive neurological impairment, often hearing cannot be preserved. Affected patients should be prepared for the possibility of progressive hearing loss and warned to avoid heights and swimming alone. At-risk individuals demonstrated not to be gene carriers by molecular genetic analysis can be excluded from further surveillance.

A notable feature of NF2 is a high prevalence of somatic mosaicism such that up to a third of people with new mutations are mosaic (Kluwe et al. 2003; Moyhuddin et al. 2003). Mosaicism should be suspected in individuals with mild disease and no detectable *NF2* mutation in blood. In cases with bilateral tumors and no detectable mutation in blood, the identification of an identical *NF2* mutation in both vestibular schwannomas is an indication of mosaicism. The risk of disease transmission from mosaic parents to offspring is low when the constitutional *NF2* mutation cannot be identified in the parent blood using standard techniques, and somatic mosaicism can cause misleading results in linkage analysis for the second generation (such that individual predicted to be at high risk on linkage analysis may have inherited a wild-type allele) (Moyhuddin et al. 2003). Conversely children who inherit a *NF2* mutation from a mosaic parent will generally be more severely affected.

The gene for NF2 maps to chromosome 22 and was identified in 1993 (Rouleau et al. 1993; Trofatter et al. 1993). No evidence of significant locus heterogeneity has been reported for classical NF2, but familial schwannomatosis (p. 6) is caused by mutations in *SMARCB1*, and mutations in this gene have occasionally been seen in patients with unilateral vestibular schwannomas and multiple central and cutaneous schwannomas or multiple meningiomas and schwannomatosis (van Munckhof et al. 2012). Mutation analysis of *NF2* must include both sequencing and analysis to detect exon deletions. Identification of germline *NF2* mutations has provided genotype–phenotype correlations such that non-mosaic patients with nonsense or frameshift mutations generally have more severe disease (Wishart type) than those with missense or splice site mutations or large deletions (though some missense mutations may be associated with a severe phenotype) (Parry et al. 1996; Ruttledge et al. 1996). For non-VIIIth nerve NF2-associated tumors (e.g., intracranial meningiomas, spinal tumors, and peripheral nerve tumors), people with constitutional *NF2* missense mutations, splice site mutations, large deletions, or somatic mosaicism had significantly fewer tumors than patients with nonsense or frameshift mutations (Baser et al. 2004; Selvanathan et al. 2010). Mosaicism is a further reason for phenotypic variability in NF2, and the high frequency of mosaicism influences molecular genetic investigation. Thus in cases of potential NF2 that fall short of the Manchester diagnostic criteria, molecular genetic analysis of tumor material can be helpful in guiding whether the patient is mosaic for a *NF2* mutation, and detailed information relating to the age at diagnosis of vestibular schwannoma and risk of mosaicism and risks to relatives have been reported (Evans et al. 2012).

The prognosis of patients with NF2 is influenced not only by genotype–phenotype correlations but also by surgical management with lower mortality in specialist centers (Baser et al. 2002a). Though surgery is the principal therapeutic intervention (with radiosurgery in some cases), there is increasing interest in the potential application of targeted nonsurgical treatments (Subbiah and Kurzrock 2012).

Neurofibromatosis: Atypical

This group comprises forms of NF that do not neatly fall into the NF1 or NF2 categories. For example, in NF3 there are features of NF1 (café-au-lait spots, cutaneous neurofibromas characteristically on the palms of the hand) and of NF2 (bilateral vestibular schwannomas, meningiomas, and spinal neurofibromas). Molecular genetic analysis of the *NF1* and *NF2* genes can be used to clarify the relationship of atypical forms of NF to NF1 and NF2. Schwannomatosis, a variant of NF2, can have a distinct pathogenesis (see above).

Nijmegen Breakage Syndrome, NBS (also known as Seemanova Syndrome II) (OMIM #251260)

This rare autosomal recessive disorder is characterized by microcephaly, growth retardation, "bird-like" face, premature ovarian failure, and humoral and cellular immunodeficiency. A characteristic feature is the marked discrepancy between the (usually) normal intelligence and severe microcephaly. The diagnosis of NBS is initially based on clinical manifestations and is confirmed by genetic analysis. There is very substantial risk of lymphoreticular malignancy – up to 50 % of patients develop lymphoma, at a median age of less than 11 years (Demuth and Digweed 2007). By age 20, 40 % of all NBS homozygotes have developed cancer (Chrzanowska et al. 2012). Laboratory findings include chromosome instability in cultured lymphocytes with frequent rearrangements involving chromosomes 7 and 14, cellular and chromosomal hypersensitivity to X-irradiation, and radio resistance of DNA replication (Taalman et al. 1989; Erola et al. 2003). Most reported cases are of eastern European (Slavic) origin, especially Czech Republic, Poland, western Russia, and the Ukraine, where a founder mutation (c.657_661del5, p.K219fsX19, in exon 6) is common. The cellular phenotype chromosome breakage and immunodeficiency features of Nijmegen breakage syndrome and AT are similar, but the clinical phenotypes are distinct. The gene for Nijmegen breakage syndrome (*NBN*, formerly *NBS1*) encodes a protein (nibrin) (Varon et al. 1998) that is phosphorylated by the ATM protein. Nibrin, together with *MRE11* and RAD50, forms a trimeric protein complex known as MRN that is involved in repairing DNA double-strand breaks. From studies of relatives of *NBN* homozygotes and from studies sequencing *NBN* in cancer cases and controls, it is clear that heterozygotes have an increased risk of tumors, including prostate and breast cancer, and melanoma (reviewed in Demuth and Digweed 2007).

Noonan Syndrome (OMIM 163950) and the RASopathies

Noonan syndrome is characterized by cardiac defects, short stature, cryptorchidism, and characteristic facial features (ptosis, hypertelorism, a low hairline, and neck webbing). The most common cardiac defects seen (85–90 % overall) are pulmonary stenosis, hypertrophic cardiomyopathy, and VSD. 65 % may have a clotting defect. It affects approximately 1 in 2.5,000 people and was originally thought to be a variant of Turner's syndrome because neck webbing and short stature were features of both. However, the karyotype is normal in Noonan syndrome (NS), and it is inherited as an autosomal dominant trait. Mutations in *PTPN11* are found in about half of patients with this condition, and the gene product, SHP2, is a component of the mitogen-activated protein kinase (MAPK) signaling pathway. More recently, germline gain-of-function mutations in other genes involved in the same Ras/MPK pathway have been found in a proportion of cases, e.g., *SHOC2, KRAS, SOS1, NRAS, BRAF*, and *RAF1* (Pandit et al. 2006). Autosomal recessive Noonan syndrome may be caused by mutations in the *SHOC2* gene.

LEOPARD syndrome (LS) (OMIM 151100), so called because of its clinical features of lentigines, ECG anomalies, ocular hypertelorism, pulmonary stenosis, abnormal genitalia, growth retardation, and deafness, is caused by gain-of-function mutations in *PTPN11* and therefore considered as a variant of Noonan syndrome (Tartaglia et al. 2006).

Germline mutations in other genes involved in the Ras/MPK pathway have been identified in children with related disorders, e.g., cardio-facio-cutaneous syndrome (CFC) (OMIM 115150) and Costello syndrome (OMIM 218040).

Preliminary studies have suggested that there is an increased risk of cancer in patients with Noonan syndrome with germline *PTPN11* mutations in older age groups, but this has not been confirmed. The main risk is for juvenile myelomonocytic leukemia. One mutation, threonine to isoleucine at position 73 in *SHP-2* (Thr73Ile), has been found in several NS patients suffering from JMML (Jongmans et al. 2011; Tartaglia et al. 2003).

CFC presents with cardiac defects, characteristic coarse facial features, hyperkeratotic skin lesions and nevi, sparse curly hair, sparse eyebrows, and severe developmental delay and is associated with germline mutations in *BRAF, KRAS, BRAF, MEK1*, or *MEK2* (Roberts et al. 2006), and Costello syndrome is characterized by cardiac defects, short stature, coarse facial features, and a significant increased risk of cancer, due to germline mutations in *HRAS* (Kerr et al. 2006).

It is thought that increased MAPK signal transduction results in cancer suscepti-bility; a germline *HRAS* mutation which encodes a p.G12V amino acid change with very high transforming potential causes severe neonatal lethal Costello syndrome. Most cases of Costello syndrome are due to a less strongly activating mutation p.G12S, which results in a 15 % lifetime risk of tumors. There is another recurrent mutation, p.G13C, which results in a milder phenotype. The lifetime risk of cancer in Costello syndrome is estimated to be 15 %, 60 % of these being rhabdomyosarcoma, which tend to occur in childhood, and others commonly being neuroblastoma and bladder cancer. The bladder cancer may occur as early as the second decade of life.

The risk of rhabdomyosarcoma in Costello syndrome is similar to that in Beckwith–Wiedemann syndrome, which may justify screening. Based on the rec-ommendations for screening BWS patients, it has been suggested that children with Costello syndrome be offered screening by ultrasound examination of the abdomen and pelvis 3–6 monthly until 10 years of age for rhabdomyosarcoma and abdominal neuroblastoma, urine catecholamine metabolite analysis 6–12 monthly until 5 years of age for neuroblastoma, and annual urinalysis for hematuria for bladder carci-noma after 10 years of age (Gripp et al. 2002).

Noonan, CFC, and Costello syndromes, together with neurofibromatosis type 1 and Noonan syndrome with multiple lentigines (LEOPARD syndrome), caused by germline mutations in the genes in the Ras/MAPK pathway, are becoming known as the RASopathies, and a RASopathy patient/family support group has been pro-posed, but the patient groups remain separate as the issues are all rather different for the different conditions.

Perlman Syndrome (OMIM 267000)

This rare disorder is an autosomal recessively inherited congenital overgrowth syn-drome with phenotypic similarities to Beckwith–Wiedemann syndrome. Affected children are large at birth and hypotonic and have organomegaly, characteristic facial dysmorphisms (inverted V-shape upper lip, prominent forehead, deep set eyes, broad flat nasal bridge, low set ears), renal anomalies (nephromegaly and hydronephrosis), frequent neurodevelopmental delay, and high neonatal mortality (Perlman 1986; Greenberg et al. 1988). Perlman syndrome is associated with a very high risk of Wilms tumor (64 % incidence in infants surviving beyond the neonatal period), an earlier age at diagnosis than in sporadic cases (<2 years and 3–4 years, respectively), and a high frequency of bilateral tumors (55 %). Histological examination of the kidneys in children with Perlman syndrome shows frequent nephroblastomatosis (an important precursor lesion for Wilms tumor).

Perlman syndrome is caused by germline inactivating mutations in *DIS3L2* (a homologue of the yeast *Dis3* gene). Dis3 is a critical component of the evolution-arily conserved exosome complex, and it has been suggested that the inactivation of *DIS3L2* leads to disordered RNA metabolism with aberrant expression of mitotic checkpoint proteins (Astuti et al. 2012; Greenberg et al. 1986).

Peutz–Jeghers Syndrome (PJS) (OMIM 602216, OMIM 175200)

PJS is a rare autosomal dominant inherited hamartoma cancer syndrome character- ized by tiny pigmented mucocutaneous macules on the skin and GI hamartomatous polyps and a high risk of GI, breast, and pancreatic carcinomas (Hemminki et al. 1997; Eng et al. 2001). Germline mutations in *STK11* on chromosome 19p13 are found in most classical cases of PJS, but a very small proportion of cases do not have detectable mutations in this gene (de Leng et al. 2007; Volikos et al. 2006).

Clinical Features

The presence of melanin spots on the lips, perioral region, and buccal mucosa is pathognomonic for PJS and probably occurs in 95 % of such individuals (Peutz 1921; Jeghers et al. 1949). These tiny macules can also occur as black or bluish spots on the hands (especially the palms), arms, feet (especially plantar areas), legs, genitalia, and anus. The skin pigmentation is present from early childhood and may fade after the age of 25 years. The absence of the pigmented spots therefore does not exclude the diagnosis of PJS (Lampe et al. 2003). Most patients present because of symptomatology related to their GI hamartomatous polyps, although polyps can occur in the nasal mucosa, bladder, uterus, and gallbladder as well. They can present with episodes of colicky abdominal pain from childhood (usually the second decade). Intussusception and obstruction are not uncommon complications, and rectal bleeding, severe enough to present with anemia, may occur. The distribution of polyps is most commonly in the small intestine (60–90 %), but also in the colon (50–64 %), stomach (49 %), and rectum (32 %) (Jeghers et al. 1949). The polyps are broad-based hamartomas of the smooth muscle that extend into the lamina propria. Many show histological features of "pseudoinvasion." Nevertheless, adenomatous change may develop within the polyps, and there is an increased risk of malignancy (relative risk 13), and mortality from cancer as high as 40 % by 50 years of age has been quoted for this condition (Boardman et al. 1998; Giardiello et al. 1987; Lim et al. 2004). In the absence of the characteristic melanin spots, the histopathology of the polyps is critical in making the diagnosis of PJS, as the PJS polyp has a diagnos- tically useful central core of smooth muscle that extends in a tree-like manner ("arborization") into the superficial epithelial layer. There is frond-like elongated epithelium and cystic gland dilatation extending to the muscularis propria with arborizing smooth muscle. Thus invagination of the epithelial layer occurs, essen- tially trapping these cells within the smooth muscle component, and causing "pseu- doinvasion" of the bowel wall that can be misdiagnosed as cancer, but has no evidence of cytological atypia. This involvement of the three tissue layers predis- poses to intussusception and the formation of the distinctive lobulated PJS polyp. Nonetheless, the operational clinical diagnostic criteria for PJS are as follows:

1. Two or more histologically confirmed PJS polyps
2. Any number of PJS polyps or characteristic mucocutaneous pigmentation, with a positive family history of PJS
3. Any number of PJS polyps with characteristic mucocutaneous pigmentation (Aretz et al. 2005; Aaltonen et al. 1998)

In addition to an increased risk of GI cancer, extraintestinal cancers are overrepresented in PJS as well (Giardiello et al. 1987). Invasive ductal carcinomas of the breast and pancreatic adenocarcinomas are significantly associated with PJS (Boardman et al. 1998). Nonmalignant tumors associated with this syndrome include ovarian sex cord tumors and testicular (Sertoli cell) tumors. The histology of these tumors is intermediate between granulosa cell tumors and Sertoli cell tumors. They are common in this syndrome, and rarely malignant, although at least one such malignancy has been described. The clinical effects are mainly due to the hyperestrogenization in females and can give rise to adenoma malignum of the cervix, which can be very malignant. Many of these tumors occur in young adults, and the Sertoli and sex cord tumors may occur in prepubertal boys, causing sexual precocity and gynecomastia. Sertoli cell tumors of the ovary may occur, and ovarian sex cord tumors are common, bilateral and multifocal.

The relative risks of all cancers in PJS are high, assessed as 3 % by age of 30 years, 19 % by 40 years, 32 % by 50 years, 63 % by 60 years, and 81 % by age of 70 years. The respective risks of GI cancer (esophagus, stomach, small bowel, colorectum, and pancreas) are 1, 10, 18, 42, and 66 % and of gynecological cancer 3, 6, 13, and 13 % overall, and the breast cancer risks are 8 % by 40 years of age, 11 % by 50 years, and 32 % by 50 years of age. The risk of pancreatic cancer may reach 5 % by age 40 years and 8 % by 60 years (Lim et al. 2003, 2004).

Genetics

Germline loss-of-function mutations in *STK11*, on19p13.3, encoding a multifunctional nuclear serine–threonine kinase, were found in a proportion of PJS individuals and kindreds (Hemminki et al. 1997, 1998; Jenne et al. 1998). *STK11* mutations have been found in 80–96 % of cases, leading to the suggestion of either locus heterogeneity or the presence of large deletions and promoter mutations, which have not been systematically analyzed. There is no clear genotype–phenotype association; current evidence suggests that it is unlikely that there is another major PJS locus.

STK11 has nine exons, and the normal protein product acts as a tumor suppressor, a notable role for a protein kinase. Studies show that biallelic inactivation of *STK11* in the tumor, either through germline mutation plus somatic mutation or more commonly promoter hypermethylation of the wild-type allele, causes hamartomatous polyps to develop. The gene product is a serine–threonine kinase which regulates cell proliferation, partly via G1 cell-cycle arrest. It also plays a role in cell polarity and WNT signaling and is a negative regulator of mTOR in the TSC pathway.

Genetic and Medical Management

As with other inherited cancer syndromes, patients with or suspected to have PJS should be referred to clinical cancer genetic consultation. The presence of a germ-line *STK11* mutation is diagnostic of PJS. However, failure to find a mutation in an individual who meets the clinical diagnostic criteria for PJS does not exclude the diagnosis, and such individuals should be managed like anyone with PJS and/or germline *STK11* mutation.

Initial follow-up and management in PJS is aimed at detecting polyps in the bowel to prevent complications arising such as intussusception and intestinal obstruction. Later in adult life, screening is done to detect precancerous lesions and early cancer. Suggested protocols are baseline colonoscopy and upper GI endoscopy at 8 years and if no polyps are detected, initiating further small bowel video capsule endoscopies and colonoscopies at 18 years, 3 yearly. If polyps are detected at 8 years of age, 3-yearly screening is recommended from that age. It is also recommended that after the age of 50 years, the frequency is increased to every 12 months due to the rapid increase in cancer risk after this age. If video capsule endoscopies are not available, barium meal and follow-through in adults or MRI can be alternatives. If a laparotomy is being performed, endoscopic polypec-tomy ("on table enteroscopy and polypectomy") should be considered. Screening for breast cancer by MRI annually from 25 years should be performed if possible, and cervical smears with liquid-based cytology are advised in adult women. However, screening for pancreatic or other cancers is not of proven benefit and is not recommended (Beggs et al. 2010). Treatment with MTOR inhibitors such as Rapamycin is under development with some initial indications of success.

Laparotomy may be required for suspicious symptoms. Polypectomy should be as complete as possible and can be performed at endoscopy. Surveillance for extraintestinal malignancy includes mammography, yearly gynecological evalua-tion and pelvic ultrasound, and 3-yearly cervical smears. Testicular ultrasound is suggested for males with feminizing features because of the risk of feminizing Sertoli cell tumors of the testis.

Pleuropulmonary Blastoma – Familial Tumor Dysplasia Syndrome (PPB-FTDS) (OMIM #601200, #138800)

Pleuropulmonary blastoma (PPB) is a rare lung tumor which presents in children under the age of 72 months at one of three stages – type 1, a bland-looking, but malignant, cyst; type 2, a partly solid, partly cystic lesion; and type 3, an entirely solid, highly malignant sarcoma-like lesion (Priest et al. 1997). It is the sentinel lesion of the PPB-FTDS, also known as the DICER1 syndrome. Other character-istic features of this rare syndrome include lung cysts (essentially a quiescent or regressed form of PPB), multinodular goiter, ovarian sex cord–stromal tumors (particularly Sertoli–Leydig cell tumor), cystic nephroma, embryonal rhabdomyo-sarcoma, and other very rare manifestations including pituitary blastoma, ciliary body medulloepithelioma, pineoblastoma, other primitive neuroectodermal tumors, juvenile intestinal polyps, adult-onset pleomorphic sarcoma, Wilms tumor, and possibly pulmonary sequestration (Priest et al. 1996; Hill et al. 2009; Foulkes et al. 2011; Rio Frio et al. 2011; Slade et al. 2011). Causative germline mutations in *DICER1*, a microRNA processing-RNase III-type endoribonuclease that is cru-cial for embryogenesis and early development (Bernstein et al. 2003), have been reported thus far in about 50 families (Hill et al. 2009; Bahubeshi et al. 2010; Foulkes et al. 2011; Rio Frio et al. 2011; Slade et al. 2011). Most of the germline mutations appear to truncate or otherwise disable the protein. In contrast, the sec-ond hits in the tumor, nearly all involve the RNase IIIb domain (Heravi-Moussavi et al. 2012) and apparently result in a failure to process 5′ mature miRNAs (Gurtan et al. 2012).

Porphyria

There are several forms of porphyria – inborn errors of porphyrin metabolism with sunlight-sensitive dermatological eruptions and abnormal porphyrin excretion pat-terns – most of which are inherited as autosomal dominant traits. Congenital eryth-ropoietic porphyria is an autosomal recessive trait. Clinical and molecular aspects of the different porphyrias are reviewed by Kauppinen (2005). Siderosis of the liver develops in the hepatic porphyrias and can lead to inflammation and fibrosis, with the risk of hepatomas developing, particularly in porphyria cutanea tarda and var-iegate porphyria (Gisbert et al. 2004). The dermatological features of these two types are bullae and fragile skin in sun-exposed areas, with hyperpigmentation, hypertrichosis, photosensitivity, erosions, milia, and sclerodermoid areas. Treatment is by phlebotomy and chloroquine. Many of the genes underlying the porphyrias – notably coproporphyria, acute intermittent, erythropoietic, and varie-gate porphyria (Martasek et al. 1994; Ostasiewicz et al. 1995; Meissner et al. 1996) – have been delineated, and it is possible to detect germline mutations in these in affected probands. In a study of 650 patients with acute intermittent porphyria followed up for 7 years, 7 were diagnosed with hepatocellular cancer (3 asymptom-atic), with an overall standardized rate ratio of 36 (95 % CI, 14–74). The occur-rence of cancer was not related to the specific heme biosynthetic abnormality, but heme precursors were significantly increased (and melatonin decreased) in cancer cases (Andant et al. 2000). From a follow-up study of 39 patients with porphyria cutanea tarda on surveillance with 6-monthly ultrasound and CA125 measure-ments, on treatment with phlebotomies resulting in clinical remission, only one patient developed hepatocellular cancer (cumulative incidence 0.26 %), and this patient was an alcoholic with hepatitis C virus (HCV) infection (Gisbert et al. 2004) The authors concluded that the risk of hepatocellular carcinoma was relatively low in such patients, but that the risk increased with HCV infection and advanced fibro-sis/cirrhosis. Other studies reported a relative risk of 5.3 (Fracanzani et al. 2001). It has been recommended that PCT patients should have liver biopsies to determine the presence of such factors and surveillance if they were present. The percentage of hepatocellular cancer attributable to HCV infection may be 25 %, and most develop in cirrhotic livers; surveillance should be by 6-monthly screening in such high-risk patients (Montalto et al. 2002). Other genetic factors increasing the risk for hepatocellular cancer are hemochromatosis, glycogen storage diseases 1A and 1b, tyrosinemia, and alpha-1 antitrypsin deficiency (Dragani 2010) (see p. 53). Patients with porphyria should be checked for their hepatitis and hemochromatosis status as these likely increase the risk of neoplasia.

Rhabdoid Tumor Predisposition Syndrome 1 (OMIM #609322)

Rhabdoid tumors are malignant, aggressive neoplasms that usually arise in infancy and early childhood. When these tumors occur in the brain and spinal cord, they are referred to as atypical teratoid/rhabdoid tumor (AT/RT), and when they arise in the kidney and/or soft tissues, they are termed malignant rhabdoid tumor (MRT) or extra-cranial rhabdoid tumor. Homozygous deletions on chromosome 22q, involving the *SNF5/INI1* gene (sucrose nonfermenting 5/integrase interactor 1), now known as *SMARCB1/BAF47*, were reported in cell lines derived from malignant rhabdoid tumors (Versteege et al. 1998). The SMARCB1 protein and other family members such as BRG1/SMARCA4 (see below) and ARID1A/SMARCF1 are involved in chromatin remodeling (Wilson and Roberts 2011). Subsequently, germline mutations were identified in children with ATRT and MRT (Sevenet et al. 1999; Biegel et al. 1999; Taylor et al. 2000). One-third of children with ATRT/MRT carry germline *SMARCB1* mutations, and in about a quarter of cases, transmission from parent to child is reported, implying a less aggressive phenotype in the parent (Eaton et al. 2011). Compared to sporadic cases (untested or negative for *SMARCB1* mutations), familial cases, mostly with germline *SMARCB1* mutations, had earlier onset of more aggressive, widespread disease that was more likely to be fatal (Bruggers et al. 2011). An antibody to BAF47 (encoded by *SMARCB1*) is available and can be used as a screening step prior to germline mutation analysis, since *SMARCB1* appears to be a classical 'two-hit' tumor suppressor (Roberts and Biegel 2009). Germline *SMARCB1* mutations can also result in familial schwannomatosis, and occasionally, both ATRT and schwannomatosis have been reported in the same family (Carter et al. 2012).

Rhabdoid Tumor Predisposition Syndrome 2 (OMIM #613325)

Investigation of two sisters with ATRT/MRT who did not show abnormal BAF47/SMARCB1/INI1 immunohistochemical staining or germline or somatic mutations in *SMARCB1* led to the identification of germline mutations in the partner molecule

BRG1/SMARCA4 (Schneppenheim et al. 2010). As for SMARCB1, immunohisto-chemical testing showed loss of BRG1/SMARCA4 in the tumor. The mutation was transmitted from an unaffected father. A second family containing a nine-month-old boy with an ATRT and a germline mutation in *SMARCA4* has also been reported (Hasselblatt et al. 2011). Therefore testing of *SMARCA4* might be indicated if the immunohistochemical staining of an ATRT/MRT for BAF47/INI1 is normal. The full spectrum of diseases associated with germline *SMARCA4* mutations remains to be determined.

Rothmund–Thomson Syndrome (OMIM 268400)

This rare autosomal recessive disorder is characterized by atrophy, pigmentation, and telangiectasia of the skin associated with juvenile zonular cataracts and short stature. The dermal erythematous lesions may be present at birth and have usually appeared by the first 6 months of life. They begin on the face and spread to involve the whole of the body. The skin atrophy, pigmentation, and telangiectasia develop from the 3rd to the 6th month of life, particularly on extensor surfaces of the hands, arms, legs, and buttocks, and are worst over exposed surfaces. This inflammatory stage is followed by skin atrophy with pigmentation anomalies. Bilateral cataracts develop at 4–7 years, and there may be alopecia. Warty dyskeratosis is seen, and squamous cell carcinoma may develop in the skin in adulthood; multiple Bowen disease has been described (Haneke and Gutschmidt 1979; Kitao et al. 1999). There are two case reports of oral squamous cell carcinoma (Dahele et al. 2004). Associated abnormalities that may occur include sparse hair or alopecia, atrophic nails, micro-dontia or other dental malformations, hypogonadism, small saddle nose, hypoplas-tic thumbs, forearm reduction defects, small hands and feet, and osteoporosis or sclerosis.

Osteogenic sarcoma has been described in a proportion of patients (32 % in one series, mean age 11.5 years), and skin malignancy may also occur (Starr et al. 1985; Wang et al. 2001). Myelodysplasia and fibrosarcoma have also been described in this condition (Naryan et al. 2001). A subset of cases are due to bial-lelic mutations in the *RECQL4* helicase, and those with truncating mutations may be at higher risk of osteosarcoma (Wang et al. 2003a). In a 25-year retrospective study of 938 individuals with osteosarcoma, 66 had multiple primary cancers. One of these cases had Rothmund–Thompson syndrome, illustrating the rarity of this condition in patients ascertained by a diagnosis of osteosarcoma (Hauben et al. 2003).

Patients with Rothmund–Thompson syndrome have an increased risk of second malignant tumor – almost 20 % of Rothmund–Thompson syndrome patients being for a primary tumor (osteosarcoma, soft tissue sarcoma, or hematological neoplasia) developed a second malignancy (Stinco et al. 2008).

Severe Combined Immunodeficiency Disease (OMIM 102700)

This comprises a heterogeneous group of disorders characterized by severe cell-mediated and humoral immunodeficiency. Autosomal recessive and X-linked forms (the most common form in males) occur. Although infection is the most common cause of death, there is also an increased risk of lymphoma (see p. 153). Following the mapping of X-linked severe combined immunodeficiency disease to Xq13.1, mutations in the interleukin-2 receptor chain gene were identified (Noguchi et al. 1993; Puck et al. 1993). Mutations are heterogeneous and molecular genetic analysis is technically demanding (Puck et al. 1997, 1997). An atypical form is also recognized. At least eight autosomal genes are implicated in recessive SCID including adenosine deaminase, CD3 delta and CD3 epsilon chain, CD45, IL-7 receptor alpha chain, JAK3 and RAG1/RAG2 deficiencies, and Artemis mutations (Buckley 2004a, b). There is no evidence that heterozygotes for autosomal recessive causes of the disease (including adenosine deaminase deficiency) are at increased risk for cancer (Morrell et al. 1987). A recent Australian survey of SCID recorded an incidence of 1.8 per 100,000 births. Of 33 cases identified over a 6-year period, 26 were classical SCID and 7 were atypical. Of the classical cases, the causative genes/syndromes were IL2RG ($n = 13$), ADA (4), IL-7 receptor alpha chain (1), Omenn syndrome (2), and DiGeorge syndrome (2), and 4 were autosomal recessive, not otherwise defined (Yee et al. 2008).

Shwachman–Diamond Syndrome (OMIM 260400)

This is a rare autosomal recessive disease characterized by exocrine pancreatic insufficiency, skeletal abnormalities (e.g., metaphyseal dysostosis), growth retardation, recurrent infections, and hematological abnormalities (neutropenia, hypoplastic anemia, thrombocytopenia, or pancytopenia) (Dror and Freedman 1999) (see Table 11.12 for diagnostic criteria). The risk of leukemia in Shwachman–Diamond syndrome was calculated to increase 27-fold (Woods et al. 1981). A range of leukemic types have been described in this condition including ALL, AML, chronic myeloid leukemia (CML), and erythroleukemia. Although the risk of leukemic transformation had been considered to be 5–10 %, Smith et al. (1996) suggested that this was an underestimate. The Shwachman–Diamond syndrome gene maps to 7q11 and encodes a protein of 250 amino acids (Boocock et al. 2003). Most mutations appeared to result from gene conversion events with a pseudogene.

There is no apparent prognostic significance to genotype analysis. Patients with Shwachman–Diamond syndrome with very early symptoms or cytopenia at diagnosis are considered at a high risk of severe hematological complications (Donadieu et al. 2012). When comparing Shwachman–Diamond syndrome with other inherited bone marrow failure syndromes such as Diamond–Blackfan, Fanconi anemia, Kostmann syndrome, and dyskeratosis congenita, one of the main differences between

Table 11.12 Diagnostic criteria for Shwachman–Diamond syndrome

Fulfilling at least two of the following criteria (1–4)
1. At least two of the following:
(a) Chronic cytopenia(s) detected on at least two occasions over at least 3 months
(b) Reduced marrow progenitors (granulocyte–monocyte colony-forming units, erythroid burst forming units, and granulocyte, erythroid, monocyte, megakaryocyte colony-forming units)
(c) Persistent elevation of hemoglobin F (on at least two occasions over at least 3 months apart)
(d) Persistent red blood cell macrocytosis (on at least two occasions over at least 3 months apart) (not caused by hemolysis or a nutritional deficiency)
2. At least one of the following:
(a) Evidence of pancreatic lipomatosis (e.g., by ultrasound, computed tomography, magnetic resonance imaging, or pathological examination of the pancreas e.g. by autopsy)
(b) Reduced levels of at least two pancreatic enzymes adjusted to age (fecal elastase, serum trypsinogen, serum isoamylase, or duodenal enzymes following stimulation test)
3. Positive genetic testing (*SBDS* and others once they become available)
4. First-degree family history of Shwachman–Diamond syndrome

Adapted from Hashmi et al. (2011)

Shwachman–Diamond syndrome and the other types of inherited bone marrow failures was that the combination of isolated neutropenia and high HbF or MCV was more likely to present at time of diagnosis in Shwachman–Diamond syndrome, whereas severe neutropenia and thrombocytopenia are less common at presentation (Hashmi et al. 2011).

Simpson–Golabi–Behmel Syndrome (OMIM 312870)

An X-linked congenital overgrowth syndrome with some expression in carrier females, Simpson–Golabi–Behmel syndrome is characterized by prenatal and postnatal overgrowth, coarse facies with hypertelorism and a midline groove of the lower lip, and a variety of developmental defects including cleft lip and palate, polydactyly, supernumerary nipples, congenital heart disease, and cryptorchidism. Mental retardation is not usually a feature. Simpson–Golabi–Behmel syndrome must be distinguished from other overgrowth syndromes, in particular Beckwith–Wiedemann syndrome (BWS) (p. 221). There is an increased risk of embryonal tumors, and screening for Wilms tumor may be offered as described for BWS (renal ultrasonography every 3–4 months until age 7 years) (Scott et al. 2006).

Simpson–Golabi–Behmel syndrome is caused by mutations in the glypican 3 (*GPC3*) gene, which maps to Xq26 (Hughes-Benzie et al. 1996; Pilia et al. 1996; Brzustowicz et al. 1999). In addition, a second locus (*SGBS2*) was mapped to Xp22 in a family considered to have a severe form of Simpson–Golabi–Behmel syndrome, and a mutation in the *OFD1* gene was subsequently found in this family (making SGBS2 allelic with oral–facial–digital type I syndrome) (Budny et al. 2006). Li et al. (2001) suggested that hepatoblastoma and nephroblastomatosis are part of the Simpson–Golabi–Behmel syndrome phenotype and identified *GPC3* deletion in two patients previously diagnosed as Sotos syndrome and Perlman syndrome.

Sotos Syndrome (OMIM 117550)

The cardinal features of this congenital overgrowth disorder are a characteristic facial appearance (high and broad forehead, frontotemporal hair sparsity, and prominent chin), learning disability (mostly mild–moderate), and prenatal and childhood overgrowth (tall stature and macrocephaly). In most cases bone age is advanced. Neonatal jaundice and/or feeding difficulties are common. About 25 % of children will have congenital anomalies involving the heart (e.g., septal defects or more complex congenital heart defects), kidney (vesicoureteic reflux or structural anomalies), or spine (scoliosis) (Baujat and Cormier-Daire 2007; Tatton-Brown et al. 2007).

Sotos syndrome must be differentiated from other congenital overgrowth syndromes particularly Weaver syndrome but also Beckwith–Wiedemann syndrome, Bannayan–Riley–Ruvalcaba syndrome, and Simpson–Golabi–Behmel syndrome. A clinical diagnosis of Sotos syndrome can be confirmed by detecting inactivating mutations in the *NSD1* (nuclear receptor set domain protein-1) (Tatton-Brown et al. 2005). Most cases have intragenic *NSD1* mutations, but microdeletions can occur, and these are the most common cause of Sotos syndrome in cases from Japan. A few patients with Sotos-like features but no mutation in *NSD1* have been reported to harbor *NFIX* alterations (Yoneda et al. 2012). Most cases appear to be sporadic and arise from a de novo mutation, but familial cases are inherited in an autosomal dominant manner.

Although there is reported to be an increased relative risk of neural crest tumors and sacrococcygeal teratomas, the absolute risk of tumors has been estimated to be < 3 %, and no specific screening is recommended (other than annual clinical review) (Tatton-Brown et al. 2007).

Tuberous Sclerosis (Tuberose Sclerosis) (OMIM 191100 and 191092)

This is an autosomal dominant hamartomatous disorder with an incidence of approximately 1 per 12,000 live births. New mutations account for 70 % of cases, and the mutation rate is 2.5×10^{-5}/haploid genome. Most serious morbidity is caused by the CNS lesions, which produce mental retardation and epilepsy, but renal angiomyolipomas can occasionally be life threatening, and RCC may occur at an increased rate, albeit infrequently (Washecka and Hanna 1991). Tuberous sclerosis is a multisystem disorder and the clinical features are diverse (Lendvay and Marshall 2003):

Skin: Hypopigmented oval or "ash leaf" patches (80–90 %), facial angiofibromas (adenoma sebaceum, 40–90 %), Shagreen patches (20–40 %), forehead fibrous plaque (25 %), periungual fibromas (Koenen tumors) (15–50 %), and molluscum fibrosum pendulum (23 %).

Eyes: Hamartomas of the retina or optic nerve occur in about 50 % of patients with tuberous sclerosis. Just under half of these are calcified. Most retinal lesions do not grow, and although visual impairment from retinal or optic nerve astrocytoma is recorded, it is a rare complication (Robertson 1988).

CNS: Epilepsy (approximately 80 % of patients), mental retardation (50 %), and giant cell astrocytomas (5–10 %) are important features. Although MRI scanning demonstrates cortical tubers more easily than CT scanning, the latter is more sensitive in detecting small areas of intracranial calcification. Intracranial tumors are usually benign astrocytomas (subependymal nodules), which often calcify and are typically situated around the lateral aspects of the lateral ventricles. Infrequently, malignant giant cell astrocytomas develop from these subependymal nodules, most commonly near the foramen of Monro and resulting in bilateral (but often asymmetric) obstructive hydrocephalus. Less often, the tumor occurs at the frontal or temporal horns of the lateral ventricle or in the third ventricle. On CT scan, giant cell astrocytomas have a mixed pattern with foci of calcification and areas of vascularity showing enhancement with intravenous contrast. Most tumors are slow growing and distant metastases have not been reported. Subependymal giant cell astrocytomas can be demonstrated in about 8 % of patients, and although the proportion of tuberous sclerosis patients who develop intracranial hypertension is not accurately defined, it is estimated to be less than 3 % (Gomez 1988).

Teeth: Enamel "pits" due to enamel hypoplasia (70 %); however, these are very common in the general population and are not of any diagnostic value.

Kidney: Renal lesions occur in up to 75 % of cases and are a major cause of morbidity and mortality in older patients, and their importance has increased with the advent of more effective seizure control. The most frequent renal complications of tuberous sclerosis are angiomyolipomas (49 %) and renal cysts (32 %) (Cook et al. 1996). Angiomyolipomas are frequently multiple and bilateral. Most patients with a single angiomyolipoma do not have tuberous sclerosis, and patients with non-tuberous sclerosis-associated angiomyolipomas are usually middle-aged or elderly women (Robbins and Bernstein 1988). Angiomyolipomas in tuberous sclerosis patients present earlier (mean 32 versus 54 years) in non-tuberous sclerosis cases (Steiner et al. 1993). Most angiomyolipomas are asymptomatic, and although severe hemorrhage may occur, there is no indication to treat asymptomatic tumors. There is no convincing evidence for malignant transformation occurring in an angiomyolipoma (Robbins and Bernstein 1988). Angiomyolipomas consist of disorganized smooth muscle cells, adipose tissue, and aberrant blood vessels, which do not have an internal elastic lamina and are prone to rupture. Larger tumors tend to be symptomatic, and whereas small asymptomatic lesions may be kept under surveillance, it has been 1 that symptomatic angiomyolipomas ≥4 cm are investigated (angiography) and treated (embolization or renal sparing surgery). Renal cystic disease is the second most common renal manifestation, and renal cysts tend to occur at a younger age than angiomyolipomas. Severe renal cystic disease may result from a contiguous deletion of the *TSC2* (see below) and *PKD1* (autosomal dominant adult-onset polycystic kidney disease) genes (Brook-Carter et al. 1994; Sampson et al. 1997).

The risk of RCC in tuberous sclerosis is controversial (Tello et al. 1998), but although it appears to affect only a minority of cases (2 %), those cases reported were frequently bilateral (43 %), with an early age at onset (median 28 years) (Washecka and Hanna 1991).

GI: Benign, small, adenomatous rectal polyps.

Bones: Cysts (60 %), areas of periosteal new bone/sclerosis (60 %). However, these findings are of no diagnostic value.

Cardiac: Rhabdomyomas are present in most infants with tuberous sclerosis. Thereafter many regress and echocardiographically demonstrable lesions occur in only about 30 % of adult patients. Obstructive symptoms or rhabdomyoma-induced arrhythmias are rare, and the likelihood of spontaneous regression favors conservative management in most cases.

Lungs: A specific feature of tuberous sclerosis is lymphangioleiomyomatosis (LAM) caused by an overgrowth of atypical smooth muscle cells. It is nearly always restricted to women and is very rare in the general population (1 per million) (Johnson and Tattersfield 2002) Honeycomb fibros is also seen but is rare.

Conventional diagnostic criteria for tuberous sclerosis are shown in Table 11.13. The manifestations of tuberous sclerosis can be mild and easily overlooked, so that the assessment of at-risk relatives must be performed assiduously. In addition to careful examination of the skin (including Wood's lamp examination) and nails, further examinations usually indicated include brain CT or MRI scans, renal ultrasound, specialist eye examination, and echocardiogram (in children). Dental pits are more common in patients with tuberous sclerosis, but their usefulness as a diagnostic feature is limited because many normal persons have small numbers of these. Truly non-penetrant gene carriers are extremely unusual, so that the risk to individuals with negative investigations as outlined above will be small. A frequent diagnostic problem occurs in assessing the significance of a single ambiguous lesion (e.g., ash leaf patch or equivocal CT scan finding) in an at-risk individual. Parents of a child with tuberous sclerosis who have been fully investigated with negative results should be given a 2 % recurrence risk for tuberous sclerosis in further children, because of the possibility of germline mosaicism or non-penetrance.

The presence of locus heterogeneity in tuberous sclerosis is firmly established, with two genes (*TSC1* and *TSC2*, respectively) mapped at 9q34 and 16p13.3 adjacent to the autosomal dominant polycystic kidney locus (APKD1). The *TSC2* gene was isolated first, and the *TSC1* gene was cloned 10 years after the initial mapping to chromosome 9 (van Slegtenhorst et al. 1997). Loss of heterozygosity at *TSC1* or *TSC2* is observed in hamartomas from tuberous sclerosis patients, consistent with both genes having a tumor suppressor function (Sepp et al. 1996). Half of familial cases are linked to *TSC1* and half to *TSC2*, but 80 % of sporadic cases have *TSC2* mutations (Jones et al. 1999). The proteins specified by the *TSC1* and *TSC2* genes

Table 11.13 Diagnostic criteria for tuberous sclerosis. A diagnosis of tuberous sclerosis is suggested if a single primary or two secondary diagnostic features are present

Primary features	Secondary features
Classical shagreen patch	Ash leaf patch (hypomelanotic macules)
Ungual fibroma	Gingival fibroma
Retinal hamartoma	Bilateral polycystic kidney
Facial angiofibromas	Cardiac rhabdomyoma
Subependymal glial nodule (on CT scan)	Cortical tuber
	Radiographic "honeycomb" lungs
Renal angiomyolipoma	Infantile spasms
Lymphangioleiomyomatosis (lung)	Myoclonic, tonic, or atonic seizures
	First-degree relative with tuberous sclerosis
	Forehead fibrous plaque
	Giant cell astrocytoma

After Gomez (1988)

(hamartin and tuberin, respectively) interact directly with, and mutations affecting either gene result in the tuberous sclerosis phenotype (Hodges et al. 2001). Hamartin or tuberin inactivation leads to dysregulation of the mammalian target of rapamycin (mTOR) and abnormal cell growth (Inoki et al. 2005). This finding suggests that inhibitors of mTOR (e.g., rapamycin) have a potential role in tuberous sclerosis therapy.

Large kindreds with tuberous sclerosis are unusual, and in most cases reliable presymptomatic or prenatal diagnosis using linked DNA markers is not usually feasible. Molecular diagnosis by direct mutation analysis is possible, but the *TSC2* gene is very large and mutations are heterogeneous and so molecular diagnosis may not be available. All parents of apparently isolated cases of tuberous sclerosis should undergo detailed clinical examination (including examination of nails and Wood's light), a CT or MRI brain scan, and renal and liver ultrasound examination. If these investigations are negative, the recurrence risk is reduced to approximately 2 %.

The clinical features of germline mutations in *TSC1* and *TSC2* appear similar, except that the presence of severe renal cystic disease is strongly correlated with deletions of both *TSC2* and *APKD1* genes (Brook-Carter et al. 1994), and intellectual disability is more frequent in sporadic cases, which are mostly caused by *TSC2* mutations. Renal carcinoma has been described in families linked to *TSC1* and to *TSC2*, and although RCC is uncommon in tuberous sclerosis, a germline mutation in rat *TSC2* gene is responsible for the Eker rat model of hereditary renal carcinoma (Kobayashi et al. 1995).

The investigation of asymptomatic at-risk relatives has been described. For unequivocally affected individuals, management is directed towards the active clinical problems; however, regular surveillance of asymptomatic angiomyolipomas may be undertaken, particularly if large (>4 cm). Symptomatic angiomyolipomas may be investigated by angiography and, particularly if larger than 4 cm. Diameter, embolization or renal sparing surgery performed.

Turcot Syndrome (OMIM 276300 and 175100)

The association of multiple polyps of the colon with malignant tumors of the CNS is known as Turcot syndrome (Turcot et al. 1959). The condition seems to be rare. The colorectal polyps are characteristically not as numerous as in FAP (fewer than 100), and are larger, developing in the second decade of life, but the brain tumors may occur in childhood. Medulloblastomas and glioblastomas predominate. Café-au-lait spots and pigmented spots have been noted (Itoh and Ohsato 1985), and sebaceous cysts and BCC may occur (Michels and Stevens 1982).

Despite original suggestions that the condition was only an autosomal recessive trait, it is clearly autosomal dominant in some families (Costa et al. 1987; Kumar et al. 1989). Current evidence suggests that in some families, Turcot syndrome is allelic with FAP, especially where medulloblastomas predominate, and truncating germline *APC* mutations have been found in families with autosomal dominant Turcot syndrome (Hamilton et al. 1995). In other Turcot families (particularly those with glioblastomas), germline mismatch repair gene mutations have been reported (Tops et al. 1992; Liu et al. 1995). In these families, genomic instability was demonstrated in the brain and colonic tumors of affected individuals (Paraf et al. 1997). This has also been seen in normal tissue from patients with Turcot syndrome, perhaps suggesting that the single mutation in *PMS2* identified in this report was actually accompanied by another, hidden mutation (Miyaki et al. 1997). Clear evidence for autosomal recessive Turcot syndrome was provided by the report of two siblings who were diagnosed with a brain tumor and a colorectal cancer, respectively, at very young ages (De Rosa et al. 2000; Giunti et al. 2009). The authors identified two germline mutations in *PMS2* in the two children: 1221delG and 2361delCTTC, both of which were inherited from the patient's unaffected parents. A literature review of individuals with café-au-lait spots and early-onset colorectal cancer revealed excesses of early-onset brain tumors and lymphoma and/or leukemia. Several could be accounted for by homozygous mutations in *PMS2* or heterozygous mutations in *MLH1* (Trimbath et al. 2001a, b), and the condition is now known as constitutional mismatch repair deficiency syndrome (CMMRD), due to biallelic mutations in *MSH2, MLH1, MSH6,* and *PMS2* (p. 232). Other tumors have been reported in children with this condition including rhabdomyosarcoma and nephroblastomas; there is a suggestion that the MMR mutations causing this condition are less penetrant than those causing the usual type of Lynch syndrome because of the relatively low incidence of Lynch syndrome-type cancers in the families of affected children (Ostergaard et al. 2005; Giunti et al. 2009a, b).

Homozygous *PMS2* mutations occur in some children with brain tumors, but these cases are not strictly Turcot syndrome, as the supratentorial primitive neuroectodermal tumors (PNETs) that occur (along with café-au-lait lesions and susceptibility to hematological malignancies) (De Vos et al. 2004) are not usually associated with a personal on family history of colorectal cancer. However, De Vos et al. identified two germline *PMS2* mutations in the two siblings who were described by Turcot in 1959. Previously, a single *PMS2* mutation p.Arg134X had been identified in the two affected sibs and their father (Hamilton et al. 1995;

Trimbath et al. 2001), and although the parents were unaffected, it was assumed to be a dominantly inherited disorder in that family. The identification of another mutation, 2184delTC, and its presence in the mother, confirms the original Turcot pedigree as an example of autosomal recessive Turcot syndrome. This stresses the need for genomic analysis of *PMS2* in families with childhood supratentorial PNETs and/or other brain tumors, particularly if café-au-lait spots are present. Surveillance of first-degree relatives at risk for Turcot syndrome should include regular colonoscopies from age of 25 years in cases associated with Lynch syndrome or surveillance appropriate for FAP if this is the underlying condition.

Turner Syndrome

Turner syndrome (TS) is due to complete or partial X-chromosome monosomy. The main risk of cancer in this syndrome is for gonadoblastoma, in cases with evidence of some Y chromosome lineage. However, the risk may only be 7–10 % and may have been overestimated in the past (Gravholt et al. 2000). The cumulative risk has been found to be 7.9 % by age 25 in this group of patients (Schoemaker et al. 2008). The risk of breast cancer is significantly decreased in TS (SIR 0.3 [0.2–0.6]). Tumors of the CNS, especially meningioma and childhood brain tumors, appear to occur with increased risk in TS (meningioma SIR 12.0 [4.8–24.8], childhood brain tumors 10.3 [2.1–30.1], cancers of the bladder and urethra 4.0 [1.3–9.2] and eye 10.5 [1.3–37.9]), and there may also be increased risks of melanoma, SIR 2.2 (95 % CI 1.0–4.4), and of corpus uteri cancer especially at ages 15–44 years (SIR 8.0 [1.6–23.2], compared with the general population, with a cumulative risk of 7.9 % (95 % CI 3.1–19.0) by age 25 years in this group (Schoemaker et al. 2008).

Tylosis (Keratosis Palmaris et Plantaris) (OMIM 148500)

This autosomal dominant condition is characterized by a diffuse keratoderma of the palms and soles developing from the age of 5 years (typically around puberty). It is associated with a very high risk of developing cancer of the esophagus (95 % risk by the age of 60 years) (Harper et al. 1970). Oral leukoplakia also occurs and there is a risk of squamous carcinoma of the lip and mouth. The differential diagnosis from the more common diffuse palmoplantar keratoderma, which carries no increased risk of carcinoma of the esophagus, is that in the latter condition, lesions develop in infancy and are well established by 6–12 months of life. The incidence of esophageal cancer in gene carriers (heterozygotes) reaches 95 % by the age of 63 years, and the mean age at onset of the cancer is 45 years. Prophylactic esophagectomy with interposition of a segment of colon has been suggested for affected individuals. If prophylactic esophagectomy has not been performed, then annual esophagoscopy is recommended, and immediate esophagectomy is advisable if dysplasia is detected. The gene for this condition has been mapped to chromosome 17q, but distal to the keratin gene cluster on 17q (Hennies et al. 1995; Kelsell et al. 1996), mutations of which are responsible for some forms of diffuse, focal, and epidermolytic palmoplantar keratosis. Finally, the tylosis gene itself was identified as *RHBDF2*. It encodes an inactive rhomboid protease (Blaydon et al. 2012).

A separate disorder of increased UVA sensitivity has been described, in which there is an autosomal dominant predisposition to the development of cutaneous pigmented keratoses in sun-exposed skin associated with the development of carcinoma of the uterus and other internal malignancies (clinically more apparent in females) (Atherton et al. 1989). Fibroblasts from affected individuals demonstrated an increased frequency of single-strand breaks in DNA following exposure to long-wave UVA.

Von Hippel–Lindau Syndrome (OMIM 193300)

This is an autosomal dominant disorder with a minimal birth incidence of 1 per 35 000 (Maher et al. 1991). A wide variety of tumors have been reported in von Hippel–Lindau (VHL) disease, but the most frequent manifestations are retinal angioma (60 % of patients); cerebellar (60 %), spinal (13–44 %), and brain stem hemangioblastomas (18 %); renal cell carcinoma (RCC) (28 %); and pheochromocytoma (7–20 %) (Maher et al. 1990b; Maher and Yates 1991; Green et al. 1986). Renal, pancreatic, and epididymal cysts are also frequent findings. Other less frequent complications include pancreatic tumors (nonsecretory endocrine neuroectodermal tumors), endolymphatic sac tumors (ELST), and broad ligament cystadenoma (Maher et al. 2011). Clinical penetrance is age dependent and almost complete by the age of 60 years (0.19 at age of 15 years, 0.52 at 25 years, and 0.91 at 45 years). The mean age at clinical diagnosis is 26 years (though rarely retinal angiomas can present in infancy), and age at diagnosis of complications is earlier in at-risk relatives under routine surveillance (see later). There is a high probability of a patient with VHL disease developing a major complication (the risk lifetime risks of cerebellar hemangioblastoma, retinal angioma, and RCC are each >70 %) (Ong et al. 2007). Nevertheless, the expression of VHL disease is very variable, and, notably for pheochromocytoma, marked interfamilial variability also occurs.

Clinical diagnostic criteria for VHL disease are (1) for isolated cases, two or more hemangioblastomas (retinal or CNS) or a single hemangioblastoma in association with a visceral tumor or endolymphatic sac tumour (ELST) or (2) if there is a family history of retinal or CNS hemangioblastoma, only one hemangioblastoma, ELST, or visceral tumor is required for the diagnosis (small numbers of visceral cysts do not provide an unequivocal diagnosis in familial cases). Up to 20 % of probands represent *de novo* mutations, and diagnosis in isolated cases is often delayed because they are only recognized when two complications have developed (whereas familial cases can be diagnosed after a single manifestation).

Nevertheless, increasingly the diagnosis is made by molecular genetic analysis after screening of individuals with an isolated manifestation (e.g., hemangioblastoma, pheochromocytoma).

Cerebellar Hemangioblastoma (See p. 4)

This is the joint most frequent complication (with retinal angiomatosis) of VHL disease. Approximately 30 % of cerebellar hemangioblastomas occur as part of VHL disease, and evidence of VHL disease should be sought in all patients with apparently sporadic cerebellar hemangioblastoma. Tumors complicating VHL disease occur, on average, at a younger age than sporadic cerebellar hemangioblastomas (see p. 4), and in about 20 % of cases the tumors are multiple or recurrent. CT scanning demonstrates a contrast-enhancing mass, but MRI scanning is more sensitive and is preferred – particularly for surveillance. These tumors are benign, may be cystic or solid, and the histological appearance is identical to that of a retinal angioma (hemangioblastoma). Approximately 4 % of patients with apparently sporadic cerebellar hemangioblastoma have a germline VHL gene mutation (Hes et al. 2000). In view of the risk of false-negative mutation analysis and somatic mosaicism, apparently sporadic early-onset cases may be kept under review in case evidence of VHL disease develops later. Surgery is usually performed when a hemangioblastoma becomes symptomatic. Stereotaxic radiotherapy may be occasionally an option for small non-cystic hemangioblastomas that are not amenable to standard surgery (Patrice et al. 1996).

Spinal Cord Hemangioblastoma

This is the second most frequent site for CNS hemangioblastomas. Pain is the most common symptom and may be followed by sensory loss and signs of cord compression. MRI scanning is the preferred method of investigation. Symptomatic lesions should be excised, and although the prognosis can be good, if diagnosis is delayed or surgery difficult, paraplegia may result. Medical treatment with anti-angiogenic agents may be considered if conventional surgery is not possible (though CNS tumors are less likely to respond than renal or pancreatic tumors).

Brain Stem Hemangioblastoma

These are symptomatic in 18 % of patients, most often in the dorsal medulla and craniocervical junction (Filling-Katz et al. 1991). Supratentorial hemangioblastomas are rare. Many CNS hemangioblastomas detected by MRI scanning are asymptomatic. Though the detection of CNS tumors is helpful in determining carrier status, surgery is usually only performed for symptomatic tumors.

Retinal Angiomatosis (See Fig. 11.8)

This is often the earliest manifestation of VHL disease (Maher et al. 1990a). Retinal angiomas are frequently asymptomatic and most occur in the peripheral retina. They have been reported in infancy and in the ninth decade, but the risk of retinal angioma before the age of 5 years is less than 1 % and mean age at diagnosis is 25 years. Early detection of retinal angiomas facilitates treatment and prevents blindness. Direct and indirect ophthalmoscopy should be performed on all patients and at-risk relatives (see Table 11.14). Fluorescein angioscopy can improve the detection of small lesions.

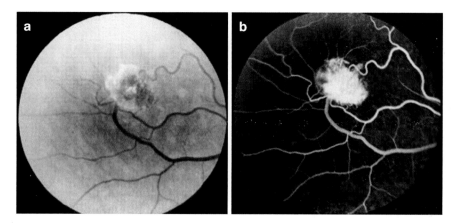

Fig. 11.8 VHL disease: (**a**) moderate-sized retinal angioma and (**b**) fluorescein angiogram of the same lesion (Reproduced with permission from Cambridge University Press)

Table 11.14 Typical screening protocol for VHL disease in affected patients and at-risk relatives

Affected patient or gene carrier
Annual physical examination and urine testing
Annual direct and indirect ophthalmoscopy
MRI brain scan every 3 years to 50 years of age and every 5 years thereafter
Annual abdominal MRI scan
Annual 24-h urine collection for catecholamines and VMAs (plasma metanephrines more sensitive)
At-risk relative
Annual physical examination and urine testing
MRI brain scan every 3 years from 15 to 40 years of age and then every 5 years until 60 years of age
Annual renal MRI or ultrasound scan from16 to 65 years of age
Annual 24-h urine collection for catecholamine and VMAs (plasma metanephrines more sensitive)

Renal Cell Carcinoma

In cross-sectional studies, 25–30 % of VHL patients have had clear cell RCC (Maher et al. 1990a). The risk of RCC in VHL disease was initially underestimated because the mean age at RCC diagnosis (44 years) is older than for retinal angioma (25 years) and cerebellar hemangioblastoma (29 years), but since emerging as the leading cause of mortality in VHL disease (Maher et al. 1990a), the importance of presymptomatic renal surveillance has been recognized. The clinical presentation and risk of metastasis in RCC complicating VHL disease are similar to those of sporadic nonfamilial tumors. However, tumors in VHL disease occur at an earlier age and are often multiple and bilateral. Renal cysts may be detected in the second decade, and RCC has been detected as early as age of 16 years. RCC may arise from the wall of renal cysts, and complex cysts require careful follow-up. Renal tumors and cysts may be detected by ultrasonography or computer tomography, but MRI scanning is preferred for routine screening as it is more sensitive than ultrasonography and avoids repeated radiation exposure. The management of renal cancer in VHL disease is motivated by a conservative nephron-sparing approach. Thus it is usual to follow small asymptomatic tumors by serial imaging until they reach about 3 cm diameter. At that stage, conservative renal surgery is performed with the aim of conserving functioning renal tissue for as long as possible. Follow-up of VHL patients treated by nephron-sparing surgery reveals a high incidence of local recurrence from new primary tumors, but a low risk of distant metastasis. In contrast, 25 % of VHL patients with more advanced RCC (>3 cm) develop metastatic disease (Walther et al. 1999a). Repeated partial nephrectomies may eventually compromise renal function, and in such cases dialysis is instigated – though renal transplantation is also an option. It appears that immunosuppression does not affect adversely the underlying course of VHL disease, and the prognosis of VHL patients after transplantation appears similar to that of other comparable groups (Goldfarb et al. 1998).

Pheochromocytoma

There are clear interfamilial differences in predisposition to pheochromocytoma in VHL disease. In a minority of families, pheochromocytoma is the most frequent complication of this disease but in other families it is rare (Maher et al. 2011). VHL disease has been subclassified according to the presence (type 2) or absence (type 1) of pheochromocytoma. In most cases, pheochromocytoma-positive VHL families also have a high incidence of renal cancer (type 2B), but in some type 2 VHL disease families, pheochromocytoma is common and renal carcinoma is rare (type 2A). In addition rare *VHL* missense mutations may cause a familial pheochromocytoma-only phenotype (type 2C) (Woodward et al. 1997). Up to 11 % of patients with apparently sporadic pheochromocytoma may have a germline *VHL* mutation (Neumann et al. 2002). Both adrenal and extra-adrenal pheochromocytomas can occur in VHL disease. Pheochromocytoma in VHL disease patients is usually associated with missense mutations (see below), and although the overall risk of malignancy in pheochromocytomas is ~10 %, the rate in VHL disease appears to be lower (~5 %).

Pancreas

Pancreatic cysts and tumors are relatively common features of VHL disease. Multiple cysts are the most frequent pancreatic manifestation and are present in most older patients. However pancreatic cysts rarely impair pancreatic function. Pancreatic tumors occur in ~10 % of cases. A high frequency of that malignancy has been reported in VHL-associated islet cell tumors, and surgery is indicated in tumors with a diameter of 3 cm or more (Libutti et al. 1998).

Endolymphatic Sac Tumors (ELSTs)

ELSTs have only been recognized as a specific component of VHL disease relatively recently. In a large survey of VHL patients using MRI and CT scans, Manski et al. (1997) found that 11 % of patients with VHL disease had an ELST. Hearing loss is the most common symptom of ELST, but tinnitus and vertigo also occur in many cases. Hence an ELST should be considered in all VHL patients who complain of hearing loss. However ELSTs are frequently asymptomatic and surgical intervention is not always indicated.

Molecular Genetics

The VHL disease gene maps to chromosome 3p25 and was isolated in 1993 (Latif et al. 1993). Germline mutations may be detected in ≥95 % of patients, and genotype–phenotype correlations have been described such that large deletions and protein-truncating mutations are associated with a low risk of pheochromocytoma, and specific missense mutations may produce a high risk of pheochromocytoma (type 2 families). Families with a high frequency of pheochromocytoma (types 2A, 2B, and 2C) usually have a surface missense mutation, whereas type 1 families have mostly germline deletions or truncating mutations. Regular screening of patients affected by VHL disease and of at-risk relatives is important to detect tumors at an early stage and to establish the carrier status for at-risk individuals (see Table 11.14). Molecular genetic analysis enables the screening protocols to be modified according to an individual's risk so that screening frequency may be reduced or discontinued as appropriate.

Werner Syndrome (OMIM #277700)

This is a rare autosomal recessive disorder with a reported prevalence that varies from 1 in 10^5 in Japan to 1 in 10^6–10^7 outside of Japan. There also appears to be an increased incidence in Sardinia. Werner syndrome (WS) is characterized by features of premature senescence and short stature with loss of subcutaneous fat and muscle, stocky trunk and slender limbs, a thin face with beaked nose, and a high-pitched and hoarse voice. The clinical features of senescence develop from the second decade, with premature greying of the hair from the third decade, generalized hair loss, juvenile cataracts from the third decade, premature arteriosclerosis and calcification of blood vessels with coronary heart disease, osteoporosis, metastatic calcification, and scleropoikiloderma of the skin giving an aged appearance. Diabetes mellitus and hypogonadism may be associated. There may be osteoporosis with ankylosis and destruction of joints and muscle atrophy, and hyperkeratosis over bony prominences and on the soles of the feet, which may ulcerate. There may be areas of hyperpigmentation and hypopigmentation of the skin, with lentigines. The clinical diagnosis is based on the presence of four cardinal signs which are found in more than 95 % of cases. These are cataracts, characteristic skin changes (scleropoikiloderma), short stature, and greying or loss of hair. If all the cardinal signs are present after the age of 10, and two additional signs from the above list (e.g., diabetes, atherosclerosis) are present, then the diagnosis is made clinically. Mutation analysis of *WRN* is used to confirm the clinical diagnosis (Coppede 2012).

About 10 % of affected individuals develop tumors, predominantly of types uncommon in the general population, notably of connective tissue or mesenchymal origin, such as soft tissue sarcomas, osteosarcomas, uterine myosarcomas, meningiomas, and adenomas of the thyroid, parathyroid, adrenal cortex, breast, and liver (Epstein et al. 1966; Goto et al. 1996). Thyroid carcinomas and melanomas have been reported more frequently in Japanese than in Caucasian WS patients. Most WS patients die of atherosclerosis or cancer during the fourth decade of life. Cultured cells from WS patients show chromosome instability and hypersensitivity to DNA cross-linking agents (Moser et al. 2000).

WS is caused by loss-of-function mutations in a gene (*WRN*, *RECQL2*) at chromosome 8p12 that encodes a protein, WRN, which is a member of the RECQ DNA helicase family (Yu et al. 1996; Nishijo et al. 2004). In culture, cells from WS patients show increased chromosomal aberrations, premature senescence, and telomere shortening. Defects in DNA replication are observed. Most mutations result in absence of the WRN protein, although some deleterious missense mutations have been reported (Coppede 2012).

Chen et al. (2003) found that 20 % of patients referred to an international registry for molecular diagnosis of Werner syndrome had wild-type WRN mutation analysis. Sequence analysis of the *LMNA* gene (which is mutated in a rare childhood syndrome of premature aging, Hutchinson–Gilford syndrome, and other disorders) in this subset revealed a heterozygous *LMNA* missense mutation in 15 % of cases. This atypical form of WS typically has an earlier onset of aging phenotypes than *RECQL2*-associated classical WS cases but lacks cataracts and diabetes.

Experiments in mice suggest that the short stature seen in WS and related progeroid conditions is a result of suppression of the somatotropic axis in response to excessive DNA damage – the so-called survival response. It seems likely that genome maintenance, premature aging, and predisposition to cancer are tightly linked (Hoeijmakers 2009).

Wiskott–Aldrich syndrome, OMIM #301000; X-Linked Thrombocytopenia, #313900; Intermittent X-Linked Thrombocytopenia, #313900; and X-Linked Neutropenia, #300299

All the above conditions are caused by mutations in the gene *WASP*; which condition develops depends on the type and/or position of the mutations found in *WASP* (see below). The classic X-linked recessive disorder, Wiskott–Aldrich syndrome (WAS), is rare – its incidence is between 1 and 10 per million persons. It is characterized by immunodeficiency, eczema, and microthrombocytopenia. The typical presentations (often at birth) include mucocutaneous petechiae, bruising, and bloody diarrhea. Severe eczema often develops in infancy or childhood. Hepatosplenomegaly can occur. Complications include susceptibility to pyogenic infection (especially otitis media and pneumonia), arthritis, autoimmune disease, and lymphoma. Death in childhood may occur from overwhelming bacterial or viral infections. Eczema can be complicated by molluscum contagiosum, herpes simplex, and bacterial infections (Thrasher 2009). Patients have small platelets, and the immunodeficiency involves both T cell and B cell function. There is low antigen-induced lymphocyte proliferation, with low IgM and defective antibody production. There is progressive loss of lymphoid elements normally found in the thymus, spleen, lymph nodes, etc. Malignancy of the reticuloendothelial system, lymphomas, and lymphomatoid granulomatosis are common, being the cause of death in about 10 % of cases (ten Bensel et al. 1964). However, by the age of 30 years, the risk of non-Hodgkin lymphoma approaches 100 %. The basic defect underlying all four disorders is dysregulated actin polymerization in hematopoietic cells on account of loss or inappropriate activity of the WAS protein, WASP.

The *WASP* gene was identified in 1994 (Derry et al. 1994a, b). Since then, numerous *WASP* mutations have been characterized, including a small number of hot spot mutations (~25 % of all identified mutations) and genotype–phenotype correlations have also been characterized. *WASP* mutations may result in four distinct phenotypes: the classic WAS triad of thrombocytopenia/small platelets, recurrent infections as a result of immunodeficiency, and eczema; the milder X-linked thrombocytopenia (XLT) variant, where eczema, immune deficiency, infection, and cancer may or may not occur; intermittent XLT, where microthrombocytopenia may be the sole manifestation; and X-linked neutropenia (XLN) where congenital neutropenia and associated infections are the only manifestations. Persons with a normal-sized but mutated protein (usually reduced in quantity), associated with a missense mutation in exons 1–3 (or in-frame deletions elsewhere in *WASP*), nearly always have XLT. Missense mutations that disrupt autoinhibition cause XLN, whereas other missense mutations can cause IXLT (Thrasher 2009). Those with mutations leading to complete loss of protein expression or expression of a truncated protein have a more severe classical WAS phenotype and a higher risk of malignancy (Imai et al. 2004; Jin et al. 2004). Treatment of severely affected children is with intravenous immunoglobulins (even if total IgG levels are normal) and prompts hematopoietic stem cell transplantation.

X-Linked Lymphoproliferative Disorder (Duncan Disease) (OMIM 308240)

This condition affects about 3 per million males, and the gene has been mapped to Xq25. Affected males are susceptible to severe infectious mononucleosis infections (fatal in 50 %, often in childhood), and 25 % develop malignant lymphoma, typically Burkitt-type non-Hodgkin lymphoma in the ileocecal region, but CNS, hepatic, and renal lymphomas are also common. Systemic vasculitis is a rare complication (Dutz et al. 2001). X-linked lymphoproliferative disorder is caused by mutations in the SH2 domain protein 1A (*SH2D1A*) gene (Sumegi et al. 2000). At least one-quarter of all mutations are missed by direct sequencing, so there may be a role for other, function-based assays in definite cases or in possible heterozygotes (Tabata et al. 2005).

Xeroderma Pigmentosum (OMIM #278700, 610651, 278720, 278730, 278740, 278760, 278780, and variant 278750)

This is a heterogeneous group of autosomal recessive disorders with a prevalence of about 1 in 70,000 of the population. It is characterized by hypersensitivity to UV light and a high incidence of UV-induced skin cancers. Clinical onset is before the age of 18 months in 50 %. Freckle-like skin lesions with erythema develop in sun-exposed skin in the first few years of life, and there may be extreme sunlight sensitivity (see Fig. 11.6). Macules of increased pigmentation develop on the skin and mucous membranes, and achromic areas may also occur. Subsequently, there is an atrophic and telangiectatic stage in which the skin becomes dry and scaly, with atrophy and spotted dyschromia. Hyperkeratotic plaques, keratomas, keratoacanthomas, fibromas, angiomyomas, cutaneous horns, and other benign tumors ensue, and there may be facial ulcerations. Multiple malignant basal and squamous cell carcinomas and malignant melanoma develop in sun-exposed areas; the risk for malignancy is up to 2,000-fold increase above normal. The median age at onset for skin cancer in XP has been estimated to be 8 years, compared with 60 years in the general population. Squamous cell carcinomas, sarcomas, melanomas, and epitheliomas may develop in the eyes and mucous membranes, and squamous cell carcinomas of the tongue and oropharynx may occur, with a relative risk of 10,000 times normal. Other malignant tumors may develop, including neurinomas, sarcomas, and adenocarcinomas. It has been suggested that there is also a 10–20-fold increased incidence of internal neoplasms, such as lung, uterine, brain, breast, or testicular tumors in XP. Actinic damage to the eyes may cause keratitis and conjunctivitis, which can lead to symblepharon and neoplasia, particularly at the corneoscleral junction. Entropion and ectropion may occur. Death results from disseminated tumors, usually by the second or third decade (Giannelli and Pawsey 1976; Kraemer and Slor 1985).

De Sanctis–Cacchione syndrome emphasized neurological involvement in a subgroup of XP patients. Neurological complications are variable and include progressive mental deficiency, microcephaly, ataxia, choreoathetosis, spasticity, sensorineural deafness, and lower motor neuron and cranial nerve damage. Onset of these neurological abnormalities may be in infancy or later in childhood and may be mild or severe. They develop in about 18 % of cases of XP (Kraemer and Slor 1985). They can occur in any subgroup of XP but do so most commonly in complementation group D (XPD) (see below). Loss or absence of neurons may be demonstrated in the cerebrum or cerebellum at autopsy in these cases. The karyotype is normal, but there is hypersensitivity to chromosomal damage after exposure to UV light.

Different subgroups (complementation groups) of XP are described, each with a different type of mutation reducing the capacity for excision repair of UV-induced DNA damage (Giannelli 1986). These subgroups are associated with different clinical severity. Complementation group A (XPA) includes cases of all degrees of clinical severity, with and without neurological complications; group C (XPC) is the most commonly described; and most are neurologically normal. Cockayne syndrome with XP has been described in single cases (Neilan et al. 2008). The molecular bases for these conditions have been delineated and are due to various defects in solar-induced DNA damage. These defects comprise lack of a functional helicase, endonuclease, or lesion-recognizing protein involved in the initial steps of nucleotide excision repair. Different enzyme defects are found in the different complementation groups. They include proteins involved in recognition of photoproducts (XPE), and of other DNA defects such as pyrimidine dimers (XPA), DNA helicases (XPB, XPD), and endonucleases that perform two incisions (XPG), and single-strand-binding proteins (XPC) (Boulikas 1996; Chu and Mayne 1996). Prenatal diagnosis by chorionic villus sampling is becoming available in those families in which the mutation can be defined at the DNA level.

Mutations in eight genes may cause XP. The genes for group A and group C xeroderma pigmentosum (XPA and XPC) are involved solely in nucleotide excision repair, whereas the XPB and XPD proteins are both components of transcription factor TFIIH, which is involved in nucleotide excision repair, in basal transcription and in activated transcription (Lehmann 2003). All bona fide patients with XPE have a mutation in the *DDB2* gene that encodes the smaller subunit of the heterodimeric damaged DNA-binding protein. XP group F (XPF) is caused by mutations in the *ERCC4* gene and group G (XPG) by mutations in *ERCC5*.

XP variant (XP-V) is indistinguishable from XP clinically, except the neurological features do not develop. Unlike other XP cells belonging to XPA to XPG,

XP-V cells have normal nucleotide excision repair processes, but have defective replication of UV-damaged DNA. This form of XP is caused by mutations in the DNA polymerase eta gene (*POLH*) (Masutani et al. 1999). Suggestions of an increased risk of lung cancer in heterozygote carriers (for all relatives: relative risk, 1.93) (Swift and Chase 1979) have prompted association studies of XP gene variants and lung cancer risk with mixed results (Marin et al. 2004; Benhamou and Sarasin 2005).

Treatment is by protection from sunlight and careful surveillance, with early excision of tumors. Avoidance of UV light should be instigated in childhood, when the apparent health of young children makes this difficult. The use of an UV light meter can be helpful. It is interesting that spontaneous regression of malignant melanoma has been described to occur in XP, although the mechanism for this is not understood (Lynch et al. 1978). Information for patients and their families is available from the xeroderma pigmentosum society (http://www.xps.org).

Prenatal diagnosis of XP has been accomplished by demonstrating abnormal levels of DNA repair capacity on measurement of unscheduled DNA synthesis in UV-irradiated fetal amniocytes (Aras et al. 1985) or by mutation analysis.

A separate disorder of increased UVA sensitivity has been described, in which there is an autosomal dominant predisposition to the development of cutaneous pigmented keratoses in sun-exposed skin associated with the development of carcinoma of the uterus and other internal malignancies (clinically more apparent in females) (Atherton et al. 1989). Fibroblasts from affected individuals demonstrated an increased frequency of single-strand breaks in DNA following exposure to long-wave UVA.

References

Aaltonen LA, Salovaara R, Kristo P, Canzian F, Hemminki A, Peltomaki P, Chadwick RB, Kaariainen H, Eskelinen M, Jarvinen H, Mecklin JP, Delachapelle A, Percesepe A, Ahtola H, Harkonen N, Julkunen R, Kangas E, Ojala S, Tulikoura J, Valkamo E. Incidence of hereditary nonpolyposis colorectal cancer and the feasibility of molecular screening for the disease. New Engl J Med. 1998;338(21):1481–7.

Aarnio M, Mecklin J-P, Aaltonen LA, et al. Life-time risk of different cancers in hereditary nonpolyposis colorectal cancer (HNPCC) syndrome. Int J Cancer. 1995;64:430–3.

Aarnio M, Sanikala R, Pukkala E, et al. Cancer risk in mutation carriers of DNA-mismatch repair genes. Int J Cancer. 1999;81:214–8.

Agarwal SK, Guru SC, Heppner C, et al. Menin interacts with the AP1 transcription factor JunD and represses JunD-activated transcription. Cell. 1999;96:143–52.

Agarwal SK, Novotny EA, Crabtree JS, et al. Transcription factor JunD, deprived of menin, switches from growth suppressor to growth promoter. Proc Natl Acad Sci U S A. 2003;100:10770–5.

Agarwal SK, Mateo CM, Marx SJ. Rare germline mutations in cyclin-dependent kinase inhibitor genes in MEN1 and related states. J Clin Endocrinol Metab. 2009;94:1826–34.

Akiyama Y, Satoh H, Yamada T, et al. Germline mutations of the HMSH6/9 TBP gene in an atypical hereditary nonpolyposis colorectal cancer kindred. Cancer. 1997;57:3920–3.

Aktan-Collan K, Mecklin J-P, Jarvinen H, et al. Predictive genetic testing for hereditary nonpolyposis colorectal cancer: uptake and long-term satisfaction. Int J Cancer. 2000;89:44–50.

Aktas D, Koc A, Boduroglu K, Hicsonmez G, Tuncbilek E. Myelodysplastic syndrome associated with monosomy 7 in a child with Bloom syndrome. Cancer Genet Cytogenet. 2000;116(1): 44–6.

Albrechts AE, Rapini RP. Malignancy in Maffucci's syndrome. Dermatol Clin. 1995;13:73–8.

Alrashdi I, Bano G, Maher ER, Hodgson SV. Carney triad versus Carney Stratakis syndrome: two cases which illustrate the difficulty in distinguishing between these conditions in individual patients. Fam Cancer. 2010;9:443–7.

Al-Tassan N, Chmiel NH, Maynard J, et al. Inherited variants of MYH associated with somatic G:C-T:A mutations in colorectal tumors. Nat Genet. 2002;30(2):227–32.

Alter BP. The bone marrow failure syndromes. In: Nathan DG, Oski, FS, editors, Haematology of infancy and childhood. 3rd ed. Philadelphia: W.B. Saunders; 1987.

Alter BP. Cancer in Fanconi anemia, 1927–2001. Cancer. 2003;97:425–40.

Alter BP, Greene MH, Velazquez I, Rosenberg PS. Cancer in Fanconi anemia. Blood. 2003;101:2072.

Amary MF, Damato S, Halai D, Eskandarpour M, Berisha F, Bonar F, McCarthy S, Fantin VR, Straley KS, Lobo S, Aston W, Green CL, Gale RE, Tirabosco R, Futreal A, Campbell P, Presneau N, Flanagan AM. Ollier disease and Maffucci syndrome are caused by somatic mosaic mutations of IDH1 and IDH2. Nat Genet. 2011;43(12):1262–5.

Andant C, Puy H, Bogard C, et al. Hepatocellular carcinoma in patients with acute hepatic porphyria: frequency of occurrence and related factors. J Hepatol. 2000;32:933–9.

Aoki Y, Niihori T, Kawame H, Kurosawa K, Ohashi H, Tanaka Y, Filocamo M, Kato K, Suzuki Y, Kure S, Matsubara Y. Germline mutations in HRAS proto-oncogene cause Costello syndrome. Nat Genet. 2005;37:1038–40.

Aras S, Bohnert E, Fischer E, Jung EG. Prenatal exclusion of xeroderma pig-mentosa (XP-D) by amniotic cell analysis. Photodermatology. 1985;2:181–3.

Aretz S, Uhlhaas S, Goergens H, Siberg K, Vogel M, Pagenstecher C, Mangold E, Caspari R, Propping P, Friedl W. MUTYH-associated polyposis: 70 of 71 patients with biallelic mutations present with an attenuated or atypical phenotype. Int J Cancer. 2006;119(4):807–14. http://www.ncbi.nlm.nih.gov/pubmed/16557584.

Aretz S, Stienen D, Uhlhaas S, Stolte M, Entius MM, Loff S, Back W, Kaufmann A, Keller KM, Blaas SH, Siebert R, Vogt S, Spranger S, Holinski-Feder E, Sunde L, Propping P, Friedl W. High proportion of large genomic deletions and a genotype phenotype update in 80 unrelated families with juvenile polyposis syndrome. J Med Genet. 2007;44(11):702–9. Epub 2007 Sep 14.

Aretz S, Tricarico R, Papi L, Spier I, Pin E, Horpaopan S, Cordisco EL, Pedroni M, Stienen D, Gentile A, Panza A, Piepoli A, deLeon MP, Friedl W, Viel A, Genuardi M. MUTYH-associated polyposis (MAP): evidence for the origin of the common European mutations p.Tyr179Cys and p.Gly396Asp by founder events. Eur J Hum Genet. 2013 Jan 30. doi:10.1038/ejhg.2012.309.

Aretz S, Stienen D, Uhlhaas S, Loff S, Back W, Pagenstecher C, McLeod DR, Graham GE, Mangold E, Santer R, Propping P, Friedl W. High proportion of large genomic STK11 deletions in Peutz-Jeghers syndrome. Hum Mutat. 2005;26:513–9.

Arvanitis ML, Jagleman DG, Fazio VW, et al. Mortality in patients with familial adenomatous polyposis. Dis Colon Rectum. 1990;33:639–42.

Astuti D, Morris MR, Cooper WN, Staals RH, Wake NC, Fews GA, Gill H, Gentle D, Shuib S, Ricketts CJ, Cole T, van Essen AJ, van Lingen RA, Neri G, Opitz JM. RumpP, Stolte-Dijkstra I, Müller F, Pruijn GJ, Latif F, Maher ER. Germline mutations in DIS3L2 cause the Perlman syndrome of overgrowth and Wilms tumor susceptibility. Nat Genet. 2012;44(3):277–84.

Atherton DJ, Botcherby PK, Francis AJ, et al. Familial keratoses of actinic distribution associated with internal malignancy and cellular hypersensitivity to UVA. Br J Dermatol. 1989;120:671–81.

Athma P, Rappaport R, Swift M. Molecular genotyping shows that ataxia-telangiectasia heterozygotes are predisposed to breast cancer. Cancer Genet Cytogenet. 1996;92:130–4.

Attard-Montalto SP, Schuller I, Lastowska MA, et al. Non-Hodgkin's lymphoma and Klinefelter syndrome. Pediatr Haematol Oncol. 1994;11:197–200.

Auerbach AD. Fanconi anemia diagnosis and the diepoxybutane (DEB) test. Exp Hematol. 1993;21:731–3.

Auerbach AD, Sagi M, Adler B. Fanconi anemia: prenatal diagnosis in 30 fetuses at risk. Pediatrics. 1985;76:794–800.

Bader JL, Miller RW. Neurofibromatosis and childhood leukemia. J Pediatr. 1978;92:925–9.

Bahubeshi A, Bal N, Frio TR, Hamel N, Pouchet C, Yilmaz A, Bouron-Dal SD, Williams GM, Tischkowitz M, Priest JR, Foulkes WD. Germline DICER1 mutations and familial cystic nephroma. J Med Genet. 2010;47:863–6.

Baldinu P, Cossu A, Manca A, et al. Microsatellite instability and mutation analysis of candidate genes in unselected Sardinian patients with endometrial carcinoma. Cancer. 2002;94: 3157–68.

Bandipalliam P. Syndrome of early onset color cancer, hematologic malignancies and features of neurofibromatosis in HNPCC families with homozygous mismatch repair gene mutations. Fam Cancer. 2005;4(4):323–33.

Barana D, van der Wijnen KH, Longa J, Radice ED, Cetto P, Fodde GL, Oliani C. Spectrum of genetic alterations in Muir–Torre syndrome is the same as in HNPCC. Am J Med Genet A. 2004;125(3):318–9.

Bardram L, Stage JG. Frequency of endocrine disorders in patients with the Zollinger–Ellison syndrome. Scand J Gasteroenterol. 1985;20:233–8.

Barrow PJ, Ingham S, O'Hara C et al. The spectrum of urological malignancy in Lynch syndrome. Fam Cancer 2012. In press

Barrow E, Robinson L, Alduaij W, et al. Cumulative lifetime incidence of extracolonic cancers in Lynch syndrome: a report of 121 families with proven mutations. Clin Genet. 2009;75(2): 141–9.

Barrow PJ, Ingham S, O'Hara C, et al. The spectrum of urological malignancy in Lynch syndrome. Fam Cancer. 2013;12:57–63.

Bartkova J, Horejsi Z, Koed K, Kramer A, Tort F, Zieger K, Guldberg P, Sehested M, Nesland JM, Lukas C, Orntoft T, Lukas J, Bartek J. DNA damage response as a candidate anti-cancer barrier in early human tumorigenesis. Nature. 2005;434:864–70.

Bartkova J, Tommiska J, Oplustilova L, Aaltonen K, Tamminen A, Heikkinen T, Mistrik M, Aittomäki K, Blomqvist C, Heikkilä P, Lukas J, Nevanlinna H, Bartek J. Aberrations of the MRE11-RAD50-NBS1 DNA damage sensor complex in human breast cancer: MRE11 as a candidate familial cancer-predisposing gene. Mol Oncol. 2008;2(4):296–316.

Baser ME, Friedman JM, Aeschliman D, Joe H, Wallace AJ, Ramsden RT, Evans DG. Predictors of the risk of mortality in neurofibromatosis 2. Am J Hum Genet. 2002a;71:715–23.

Baser ME, Friedman JM, Wallace AJ, Ramsden RT, Joe H, Evans DGR. Evaluation of clinical diagnostic criteria for neurofibromatosis 2. Neurology. 2002b;59:1759–65.

Baser ME, Kuramoto L, Joe H, Friedman JM, Wallace AJ, Gillespie JE, Ramsden RT, Evans DG. Genotype–phenotype correlations for nervous system tumors in neurofibromatosis 2: a population-based study. Am J Hum Genet. 2004;75:231–9.

Baujat G, Cormier-Daire V. Sotos syndrome. Orphan J Rare Dis. 2007;2:36. doi:10.1186/1750-1172-2-36.

Bazzi W, Renon M, Vercherat C, Hamze Z, Lacheretz-Bernigaud A, Wang H, Blanc M, Roche C, Calender A, Chayvialle JA, Scoazec JY, Cordier-Bussat M. MEN1 missense mutations impair sensitization to apoptosis induced by wild-type menin in endocrine pancreatic tumor cells. Gastroenterology. 2008;135:1698–709.

Beggs AD, Latchford AR, Vasen HF, Moslein G, Alonso A, Aretz S, Bertario L, Blanco I, Bülow S, Burn J, Capella G, Colas C, Friedl W, Møller P, Hes FJ, Järvinen H, Mecklin JP, Nagengast FM, Parc Y, Phillips RK, Hyer W, Ponz de Leon M, Renkonen-Sinisalo L, Sampson JR, Stormorken A, Tejpar S, Thomas HJ, Wijnen JT, Clark SK, Hodgson SV. Peutz-Jeghers syndrome: a systematic review and recommendations for management. Gut. 2010;59(7):975–86.

Benhamou S, Sarasin A. ERCC2 /XPD gene polymorphisms and lung cancer: a HuGE review. Am J Epidemiol. 2005;161:1–14.

Bennett KL, Mester J, Eng C. Germline epigenetic regulation of KILLIN in Cowden and Cowden-like syndrome. JAMA. 2010;304:2724–31.

Berends MJ, Wu Y, Sijmons RH, Mensink RG, van Der ST, Hordijk-Hos JM, de Vries EG, Hollema H, Karrenbeld A, Buys CH, van der Zee AG, Hofstra RM, Kleibeuker JH. Molecular and clinical characteristics of MSH6 variants: an analysis of 25 index carriers of a germline variant. Am J Hum Genet. 2002;70(1):26–37.

Bernstein E, Kim SY, Carmell MA, Murchison EP, Alcorn H, Li MZ, Mills AA, Elledge SJ, Anderson KV, Hannon GJ. Dicer is essential for mouse development. Nat Genet. 2003;35:215–7.

Bertherat J, Hovath A, Groussin L, Grabar S, Biokos S, Cazabat L, Libe R, Rene-Corail F, Stergiopoulos T, Bourdeau I, Bei T, Clauser E, Calender A, Kirschner LS, Bertagna X, Carney JA, Stratakis CA. Mutations in regulatory subunit type 1A of cyclic adenosine 5'-monophosphate-dependent protein kinase (PRKAR1A): phenotype analysis in 353 patients and 80 different genotypes. J Clin Endocrinol Metab. 2009;94:2085–91.

Bertola DR, Cao H, Albano LM, Oliveira DP, Kok F, Marques-Dias MJ, Kim CA, Hegele RA. Cockayne syndrome type A: novel mutations in eight typical patients. J Hum Genet. 2006;51(8):701–5.

Bevan S, Woodford-Richens K, Rozen P, et al. Screening SMAD1, SMAD2, SMAD3 and SMAD5 for germline mutations in juvenile polyposis syndrome. Gut. 1999;45:406–8.

Biegel JA, Zhou JY, Rorke LB, Stenstrom C, Wainwright LM, Fogelgren B. Germ-line and acquired mutations of INI1 in atypical teratoid and rhabdoid tumors. Cancer Res. 1999;59:74–9.

Bignami M, Casorrlli I, Karran P, et al. Mismatch repair and response to DNA-damaging antitumor therapies. Eur J Cancer. 2003;39:2142–9.

Birch JM, Hartley AL, Blair V, et al. The Li–Fraumeni cancer family syndrome. J Pathol. 1990;161:1–2.

Birch JM, Hartley AL, Tricker KJ, et al. Prevalence and diversity of constitutional mutations in the p53 gene among 21 Li–Fraumeni families. Cancer Res. 1994;54:1298–304.

Birch JM, Blair V, Kelsey AM, Evans DG, Harris M, Tricker KJ, Varley JM. Cancer phenotype correlates with constitutional TP53 genotype in families with the Li–Fraumeni syndrome. Oncogene. 1998;17:1061–8.

Birch JM, Alston RD, McNally RJQ, et al. Relative frequency and morphology of cancers in carriers of germline *TP53* mutations. Oncogene. 2001;20:4621–8.

Birt AR, Hogg GR, Dube WJ. Hereditary multiple fibrofolliculomas with trichodiscomas and acrochordons. Arch Dermatol. 1977;113(12):1674–7.

Blaydon DC, Etheridge SL, Risk JM, Hennies HC, Gay LJ, Carroll R, Plagnol V, McRonald FE, Stevens HP, Spurr NK, Bishop DT, Ellis A, Jankowski J, Field JK, Leigh IM, South AP, Kelsell DP. RHBDF2 mutations are associated with tylosis, a familial esophageal cancer syndrome. Am J Hum Genet. 2012;90:340–6.

Bliek J, Alders M, Maas SM, Oostra RJ, Mackay DM, van der Lip K, Callaway JL, Brooks A, van't Padje S, Westerveld A, Leschot NJ. Mannens MM. Lessons from BWS twins: complex maternal and paternal hypomethylation and a common source of haematopoietic stem cells. Eur J Hum Genet. 2009;17(12):1625–34.

Bloom D. The syndrome of congenital telangiectatic erythema and stunted growth. J Pediatr. 1966;68:103–13.

Boardman LA, Thibodeau SN, Schaid DJ, et al. Increased risk for cancer in patients with the Peutz–Jeghers syndrome. Ann Int Med. 1998;128:896–9.

Boland, et al. A National Cancer Institute Workshop on Microsatellite for cancer detection and familial predisposition: development of international criteria for determination of microsatellite instability in colorectal cancer. Cancer Res. 1998;58:5248–57.

Bolino A, Schuffenecker I, Luo Y, et al. *RET* mutations in exons 13 and 14 of FMTC patients. Oncogene. 1995;10:2415–9.

Bonadona V, et al. Cancer risks associated with germline mutations in *MLH1, MSH2*, and *MSH6* genes in Lynch Syndrome. JAMA. 2011;305:2302–10.

Boocock GRB, Morrison JA, Popovic M, Richards N, Ellis L, Durie PR, Rommens JM. Mutations in SBDS are associated with Shwachman–Diamond syndrome. Nat Genet. 2003;33: 97–101.

Boria I, Garelli E, Gazda HT, Aspesi A, Quarello P, Pavesi E, Ferrante D, Meerpohl JJ, Kartal M, DaCosta L, Proust A, Leblanc T, Simansour M, Dahl N, Fröjmark AS, Pospisilova D, Cmejla R, Beggs AH, Sheen MR, Landowski M, Buros CM, Clinton CM, Dobson LJ, Vlachos A,

Atsidaftos E, Lipton JM, Ellis SR, Ramenghi U, Dianzani I. The ribosomal basis of Diamond-Blackfan anemia: mutation and database update. Hum Mutat. 2010;31:1269–79.

Bougeard G, Charbonnier F, Moerman A, et al. Early onset brain tumor and lymphoma in MSH2 deficient children. Am J Hum Genet. 2003;72:213–6.

Bougeard G, Sesboue R, Baert-Desurmont S, Vasseur S, Martin C, Tinat J, Brugieres L, Chompret A, de Paillerets BB, Stoppa-Lyonnet D, Bonaiti-Pellie C, Frebourg T. Molecular basis of the Li-Fraumeni syndrome: an update from the French LFS families. J Med Genet. 2008;45: 535–8.

Boulikas T. Xeroderma pigmentosum and molecular cloning of DNA repair genes. Anticancer Res. 1996;16:693–708.

Boyd KP, Korf BR, Theos A. Neurofibromatosis type 1. J Am Acad Dermatol. 2009;61:1–14.

Brand R, Nielsen M, Lynch H, Infante E. MUTYH-associated polyposis. In: Pagon RA, Bird TD, Dolan CR, Stephens K, Adam MP, editors. GeneReviews™ [Internet]. Seattle: University of Washington, Seattle; 1993–2012 Oct 04.

Brandi ML, Marx SJ, Aurbach GD, Fitzpatrick LA. Familial multiple endocrine neoplasia type 1. A new look at pathophysiology. Endocrinol Rev. 1987;8:391–405.

Brandi M, Gagel R, Angeli A, Bilezikian J, Beck-Peccoz P, Bordi C, Conte-Devolx B, Falchetti A, Gheri R, Libroai A, Lips C, Lombardi G, Mannelli M, Pacini F, Ponder B, Raue F, Skosgeid B, Tamburrano G, Thakker R, Thompson N, Tommasetti P, Tonelli F, Wells S, Marx S. Guidelines for diagnosis and therapy of MEN type 1 and type 2. J Clin Endocrinol Metab. 2001;86:5658–71.

Brook-Carter PT, Peral B, Ward CJ, Thompson P, Hughes J, Maheshwar MM, Nellist M, Gamble V, Harris PC, Sampson JR. Deletion of the TSC2 and PKD1 genes associated with severe infantile polycystic kidney disease – a contiguous gene syndrome. Nat Genet. 1994;8:328–32.

Brosens LA, Keller JJ, Offerhaus GJ, et al. Prevention and management of duodenal polyps in familial adenomatous polyposis. Gut. 2005;54:1034–43.

Bruggers CS, Bleyl SB, Pysher T, Barnette P, Afify Z, Walker M, Biegel JA. Clinicopathologic comparison of familial versus sporadic atypical teratoid/rhabdoid tumors (AT/RT) of the central nervous system. Pediatr Blood Cancer. 2011;56:1026–31.

Brzustowicz LM, Farrell S, Khan MB, Weksberg R. Mapping of a new SGBS locus to chromosome Xp22 in a family with a severe form of Simpson-Golabi-Behmel syndrome. Am J Hum Genet. 1999;65:779–83.

Bubb VJ, Curtis LJ, Cunningham C, Dunlop MG, Carothers AD, Morris RG, White S, Bird CC, Wyllie AH. Microsatellite instability and the role of hMSH2 in sporadic colorectal cancer. Oncogene. 1996;12(12):2641–9.

Buckley RH. The multiple causes of human SCID. J Clin Invest. 2004a;114:1409–11.

Buckley RH. Molecular defects in human severe combined immunodeficiency and approaches to immune reconstitution. Annu Rev Immunol. 2004b;22:625–55.

Budny B, Chen W, Omran H, Fliegauf M, Tzschach A, Wisniewska M, Jensen LR, Raynaud M, Shoichet SA, Badura M, Lenzner S, Latos-Bielenska A, Ropers H-H. A novel X-linked recessive mental retardation syndrome comprising macrocephaly and ciliary dysfunction is allelic to oral-facial-digital type I syndrome. Hum Genet. 2006;120:171–8.

Bunyan DJ, Shea-Simmonds J, Reck AC, et al. Genotype/phenotype correlations of new causative APC gene mutations in patients with familial adenomatous polyposis. J Med Genet. 1995;32:728–31.

Burgess JR, Harle RA, Tucker P, et al. Adrenal lesions in a large kindred with multiple endocrine neoplasia type 1. Arch Surg. 1996;131:699–702.

Burn J, Chapman P, Delhanty J, et al. The UK northern region genetic register for familial adenomatous polyposis coli: use of age of onset, CHRPE and DNA markers in risk calculations. J Med Genet. 1991;28:289–96.

Burn J, Bishop DT, Chapman PD, Elliott F, Bertario L, Dunlop MG, Eccles D, Ellis A, Evans DG, Fodde R, Maher ER, Möslein G, Vasen HF, Coaker J, Phillips RK, Bülow S, Mathers JC, International CAPP Consortium. A randomized placebo-controlled prevention trial of aspirin and/or resistant starch in young people with familial adenomatous polyposis. Cancer Prev Res (Phila). 2011;4(5):655–65. doi:10.1158/1940-6207.CAPR-11-0106.

Butler MG, Dasouki MJ, Zhou XP, Talebizadeh Z, Brown M, Takahashi TN, Miles JH, Wang CH, Stratton R, Pilarski R, Eng C. Subset of individuals with autism spectrum disorders and macrocephaly associated with germline mutations in the PTEN tumour suppressor gene. J Med Genet. 2005;42:318–21.

Cahill DP, Lengauer C, Yu J, Riggins GJ, Willson JK, Markowitz SD, Kinzler KW, Vogelstein B. Mutations of mitotic checkpoint genes in human cancers. Nature. 1998;392(6673):300–3.

Cairney AEL, Andrews M, Greenberg M, Smith D, Weksberg R. Wilms' tumor in three patients with Bloom syndrome. J Pediatr. 1987;111:414–6.

Cairns SR, Scholefield JH, Steele RJ, Dunlop MG, Thomas HJ, Evans GD, Eaden JA, Rutter MD, Atkin WP, Saunders BP, Lucassen A, Jenkins P, Fairclough PD, Woodhouse CR, British Society of Gastroenterology; Association of Coloproctology for Great Britain and Ireland. Guidelines for colorectal cancer screening and (update from 2002) surveillance in moderate and high risk groups. Gut. 2010;59:666–89.

Calin G, Herlea V, Barbanti-Brodano G, Negrini M. The coding region of the Bloom syndrome BLM gene and of the CBL proto-oncogene is mutated in genetically unstable sporadic gastrointestinal tumors. Cancer Res. 1998;58(17):3777–81.

Calin GA, Gafa R, Tibiletti MG, Herlea V, Becheanu G, Cavazzini L, Barbanti-Brodano G, Nenci I, Negrini M, Lanza G. Genetic progression in microsatellite instability high (MSI-H) colon cancers correlates with clinico-pathological parameters: a study of the TGRbetaRII, BAX, hMSH3, hMSH6, IGFIIR and BLM genes. Int J Cancer. 2000;89(3):230–5.

Carney JA, Go VL, Sizemore GW, Hayles AB. Alimentary-tract ganglioneuromatosis. A major component of the syndrome of multiple endocrine neoplasia, type 2b. New Engl J Med. 1976;295:1287–91.

Carney JA, Gordon H, Carpenter PC, Shenoy BV, Go VL. The complex of myxomas, spotty pigmentation and endocrine overactivity. Medicine. 1985;64:270–83.

Carney JA, Hruska LS, Beauchamp GD, Gordon H. Dominant inheritance of the complex of myxomas, spotty pigmentation and endocrine overactivity. Mayo Clin Proc. 1986;61:165–72.

Carpten JD, Robbins CM, Villablanca A, et al. HRPT 2, encoding parafibromin is mutated in hyperparathyroidism – Jaw tumor syndrome. Nat Genet. 2002;32:676–80.

Carter JM, O'Hara C, Dundas G, Gilchrist D, Collins MS, Eaton K, Judkins AR, Biegel JA, Folpe AL. Epithelioid malignant peripheral nerve sheath tumor arising in a schwannoma, in a patient with "neuroblastoma-like" schwannomatosis and a novel germline SMARCB1 mutation. Am J Surg Pathol. 2012;36:154–60.

Cascon A, Huarte-Mednicoa CV, Learndro-Garcia L, Leton R, Suela J, Santana A, Costa MB, Comino-Mendez I, Landa I, Sanchez L, Rodrigues AC, Cigudosa JC, Robledo M. Detection of the first gross CDC73 germline deletion in an HPT-JT syndrome family. Gene Chrom Cancer. 2011;50:922–9.

Celentano V, Luglio G, Antonelli G, Bucci L. Prophylactic surgery in Lynch Syndrome. Techn Coloproctol. 2011;15:129–34.

Chandrasekharappa SC, Guru SC, Manickam P, et al. Positional cloning of the gene for multiple endocrine neoplasia type 1 (MEN 1) gene. Science. 1997;276:404–7.

Chang S, Prados MG. Identical twins with Ollier's disease and intracranial gliomas: case report. Neurosurgery. 1994;34:903–6.

Chen JD, Morrison CD, Zhang C, Kahnoski K, Carpten JD, Teh BT. Hyperparathyroidism-jaw tumor syndrome. J Int Med. 2003;253:634–42.

Chernin G, Vega-Warner V, Schoeb DS, Heeringa SF, Ovunc B, Saisawat P, Cleper R, Ozaltin F, Hildebrandt F. Members of the GPN Study Group. Genotype/phenotype correlation in nephrotic syndrome caused by WT1 mutations. Clin J Am Soc Nephrol. 2010;5(9):1655–62.

Chessa L. Six novel ATM mutations in Italian patients with classical ataxia-telangiectasia. Hum Mutat. 2003;21:450.

Chompret A, Brugières L, Ronsin M, Gardes M, Dessarps-Freichey F, Abel A, Hua D, Ligot L, Dondon MG, Bressac-de Paillerets B, Frébourg T, Lemerle J, Bonaïti-Pellié C, Feunteun J. P53 germline mutations in childhood cancers and cancer risk for carrier individuals. Br J Cancer. 2000;82:1932–7.

Choufani S, Shuman C, Weksberg R. Beckwith-Wiedemann syndrome. Am J Med Genet C Semin Med Genet. 2010;154C(3):343–54. Review. PubMed PMID: 20803657.

Christian JE, Ballon SC. Ovarian fibrosarcoma associated with Maffucci's syndrome. Gynaecol Oncol. 1990;37:290–1.

Chrzanowska KH, Gregorek H, Dembowska-Baginska B, Kalina MA, Digweed M. Nijmegen breakage syndrome (NBS). Orphanet J Rare Dis. 2012;7:13.

Chu G, Mayne L. Xeroderma pigmentosum, Cockayne syndrome and trichothiodystrophy: do the genes explain the disease? Trend Genet. 1996;12:187–92.

Church J. In which patients do I perform IRA and why? Fam Cancer. 2006;5(3):237–40. discussion 262–2.

Clark RD, Hutter JJ. Familial neurofibromatosis and juvenile chronic myelogenous leukemia. Hum Genet. 1982;60:230–2.

Clark AJ, Barnetson SM, Farrington SM, Dunlop MG. Prognosis I DNA mismatch repair deficient colorectal cancer: are all MSI tumors equivalent? Fam Cancer. 2004;3:85–91.

Clericuzio CL, Martin RA. Diagnostic criteria and tumor screening for individuals with isolated hemihyperplasia. Genet Med. 2009;11(3):220–2.

Coburn MC, Pricolo VE, DeLuca FG, Bland KI. Malignant potential in intestinal juvenile polyposis syndromes. Ann Surg Oncol. 1995;2:386–91.

Cohen PR, Kohn SR, Kurzrock R. Association of sebaceous gland tumors and internal malignancy: the Muir–Torre syndrome. Am J Med. 1991;90:606–13.

Cook JA, Oliver K, Mueller RF, et al. A cross-sectional study of renal involvement in tuberous sclerosis. J Med Genet. 1996;33:480–4.

Cooper WN, Luharia A, Evans GA, et al. Molecular subtypes and phenotypic expression of Beckwith–Wiedemann syndrome. Eur J Hum Genet. 2005;13:1025–32.

Coppede F. Premature aging syndrome. Adv Exp Med Biol. 2012;724:317–31.

Coppes MJ, Huff V, Pelletier J. Denys–Drash syndrome: relating a clinical disorder to genetic alterations in the tumor suppressor gene WT1. J Pediatr. 1993;123:673–8.

Corbetta S, Pizzocaro A, Peracchi M, et al. Multiple endocrine neoplasia type 1 in patients with recognized pituitary tumors of different types. Clin Endocrinol. 1997;47:507–12.

Corrao, G., Corazza, G.R., Bagnardi, V., Brusco, G., Ciacci, C., Cottone, M., Sategna Guidetti, C., Usai, P., Cesari, P., Pelli, M.A., Loperfido, S., Volta, U., Calabro, A. & Certo, M. Club del Tenue Study Group. Mortality in patients with coeliac disease and their relatives: a cohort study. Lancet. 2001;358(9279):356–61.

Costa OL, Silva DM, Colnago FA, Vieira MS, Musso CM. Turcot syndrome. Autosomal dominant or recessive transmission? Dis Colon Rectum. 1987;30:391–4.

Crabtree MD, Tomlinson IP, Hodgson SV, et al. Explaining variation in familial adenomatous polyposis: relationship between genotype and phenotype and evidence for modifier genes. Gut. 2002;51:420–3.

Crabtree M, Sieber OM, Lipton L, Hodgson SV, Lamlum H, Thomas HJ, Neale K, Phillips RK, Heinimann K, Tomlinson IP. Refining the relation between 'first hits' and 'second hits' at the APC locus: the 'loose fit' model and evidence for differences in somatic mutation spectra among patients. Oncogene. 2003;27:4257–65.

Crabtree MD, Fletcher C, Churchman M, Hodgson SV, Neale K, Phillips RK, Tomlinson IP. Analysis of candidate modifier loci for the severity of colonic familial adenomatous polyposis, with evidence for the importance of the N-acetyl transferases. Gut. 2004;53:271–6.

Dahele MR, et al. A patient with Rothmund–Thomson syndrome and tongue cancer – experience of radiation toxicity. Clin Oncol (R Coll Radiol). 2004;16(5):371–2.

Dasouki MJ, Ishmael H, Eng C. Macrocephaly, macrosomia and autistic behavior due to a de novo PTEN germline mutation. Am. J. Hum. Genet. 2001;69S:280 [Abstract 564].

DeBaun MR. Screening for cancer in children with Costello syndrome. Am J Med Genet. 2002;108:88–90.

DeBaun MR, Niemitz EL, McNeil DE, Brandenburg SA, Lee MP, Feinberg AP. Epigenetic alterations of H19 and LIT1 distinguish patients with Beckwith– Wiedemann syndrome with cancer and birth defects. Am J Hum Genet. 2002;70:604–11.

Debinski HS, Spigelman AD, Hatfield A, et al. Upper Intestinal surveillance in FAP. Eur J Cancer. 1995;31A(7–8):1149–53.

De la Chapelle A. Genetic predisposition to colorectal cancer. Nat Rev Cancer. 2004;4:769–80.

De la Torre C, Pincheria J, Lopez-Saez JF, et al. Human syndromes with genomic instability and multiprotein machines that repair DNA double-strand breaks. Histol Histopathol. 2003;18:225–43.

de Leng WW, Jansen M, Carvalho R, Polak M, Musler AR, Milne AN, Keller JJ, Menko FH, de Rooij FW, Iacobuzio-Donahue CA, Giardiello FM, Weterman MA, Offerhaus GJ. Genetic defects underlying Peutz-Jeghers syndrome (PJS) and exclusion of the polarity-associated MARK/Par1 gene family as potential PJS candidates. Clin Genet. 2007;72(6):568–73. Epub 2007 Oct 9.

De Raedt T, Brems H, Wolkenstein P, Vidaud D, Pilotti S, Perrone F, Mautner V, Frahm S, Sciot R, Legius E. Elevated risk for MPNST in NF1 microdeletion patients. Am J Hum Genet. 2003;72:1288–92.

De Rosa M, Fasano C, Panariello L, et al. Evidence for a recessive inheritance of Turcot's syndrome caused by compound heterozygous mutations within the PMS2 gene. Oncogene. 2000;19:1719–23.

De Vos M, Hayward BE, Picton S, Sheridan E, Bonthron DT. Novel PMS2 pseudogenes can conceal recessive mutations causing a distinctive childhood cancer syndrome. Am J Hum Genet. 2004;74(5):954–64.

DeBaun MR, Niemitz EL, Feinberg AP. Association of in vitro fertilization with Beckwith–Wiedemann syndrome and epigenetic alterations of LIT1 and H19. Am J Hum Genet. 2003;72:156–60.

Decker RA, Peacock ML, Borst MJ, Sweet JD, Thompson NW. Progress in genetic screening of multiple endocrine neoplasia type 2A: is calcitonin testing obsolete? Surgery. 1995;118:257–64.

Dempsey-Robertson M, Wilkes D, Stall A, Bush P. Incidence of abdominal tumors in syndromic and idiopathic hemihypertrophy/isolated hemihyperplasia. J Pediatr Orthop. 2012;32:322–6.

Demuth I, Digweed M. The clinical manifestation of a defective response to DNA double-strand breaks as exemplified by Nijmegen breakage syndrome. Oncogene. 2007;26:7792–8.

Derenoncourt AN, Castro Magana M, Jones KL. Mediastinal teratoma and precocious puberty in a boy with mosaic Klinefelter syndrome. Am J Med Genet. 1995;55:38–42.

Derry JM, Ochs HD, Francke U. Isolation of a novel gene mutated in Wiskott-Aldrich syndrome. Cell. 1994a;78:635–44. Erratum in: Cell. 1994;79(5):following 922.

Derry JM, Ochs HD, Francke U. Isolation of a novel gene mutated in Wiskott– Aldrich syndrome. Cell. 1994b;75:635–44.

DeVivo I, Gertig D, Nagase S, et al. Novel germline mutations in the PTEN tumor suppressor gene found in women with multiple cancers. J Med Genet. 2000;37:336–41.

DiFiore F, Charbonnier F, Martin C, et al. Screening for genomic rearrangements of the MMR genes must be included in the routine diagnosis of HNPCC. J Med Genet. 2004;41:18–20.

Diller L, Sexsmith E, Gottlieb A, et al. Germline p53 mutations are frequently detected in young children with rhabdomyosarcoma. J Clin Invest. 1995;95:1606–11.

Distante S, Nasoulias S, Somers GR, et al. Familial adenomatous polyposis in a 5 year old child: a clinical pathological and molecular genetic study. J Med Genet. 1996;33:157–60.

Dobru D, Seuchea N, Dorin M, Careinau V. Blue Rubber Bleb syndrome: a case report and literature review. Rom J Gastro. 2004;13:237–40.

Domchek SM, Tang J, Stopfer J, Lilli DR, Hamel N, Tischkowitz M, Monteiro AN, Messick TE, Powers J, Yonker A, Couch FJ, Goldgar DE, Davidson HR, Nathanson KL, Foulkes WD, Greenberg RA. Biallelic deleterious BRCA1 mutations in a woman with early-onset ovarian cancer. Cancer Discov. 2013;3(4):399–405.

Donadieu J, Fenneteau O, Beaupain B, Beaufils S, Bellanger F, Mahlaoui N, Lambilliotte A, Aladjidi N, Bertrand Y, Mialou V, Perot C, Michel G, Fouyssac F, Paillard C, Gandemer V, Boutard P, Schmitz J, Morali A, Leblanc T, Bellanne-Chantelot C. Classification and risk factors of hematological complications in a French national cohort of 102 patients with Shwachman-Diamond syndrome. Haematologica. 2012;(9):1312–9. doi:10.3324/haematol.2011.057489.

Dragani TA. Risk of HCC: genetic heterogeneity and complex genetics. J Hepatol. 2010;52: 252–7.

Draptchinskaia N, Gustavsson P, Andersson B, Pettersson M, Willig TN, Dianzani I, Ball S, Tchernia G, Klar J, Matsson H, Tentler D, Mohandas N, Carlsson B, Dahl N. The gene encoding ribosomal protein S19 is mutated in Diamond-Blackfan anemia. Nat Genet. 1999;21(2):169–75.

Dreijerink KM, Lips CJ. Diagnosis and management of multiple endocrine neoplasia tye 1 (MEN1). Heredit Cancer Clin Pract. 2005;3:1–6.

Dror Y, Freedman MH. Shwachman-Diamond syndrome: An inherited preleukemic bone marrow failure disorder with aberrant hematopoietic progenitors and faulty marrow microenvironment. Blood. 1999;94(9):3048–54.

Duker NJ. Chromosome breakage syndromes and cancer. Am J Med Genet. 2002;115:125–9.

Dunlop MG. Guidance on gastroenterological surveillance for hereditary non-polyposis colorectal cancer, familial adenomatous polyposis, juvenile polyposis and Peutz–Jeghers syndrome. Gut. 2002;51(Suppl. V):v21–7.

Dunlop MG, Farrington SM, Carothers AD, Wyllie AH, Sharp L, Burn J, Liu B, Kinzler KW, Vogelstein B. Cancer risk associated with germline DNA mismatch repair gene mutations. Hum Mol Genet. 1997;6(1):105–10.

Dutz JP, Benoit L, Wang X, Demetrick DJ, Junker A, de Sa D, Tan R. Lymphocytic vasculitis in X-linked lymphoproliferative disease. Blood. 2001;97:95–100.

Easton DF, Ponder MA, Cummings T, et al. The clinical and age-at-onset distribution for the MEN-2 syndrome. Am J Hum Genet. 1989;44:208–15.

Eaton KW, Tooke LS, Wainwright LM, Judkins AR, Biegel JA. Spectrum of SMARCB1/INI1 mutations in familial and sporadic rhabdoid tumors. Pediatr Blood Cancer. 2011;56:7–15.

Eeles RA. Germline mutations in the TP53 gene. Cancer Surv. 1995;25:101–24.

Eerola I, Boon LM, Mulliken JB, et al. Capillary malformation–arteriovenous malformation, a new clinical and genetic disorder caused by RASA1 mutations. Am J Hum Genet. 2003;73: 1240–9.

Elliott ML, Maher ER. Syndrome of the month: Beckwith–Wiedemann syndrome. J Med Genet. 1994;31:560–4.

Ellis NA, German J. Molecular genetics of Bloom's syndrome. Hum Mol Genet. 1996;5:1457–63.

Ellis NA, Groden J, Ye TZ, Straughen J, Kennon DJ, Ciocci S, Proytcheva M, German J. The Bloom's syndrome gene product is homologous to RecQ helicases. Cell. 1995;83(4): 655–66.

Elsaleh HIB, et al. Microsatellite instability is a predictive marker for survival benefit from adjuvant chemotherapy in a population-based series of stage III colorectal carcinoma. Clin. Colorectal Cancer. 2001;1:103–9.

Eng C. RET proto-oncogene in the development of human cancer. J Clin Oncol. 1999;17:380–93.

Eng C. Familial papillary thyroid cancer – many syndromes, too many genes? J Clin Endocrinol Metab. 2000a;85:1755–7.

Eng C. Will the real Cowden syndrome please stand up: revised diagnostic criteria. J Med Genet. 2000b;37:828–30.

Eng C. News and views: to be or not to BMP. Nat Genet. 2001;28:105–7.

Eng C. Mendelian genetics of rare-and not so rare-cancers. Ann N Y Acad Sci. 2010;1214:70–82.

Eng C, Parsons R. Cowden syndrome. In: Vogelstein B, Kinzler KW, editors. The genetic basis of human cancer. New York: McGraw-Hill; 1998. p. 519–26.

Eng C, Peacocke M. PTEN and inherited hamartoma-cancer syndromes. Nat Genet. 1998;19:223.

Eng C, Smith DP, Mulligan LM, et al. Point mutation within the tyrosine kinase domain of the RET proto-oncogene in multiple endocrine neoplasia type 2B and related sporadic tumors. Hum Mol Genet. 1994;3:237–41.

Eng C, Mulligan LM, Smith DP, et al. Mutation in the RET proto-oncogene in sporadic medullary thyroid carcinoma. Gene Chrom Cancer. 1995a;12:209–12.

Eng C, Smith DP, Mulligan LM, et al. A novel point mutation in the tyrosine kinase domain of the RET proto-oncogene in sporadic medullary thyroid carcinoma and in a family with FMTC. Oncogene. 1995b;10:509–13.

Eng C, Clayton D, Schuffenecker I, et al. The relationship between specific *RET* proto-oncogene mutations and disease phenotype in multiple endocrine neoplasia type 2: International *RET* Mutation Consortium analysis. J Am Med Assoc. 1996a;276:1575–9.

Eng C, Mulligan LM, Healey CS, et al. Heterogeneous mutation of the *RET* proto-oncogene in subpopulations of medullary thyroid carcinoma. Cancer Res. 1996b;56:2167–70.

Eng C, Schneider K, Fraumeni JF, Li FP. Third International Workshop on collaborative interdisciplinary studies of *p53* and other predisposing genes in Li–Fraumeni syndrome. Cancer Epidemiol Biomark Prev. 1997;6:379–83.

Eng C, Hampel H, de la Chapelle A. Genetic testing for cancer predisposition. Annu Rev Med. 2001;52:371–400.

Eng C, Kiuru M, Fernandez MJ, Aaltonen LA. A role for mitochondrial enzymes in inherited neoplasia and beyond. Nat Rev Cancer. 2003;3:193–202.

Engel JR, Smallwood A, Harper A, Higgins MJ, Oshimura M, Reik W, Schofield PN, Maher ER. Epigenotype-phenotype correlations in Beckwith– Wiedemann syndrome. J Med Genet. 2000;37:921–6.

Engel C, Loeffler M, Steinke V, et al. Risks of less common cancers in proven mutation carriers with Lynch syndrome. J Clin Oncol. 2012;30:4409–15.

Epstein CJ, Martin GM, Schultz AL, et al. Werner's syndrome. Medicine. 1966;45:177–221.

Erlic Z, Hoffmann MM, Sullivan M, Franke G, Peczkowska M, Harsch I, Schott M, Gabbert HE, Valimaki M, Preuss SF, Hasse-Lazar K, Wailgorski D, Robledo M, Januszewicz A, Eng C, Neumann HPH. Pathogenicity of DNA variants and double mutations in multiple endocrine neoplasia type 2 and von Hippel-Lindau disease. J Clin Endocrinol Metab. 2010;95:308–13.

Evans DG. Are we ready for targeted early breast cancer detection strategies in women with NF1 aged 30-49 years? Am J Med Genet. 2012;Part A 158A:3054–5.

Evans DG, Howard E, Giblin C, Clancy T, Spencer H, Huson SM, Lalloo F. Birth incidence and prevalence of tumor-prone syndromes: estimates from a UK family genetic register service. Am J Med Genet A. 2010;152A:327–32.

Evans DG, Raymond FL, Barwell JG, Halliday D. Genetic testing and screening of individuals at risk of NF2. Clin Genet. 2012;82:416–24.

Evans DGR, Huson S, Donnai D, et al. A clinical study of type 2 neurofibromatosis. Q J Med. 1992;84:603–18.

Evans DRG, Ladisans EJ, Rimmer S, Burnell LD, Thakker N, Farndon PA. Complications of the nevoid basal cell carcinoma syndrome: results of a population based study. J Med Genet. 1993;30:460–4.

Evans DG, Mason S, Huson SM, Ponder M, Harding AE, Strachan T. Spinal and cutaneous schwannomatosis is a variant form of type 2 neurofibromatosis: a clinical and molecular study. J Neurol Neurosurg Psychiat. 1997;62:361–6.

Evans DG, Baser ME, McGaughran J, Sharif S, Howard E, Moran A. Malignant peripheral nerve sheath tumors in neurofibromatosis 1. J Med Genet. 2002;39:311–4.

Evans DGR, Lalloo F, Wallace A, Rahman N. Update on the Manchester Scoring System for BRCA1 and BRCA2 testing. J Med Genet. 2005;42:e39. doi:10.1136/jmg.2005.031989.

Fackenthal J, Marsh DJ, Richardson AL, et al. Male breast cancer in Cowden syndrome patients with germline *PTEN* mutations. J Med Genet. 2001;38:159–64.

Falchetti A, Marini F, Brandi ML. Multiple endocrine neoplasia type 1. Gene Reviews. Pagon RA, Bird TD, Dolan CR, Stephens K. Seattle: University of Washington Press; 2010.

Farndon JR, Leight GS, Dilley WG, et al. Familial medullary thyroid carcinoma without associated endocrinopathies: a distinct clinical entity. Br J Surg. 1986;73:278–81.

Farndon PA, Del Mastro RG, Evans DGR, et al. Location of gene for Gorlin syndrome. Lancet. 1992;339:581–2.

Farrington SM, McKinley AJ, Carothers AD, Cunningham C, Bubb VJ, Sharp L, Wyllie AH, Dunlop MG. Evidence for an age-related influence of microsatellite instability on colorectal cancer survival. Int J Cancer. 2002;98(6):844–50.

Fearon ER. Human cancer syndromes: clues on the origin and nature of cancer. Science. 1997;278:1043–50.

Felix CA, Slavc L, Dunn M, et al. *p53* gene mutations in pediatric brain tumors. Med Pediatr Oncol. 1995;25:431–6.

Fenton PA, Clarke SEM, Owen W, et al. Cribriform variant papillary thyroid cancer: a characteristic of familial adenomatous polyposis. Thyroid. 2001;11:193–7.

Ferguson A, Kingstone K. Coeliac disease and malignancies. Acta Paediatr Suppl. 1996;412: 78–81.

Figueiredo BC, Sandrini R, Zambetti GP, et al. Penetrance of adrenocortical tumor associated with the germline TP53 R337H mutation. J Med Genet. 2006;43(1):91–6.

Filling-Katz MR, Choyke P, Patronas N, et al. Central nervous involvement in von Hippel–Lindau disease. Neurology. 1991;41:41–6.

Fiorentino DF, Nguyen JC, Egbert BM, Swetter SM. Muir–Torre syndrome: confirmation of diagnosis by immunohistochemical analysis of cutaneous lesions. J Am Acad Dermatol. 2004;50(3):476–8.

Floy KM, Hess RO, Meisner LF. DNA polymerase alpha defect in the N syndrome. Am J Med Genet. 1990;35:301–5.

Fodde R, Kuipers J, Smits R, et al. Mutations in the APC tumor suppressor gene cause chromosome instability. Nat Cell Biol. 2001;3:433–8.

Fong LY, Fidanza V, Zanesi N, Lock LF, Siracusa LD, Mancini R, Siprashvili Z, Ottey M, Martin SE, Druck T, McCue PA, Croce CM, Huebner K. Muir–Torre-like syndrome in Fhit-deficient mice. Proc Natl Acad Sci USA. 2000;97(9):4742–7.

Foulkes WD. Review: a tale of four syndromes: familial adenomatous polyposis, Gardner syndrome, attenuated APC and Turcot syndrome. Q J Med. 1995;88:853–63.

Foulkes WD, Thiffault I, Gruber SB, et al. The founder mutation MSH2* 1906G-C is an important cause of hereditary nonpolyposis colorectal cancer in the Ashkenazi Jewish population. Am J Hum Genet. 2002;71:1395–412.

Foulkes WD, Bahubeshi A, Hamel N, Pasini B, Asioli S, Baynam G, Choong CS, Charles A, Frieder RP, Dishop MK, Graf N, Ekim M, Bouron-Dal SD, Arseneau J, Young RH, Sabbaghian N, Srivastava A, Tischkowitz MD, Priest JR. Extending the phenotypes associated with DICER1 mutations. Hum Mutat. 2011;32:1381–4.

Fracanzani AL, Taioli E, Sampietro M, Fatta E, Bertelli C, Fiorelli G, Fargion S. Liver cancer risk is increased in patients with porphyria cutanea tarda in comparison to matched control patients with chronic liver disease. J Hepatol. 2001;35:498–503.

Frank-Raue K, Rybicki LA, Erlic Z, Schweizer H, Winter A, Milos I, Toledo SP, Toledo RA, Tavares MR, Aleviazaki M, Mian C, Siggelkow H, Hufner M, Wohlik N, Opocher G, Dvorakova S, Bendlova B, Czewertynska M, Skasko E, Barontini M, Sanso G, Vorlander C, Maia AL, Patocs A, Links TP, de Groot JW, Kersents MN, Valk GD, Miehle K, Musholt TJ, Biarnes J, Damjanovic S, Muresan M, Wuster C, Fassnacht M, Peczkowska M, Fauth C, Golcher H, Walter MA, Pichl J, Raue F, Eng C, Neumann HPH. Risk profiles and penetrance estimations in multiple endocrine neoplasia type 2A caused by germline RET mutations located in exon 10. Hum Mutat. 2011;32:51–8.

Frebourg T, Barbier N, Yan YX, et al. Germline p53 mutations in 15 families with Li–Fraumeni syndrome. Am J Hum Genet. 1995;56:608–15.

Freedman MH, Bonilla MA, Fier C, Bolyard AA, Scarlata D, Boxer LA, Brown S, Cham B, Kannourakis G, Kinsey SE, Mori PG, Cottle T, Welte K, Dale DC. Myelodysplasia syndrome and acute myeloid leukemia in patients with congenital neutropenia receiving G-CSF therapy. Blood. 2000;96:429–36.

Friedl W, Kruse R, Uhlhaas S, et al. Frequent 4-bp deletion in exon 9 of the *SMAD4/ MADH4* gene in familial juvenile polyposis patients. Gene Chrom Cancer. 1999;25:403–6.

Friedl W, Uhlhaas S, Schulmann K, et al. Juvenile polyposis: massive gastric polyposis is more common in MADH4 mutation carriers than in BMPR1A mutation carriers. Hum Genet. 2002;111:108–11.

Fukhro, et al. Blue rubber bleb nevus syndrome and gastrointestinal haemorrhage: which treatment? Eur J Paed Surg. 2002;12:129–33.

Gaglia P, Atkin WS, Whitelaw S, et al. Variables associated with the risk of colorectal adenomas in asymptomatic patients with a family history of colorectal cancer. Gut. 1995;36:385–90.

Gallione CJ, Pasyk KA, Boon LN, et al. A gene for familial venous malformation maps to chromosome 9p in a second large kindred. J Med Genet. 1995;32:197–9.

Gammon A, Jasperson K, Kohlman W, Burt RW. Hamartomatous polyposis syndromes. Best Pract Res Clin Gastroenterol. 2009;23:219–31.

Ganslandt O, Buchfelder M, Grabenauer GG. Primary spinal germinoma in a patient with concomitant Klinefelter's syndrome. Br J Neurosurg. 2000;14:252–5.

Garber JE, Goldstein AM, Kantor AF, et al. Follow-up study of twenty-four families with Li–Fraumeni syndrome. Cancer Res. 1991;51:6094–7.

Gardner E, Papi L, Easton DF, et al. Genetic linkage studies map the multiple endocrine neoplasia type 2 loci to a small interval on chromosome 10q11.2. Hum Mol Genet. 1993;2: 241–6.

Gaujoux S, Tissier F, Ragazzon B, et al. Pancreatic ductal and acinar cell neoplasms in Carney Complex: a possible new association. J Clin Endo Metab. 2011;96:E1888–95.

Gazda H, Lipton JM, Willig TN, Ball S, Niemeyer CM, Tchernia G, Mohandas N, Daly MJ, Ploszynska A, Orfali KA, Vlachos A, Glader BE, Rokicka-Milewska R, Ohara A, Baker D, Pospisilova D, Webber A, Viskochil DH, Nathan DG, Beggs AH, Sieff CA. Evidence for linkage of familial Diamond–Blackfan anemia to chromosome 8p23.3–p22 and for non-19q non-8p disease. Blood. 2001;97(7):2145–50.

Gazda HT, Sheen MR, Vlachos A, Choesmel V, O'Donohoe M-F, Schneider H, Darras N, Hasman C, Sieff CA, Newburger PE, Ball SE, Niewiadomska E, Matysiak M, Zaucha JM, Glader B, Niemeyer C, Meerpohl JJ, Atsidaftos E, Lipton JM, Gleizes PE, Beggs AH. Ribosomal protein L5 and L11 mutations are associated with cleft palate and abnormal thumbs in Diamond-Blackfan anemia patients. Am J Hum Genet. 2008;83:769–80.

Giannelli F, Pawsey SA. DNA repair synthesis in human heterokaryons. III. The rapid and slow complementing varieties of xeroderma pigmentosum. J Cell Sci. 1976;20:207–13.

Giannelli F. DNA maintenance and its relation to human pathology. J Cell Sci Suppl. 1986;4:383–416.

Giardiello FM, Welsh SB, Hamilton SR, et al. Increased risk of cancer in the Peutz–Jeghers syndrome. New Engl J Med. 1987;316:1511–4.

Gicquel C, Gaston V, Mandelbaum J, Siffro J-P, Flahault A, Le Bouc Y. In vitro fertilization may increase the risk of Beckwith–Wiedemann syndrome related to abnormal imprinting of the KCNQ1OT gene. Am J Hum Genet. 2003;72:1338–41.

Gimm O, Marsh DJ, Andrew SD, et al. Germline dinucleotide mutation in codon 883 of the RET proto-oncogene in multiple endocrine neoplasia type 2B without codon 918 mutation. J Clin Endocrinol Metab. 1997;82:3902–4.

Giraud S, Zhang CX, Serova-Sinilnikova O, et al. Germ-line mutation analysis in patients with multiple endocrine neoplasia type 1 and related disorders. Am J Hum Genet. 1998;63: 455–67.

Gisbert JP, Garcia-Buey L, Alonso A. Hepatocellular carcinoma risk in patients with porphyria cutanea tarda. Eur J Gastroenterol Hepatol. 2004;16:689–92.

Giunti L, Cetica V, Ricci U, Giglio S, Sardi I, Paglierani M, Andreucci E, Sanzo M, Forni M, Buccoliero AM, Genitori L, Genuardi M. Type A microsatellite instability in pediatric gliomas as an indicator of Turcot syndrome. Europ J Hum Genet. 2009a;27:919–27.

Giunti L, Cetica V, Ricci U, Giglio S, Sardi I, Paglierani M, Andreucci E, Sanzo M, Forni M, Buccoliero AM, Genitori L, Genuardi M. Type A microsatellite instability in pediatric gliomas as an indicator of Turcot syndrome. Eur J Hum Genet. 2009b;17(7):919–27.

Goldfarb DA, Neumann HPH, Penn I, Novick AC. Results of renal transplantation in patients with renal cell carcinoma in Von Hippel–Lindau disease. Transplantation. 1998;64:1726–9.

Gomes MC, Kotsopoulos J, de Almeida GL, Costa MM, Vieira R, Filho FA, Pitombo MB, Paulo Roberto FL, Royer R, Zhang P, Narod SA. The R337H mutation in TP53 and breast cancer in Brazil. Hered Cancer Clin Pract. 2012;10:3.

Gomez MR, editor. Tuberous Sclerosis. New York: Raven Press; 1988.

Gonzalez KD, Noltner KA, Buzin CH, Gu D, Wen-Fong CY, Nguyen VQ, Han JH, Lowstuter K, Longmate J, Sommer SS, Weitzel JN. Beyond Li Fraumeni Syndrome: clinical characteristics of families with p53 germline mutations. J Clin Oncol. 2009;27:1250–6.

Gorlin RJ. Nevoid basal-cell carcinoma syndrome. Medicine. 1987;66:98–113.

Gorlin RJ. Nevoid basal cell carcinoma syndrome. Dermatol Clin. 1995;13:113–25.

Gorlin RJ, Sedano HO, Vickers RA, Cervenka J. Multiple mucosal neuromas, phaeochromocytoma and medullary carcinoma of the thyroid – a syndrome. Cancer. 1968;22:293–9.

Gorlin RJ, Cohen MM, Condon LM, Burke BA. Bannayan-Riley-Ruvalcaba syndrome. Am J Med Genet. 1992;44:307–14.

Goss KH, Risinger MA, Kordich JJ, Snaz MM, Straughen LE, Capobianco AJ, German J, Boivin GP, Groden J. Enhanced tumor formation in mice heterozygous for Blm mutation. Science. 2002;297(5589):2051–3.

Goto M, Miller RW, Ishikawa Y, Sugano H. Excess of rare cancers in Werner syndrome (adult progeria). Cancer Epidemiol Biomark Prev. 1996;5(4):239–46.

Graham Jr JM, Anayne-Yeboa K, Raams A, et al. Cerebro-oculo-facio-skeletal syndrome with a nucleotide excision repair defect and a mutated XPD gene, with prenatal diagnosis in a triplet pregnancy. Am J Hum Genet. 2001;69:291–300.

Graham RB, Nolasco M, Peterlin B, Garcia CK. Nonsense mutations in folliculin presenting as isolated familial spontaneous pneumothorax in adults. Am J Respir Crit Care Med. 2005;172(1):39–44.

Gravholt CH, Fedder J, Naeraa RW, Müller J. Occurrence of Gonadoblastoma in Females with Turner Syndrome and Y Chromosome Material: A Population Study. J Clin Endocrinol Metab. 2000;85(9):3199–202.

Green JS, Bowmer MI, Johnson GJ. Von Hippel–Lindau disease in a Newfoundland kindred. Can Med Assoc J. 1986;134:133–46.

Greenberg F, Stein F, Gresnik MV, et al. The Perlman nephroblastomatosis syndrome. Am J Med Genet. 1986;24:101–10.

Greenberg F, Copeland K, Gresik MV. Expanding the spectrum of the Perlman syndrome. Am J Med Genet. 1988;29:773–6.

Griffiths DFR, Williams GT, Wilhaus ED. Duodenal carcinoid tumors, phaeochromocytoma and neurofibromatosis. Islet cell tumor, phaeochromocytoma and von Hippel–Lindau complex: two distinctive neuroendocrine syndromes. Q J Med. 1987;64:769–82.

Grignon DJ, Shum DT, Bruckschwaiger O. Transitional cell carcinoma in the Muir–Torre syndrome. J Urol. 1987;38:406–8.

Grindedal EM, Moller P, Eeles R, et al. Germ-line mutations in mismatch repair genes associated with prostate cancer. Cancer Epidemiol Biomarkers Prev. 2009;18(9):2460–7.

Gripp KW, Lin AE. Costello syndrome: a Ras/mitogen activated protein kinase pathway syndrome (rasopathy) resulting from HRAS germline mutations. Genet Med. 2012;14(3):285–92.

Gripp KW, Scott Jr CI, Nicholson L, et al. Five additional Costello patients with rhabdomyosarcoma: proposal for a tumour screening protocol. Am J Med Genet. 2002;108:80–7.

Gripp KW, Stabley DL, Nicholson L, Hoffman JD, Sol-Church K. Somatic mosaicism for an HRAS mutation causes Costello syndrome. Am J Med Genet. 2006;140A:2163–9.

Groet J, McElwain S, Spinelli M, et al. Acquired mutations in GATA1 in neonates with Down's syndrome with transient myeloid disorders. Lancet. 2003;361:1617–20.

Groves CJ, Saunders BP, Spigelman AD, Phillips RK. Duodenal cancer in patients with familial adenomatous polyposis (FAP); results of a 10 year prospective study. Gut. 2002;50:636–41.

Gruber SB, Ellis NA, Rennert G, Offit K, Scott KK, Almog R, Kolachana P, Bonner JD, Kirchhoff T, Tomsho LP, Nafa K, Pierce H, Low M, Satagopan J, Rennert H, Huang H, Greenson JK, Groden J, Rapaport B, Shia J, Johnson S, Gregersen PK, Harris CC, Boyd J. BLM heterozygosity and the risk of colorectal cancer. Science. 2002;297(5589):2013.

Grundy P, Telzerow P, Paterson MC, et al. Chromosome 11 uniparental disomy predisposing to embryonal neoplasms. Lancet. 1991;338:1079–80.

Gryfe R, Kim H, Hsieh ETK, Aronson MD, Holowaty EJ, Bull SB, Redston M, Gallinger S. Tumor microsatellite instability and clinical outcome in young patients with colorectal cancer. New Engl J Med. 2000;342(2):69–77.

Gurtan AM, Lu V, Bhutkar A, Sharp PA. In vivo structure-function analysis of human Dicer reveals directional processing of precursor miRNAs. RNA. 2012;18:1116–22.

Gustavsson P, Willig T-N, van Hareingen A, et al. Diamond–Blackfan anemia: genetic homogeneity for a gene on chromosome 19q13 restricted to 1.8Mb. Nat Genet. 1997;16:368–71.

Hahn H, Wickling C, Zaphiropoulous PG, et al. Mutations of the human homologue of *Drosophila* patched in the nevoid basal cell carcinoma syndrome. Cell. 1996;85:841–51.

Hahnloser D, Petersen GM, Rabe K, et al. The APC E1317Q variant in adenomatous polyps and colorectal cancers. Cancer Epidemiol Biomark Prev. 2003;12:1023–8.

Hammami MM, al-Zahrani A, Butt A, Vencer LJ, Hussain SS. Primary hyperparathyroidism-associated polyostotic fibrous dysplasia: absence of McCune–Albright syndrome mutations. J Endocrinol Invest. 1997;20:552–8.

Hamilton SR, Liu B, Parsons RE, et al. The molecular basis of Turcot's syndrome. New Engl J Med. 1995;332:839–47.

Haneke E, Gutschmidt E. Premature multiple Bowen's disease in poikiloderma congenitale with warty hyperkeratoses. Dermatologica. 1979;158:384–8.

Hanks S, Coleman K, Reid S, Plaja A, Firth H, Fitzpatrick D, Kidd A, Mehes K, Nash R, Robin N, Shannon N, Tolmie J, Swansbury J, Irrthum A, Douglas J, Rahman N. Constitutional aneuploidy and cancer predisposition caused by biallelic mutations in BUB1B. Nat Genet. 2004;36(11):1159–61.

Hanssen AMN, Fryns JP. Cowden syndrome. J Med Genet. 1995;32:117–9.

Happle R. The McCune Albright syndrome: a lethal gene surviving by mosaicism. Clin Genet. 1989;29:321–4.

Harper PS, Harper RM, Howel-Evans AW. Carcinoma of the oesophagus with tylosis. Q J Med. 1970;39(155):317–33.

Harris WR. Chondrosarcoma complicating total hip arthroplasty in Maffucci's syndrome. Clin Orthop. 1990;260:212–4.

Hartley AL, Birch JM, Marsden HB, Harris M, Blair V. Neurofibromatosis in children with soft tissue sarcoma. Pediatr Hematol Oncol. 1988;5:7–16.

Harwood CA, McGregor JM, Swale VJ, Proby CM, Leigh IM, Newton R, Khorshid SM, Cerio R. High frequency and diversity of cutaneous appendageal tumors in organ transplant recipients. J Am Acad Dermatol. 2003;48(3):401–8.

Hashmi SK, Allen C, Klaassen R, Fernandez CV, Yanofsky R, Shereck E, Champagne J, Silva M, Lipton JH, Brossard J, Samson Y, Abish S, Steele M, Ali K, Dower N, Athale U, Jardine L, Hand JP, Beyene J, Dror Y. Comparative analysis of Shwachman-Diamond syndrome to other inherited bone marrow failure syndromes and genotype-phenotype correlation. Clin Genet. 2011;79:448–58.

Hasle H. Pattern of malignant disorders in individuals with Down's syndrome. Lancet Oncol. 2001;2:429–36.

Hasle H, Mellengaard A, Nielson J, Hanses J. Cancer incidence in men with Klinefelter syndrome. Br J Cancer. 1995;71:416–20.

Hasle H, Hammerstrup Clemensau I, Mikkelson M. Risks of leukaemia and other tumours in individuals with Downs syndrome. Lancet. 2000;355:165–9.

Hasselblatt M, Gesk S, Oyen F, Rossi S, Viscardi E, Giangaspero F, Giannini C, Judkins AR, Fruhwald MC, Obser T, Schneppenheim R, Siebert R, Paulus W. Nonsense mutation and inactivation of SMARCA4 (BRG1) in an atypical teratoid/rhabdoid tumor showing retained SMARCB1 (INI1) expression. Am J Surg Pathol. 2011;35:933–5.

Hatada I, Ohashi H, Fukushima Y, et al. An imprinted gene p57^{KIP2} is mutated in Beckwith–Wiedemann syndrome. Nat Genet. 1996;14:171–3.

Hauben EI, et al. Multiple primary malignancies in osteosarcoma patients. Incidence and predictive value of osteosarcoma subtype for cancer syndromes related with osteosarcoma Eur J Hum Genet. 2003;11(8):611–8.

Hayward BE, De Vos M, Sheridan E, Bonthron DT. PMS2 mutations in HNPCC. Clin Genet. 2004;66(6):566–7.

Heald B, Hilden JM, Zbuk KM, Norton A, Vyas P, Theil KS, Eng C. Severe TMD/AMKL with *GATA1* mutation in a stillborn fetus with Down syndrome. Nature Clin Pract Oncol. 2007;4:433–8.

Heald B, Mester J, Rybicki LA, Orloff MS, Burke CA, Eng C. Frequent gastrointestinal polyps and colorectal cancer in prospective series of *PTEN* mutation carriers. Gastroenterology. 2010;139:1927–33.

Heikkinen K, Rapakko K, Karppinen SM, Erkko H, Knuutila S, Lundan T, Mannermaa A, Borresen-Dale AL, Borg A, Barkardottir RB, Petrini J, Winqvist R. RAD50 and NBS1 are breast cancer susceptibility genes associated with genomic instability. Carcinogenesis. 2006;27:1593–9.

Heiskanen I, Luostarinen T, Jarvinen HJ. Impact of screening examinations on survival in familial adenomatous polyposis. Scand J Gastroenterol. 2000;35(12):1284–7.

Hemminki A, Tomlinson I, Markie D, et al. Localisation of a susceptibility locus for Peutz-Jeghers syndrome to 19p using comparative genomic hybridization and targeted linkage analysis. Nat Genet. 1997;15:87–90.

Hemminki A, Markie D, Tomlinson I, et al. A serine/threonine kinase gene defective in Peutz–Jeghers syndrome. Nature. 1998;391:184–7.

Hennies H-C, Hagedorn M, Rais A. Palmoplantar keratoderma in association with carcinoma of the esophagus maps to chromosome 17q distal to the keratin gene cluster. Genomics. 1995;29:537–40.

Heravi-Moussavi A, Anglesio MS, Cheng SW, Senz J, Yang W, Prentice L, Fejes AP, Chow C, Tone A, Kalloger SE, Hamel N, Roth A, Ha G, Wan AN, Maines-Bandiera S, Salamanca C, Pasini B, Clarke BA, Lee AF, Lee CH, Zhao C, Young RH, Aparicio SA, Sorensen PH, Woo MM, Boyd N, Jones SJ, Hirst M, Marra MA, Gilks B, Shah SP, Foulkes WD, Morin GB, Huntsman DG. Recurrent somatic DICER1 mutations in nonepithelial ovarian cancers. N Engl J Med. 2012;366:234–42.

Herera L, Kakatis S, Gibas L. Gardner syndrome in a man with an interstitial deletion of 5q. Am J Med Genet. 1986;25:473–6.

Herman GE, Butter E, Enrile B, Pastore M, Prior TW, Sommer A. Increasing knowledge of germ-line PTEN mutations: two additional patients with autism and macrocephaly. Am J Med Genet A. 2007;143:589–93.

Hes FJ, McKee S, Taphoorn MJB, Rehal P, van der Luijt RB, McMahon R, van der Smagt JJ, Dow D, Zewald RA, Whittaker J, Lips CJM, MacDonald F, Pearson PL, Maher ER. Cryptic von Hippel–Lindau disease: germline mutations in patients with haemangioblastoma only. J Med Gen. 2000;37:939–43.

Hill DA, Ivanovich J, Priest JR, Gurnett CA, Dehner LP, Desruisseau D, Jarzembowski JA, Wikenheiser-Brokamp KA, Suarez BK, Whelan AJ, Williams G, Bracamontes D, Messinger Y, Goodfellow PJ. DICER1 mutations in familial pleuropulmonary blastoma. Science. 2009;325:965.

Hirsch B, Shimamura A, Moreau L, Baldinger S, Hag-alshiekh M, Bostrom B, Sencer S, D'Andrea AD. Association of biallelic BRCA2/FANCD1 mutations with spontaneous chromosomal instability and solid tumors of childhood. Blood. 2004;103:2554–9.

Hirschman BA, Pollack BH, Tomlinson GE, et al. The spectrum of APC mutations in children with hepatoblastoma from familial adenomatous polyposis kindreds. J Paediatrics. 2005;147: 263–6.

Hitchins MP, Ward RL. Constitutional (germline) MLH1 epimutation as an aetiological mechanism for hereditary non-polyposis colorectal cancer. J Med Genet. 2009;46:793–802.

Hitzler JK, Zipursky A. Origins of leukaemia in children with Down syndrome. Nat Rev Cancer. 2004;5:11–20.

Hobert J, Eng C. PTEN hamartoma tumor syndrome - an overview. Genet Med. 2009;11:687–94.

Hodges AK, Li S, Maynard J, Parry L, Braverman R, Cheadle JP, DeClue JE, Sampson JR. Pathological mutations in TSC1 and TSC2 disrupt the interaction between hamartin and tuberin. Hum Mol Genet. 2001;10:2899–905.

Hodgson SV, Bishop DT, Jay B. Genetic heterogeneity of congenital hyper-trophy of the retinal pigment epithelium (CHRPE) in families with familial adenomatous polyposis. J Med Genet. 1994;31:55–8.

Hodgson SV, Bishop DT, Dunlop MG, et al. Suggested screening guidelines for familial colorectal cancer. J Med Screening. 1995;2:45–51.

Hoeijmakers JH. DNA damage, aging, and cancer. N Engl J Med. 2009;361:1475–85.

Holbach LM, von Moller A, Decker C, Junemann AG, Rummelt-Hofmann C, Ballhausen WG. Loss of fragile histidine triad (FHIT) expression and microsatellite instability in periocular sebaceous gland carcinoma in patients with Muir–Torre syndrome. Am J Ophthalmol. 2002;134(1):147–8.

Hornstein OP, Knickenberg M. Perifollicular fibromatosis cutis with polyps of the colon–a cutaneo-intestinal syndrome sui generis. Arch Dermatol Res. 1975;253:161–75.

Houlston RS, Ford D. Genetics of coeliac disease. Q J Med. 1996;89:737–43.

Hovhannisyan Z, Weiss A, Martin A, Wiesner M, Tollefsen S, Yoshida K, Ciszewski C, Curran SA, Murray JA, David CS, Sollid LM, Koning F, Teyton L, Jabri B. The role of HLA-DQ8 beta-57 polymorphism in the anti-gluten T-cell response in coeliac disease. Nature. 2008;456:534–8.

Howdle PD, Jalal PK, Holmes GK, Houlston RS. Primary small-bowel malignancy in the UK and its association with coeliac disease. QJM. 2003;96:345–53.

Howe JR, Norton JA, Wells SA. Prevalence of pheochromocytoma and hyperparathyroidism in multiple endocrine neoplasia type 2A: results of long-term follow-up. Surgery. 1993;114:1070–7.

Howe JR, Roth S, Ringold JC, et al. Mutations in the *SMAD4/DPC4* gene in juvenile polyposis. Science. 1998;280:1086–8.

Howe JR, Blair JA, Sayed MG, et al. Germline mutations of *BMPR1A* in juvenile polyposis. Nat Genet. 2001;28:184–7.

Howell VM, Haven CJ, Kahnoski K, et al. *HRPT2* mutations are associated with malignancy in sporadic parathyroid tumors. J Med Genet. 2003;40:657–63.

Howlett NG, Taniguchi T, Olson S, Cox B, Waisfisz Q, De Die-Smulders C, Persky N, Grompe M, Joenje H, Pals G, Ikeda H, Fox EA, D'Andrea AD. Biallelic inactivation of BRCA2 in Fanconi anemia. Science. 2002;297:606–9.

Hoyme HE, Seaver LH, Jones KL, Procopio F, Crooks W, Feingold M. Isolated hemihyperplasia (hemihypertrophy): report of a prospective multicenter study of the incidence of neoplasia and review. Am J Med Genet. 1998;79:274–8.

Hu M, Zhang GY, Arbuckle S, Graf N, Shun A, Silink M, Lewis D, Alexander SI. Prophylactic bilateral nephrectomies in two pediatric patients with missense mutations in the WT1 gene. Nephrol Dial Transplant. 2004;19(1):223–6.

Huang RL, Chao CF, Ding DC, et al. Multiple epithelial and non-epithelial tumors in hereditary non-polyposis colorectal cancer: characterisation of germline and somatic mutations of the MSH2 gene and heterogeneity of replication error phenotypes. Cancer Genet Cytogenet. 2004;153:108–14.

Hughes-Benzie RM, Pilia G, Xuan JY, et al. Simpson–Golabi–Behmel syndrome: genotype/phenotype analysis of 18 affected males from 7 unrelated families. Am J Med Genet. 1996;66:227–34.

Huson SM, Harper PS, Compston DAS. Von Recklinghausen neurofibromatosis. Brain. 1988;111:1355–81.

Huson SM, Compston DAS, Harper PS. A genetic study of von Recklinghausen neurofibromatosis in south east Wales. II Guidelines for genetic counselling J Med Genet. 1989;26:712–21.

Hwang SL, Lozano G, Amos CL, Strong LC. Germline *p53* mutations in a cohort with childhood sarcoma: sex differences in cancer risk. Am J Hum Genet. 2003;72:975–83.

Hyer W, Fell JM. Screening for familial adenomatous polyposis. Arch Dis Child. 2001;84:377–80.

Ilyas M, Tomlinson I. The interactions of APC. E-cadherin and beta-catenin in tumor development and progression J Pathol. 1997;182(2):128–32.

Imai K, Morio T, Zhu Y, Jin Y, Itoh S, Kajiwara M, Yata J, Mizutani S, Ochs HD, Nonoyama S. Clinical course of patients with WASP gene mutations. Blood. 2004;103:456–64.

Inoki K, Corradetti MN, Guan KL. Dysregulation of the TSC-mTOR pathway in human disease. Nat Genet. 2005;37:19–24.

Ismail SMI, Walker SM. Bilateral virilising sclerosing stromal tumors of the ovary in a pregnant woman with Gorlin's syndrome: implications for pathogenesis of ovarian stromal neoplasms. Histopathology. 1990;17:159–63.

Itoh H, Ohsato K. Turcot syndrome and its characteristic colonic manifestations. Dis. Colon Rectum. 1985;28:399–402.

Jacobs I, Lancaster J. The molecular genetics of sporadic and familial epithelial ovarian cancer. Int J Gynaecol Cancer. 1996;6:337–55.

Jacobs KB, Yeager M, Zhou W, et al. Detectable clonal mosaicism and its relationship to aging and cancer. Nat Genet. 2012;44:651–8.

Jacquemont S, Boceno M, Rival JM, Mechinaud F, David A. High risk of malignancy in mosaic variegated aneuploidy syndrome. Am J Med Genet. 2002;109(1):17–21.

Jadresic L, Wadey RB, Buckle B, Barratt TM, Mitchell CD, Cowell JK. Molecular analysis of chromosome region 11p13 in patients with Drash syndrome. Hum Genet. 1991;86: 497–501.

Jain D, Hui P, McNamara J, Schwartz D, German J, Reyes-Mugica M. Bloom syndrome in sibs: first reports of hepatocellular carcinoma and Wilms tumor with documented anaplasia and nephrogenic rests. Pediatr Dev Pathol. 2001;4(6):585–9.

Jarvinen HJ, Mecklin JP, Sistonen P. Screening reduces colorectal cancer rate in families with hereditary nonpolyposis colorectal cancer. Gastroenterology. 1995;108:1405–11.

Jarvinen HJ, Aarnio M, Mustonen H, Aktan-Collan K, Aaltonen LA, Peltomaki P, de La CA, Mecklin JP. Controlled 15-year trial on screening for colorectal cancer in families with hereditary nonpolyposis colorectal cancer. Gastroenterol. 2000;118:829–34.

Jass JR. Colorectal adenoma progression and genetic change: is there a link? Ann Med. 1995;27:301–6.

Jass JR. HNPCC and sporadic colorectal cancer: a review of the morphological similarities and differences. Fam Cancer. 2004;3(2):93–100.

Jass JR, Williams CB, Bussey HJR, Morson BC. Juvenile polyposis – a pre-cancerous condition. Histopathology. 1988;13:619–30.

Jeghers H, McKusick VA, Katz KH. Generalised intestinal polyposis and melanin spots of the oral mucosa, lips and digits. New Engl J Med. 1949;241(31–6):993–1005.

Jenne DE, Reimann H, Nezu J-I, et al. Peutz–Jeghers syndrome is caused by mutations in a novel serine threonine kinase. Nat Genet. 1998;18:38–44.

Jensen UB, Sunde L, Timshel S, Halvarsson B, Nissen A, Bernstein I, Nilbert M. Mismatch repair defective breast cancer in the hereditary nonpolyposis colorectal cancer syndrome. Breast Cancer Res Treat. 2009;120:777–82.

Jin Y, Mazza C, Christie JR, Giliani S, Fiorini M, Mella P, Gandellini F, Stewart DM, Zhu Q, Nelson DL, Notarangelo LD, Ochs HD. Mutations of the Wiskott–Aldrich Syndrome Protein (WASP): hotspots, effect on transcription, and translation and phenotype/genotype correlation. Blood. 2004;104:4010–9.

Johnson JA. Ataxia telangiectasia and other—fetoprotein-associated disorders. In: Lynch HT, Hirayama T, editors. Genetic epidemiology of cancer. Boca Raton: CRC Press; 1989. p. 145–57.

Johnson SR, Tattersfield AE. Lymphangioleiomyomatosis Semin Respir Crit Care Med. 2002;23(2):85–92.

Johnson RL, Rothman AL, Xie J, et al. Human homolog of patched, a candidate gene for the basal cell nevus syndrome. Science. 1996;272:1668–71.

Jonasdottir TJ, Mellersh CS, Moe L, Heggebo R, Gamlem H, Ostrander EA, Lingaas F. Genetic mapping of a naturally occurring hereditary renal cancer syndrome in dogs. Proc Natl Acad Sci USA. 2000;97(8):4132–7.

Jones AC, Shyamsundar MM, Thomas MW, Maynard J, Idziaszczyk S, Tomkins S, Sampson JR, Cheadle JP. Comprehensive mutation analysis of TSC1 and TSC2- and phenotypic correlations in 150 families with tuberous sclerosis. Am J Hum Genet. 1999;64:1305–15.

Jongmans MCJ, van der Burgt I, Hoogerbrugge PM, et al. Cancer risk in patients with Noonan syndrome carrying a PTPN11 mutation. Eur J Hum Genet. 2011;19:870–4.

Kaneko H, Isogai K, Fukao T, Matsui E, Kasahara K, Yachie A, Seki H, Koizumi S, Arai M, Utunomiya J, Miki Y, Kando N. Relatively common mutations of the Bloom syndrome gene in the Japanese population. Int J Mol Med. 2004;14(3):439–42.

Kanter WR, Eldridge R, Fabricant R, Allen JC, Koerber T. Central neurofibromatosis with bilateral acoustic neuroma: genetic, clinical and biochemical distinctions from peripheral neurofibromatosis. Neurology. 1980;30:851–9.

Karnik SK, Hughes CM, Gu X, Rozenblatt-Rozen O, McLean GW, Xiong Y, Meyerson M, Kim SK. Menin regulates pancreatic islet growth by promoting histone methylation and expression of genes encoding p27Kip1 and p18INK4c. Proc Natl Acad Sci U S A. 2005;102: 14659–64.

Kastrinos F, Mukherjee B, Tayob N, et al. Risk of pancreatic cancer in families with Lynch syndrome. JAMA. 2009;302(16):1790–5.

Kauppinen R. Porphyrias. Lancet. 2005;365:241–52.

Kelsell DP, Risk JM, Leigh IM, et al. Close mapping of the focal non-epidermolytic palmoplantar keratoderma (PPK) locus associated with esophageal cancer (TOC). Hum Mol Genet. 1996;5:857–60.

Kerr B, Delrue M-A, Sigaudy S, Perveen R, Marche M, Burgelin I, Stef M, Tang B, Eden OB, O'Sullivan J, De Sandre-Giovannoli A, Reardon W, and 14 others. Genotype-phenotype correlation in Costello syndrome: HRAS mutation analysis in 43 cases. J Med Genet. 2006;43:401–5.

Kersey JH, Shapiro RS, Filipovich AH. Relationship of immunodeficiency to lymphoid malignancy. Pediatr Infect Dis J. 1988;7:510–2.

Keung Y-K, Buss D, Chauvenet A, Pettenati M. Haematologic malignancy and Klinefelter syndrome: a chance association? 2002.

Kim SJ. Blue rubber bleb nevus syndrome with central nervous syndrome involvement. Ped Neurol. 2000;22:410–2.

Kim H, Lee JE, Cho EJ, Liu JO, Youn HD. Menin, a tumor suppressor, represses JunD-Mediated Transcriptional Activity by Association with an mSin3A-Histone Deacetylase Complex. Cancer Res. 2003;63:6135–9.

Kimonis VE, Mehta SG, DiGiovanna JJ, Bale SJ, Pastakia B. Radiological features in 82 patients with nevoid basal cell carcinoma (NBCC or Gorlin) syndrome. Genet Med. 2004;6(6): 495–502.

Kirschner LS, Carney JA, Pack SD, et al. Mutations in the gene encoding the protein kinase A type 1-alpha regulatory subunit in patients with Carney complex. Nat Genet. 2000a;26:89–92.

Kirschner LS, Sandrini F, Monbo J, Lin JP, Carney JA, Stratakis CA. Genetic heterogeneity and spectrum of mutations of the PRKAR1A gene in patients with the Carney complex. Hum Mol Genet. 2000b;9:3037–46.

Kitao S, Shimamoto A, Goto M, et al. Mutations in RECQL4 cause a subset of Rothmund–Thomson syndrome. Nat Genet. 1999;22:82–4.

Klamt B, Koziell A, Poulat F, Wieacker P, Scambler P, Berta P, Gessler M. Frasier syndrome is caused by defective alternative splicing of WT1 leading to an altered ratio of WT1 $_3/_3$ KTS splice isoforms. Hum Mol Genet. 1998;7(4):709–14.

Klarsov L, Holck S, Bernstein I, et al. Challenges in the identification of MSH6-associated colorectal cancer: rectal location, less typical histology, and a subset with retained mismatch repair function. Am J Surg Path. 2011;35:1391–9.

Klein C, Grudzien M, Appaswamy G, Germeshausen M, Sandrock I, Schaffer AA, Rathinam C, Boztug K, Schwinzer B, Rezaei N, Bohn G, Melin M, Carlsson G, Fadeel B, Dahl N, Palmblad J, Henter JI, Zeidler C, Grimbacher B, Welte K. HAX1 deficiency causes autosomal recessive severe congenital neutropenia (Kostmann dissase). Nat Genet. 2007;39:86–92.

Kloos RT, Eng C, Evans DB, Francis GL, Gagel R, Gharib H, Moley JF, Pacini F, Ringel MD, Schlumberger M, Wells SA. Medullary thyroid carcinoma: Management Guidelines of the American Thyroid Association. Thyroid. 2009;19:565–612.

Klusmann JH, Reinhardt D, Hasle H, Kaspers GJ, Creutzig U, Hahlen K, van den Heuvel-Eibrink MM, Zwaan CM. Janus kinase mutations in the development of acute megakaryoblastic leukemia in children with and without Down's syndrome. Leukemia. 2007;21(7):1584–7.

Kluwe L, Mautner V, Heinrich B, Dezube R, Jacoby LB, Friedrich RE, MacCollin M. Molecular study of frequency of mosaicism in neurofibromatosis 2 patients with bilateral vestibular schwannomas. J Med Genet. 2003;40:109–14.

Knudsen AL, Bülow S, Tomlinson I, Möslein G, Heinimann K, Christensen IJ, AFAP Study Group. Attenuated familial adenomatous polyposis: results from an international collaborative study. Colorectal Dis. 2010;12(10 online): e243–9. doi:10.1111/j.1463-1318.2010.02218.x.

Knudson AG, Strong LC. Mutation and cancer: neuroblastoma and phaeochromocytoma. Am J Hum Genet. 1972;24:514–32.

Kobayashi T, Hirayama Y, Kobayashi E, Kubo Y, Hino O. A germline insertion in the tuberous sclerosis (Tsc2) gene gives rise to the Eker rat model of dominantly inherited cancer. Nat Genet. 1995;9:70–4.

Kolodner RD, Hall NR, Lipford J. Structure of the human MSH2 locus and analysis of two Muir–Torre kindreds for msh2 mutations. Genomics. 1994;24:516–26.

Koopman RJJ, Happle R. Autosomal dominant transmission of the NAME syndrome (nevi, atrial myxoma, mucinosis of the skin and endocrine over activity). Hum Genet. 1991;86:300–4.

Koufos A, Grundy P, Morgan K, et al. Familial Wiedemann–Beckwith syndrome and a second Wilms' tumor locus both map to 11 p15.5. Am J Hum Genet. 1989;44:711–9.

Kovacs ME, Papp J, Szentirmay Z, et al. Deletions of the last exon of TACSTD1 constitute a distinct class of mutations predisposing to Lynch syndrome. Human Mutation. 2009;30: 197–203.

Kraemer KH, Slor H. Xeroderma pigmentosum. Clin Dermatol. 1985;3:33–69.

Kruse R, Rutten A, Schweiger N, Jakob E, Mathiak M, Propping P, Mangold E, Bisceglia M, Ruzicka T. Frequency of microsatellite instability in unselected sebaceous gland neoplasias and hyperplasias. J Invest Dermatol. 2003;120(5):858–64.

Kumar D, Blank CE, Ponder B. A family with Turcot syndrome suggesting autosomal dominant inheritance. J Med Genet. 1989;26:592 [Abstract].

Kurose K, Araki T, Matsunaka T, Takada Y, Emi M. Variant manifestation of Cowden disease in Japan: hamartomatous polyposis of the digestive tract with mutation of the *PTEN* gene. Am J Hum Genet. 1999;64:308–10.

Laiho P, Lainover V, Lahemo P, et al. Low level MSI in most colorectal cancers. Cancer Res. 2002;62:1166–70.

Laken SJ, Peterson GM, Gruber SB. Familial colorectal cancer in Ashkenazim due to a hypermutable tract in APC. Nat Genet. 1997;17:79–83.

Lalloo F, Varley J, Ellis D, et al. Prediction of pathogenic mutations in patients with early onset breast cancer by family history. Lancet. 2003;361:1101–2.

Lam WW, et al. Analysis of germline CDKN1C (p57KIP2) mutations in familial and sporadic Beckwith–Wiedemann syndrome (BWS) provides a novel genotype-phenotype correlation. J Med Genet. 1999;36(7):518–23.

Lamlum H, AlTassan N, Jaeger E, et al. APC variants in patients with multiple colorectal adenomas, with evidence of the particular importance of E1317Q. Hum Mol Genet. 2000;9:2215–21.

Lampe AK, Hampton PJ, Woodford-Richens K, Tomlinson I, Lawrence CM, Douglas FS. Laugier–Hunziker syndrome: an important differential diagnosis for Peutz-Jeghers syndrome. J Med Genet. 2003;40:E77.

Lanspa SJ, Lynch HT, Smyrk TC, et al. Colorectal adenomas in the Lynch syndromes. Results of a colonoscopy screening program Gastroenterology. 1990;98:1117–22.

Larsson C, Friedman E. Localization and identification of the multiple endocrine neoplasia type 1 disease gene. Endocrinol Metab Clin N Am. 1994;23:67–9.

Larsson C, Skosgeid B, Öberg K, Nakamura Y, Nordenskjöld M. Multiple endocrine neoplasia type 1 gene maps to chromosome 11 and is lost in insulinoma. Nature. 1988;332:85–7.

Latif F, Tory K, Gnarra J, et al. Identification of the von Hippel–Lindau disease tumor suppressor gene. Science. 1993;260:1317–20.

Lavin MF. ATM and the Mre11 complex combine to recognize and signal DNA double-strand breaks. Oncogene. 2007;26:7749–58.

Lehmann AR. DNA repair-deficient diseases, xeroderma pigmentosum, Cockayne syndrome and trichothiodystrophy. Biochimie. 2003;85:1101–11.

Lendvay TS, Marshall FF. The tuberous sclerosis complex and its highly variable manifestations. J Urol. 2003;169:1635–42.

Lengauer C, Kinzler KW, Vogelstein B. Genetic instability in colorectal cancers. Nature. 1997;386(6625):623–7.

Levanat S, Gorlin RJ, Fallet S, Johnson DR, Fantasia JE, Bale AE. A two-hit model for developmental defects in Gorlin syndrome. Nat Genet. 1996;12(1):85–7.

Levi Z, Kedar I, Barris HN, Niv Y, Geller A, Gal E, Gingold R, Morgenstern S, Heald-Leach B, Bronner MP, Eng C. Upper and lower gastrointestinal findings in PTEN mutation positive Cowden syndrome patients participating in an active surveillance program. Clin Transl Gastroenterol. 2011;2:e5.

Levitus M, Waisfisz Q, Godthelp BC, de Vries Y, Hussain S, Wiegant WW, Elghalbzouri-Maghrani E, Steltenpool J, Rooimans MA, Pals G, Arwert F, Mathew CG, Zdzienicka MZ, Hiom K, De De Winter JP, Joenje H. The DNA helicase BRIP1 is defective in Fanconi anemia complementation group J. Nat Genet. 2005;37:934–5.

Levran O, Attwooll C, Henry RT, Milton KL, Neveling K, Rio P, Batish SD, Kalb R, Velleuer E, Barral S, Ott J, Petrini J, Schindler D, Hanenberg H, Auerbach AD. The BRCA1-interacting helicase BRIP1 is deficient in Fanconi anemia. Nat Genet. 2005;37:931–3.

Lewis RA, Riccardi VM, Gerson LP, Whitford R, Axelson KA. Von Recklinghausen neurofibromatosis: II. Incidence of optic-nerve gliomata Ophthalmology. 1984;91:929–35.

Li PP, Fraumeni JF. Soft tissue sarcomas, breast cancer, and other neoplasms: a familial syndrome? Ann Int Med. 1969;71:747–52.

Li FP, Fraumeni JF, Mulvihill JJ, et al. A cancer family syndrome in 24 kindreds. Cancer Res. 1988;48:5358–62.

Li FP, Correa P, Fraumeni Jr JF. Testing for germline *p53* mutations in cancer families. Cancer Epidemiol Biomark Prev. 1991;1:91–4.

Li M, Shuman C, Fei YL, Cutiongco E, Bender HA, Stevens C, Wilkins-Haug L, Day-Salvatore D, Yong SL, Geraghty MT, Squire J, Weksberg R. GPC3 mutation analysis in a spectrum of patients with overgrowth expands the phenotype of Simpson–Golabi–Behmel syndrome. Am J Med Genet. 2001;102:161–8.

Libe R, Horvath A, Vezzosi D, Fratticci A, Coste J, Perlemoine K, Ragazzon B, Guillaud-Bataille M, Groussin L, Clauser E, Raffin-Sanson ML, Siegel J, Moran J, Drori-Herishanu L, Frauez FR, Lodish M, Nesterova M, Bertagna X, Bertherat J, Stratakis CA. Frequent phosphodiesterase 11A gene (PDE11A) defects in patients with Carney complex (CNC) caused by PRKAR1A mutations: PDE11A may contribute to adrenal and testicular tumors in CNC as a modifier of the phenotype. J Clin Endocrinol Metab. 2011;96:E208–14.

Libutti SK, Choyke PL, Bartlett DL, Vargas H, Walther M, Lubensky I, Glenn G, Linehan WM, Alexander HR. Pancreatic neuroendocrine tumors associated with von Hippel–Lindau disease: diagnostic and management recommendations. Surgery. 1998;124:1153–9.

Lightenberg MJ, Kuiper RP, van Kessel G, Hoogerbrugge N. EPCAM deletion carriers constitute a unique subgroup of Lynch syndrome patients. Fam Cancer. 2013;12:169–74.

Lim DH, Maher ER. Genomic imprinting syndromes and cancer. Adv Genet. 2010;70:145–75.

Lim W, Hearle N, Shah B, Murday V, Hodgson SV, Lucassen A, Eccles D, Talbot I, Neale K, Lim AG, O'Donohue J, Donaldson A, Macdonald RC, Young ID, Robinson MH, Lee PW, Stoodley BJ, Tomlinson I, Alderson D, Holbrook AG, Vyas S, Swarbrick ET, Lewis AA, Phillips RK, Houlston RS. Further observations on LKB1/STK11 status and cancer risk in Peutz-Jeghers syndrome. Br J Cancer. 2003;89(2):308–13.

Lim W, Olschwang S, Keller JJ, Westerman AM, Menko FH, Boardman LA, Scott RJ, Trimbath J, Giardiello FM, Gruber SB, Gille JJ, Offerhaus GJ, de Rooij FW, Wilson JH, Spigelman AD, Phillips RK, Houlston RS. Relative frequency and morphology of cancers in STK11 mutation carriers. Gastroenterology. 2004;126:1788–94.

Lim D, Bowdin SC, Tee L, Kirby GA, Blair E, Fryer A, Lam W, Oley C, Cole T, Brueton LA, Reik W, Macdonald F, Maher ER. Clinical and molecular genetic features of Beckwith-Wiedemann syndrome associated with assisted reproductive technologies. Hum Reprod. 2009;24(3):741–7.

Limaye N, Wouters V, Uebelhoer M, Tuominen M, Wirkkala R, Mulliken JB, Eklund L, Boon LM, Vikkula M. Somatic mutations in angiopoietin receptor gene TEK cause solitary and multiple sporadic venous malformations. Nature Genet. 2009;41:118–24.

Lipton LR, Johnson V, Cummings C, et al. Refining the Amsterdam Criteria and Bethesda Guidelines: testing algorithms for the prediction of mismatch repair mutation status in the familial cancer clinic. J Clin Oncol. 2004;22(24):4934–43.

Little MH, Williamson KA, Mannens M, et al. Evidence that WT1 mutations in Denys–Drash syndrome patients may act in a dominant-negative fashion. Hum Mol Genet. 1993;2:259–64.

Liu B, Nicolaides NC, Markowitz S, et al. Mismatch repair gene defects in sporadic colorectal cancers with microsatellite instability. Nat Genet. 1995;9:48–55.

Lloyd SK, Evans DG. Neurofibromatosis type 2 (NF2): diagnosis and management. Handb Clin Neurol. 2013;115:957–67.

Lodish M, Stratakis CA. The differential diagnosis of familial lentiginosis syndromes. Fam Cancer. 2011;10:481–90.

Loewinger RJ, Lichsteinstein JR, Dodson WE, Eisen AZ. Maffucci's syndrome: a mesenchymal dysplasia and multiple tumor syndrome. Br J Dermatol. 1977;96:317–22.

Lohse P, et al. Microsatellite instability, loss of heterozygosity and loss of hMLH1 and hMSH2 protein expression in endometrial carcinoma. Hum Pathol. 2002;33:347–54.

Longy M, Lacombe D. Cowden disease report of a family and review. Ann Genet. 1996;39: 35–42.

Lonn U, Lonn S, Nylen U, et al. An abnormal profile of DNA replication intermediates in Bloom's syndrome. Cancer Res. 1990;50:3141–5.

Look AT. A leukemogenic twist for GATA1. Nat Genet. 2003;32:83–4.

Loveday C, Turnbull C, Ramsay E, Hughes D, Ruark E, Frankum JR, Bowden G, Kalmyrzaev B, Warren-Perry M, Snape K, Adlard JW, Barwell J, Berg J, Brady AF, Brewer C, Brice G, Chapman C, Cook J, Davidson R, Donaldson A, Douglas F, Greenhalgh L, Henderson A, Izatt L, Kumar A, Lalloo F, Miedzybrodzka Z, Morrison PJ, Paterson J, Porteous M, Rogers MT, Shanley S, Walker L, Eccles D, Evans DG, Renwick A, Seal S, Lord CJ, Ashworth A, Reis-Filho JS, Antoniou AC, Rahman N. Germline mutations in RAD51D confer susceptibility to ovarian cancer. Nat Genet. 2011;43:879–82.

Lowy AM, Kordich JJ, Gismondi V, Varesco L, Blough RI, Groden J. Numerous colonic adenomas in an individual with Bloom's syndrome. Gastroenterol. 2001;121(2):435–9.

Lu S-L, et al. HNPCC associated with germline mutation in the TGF-beta type II receptor gene. Nat Genet. 1998;19:17–8.

Lubbe SJ, Di Bernardo MC, Chandler IP, Houlston RS. Clinical implications of the colorectal cancer risk associated with MUTYH mutation. J Clin Oncol. 2009;27(24):3975–80.

Lubs M-L, Bauer MS, Formas ME, Djokic B. Lisch nodules in neurofibromatosis type 1. New Engl J Med. 1991;324:1264–6.

Lucci-Cordisco E, Zito I, Gensini F, Genuardi M. Hereditary nonpolyposis colorectal cancer and related conditions. Am J Med Genet. 2003;122A(4):325–34.

Luo G, Santoro IM, McDaniel LD, Nishijima I, Mills M, Youssoufian H, Vogel H, Schultz RA, Bradley A. Cancer predisposition caused by elevated mitotic recombination in Bloom mice. Nat Genet. 2000;26(4):424–9.

Lynch HT, de la Chapelle A. Genetic susceptibility to nonpolyposis colorectal cancer. J Med Genet. 1999;36:801–18.

Lynch HT, Kaplan AR, Lynch JF. Klinefelter syndrome and cancer: a family study. J Am Med Assoc. 1974;229:809–11.

Lynch HT, Mulcahy GM, Harris RE, et al. Genetic and pathologic findings in a kindred with hereditary sarcoma, breast cancer, brain tumors, leukaemia, lung, laryngeal and adrenocortical carcinoma. Cancer. 1978;41:2055–64.

Lynch HT, Fusaro RM, Roberts L, Voorhees GJ, Lynch JF. Muir–Torre syndrome in several members of family with a variant of the cancer family syndrome. Br J Dermatol. 1985;113: 295–301.

Lynch HT, Ens JA, Lynch JF. The Lynch syndrome II and urological malig-nancies. J Urol. 1990a;143:24–8.

Lynch HT, Watson P, Conway TA, et al. Clinical/genetic features in hereditary breast cancer. Breast Cancer Res Treat. 1990b;15:63–71.

Lynch HT, Smyrk TC, Lanspa SJ, et al. Phenotypic variation in colorectal ade-noma/cancer expression in 2 families with hereditary flat adenoma syndromem. Cancer. 1990c;60:909–15.

Lynch HT, Smyrk TC, Watson P, et al. Genetics, natural history, tumor spectrum and pathology of hereditary non-polyposis colorectal cancer: an updated review. Gastroenterology. 1993;104:1535–49.

MacCollin M, Willett C, Heinrich B, Jacoby LB, Acierno Jr JS, Perry A, Louis DN. Familial schwannomatosis: exclusion of the NF2 locus as the germline event. Neurology. 2003;60(12): 1968–74.

Machatschek JN, Schrauder A, Helm F, et al. Acute lymphoblastic leukaemia and Klinefelter syndrome in children; two cases and review of the literature. Paed Haematol Oncol. 2004;21:621–6.

Maher ER, Reik W. Beckwith–Wiedemann syndrome imprinting in clusters revisited. J Clin Invest. 2000;105:247–52.

Maher ER, Yates JRW. Familial renal cell carcinoma – clinical and molecular genetic aspects. Br J Cancer. 1991;63:176–9.

Maher ER, Yates JRW, Ferguson-Smith MA. Statistical analysis of the two stage mutation model in von Hippel–Lindau disease and in sporadic cerebellar haeman-gioblastoma and renal cell carcinoma. J Med Genet. 1990a;27:311–4.

Maher ER, Yates JRW, Harries R, et al. Clinical features and natural history of von Hippel–Lindau disease. Q J Med. 1990b;77:1151–63.

Maher ER, Bentley E, Yates JRW, et al. Mapping of the von Hippel–Lindau disease locus to a small region of chromosome 3p by genetic linkage analysis. Genomics. 1991;10:957–60.

Maher ER, Brueton LA, Bowdin SC, Luharia A, Cooper W, Cole TR, Macdonald F, Sampson JR, Barratt CL, Reik W, Hawkins MM. Beckwith–Wiedemann syndrome and assisted reproduction technology (ART). J Med Genet. 2003;40:62–4.

Maher ER, Neumann HP, Richard S. von Hippel-Lindau disease: a clinical and scientific review. Eur J Hum Genet. 2011;19(6):617–23.

Mahmoud AAH, Yousef GM, Al-Hifzi I, Diamindos EP. Cockayne syndrome in three sisters with varying clinical presentation. Am J Med Genet. 2002;111:81–5.

Malkin D, Li FP, Strong LC, et al. Germline p53 mutations in a familial syndrome of breast cancer, sarcomas, and other neoplasms. Science. 1990;250:1233–8.

Mallory SB. Cowden Syndrome (Multiple hamartoma syndrome). Dermatal Clin. 1995;13:27–31.

Mangold E, Pagenstecher C, Leister M, Mathiak M, Rutten A, Friedl W, Propping P, Ruzicka T, Kruse R. A genotype-phenotype correlation in HNPCC: strong predominance of msh2 mutations in 41 patients with Muir–Torre syndrome. J Med Genet. 2004;41(7):567–72.

Manski TJ, Heffner DK, Glenn GM, Patronas NJ, Pikus AT, Katz D, Lebovics R, Sledjeski K, Choyke PL, Zbar B, Linehan WM, Oldfield EH. Endolymphatic sac tumors – a source of morbid hearing loss in von Hippel–Lindau disease. J Am Med Assoc. 1997;277:1461–6.

Marie PJ, de Pollack C, Chanson P, Lomri A. Increased proliferation of osteoblastic cells expressing the activating Gs alpha mutation in monostotic and polyostotic fibrous dysplasia. Am J Pathol. 1997;150:1059–69.

Marin MS, Lopez-Cima MF, Garcia-Castro L, Pascual T, Marron MG, Tardon A. Poly (AT) polymorphism in intron 11 of the XPC DNA repair gene enhances the risk of lung cancer. Cancer Epidemiol Biomark Prev. 2004;13:1788–93.

Marsh DJ, Dahia PLM, Zheng Z, et al. Germline mutations in *PTEN* are present in Bannayan–Zonana syndrome. Nat Genet. 1997;16:333–4.

Marsh DJ, Coulon V, Lunetta KL, et al. Mutation spectrum and genotype– phenotype analyses in Cowden disease and Bannayan–Zonana syndrome, two hamartoma syndromes with germline *PTEN* mutation. Hum Mol Genet. 1998;7:507–15.

Marsh DJ, Kum JB, Lunetta KL, et al. *PTEN* mutation spectrum and genotype-phenotype correlations in Bannayan–Riley–Ruvalcaba syndrome suggest a single entity with Cowden syndrome. Hum Mol Genet. 1999;8:1461–72.

Martasek P, Nordamann Y, Grandchamp B. Homozygous hereditary coporphyria caused by arginine to tryptophane substitution in coporphyrin oxidase and common intragenic polymorphisms. Hum Mol Genet. 1994;3:477–80.

Martuza RL, Eldridge RN. Neurofibromatosis 2 (bilateral acoustic neurofibromatosis). New Engl J Med. 1988;318:684–8.

Marx SJ, Simonds WF, Agarwal SK, et al. Hyperparathyroidism in hereditary syndromes: special expressions and special managements. J Bone Miner Res. 2002;17(S2):37–43.

Masciari S, Dillon DA, Rath M, Robson M, Weitzel JN, Balmana J, Gruber SB, Ford JM, Euhus D, Lebensohn A, Telli M, Pochebit SM, Lypas G, Garber JE. Breast cancer phenotype in women with TP53 germline mutations: a Li-Fraumeni syndrome consortium effort. Breast Cancer Res Treat. 2012;133(3):1125–30.

Massague J. How cells read TGF-beta signals. Nat Rev Mol Cell Biol. 2000;1:169–78.

Masutani C, Kusumoto R, Yamada A, Dohmae N, Yokoi M, Yuasa M, Araki M, Iwai S, Takio K, Hanaoka F. The XPV (xeroderma pigmentosum variant) gene encodes human DNA polymerase eta. Nature. 1999;399:700–4.

McConville CM, Stankovic T, Byrd PJ et al. Mutations associated with variant phenotypes in ataxia-telangiectasia. Am J. Hum Genet.1996;59:320–30.

Mathers JC, Mickleburgh I, Chapman PC, Bishop DT, Burn J. Concerted Action Polyp Prevention (CAPP) 1 Study. Can resistant starch and/or aspirin prevent the development of colonic neoplasia? The Concerted Action Polyp Prevention (CAPP) 1 Study. Proc Nutr Soc. 2003;62:51–7.

McDaniel LD, Chester N, Watson M, Borowsky AD, Leder P, Schultz RA. Chromosome instability and tumor predisposition inversely correlate with BLM protein levels. DNA Repair (Amst). 2003;2(12):1387–404.

McGarrity TJ, Mascari-Baker MJ, Ruggiero FM, et al. Glycogenic acanthosis associated with germline PTEN mutation positive Cowden syndrome. Am J Gastroenterol. 2003;98:1429–34.

McIntyre JF, Smith-Sorensen B, Friend SH, et al. Germline mutations of the p53 tumor suppressor gene in children with osteosarcoma. J Clin Oncol. 1994;12:925–30.

McKeen EA, Bodurtha J, Meadows AT, Douglas EG, Mulvihill JJ. Rhabdomyosarcoma complicating multiple neurofibromatosis. J Pediatr. 1978;93:992–3.

McWhinney SR, Pasini B, Stratakis CA, Consortium C-T-D. Germline mutations in the genes encoding succinate dehydrogenase subunits (SDHB, SDHC, SDHD) cause a familial form of gastrointestinal stromal tumors. N Engl J Med. 2007;357:1054–6.

Meindl A, Hellebrand H, Wiek C, Erven V, Wappenschmidt B, Niederacher D, Freund M, Lichtner P, Hartmann L, Schaal H, Ramser J, Honisch E, Kubisch C, Wichmann HE, Kast K, Deissler H, Engel C, Muller-Myhsok B, Neveling K, Kiechle M, Mathew CG, Schindler D, Schmutzler RK, Hanenberg H. Germline mutations in breast and ovarian cancer pedigrees establish RAD51C as a human cancer susceptibility gene. Nat Genet. 2010;42:410–4.

Meissner PN, Dailey TA, Hift RJ, et al. A R59W mutation in human protoporphyrinogen oxidase results in decreased enzyme activity and is prevalent in South Africans with variegate porphyria. Nat Genet. 1996;13:95–7.

Menko FH. Genetics of Colorectal Cancer for Clinical Practice. Dordrecht: Kluwer Academic; 1993. p. 58–82.

Menko FH, Kaspers GL, Meijer GA, Claes K, van Hagen JM, Gille JJ. A homozygous MSH6 mutation in a child with cafe-au-lait spots, oligodendroglioma and rectal cancer. Fam Cancer. 2004;3(2):123–7.

Menko FH, van Steensel MA, Giraud S, Friis-Hansen L, Richard S, Ungari S, Nordenskjöld M, Hansen TV, Solly J, Maher ER, European BHD Consortium. Birt-Hogg-Dubé syndrome: diagnosis and management. Lancet Oncol. 2009;10(12):1199–206. doi:10.1016/S1470-2045(09)70188-3. Review.

Mester J, Tilot AK, Rybicki LA, Frazier TW, Eng C. Analysis of prevalence and degree of macrocephaly in patients with germline PTEN mutations and of brain weight in Pten knock-in murine model. Eur J Hum Genet. 2011;19:763–8.

Meyer E, Lim D, Pasha S, Tee LJ, Rahman F, Yates JR, Woods CG, Reik W, Maher ER. Germline mutation in NLRP2 (NALP2) in a familial imprinting disorder (Beckwith-Wiedemann Syndrome). PLoS Genet. 2009;5(3):e1000423.

Michels VV, Stevens JC. Basal cell carcinoma in a patient with intestinal polyposis. Clin Genet. 1982;22:80–2.

Miyaki M, Nishio J, Konishi M, Kikuchi-Yanoshita R, Tanaka K, Muraoka M, Nagato M, Chong JM, Koike M, Terada T, Kawahara Y, Fukutome A, Tomiyama J, Chuganji Y, Momoi M,

Utsunomiya J. Drastic genetic instability of tumors and normal tissues in Turcot syndrome. Oncogene. 1997;15(23):2877–81.

Miyauchi A, Futami H, Hai N, et al. Two germline missense mutations at codons 804 and 806 of the RET proto-oncogene in the same allele in a patient with multiple endocrine neoplasia type 2B without codon 918 mutation. Jpn J Cancer Res. 1999;90(1):1–5.

Moline J, Eng C. Multiple endocrine neoplasia type 2: An overview. Genet Med. 2011;13: 755–64.

Montalto G, Cervello M, Giannitrapani L, Dantona F, Terranova A, Castagnetta LA. Epidemiology, risk factors, and natural history of hepatocellular carcinoma. Ann NY Acad Sci. 2002;963:13–20.

Moos KF, Rennie JS. Squamous cell carcinoma arising in a mandibular keratocyst in a patient with Gorlin's syndrome. Br J Oral Maxillofac Surg. 1987;25(4):280–4.

Morison IM, Becroft D, Taniguchi T, et al. Somatic overgrowth associated with over expression of insulin-like growth factor II. Nat Med. 1996;2:311–6.

Morrell D, Chase CL, Swift M. Cancer in families with severe combined immune deficiency. J Natl Cancer Inst. 1987;78:455–8.

Morrell D, Chase CL, Swift M. Cancers in 44 families with ataxia telangiectasia. Cancer Cell Cytogenet. 1990;50:119–23.

Moser MJ, Bigbee WL, Grant SG, et al. Genetic instability and hematologic disease risk in Werner syndrome patients and heterozygotes. Cancer Res. 2000;60:2492–6.

Moyhuddin A, Baser ME, Watson C, Purcell S, Ramsden RT, Heiberg A, Wallace AJ, Evans DGR. Somatic mosaicism in neurofibromatosis 2: prevalence and risk of disease transmission to offspring. J Med Genet. 2003;40:459–63.

Mueller RF. The Denys–Drash syndrome. J Med Genet. 1994;31:471–7.

Mulligan LM, Eng C, Healey CS, et al. Specific mutations of the RET proto-oncogene are related to disease phenotype in MEN 2A and FMTC. Nat Genet. 1994;6:70–4.

Muir EG, Yates-Bell AJ, Barlow KA. Multiple primary carcinomata of colon, duodenum and larynx associated with keratokanthoma of the face. Br J Surg. 1967;54:191–5.

Mulligan LM, Kwok JBJ, Healey CS, et al. Germline mutations of the RET proto-oncogene in multiple endocrine neoplasia type 2A. Nature. 1993;363:458–60.

Myrhoj T, Andersen MB, Bernstein I. Screening for urinary tract cancer with urine cytology in Lynch syndrome and familial colorectal cancer. Fam Cancer. 2008;7(4):303–7.

Nagase H, Nakamura Y. Mutations of the APC (Adenomatous Polyposis Coli) gene. Hum Mutat. 1993;2:425–34.

Nahorski MS, Lim DH, Martin L, Gille JJ, McKay K, Rehal PK, Ploeger HM, van Steensel M, Tomlinson IP, Latif F, Menko FH, Maher ER. Investigation of the Birt-Hogg-Dube tumour suppressor gene (FLCN) in familial and sporadic colorectal cancer. J Med Genet. 2010;47(6):385–90. doi:10.1136/jmg.2009.073304.

Naryan S, Fleming C, Trainer AH, Craig JA. Rothmund–Thomson syndrome with myelodysplasia. Paed Derm. 2001;18:210–2.

NCCN. NCCN practice guidelines: genetics/familial high risk cancer. Oncology. 1999;13(11A): 161–86.

Neilan EG, Delgado MR, Donovan MA, Kim SY, Jou RL, Wu B-L, Kang PB. Response of motor complications in Cockayne syndrome to carbidopa-levodopa. Arch Neurol. 2008;65:1117–21.

Nelen MR, Padberg GW, Peeters EAJ, et al. Localization of the gene for Cowden disease to 10q22–23. Nat Genet. 1996;13:114–6.

Nelen MR, van Staveren CG, Peeters EAJ, et al. Germline mutations in the PTEN/MMAC1 gene in patients with Cowden disease. Hum Mol Genet. 1997;6:1383–7.

Nelen MR, Kremer H, Konings IBM, et al. Novel PTEN mutations in patients with Cowden disease: absence of clear genotype–phenotype correlations. Eur J Hum Genet. 1999;7: 267–73.

Neumann HPH, Bausch B, McWhinney SR, Bender BU, Gimm O, Franke G, Schipper J, Klisch J, Altehoefer C, Zerres K, Januszewicz A, Eng C, Smith WM, Munk R, Manz T, Glaesker S, Apel TW, Treier M, Reineke M, Walz MK, Hoang-Vu C, Brauckhoff M, Klein-Franke A, Klose P, Schmidt H, Maier-Woelfle M, Peczkowska M, Szmigielski C, Eng C. The Freiburg-Warsaw-Columbus Pheochromocytoma Study Group. Germ-line mutations in nonsyndromic pheochromocytoma. N Engl J Med. 2002;346:1459–66.

Newey PJ, Bowl MR, Cranston T, Thakker RV. Cell division cycle protein 73 homolog (CDC73) mutations in the hyperparathyroidism-jaw tumor syndrome (HPT-JT) and parathyroid tumors. Hum Mutat. 2010;31:295–307.

Ngeow J, Mester J, Rybicki LA, Ni Y, Milas M, Eng C. Incidence and clinical characteristics of thyroid cancer in prospective series of individuals with Cowden and Cowden-like syndromes characterized by germline *PTEN, SDH* or *KLLN* alterations. J Clin Endocrinol Metab. 2011;96(12):E2063–71.

Ni Y, Zbuk KM, Sadler T, Patocs A, Lobo G, Edelman E, Platzer P, Orloff MS, Waite KA, Eng C. Germline mutations and variants in the succinate dehydrogenase genes in Cowden and Cowden-like syndromes. Am J Hum Genet. 2008;83:261–8.

Ni Y, He X, Chen J, Moline J, Mester J, Orloff MS, Ringel MD, Eng C. Germline *SDHx* variants modify breast and thyroid cancer risks in Cowden and Cowden-like syndrome via FAD/NAD-dependent destabilization of p53. Hum Mol Genet. 2012;15;21(2):300–10.

Nichols CR. Mediastinal germ cell tumors. Semin Thorac Cardiovasc Surg. 1992;4:45–50. Intracranial malignant germ cell tumors have also occasionally been described (Prall et al., 1995).

Nickerson ML, Warren MB, Toro JR, Matrosova V, Glenn G, Turner ML, Duray P, Merino M, Choyke P, Pavlovich CP, Sharma N, Walther M, Munroe D, Hill R, Maher E, Greenberg C, Lerman MI, Linehan WM, Zbar B, Schmidt LS. Mutations in a novel gene lead to kidney tumors, lung wall defects, and benign tumors of the hair follicle in patients with the Birt–Hogg–Dube syndrome. Cancer Cell. 2002;2(2):157–64.

Nicoliades NC, Papadopoulos N, Liu B, et al. Mutations of two PMS homologues in hereditary non-polyposis colorectal cancer. Nature. 1994;371:75–80.

Nilsson O, Tissell L-E, Jansson S, Ahlman H, Gimm O, Eng C. Adrenal and extra-adrenal pheochromocytomas in a family with germline *RET* V804L mutation. J Am Med Aossc. 1999;281:1587–8.

Nishijo K, et al. Mutation analysis of the RECQL4 gene in sporadic osteosarcomas. Int J Cancer. 2004;111(3):367–72.

Nobuhara Y, et al. TIE2 gain-of-function mutation in a patient with pancreatic lymphangioma associated with blue rubber-bleb nevus syndrome: report of a case. Surg Today. 2006;36: 283–6.

Noguchi M, Yi H, Rosenblatt HM, et al. Interleukin-2 receptor gamma chain mutation results in X-linked severe combined immunodeficiency in humans. Cell. 1993;73:147–57.

Norton JA, Fraker DL, Alexander HR, et al. Surgery to cure Zollinger–Ellison syndrome. New Engl J Med. 1999;341:635–44.

Nugent KP, Phillips RKS, Hodgson SV, et al. Phenotypic expression in familial adenomatous polyposis: partial prediction by mutation analysis. Gut. 1994;35:1622–4.

Nystrom-Lahti M, Kristo P, Nicolaides NC, Chang SY, Aaltonen LA, Moisio AL, Jarvinen HJ, Mecklin JP, Kinzler KW, Vogelstein B. Founding mutations and Alu-mediated recombination in hereditary colon cancer. Nat Med. 1995;1(11):1203–6.

Odent S, Atti-Bitach T, Blayau M, Mathieu M, Aug J, de Delezo AL, Gall JY, Le Marec B, Munnich A, David V, Vekemans M. Expression of the Sonic hedgehog (SHH) gene during early human development and phenotypic expression of new mutations causing holoprosencephaly. Hum Mol Genet. 1999;8(9):1683–9.

Offit K, Levran O, Mullaney B, Mah K, Nafa K, Batish SD, Diotti R, Schneider H, Deffenbaugh A, Scholl T, Proud VK, Robson M, Norton L, Ellis N, Hanenberg H, Auerbach AD. Shared genetic susceptibility to breast cancer, brain tumors, and Fanconi anemia. J Natl Cancer Inst. 2003;95:1548–51.

Okimoto K, Sakurai J, Kobayashi T, Mitani H, Hirayama Y, Nickerson ML, Warren MB, Zbar B, Schmidt LS, Hino O. A germ-line insertion in the Birt–Hogg–Dube (BHD) gene gives rise to the Nihon rat model of inherited renal cancer. Proc Natl Acad Sci USA. 2004;101:2023–7.

Olivier M, Goldgar DE, Sodha N, et al. Li–Fraumeni and related syndromes: correlation between tumor type, family structure and *TP53* genotype. Cancer Res. 2003;63:6643–50.

Olschwang S, Laurent-Puig P, et al. Germline mutations in the first 14 exons of the adenomatous polyposis coli (APC) gene. Am J Hum Genet. 1993;52:273–9.

Olschwang S, Eisinger F, Millat B. An alternative to prophylactic colectomy for colon cancer prevention in HNPCC syndrome. Gut. 2005;54:169–73.

Ombrello MJ, Remmers EF, Sun G, Freeman AF, Datta S, Torabi-Parizi P, Subramanian N, Bunney TD, Baxendale RW, Martins MS, Romberg N, Komarow H, Aksentijevich I, Kim HS, Ho J, Cruse G, Jung MY, Gilfillan AM, Metcalfe DD, Nelson C, O'Brien M, Wisch L, Stone K, Douek DC, Gandhi C, Wanderer AA, Lee H, Nelson SF, Shianna KV, Cirulli ET, Goldstein DB, Long EO, Moir S, Meffre E, Holland SM, Kastner DL, Katan M, Hoffman HM, Milner JD. Cold urticaria, immunodeficiency, and autoimmunity related to PLCG2 deletions. N Engl J Med. 2012;366:330–8.

Omura NE, Collison DW, Perry AE, Myers LM. Sebaceous carcinoma in children. J Am Acad Dermatol. 2002;47(6):950–3.

Ong KR, Woodward ER, Killick P, Lim C, Macdonald F, Maher ER. Genotype-phenotype correlations in von Hippel-Lindau disease. Hum Mutat. 2007;28(2):143–9.

Orloff MS, He X, Peterson C, Chen F, Chen JL, Mester JL, Eng C. Germline PIK3CA and AKT1 mutations in Cowden and Cowden-like syndromes. Am J Hum Genet. 2013;92:76–80.

Ostasiewicz LT, Huang JL, Wang X, et al. Human protoporphyria genetic heterogeneity at the ferrochelatase locus. Photodermatol Photoimmunol Photomed. 1995;11:18–21.

Ostergaard JR, Sunde L, Okkels H. Neurofibromatosis von Recklinghausen type I phenotype and early onset of cancers in siblings compound heterozygous for mutations in MSH6. Am J Med Genet A. 2005;139A(2):96–105.

Osterod M, et al. A global DNA repair mechanism involving the Cockayne syndrome B (CSB) gene product can prevent the in vivo accumulation of endogenous oxidative DNA base damage. Oncogene. 2002;21(54):8232–9.

Pack K, Smith-Ravin J, Phillips RKS, Hodgson SC. Exceptions to the rule: individuals with FAP-specific CHRPE and mutations in exon 6 of the APC gene. Clin Genet. 1996;50:110–1.

Palles C, Cazier JB, Howarth KM, Domingo E, Jones AM, Broderick P, Kemp Z, Spain SL, Guarino E, Salguero I, Sherborne A, Chubb D, Carvajal-Carmona LG, Ma Y, Kaur K, Dobbins S, Barclay E, Gorman M, Martin L, Kovac MB, Humphray S; CORGI Consortium; WGS500 Consortium, Lucassen A, Holmes CC, Bentley D, Donnelly P, Taylor J, Petridis C, Roylance R, Sawyer EJ, Kerr DJ, Clark S, Grimes J, Kearsey SE, Thomas HJ, McVean G, Houlston RS, Tomlinson I. Germline mutations affecting the proofreading domains of POLE and POLD1 predispose to colorectal adenomas and carcinomas. Nat Genet. 2013;45(2):136–44. doi:10.1038/ng.2503. Epub 2012 Dec 23.

Pandit B, Sarkozy A, Pennacchio LA, et al. Gain-of-function RAF mutations cause Noonan and LEOPARD syndromes with hypertrophic cardiomyopathy. Nat Genet. 2006;39:1007–12.

Pannett AA, Kennedy AM, Turner JJ, et al. Multiple endocrine neoplasia type 1 (MEN1) germline mutations in familial isolated primary hyperparathyroidism. Clin Endocrinol. 2003;58:639–46.

Pansuriya TC, van Eijk R, d'Adamo P, van Ruler MA, Kuijjer ML, Oosting J, Cleton-Jansen AM, van Oosterwijk JG, Verbeke SL, Meijer D, van Wezel T, Nord KH, Sangiorgi L, Toker B, Liegl-Atzwanger B, San-Julian M, Sciot R, Limaye N, Kindblom LG, Daugaard S, Godfraind C, Boon LM, Vikkula M, Kurek KC, Szuhai K, French PJ, Bovée JV. Somatic mosaic IDH1 and IDH2 mutations are associated with enchondroma and spindle cell hemangioma in Ollier disease and Maffucci syndrome. Nat Genet. 2011;43(12):1256–61.

Papi L, Montali E, Marconi G, Guazzelli R, Bigozzi U, Maraschio P, Zuffardi O. Evidence for a human mitotic mutant with pleiotropic effect. Ann Hum Genet. 1989;53(Pt 3):243–8.

Paraf F, Sasseville D, Watters AK, Narod S, Ginsburg O, Shibata H, Jothy S. Clinicopathological relevance of the association between gastrointestinal and sebaceous neoplasms: the Muir–Torre syndrome [Review]. Hum Pathol. 1995;26(4):422–7.

Paraf F, Jothy S, Van Meir EG. Brain tumor–polyposis syndrome. Two genetic diseases? J Clin Oncol. 1997;15:2744–58.

Park YJ, Shin K-H, Park J-G. Risk of gastric cancer in hereditary nonpolyposis colorectal cancer in Korea. Clin Cancer Res. 2000;6:2994–8.

Park DJ, Lesueur F, Nguyen-Dumont T, Pertesi M, Odefrey F, Hammet F, Neuhausen SL, John EM, Andrulis IL, Terry MB, Daly M, Buys S, Le Calvez-Kelm F, Lonie A, Pope BJ, Tsimiklis H, Voegele C, Hilbers FM, Hoogerbrugge N, Barroso A, Osorio A, Giles GG, Devilee P, Benitez J, Hopper JL, Tavtigian SV, Goldgar DE, Southey MC. Rare mutations in XRCC2 increase the risk of breast cancer. Am J Hum Genet. 2012;90:734–39.

Parker JA, Kalnins VI, Deck JHN, et al. Histopathological features of congenital fundus lesions in familial adenomatous polyposis. Can J Ophthalmol. 1990;25:159–63.

Parry DM, MacCollin MM, Kaiser-Kupfer MI, et al. Germ-line mutations in the neurofibromatosis 2 gene: correlations with disease severity and retinal abnormalities. Am J Hum Genet. 1996;59:529–39.

Parsons R, Li G-M, Langley MJ, et al. Hypermutability and mismatch repair deficiency in RER tumor cells. Cell. 1993;75:1227–36.

Pasini B, McWhinney SR, Bei T, Matyakhina L, Stergiopoulos SG, Muchow M, Boikos S, Ferrando B, Pacak K, Assié G, Baudin E, Chompret A, Ellison JW, Briere JJ, Rustin P, Gimenez-Roquelpo A-P, Eng C, Carney JA, Stratakis CA. Clinical and molecular genetics of patients with the Carney-Stratakis syndrome and germline mutations in the genes encoding succinate dehydrogenase subunits (*SDHB, SDHC, SDHD*). Eur J Hum Genet. 2008;16: 79–88.

Patrice SJ, Sneed PK, Flickinger JC, Shrieve DC, Pollock BE, Alexander III E, Larson DA, Kondziolka DS, Gutin PH, Wara WM, McDermott MW, Lunsford LD, Loeffler JS. Radiosurgery for hemangioblastoma: results of a multi-institutional experience. Int J Radiat Oncol Biol Phys. 1996;35:493–9.

Pavlovich CP, Walther MM, Eyler RA, Hewitt SM, Zbar B, Linehan WM, Merino MJ. Renal tumors in the Birt–Hogg–Dube syndrome. Am J Surg Pathol. 2002;26(12):1542–52.

Pearson T, Jansen S, Havenga C, Stones DK, Joubert G. Fanconi anemia. A statistical evaluation of cytogenetic results obtained from South African families. Cancer Genet Cytogenet. 2001; 126:52–5.

Pellegata NS, Quintanilla-Martinez L, Siggelkow H, Samson E, Bink K, Hofler H, Fend F, Graw J, Atkinson MJ. Germ-line mutations in p27Kip1 cause a multiple endocrine neoplasia syndrome in rats and humans. Proc Natl Acad Sci USA. 2006;103:15558–63.

Perlman M. Perlman syndrome: familial renal dysplasia with Wilms tumor, fetal gigantism, and multiple congenital anomalies. Am J Med Genet. 1986;25:793–5.

Peterson RD, Funkhouser JD, Tuck-Muller CM, Gatti RA. Cancer susceptibility in Ataxia Telangiectasia. Leukaemia. 1992;6 Suppl 1:8–13.

Peutz JLA. Very remarkable case of familial polyposis of mucous membrane of intestinal tract and nasopharynx accompanied by peculiar pigmentations of skin and mucous membranes (Dutch). Nederl Maandschr Geneesk. 1921;10:134–46.

Phillips RKS, Spigelman AD. Can we safely delay or avoid prophylactic colectomy in familial adenomatous polyposis (FAP)? Br J Surg. 1996;83:769–70.

Phillips RK, Wallance MH, Lynch PM, et al. A randomised, double-blind placebo controlled study of celecoxib, a selective cyclo-oxygenase 2 inhibitor, on duodenal polyposis in familial adenomatous polyposis. Gut. 2002;50:857–60.

Pilarski R, Eng C. Will the real Cowden syndrome please stand up (again)? Expanding mutational and clinical spectra of the *PTEN* hamartoma tumor syndrome. J Med Genet. 2004;41: 323–6.

Pilia G, Hughes-Benzie RM, MacKenzie A, et al. Mutations in GPC3, a glypican gene, cause the Simpson–Golabi–Behmel overgrowth syndrome. Nat Genet. 1996;12:241–7.

Pinto EM, Billerbeck AE, Villares MC, et al. Founder effect for the highly prevalent R337H mutation of tumor suppressor *p53* in Brazilian patients with adrenocortical tumors. Arq Bras Endocrinal Metabol. 2004;48(5):647–50.

Ponder BAJ, Ponder MA, Coffey R, et al. Risk estimation and screening in families of patients with medullary thyroid carcinoma. Lancet. 1988;i:397–400.

Poppe B, Van Limbergen H, Van Roy N, Vandecruys E, De Paepe A, Benoit Y, Speleman F. Chromosomal aberrations in Bloom syndrome patients with myeloid malignancies. Cancer Genet Cytogenet. 2001;128(1):39–42.

Potter NU, Sarmousakis C, Li FP. Cancer in relatives of patients with aplastic anemia. Cancer Genet Cytogenet. 1983;9:61–5.

Potter DD, Murray JA, Donohue JH, Burgart LJ, Nagorney DM, van Heerden JA, Plevak MF, Zinsmeister AR, Thibodeau SN. The role of defective mismatch repair in small bowel adenocarcinoma in celiac disease. Cancer Res. 2004;64:7073–7.

Priest JR, Watterson J, Strong L, Huff V, Woods WG, Byrd RL, Friend SH, Newsham I, Amylon MD, Pappo A, Mahoney DH, Langston C, Heyn R, Kohut G, Freyer DR, Bostrom B, Richardson MS, Barredo J, Dehner LP. Pleuropulmonary blastoma: a marker for familial disease. J Pediatr. 1996;128:220–4.

Priest JR, McDermott MB, Bhatia S, Watterson J, Manivel JC, Dehner LP. Pleuropulmonary blastoma: a clinicopathologic study of 50 cases. Cancer. 1997;80:147–61.

Puck JM, et al. The interleukin-2 receptor gamma chain maps to Xq13.1 and is mutated in X-linked severe combined immunodeficiency, SCIDX1. Hum Mol Genet. 1993;2(8):1099–104.

Puck JM, et al. Mutation analysis of IL2RG in human X-linked severe combined immunodeficiency. Blood. 1997;89(6):1968–77.

Rabin KR, Whitlock JA. Malignancy in children with trisomy 21. Oncologist. 2009;14(2):164–73.

Rajagopalan H, Nowak MA, Vogelstein B, Lengauer C. The significance of unstable chromosomes in colorectal cancer. Nat Rev Cancer. 2003;3(9):695–701.

Rapin I, Lindenbaum Y, Dicson DW, et al. Cockayne syndrome and xeroderma pigmentosum. Neurology. 2000;55:1442–9.

Reardon W, Zhou XP, Eng C. A novel germline mutation of the PTEN gene in a patient with macrocephaly, ventricular dilatation and features of VATER association. J Med Genet. 2001;38:820–3.

Reid S, Schindler D, Hanenberg H, Barker K, Hanks S, Kalb R, Neveling K, Kelly P, Seal S, Freund M, Wurm M, Batish SD, Lach FP, Yetgin S, Neitzel H, Ariffin H, Tischkowitz M, Mathew CG, Auerbach AD, Rahman N. Biallelic mutations in PALB2 cause Fanconi anemia subtype FA-N and predispose to childhood cancer. Nat Genet. 2007;39:162–4.

Renkonen-Sinisalo Z, Aarnio M, Mecklin JP, Jarvinen HJ. Surveillance improves survival of colorectal cancer in patients with HNPCC. Cancer Detect Prev. 2000;24:137–42.

Renkonen-Sinisalo L, Sipponen P, Aarnio M et al. No support for endoscopic surveillance for gastric cancer in hereditary non-polyposis colorectal cancer. Scand J Gastroenterol 2002;37(5):574–7.

Renwick A, Thompson D, Seal S, Kelly P, Chagtai T, Ahmed M, North B, Jayatilake H, Barfoot R, Spanova K, McGuffog L, Evans DG, Eccles D, Easton DF, Stratton MR, Rahman N. ATM mutations that cause ataxia-telangiectasia are breast cancer susceptibility alleles. Nat Genet. 2006;38:873–5.

Reyes CM, Allen BA, Terdiman JP, et al. Comparison of selection strategies for genetic testing of patients with hereditary non-polyposis colorectal cancer: effectiveness and cost-effectiveness. Cancer. 2002;95:1848–56.

Ribeiro RC, Sandrini F, Figueiredo B, et al. An inherited p53 mutation that con-tributes in a tissue-specific manner to pediatric adrenal cortical carcinoma. Proc Natl Acad Sci USA. 2001;98:9330–5.

Riccardi VM, Lewis RA. Penetrance of von Recklinghausen neurofibromatosis: a distinction between predecessors and descendants. Am J Hum Genet. 1988;42:284–9.

Ricciardone MD, Ozcelik T, Cevher B, Ozdag H, Tuncer M, Gurgey A, Uzunalimoglu O, Cetinkaya H, Tanyeli A, Erken E, Ozturk M. Human MLH1 deficiency predisposes to hematological malignancy and neurofibromatosis type 1. Cancer Res. 1999;59(2):290–3.

Rickard SJ, Wilson LC. Analysis of GNAS1 and overlapping transcripts identifies the parent-of-origin of mutations in patients with sporadic Albright hereditary osteodystrophy and reveals a model system in which to observe the effects of splicing mutations on translated and untranslated messenger RNA. Am J Hum Genet. 2003;72:961–74.

Rio FT, Lavoie J, Hamel N, Geyer FC, Kushner YB, Novak DJ, Wark L, Capelli C, Reis-Filho JS, Mai S, Pastinen T, Tischkowitz MD, Marcus VA, Foulkes WD. Homozygous BUB1B mutation and susceptibility to gastrointestinal neoplasia. N Engl J Med. 2010;363:2628–37.

Rio FT, Bahubeshi A, Kanellopoulou C, Hamel N, Niedziela M, Sabbaghian N, Pouchet C, Gilbert L, O'Brien PK, Serfas K, Broderick P, Houlston RS, Lesueur F, Bonora E, Muljo S, Schimke RN, Bouron-Dal SD, Arseneau J, Schultz KA, Priest JR, Nguyen VH, Harach HR, Livingston DM, Foulkes WD, Tischkowitz M. DICER1 mutations in familial multinodular goiter with and without ovarian Sertoli-Leydig cell tumors. JAMA. 2011;305:68–77.

Robbins TO, Bernstein J. Renal involvement. In: Gomez MR, editor. *Tuberous Sclerosis*. New York: Raven Press; 1988. p. 133–6.

Roberts CW, Biegel JA. The role of SMARCB1/INI1 in development of rhabdoid tumor. Cancer Biol Ther. 2009;8:412–6.

Roberts A, Allanson J, Jadico SK, Kavamura MI, Noonan J, Opitz JM, Young T. The cardiofacio-cutaneous syndrome. J Med Genet. 2006;43:833–42.

Robertson DM. Ophthalmic findings. In: Gomez MR, editor. *Tuberous Sclerosis*. Raven Press: New York; 1988. p. 89–109.

Rodriguez-Bigas MA, Boland CR, Hamilton SR, et al. A National Cancer Institute workshop on hereditary non-polyposis colorectal cancer: meeting highlights and Bethesda guidelines. J Nat Cancer Inst. 1997;89:1758–62.

Roessler E, Belloni E, Gaudenz K, Vargas F, Schere SW, Tsui LC, Muenke M. Mutations in the C-terminal domain of Sonic Hedgehog cause holoprosencephaly. Hum Mol Genet. 1997;6(11):1847–53.

Romanelli V, Nevado J, Fraga M, Trujillo AM, Mori MÁ, Fernández L, Pérez de Nanclares G, Martínez-Glez V, Pita G, Meneses H, Gracia R, García-Miñaur S, García de Miguel P, Lecumberri B, Rodríguez JI, González Neira A, Monk D, Lapunzina P. Constitutional mosaic genome-wide uniparental disomy due to diploidisation: an unusual cancer-predisposing mechanism. J Med Genet. 2011;48(3):212–6.

Rongioletti F, Hazini R, Gianotti G, Rebora A. Fibrofolliculomas, tricodiscomas and acrochordons (Birt–Hogg–Dube) associated with intestinal polyposis. Clin Exp Dermatol. 1989;14(1): 72–4.

Rosenberg PS, Greene MH, Alter BP. Cancer incidence in persons with Fanconi's anemia. Blood. 2003;101:822–5.

Rouleau GA, Merel P, Lutchman M, Sanson M, Zucman J, Marineau C, Hoang-Xuan K, Demczuk S, Desmaze C, Plougastel B, et al. Alteration in a new gene encoding a putative membrane-organizing protein causes neuro-fibromatosis type 2. Nature. 1993;63(6429):515–21.

Roy PK, Venzon DJ, Feigenbaum KM, et al. Gastric secretion in Zollinger–Ellison syndrome. Correlation with clinical expression, tumor extent and role in diagnosis – a prospective NIH study of 235 patients and a review of 984 cases in the literature. Medicine. 2001;80:189–222.

Royer-Pokora B, Beier M, Henzler M, Alam R, Schumacher V, Weirich A, Huff V. Twenty-four new cases of WT1 germline mutations and review of the literature: genotype/phenotype correlations for Wilms tumor development. Am J Med Genet A. 2004;127A(3):249–57.

Rozen P, Naiman T, Strul H, et al. Clinical and screening implications of the I1307K APC gene variant in Israeli Ashkenazi Jews with familial colorectal neoplasia. Evidence for a founder effect. Cancer. 2002;94:2561–8.

Ruttledge MH, Andermann AA, Phelan CM, et al. Type of mutation in the neurofibromatosis type 2 gene (NF2) frequently determines severity of disease. Am J Hum Genet. 1996;59:331–42.

Sampson JR, Jones N. MUTYH-associated polyposis. Best Pract Res Clin Gastroenterol. 2009;23(2):209–18.

Sampson JR, Maheshwar MM, Aspinwall R, Thompson P, Cheadle JP, Ravine D, Roy S, Haan E, Bernstein J, Harris PC. Renal cystic disease in tuberous sclerosis: role of the polycystic kidney disease 1 gene. Am J Hum Genet. 1997;61:843–51.

Sampson JR, Dolwani S, Jones S, Eccles D, Ellis A, Evans DG, Frayling I, Jordan S, Maher ER, Mak T, Maynard J, Pigatto F, Shaw J, Cheadle JP. Autosomal recessive colorectal adenomatous polyposis due to inherited mutations of MYH. Lancet. 2003;362(9377):39–41.

Sankila R, Aaltonen LA, Mecklin J-P. Better survival rates in patients with MLH1P1-associated hereditary colorectal cancer. Gastroenterology. 1996;110:682–7.

Santoro M, Carlomagno F, Romano A, et al. Activation of *RET* as a dominant transforming gene by germline mutations of MEN 2A and MEN 2B. Science. 1995;267:381–3.

Satya-Murti S, Navada S, Eames F. Central nervous system involvement in blue rubber bleb nevus syndrome. Arch Neurol. 1986;43:1184–6.

Sariozzi S, Saluto A, Taylor AM, Last JI, Trebini F, Paradiso MC, Grosso E, Funaro A, Ponzio G, Migone N, Brusco A. A late onset variant of ataxia-telangiectasia with a compound heterozygous genotype, A8030G/7481insA. J Med Genet. 2002;39:57–61.

Savitsky K, Bar-Shira A, Gilad S, et al. A single ataxia telangiectasia gene with a product similar to PI-3 kinase. Science. 1995;268:1749–53.

Scacheri PC, Davis S, Odom DT, Crawford GE, Perkins S, Halawi MJ, Agarwal SK, Marx SJ, Spiegel AM, Meltzer SJ, Collins FS. Genome-wide analysis of menin binding provides insights into MEN1 tumorigenesis. PLoS Genet. 2006;2:e51.

Scheithauer BW, Laws ER, Kovacs K, Horvath E, Randall RV, Carney JA. Pituitary adenomas of the multiple endocrine neoplasia type I syndrome. Semin Diagn Pathol. 1987;4:205–11.

Schimke RN. Genetic aspects of multiple endocrine neoplasia. Annu Rev Med. 1984;35:25–31.

Schneppenheim R, Fruhwald MC, Gesk S, Hasselblatt M, Jeibmann A, Kordes U, Kreuz M, Leuschner I, Martin Subero JI, Obser T, Oyen F, Vater I, Siebert R. Germline nonsense mutation and somatic inactivation of SMARCA4/BRG1 in a family with rhabdoid tumor predisposition syndrome. Am J Hum Genet. 2010;86:279–84.

Schoemaker MJ, Swerdlow AJ, Higgins CD, Wright AF, Jacobs PA, UK Clinical Cytogenetics Group. Cancer incidence in women with Turner syndrome in Great Britain: a national cohort study. Lancet Oncol. 2008;9(3):239–46.

Schrager CA, Schneider D, Gruener AC, Tsou HC, Peacocke M. Clinical and pathological features of breast disease in Cowden's syndrome: an underrecognised syndrome with an increased risk of breast cancer. Hum Pathol. 1997;29:47–53.

Schuffenecker I, Ginet N, Goldgar D, et al. Prevalence and parental origin of de novo RET mutations in MEN 2A and FMTC. Am J Hum Genet. 1997;60:233–7.

Schuffenecker I, Virally-Monod M, Brohet R, et al. Risk and penetrance of primary hyperparathyroidism in MEN 2A families with codon 634 mutations of the RET proto-oncogene. J Clin Endocrinol Metab. 1998;83:487–91.

Schwartz RA. Basal cell naevus syndrome and upper gastrointestinal polyposis. New Engl J Med. 1978;299:49.

Schwartz HS, Zimmerman NB, Simon MA, Wroble RR, Millar EA, Bonfiglio M. The malignant potential of enchondromatosis. J Bone Joint Surg. 1987;69A:269–74.

Scott RH, Walker L, Olsen ØE, Levitt G, Kenney I, Maher E, Owens CM, Pritchard-Jones K, Craft A, Rahman N. Surveillance for Wilms tumour in at-risk children: pragmatic recommendations for best practice. Arch Dis Child. 2006;91(12):995–9.

Seidinger AL, Mastellaro MJ, Paschoal FF, Godoy AJ, Aparecida CI, Aparecida GM, Correa RR, Brandalise SR, Dos Santos AS, Yunes JA. Association of the highly prevalent TP53 R337H mutation with pediatric choroid plexus carcinoma and osteosarcoma in southeast Brazil. Cancer. 2011;117:2228–35.

Selvanathan SK, et al. Further genotype–phenotype correlations in neurofibromatosis 2. Clin Genet. 2010;77(2):163–70.

Sepp T, Yates JR, Green AJ. Loss of heterozygosity in tuberous sclerosis hamartomas. J Med Genet. 1996;33(11):962–4.

Sevenet N, Sheridan E, Amram D, Schneider P, Handgretinger R, Delattre O. Constitutional mutations of the hSNF5/INI1 gene predispose to a variety of cancers. Am J Hum Genet. 1999;65:1342–8.

Shamseldin HE, Elfaki M, Alkuraya FS. Exome sequencing reveals a novel Fanconi group defined by XRCC2 mutation. J Med Genet. 2012;49:184–6.

Shannon KE, Gimm O, Hinze R, Dralle H, Eng C. Germline V804M in the RET proto-oncogene in two apparently sporadic cases of MTC presenting in the seventh decade of life. J Endo Genet. 1999;1:39–46.

Shattuck TM, Valimaki S, Obara T, et al. Somatic and germ-line mutations of the HRPT2 gene in sporadic parathyroid carcinoma. New Engl J Med. 2003;349:1722–9.

Shia J, Klimstra DS, Nafa K, Offit K, Guillem JG, Markowitz AJ, Gerald WL, Ellis NA. Value of immunohistochemical detection of DNA mismatch repair proteins in predicting germline mutation in hereditary colorectal neoplasms. Am J Surg Pathol. 2005;29(1):96–104.

Sidransky D, Tokino T, Helzlsouer K, Zehnbauer B, Rausch G, Shelton B, Prestigiacomo L, Vogelstein B, Davidson N. Inherited p53 gene mutations in breast cancer. Cancer Res. 1992;52:2984–6.

Sieber OM, Lipton L, Crabtree M, Heinimann K, Fidalgo P, Phillips RKS, Bisgaard M-L, Orntoft TF, Aaltonen LA, Hodgson SV, Huw DM, Thomas JW, Tomlinson PM. The multiple colorectal adenoma phenotype, familial adenomatous polyposis and germline mutations in MYH. N Engl J Med. 2003a;348:791–9.

Sieber OM, Heinimann K, Tomlinson IP. Genomic instability – the engine of tumorigenesis? Nat Rev Cancer. 2003b;3(9):701–8.

Skogseid B, Larsson C, Lindgren PG, et al. Clinical and genetic features of adrenocortical lesions in multiple endocrine neoplasia type 1. J Clin Endocrinol Metab. 1992;75:76–81.

Skogseid B, Rastad J, Öberg K. Multiple endocrine neoplasia type 1. Clinical features and screening. Endocrinol Metab Clin N Am. 1994;23:1–18.

Slade I, Bacchelli C, Davies H, Murray A, Abbaszadeh F, Hanks S, Barfoot R, Burke A, Chisholm J, Hewitt M, Jenkinson H, King D, Morland B, Pizer B, Prescott K, Saggar A, Side L, Traunecker H, Vaidya S, Ward P, Futreal PA, Vujanic G, Nicholson AG, Sebire N, Turnbull C, Priest JR, Pritchard-Jones K, Houlston R, Stiller C, Stratton MR, Douglas J, Rahman N. DICER1 syndrome: clarifying the diagnosis, clinical features and management implications of a pleiotropic tumour predisposition syndrome. J Med Genet. 2011;48:273–8.

Smith OP, Hann IM, Chessells JM, Reeves BR, Milla P. Haematological abnormalities in Shwachman–Diamond syndrome. Br J Haemat. 1996;94:279–84.

Smith DP, Houghton C, Ponder BAJ. Germline mutation of *RET* codon 883 in two cases of *de novo* MEN 2B. Oncogene. 1997;15:1213–7.

Smith JM, Kirk EPE, Theodosopoulos G, et al. Germline mutation of the tumor suppressor *PTEN* in Proteus syndrome. J Med Genet. 2002;39:937–40.

Smyrk TC, Watson P, Kaul K, et al. Tumor-infiltrating lymphocytes are a marker for microsatellite instability in colorectal cancer. Cancer. 2001;91:2417–22.

Snape K, Hanks S, Ruark E, Barros-Nunez P, Elliott A, Murray A, Lane AH, Shannon N, Callier P, Chitayat D, Clayton-Smith J, Fitzpatrick DR, Gisselsson D, Jacquemont S, Asakura-Hay K, Micale MA, Tolmie J, Turnpenny PD, Wright M, Douglas J, Rahman N. Mutations in CEP57 cause mosaic variegated aneuploidy syndrome. Nat Genet. 2011;43:527–9.

Sorensen SA, Mulvihill JJ, Nielsen A. Long-term follow-up of von Recklinghausen neurofibromatosis. New Engl J Med. 1986;314:1010–5.

Spector BD, Filipovich AH, Perry GS, Kersey JH. Epidemiology of cancer in ataxia telangiectasia. In: Bridges BA, Harnden DG, editors. Ataxia Telangiectasia: a cellular and molecular link between cancer, neuropathology and immune deficiency. Chichester: Wiley; 1982. p. 103–38.

Spigelman AD, Arese P, Phillips RKS. Polyposis: the Peutz–Jeghers syndrome. Br J Surg. 1995;82:1311–4.

Spirio L, Olschwang S, Groden J, et al. Alleles of the APC gene: an attenuated form of familial polyposis. Cell. 1993;75:951–7.

Spirio LN, Samowitz W, Robertson J, et al. Alleles of APC modulate the frequency and classes of mutations that lead to colon polyps. Nat Genetics. 1998;20:385–8.

Srivastava S, Zou Z, Pirollo K, Blattner W, Chang EH. Germ-line transmission of a mutated *p53* gene in a cancer-prone family with Li–Fraumeni syndrome. Nature. 1990;348:747–9.

Starink TM, van der Veen JPW, Arwert F, et al. The Cowden syndrome: a clinical and genetic study in 21 patients. Clin Genet. 1986;29:222–33.

Starr DG, McClure JP, Connor JM. Non-dermatological complications and genetic aspects of the Rothmund–Thomson syndrome. Clin Genet. 1985;27:102–4.

Stefanini M, Fawcett H, Botta E, Nardo T, Lehmann AR. Genetic analysis of twenty-two patients with Cockayne syndrome. Hum Genet. 1996;97:418–23.

Steinbach G, Lynch PM, Phillips RK, et al. The effect of celecoxib, a cyclooxy-genase-2 inhibitor, in familial adenomatous polyposis. New Engl J Med. 2000;342(26):1946–52.

Steiner MS, Goldman SM, Fishman EK, Marshall FF. The natural history of renal angiomyolipoma. J Urol. 1993;150:1782–6.

Stewart GS, Maser RS, Stancovic T, et al. The DNA strand double break repair gene hMRE11 is mutated in individuals with an ataxia-telangiectasia-like disorder. Cell. 1999;99:577–87.

Stiller CA, Chessells JM, Fitchett M. Neurofibromatosis and childhood leukaemia/lymphoma: a population based UKCCSG study. Br J Cancer. 1994;70:969–72.

Stinco G, Governatori G, Mattighello P, Patrone P. Multiple cutaneous neoplasms in a patient with Rothmund-Thomson syndrome: case report and published work review. J Dermatol. 2008;35(3): 154–61.

Stormorken ST, Thomas HJW, Wijnen J, Phillips R, Clark SK, de Leon Ponz M, Renkonen-Sinisalo L, Sampson JR, Hodgson A, Järvinen H, Mecklin J-P, Møller P, Myrhøi T, Nagengast FM, Parc Y, Bülow, Burn J, Capella G, Colas C, Engel C, Frayling I, Friedl W, Hes FJ, Vasen A, Möslein G, Alonso A, Aretz S, Bernstein I, Bertario L, Blanco I, Nieuwenhuis MH, Vasen HFA. Correlation between mutation site in APC and phenotype of familial adenomatous polyposis (FAP): a review of the literature. Crit Rev oncol Haematol. 2007;61(2):153–61.

Stratakis CA, Carney JA. The triad of paragangliomas, gastric stromal tumours and pulmonary chondromas (Carney triad), and the dyad of paragangliomas and gastric stromal sarcomas (Carney-Stratakis syndrome): molecular genetics and clinical implications. J Intern Med. 2009;266:43–52.

Stratakis CA, Sarlis N, Kirschner LS, et al. Paradoxical response to dexamethasone in the diagnosis of primary pigmented nodular adrenocortical disease. Ann Int Med. 1999;131:585–91.

Stratakis CA, Kirschner LS, Carney JA. Clinical and molecular features of the Carney complex diagnostic criteria and recommendations for patient evaluation. J Clin Endocrinol Metab. 2001;86:4041–6.

Subbiah V, Kurzrock R. Ewing's Sarcoma: overcoming the therapeutic plateau. Discov Med. 2012;13:405–15.

Sumegi J, Huang D, Lanyi A, Davis JD, Seemayer TA, Maeda A, Klein G, Seri M, Wakiguchi H, Purtilo DT, Gross TG. Correlation of mutations of the SH2D1A gene and Epstein–Barr virus infection with clinical phenotype and outcome in X-linked lymphoproliferative disease. Blood. 2000;9(6):3118–25.

Sun TC, Swee RG, Shives TC, Unni KK. Chondrosarcoma in Maffucci's syndrome. J Bone Joint Surg. 1985;67A:1214–9.

Sun X, Becker-Catania SG, Chun HH, et al. Early diagnosis of ataxia telangiectasia using radiosensitivity testing. J Paed. 2002;140:734–21.

Sutter C, Dallenbach-Hellweg G, Schmidt D. Molecular analysis of endometrial hyperplasia in HNPCC-suspicious patients may predict progression to endometrial carcinoma. Int J Gynecol Pathol. 2004;23(1):18–25.

Swerdlow AJ, Schoemeker J, Higgins D, et al. Cancer Incidence and mortality in men with Klinefelter Syndrome: a cohort study. JNCI. 2005;97:1204–10.

Swift M, Chase C. Cancer in families with xeroderma pigmentosum. J Natl Cancer Inst. 1979;62:1415–21.

Swift M, Caldwell RJ, Chase C. Reassessment of cancer predisposition of Fanconi anemia heterozygotes. J Natl Cancer Inst. 1980;65:863–7.

Swinburn PA, Yeong ML, Lane MR, Nicholson GI, Holdaway IM. Neurofibromatosis associated with somatostionoma: report of two patients. Clin Endocrinol. 1988;28:353–9.

Syngal S, Fox EA, Eng C, Kolodner RD, Garber JE. Sensitivity and specificity of clinical criteria for hereditary non-polyposis colorectal cancer associated mutations in MSH2 and MLH1. J Med Genet. 2000;37(9):641–5.

Taalman RDFM, Hustinx TWJ, Weemaes CMR, et al. Further delineation of the Nijmegen breakage syndrome. Am J Med Genet. 1989;32:425–31.

Tabata Y, Villanueva J, Lee SM, Zhang K, Kanegane H, Miyawaki T, Sumegi J, Filipovich AH. Rapid detection of intracellular SH2D1A protein in cytotoxic lymphocytes from patients with X-linked lymphoproliferative disease and their family members. Blood. 2005;105: 3066–71.

Tabori U, Shlien A, Baskin B, Levitt S, Ray P, Alon N, Hawkins C, Bouffet E, Pienkowska M, Lafay-Cousin L, Gozali A, Zhukova N, Shane L, Gonzalez I, Finlay J, Malkin D. TP53 alterations determine clinical subgroups and survival of patients with choroid plexus tumors. J Clin Oncol. 2010;28:1995–2001.

Taconis WK. Osteosarcoma in fibrous dysplasia. Skeletal Radiol. 1988;17:163–70.

Tan MH, Mester J, Peterson C, Yang Y, Chen JL, Rybicki LA, Milas K, Pederson H, Remzi B, Orloff MS, Eng C. A clinical scoring system for selection of patients for PTEN mutation testing is proposed on the basis of a prospective study of 3042 probands. Am J Hum Genet. 2011;88:42–56.

Tan MH, Mester JL, Ngeow J, Rybicki LA, Orloff MS, Eng C (2012) Lifetime cancer risks in individuals with germline PTEN mutations. Clin Cancer Res. 2012;15;18(2):400–7.

Tartaglia M, Niemeyer CM, Fragale A, et al. Somatic mutations in PTP11 in juvenile myelomonocytic leukaemia, myelodysplastic syndromes and acute myeloid leukaemia. Nat Genet. 2003;34:148–50.

Tartaglia M, Martinelli S, Stella L, Bocchinfuso G, Flex E, Cordeddu V, Zampino G, van der Burgt I, Palleschi A, Petrucci TC, Sorcini M, Schoch C, Foa R, Emanuel PD, Gelb BD. Diversity and functional consequences of germline and somatic PTPN11 mutations in human disease. Am J Hum Genet. 2006;78:279–90.

Tatton-Brown K, Rahman N. Sotos syndrome. Eur J Hum Genet. 2007;15(3):264–71. Epub 2006 Sep 13. http://www.ncbi.nlm.nih.gov/pubmed/16969376.

Tatton-Brown K, Douglas J, Coleman K, Baujat G, Cole TR, Das S, Horn D, Hughes HE, Temple IK, Faravelli F, Waggoner D, Turkmen S, Cormier-Daire V, Irrthum A, Rahman N, Childhood Overgrowth Collaboration. Genotype-phenotype associations in Sotos syndrome: an analysis of 266 individuals with NSD1 aberrations. Am J Hum Genet. 2005;77(2):193–204. Epub 2005 Jun 7.

Tavtigian SV, Oefner PJ, Babikyan D, Hartmann A, Healey S, Le Calvez-Kelm F, Lesueur F, Byrnes GB, Chuang SC, Forey N, Feuchtinger C, Gioia L, Hall J, Hashibe M, Herte B, McKay-Chopin S, Thomas A, Vallee MP, Voegele C, Webb PM, Whiteman DC, Sangrajrang S, Hopper JL, Southey MC, Andrulis IL, John EM, Chenevix-Trench G. Rare, evolutionarily unlikely missense substitutions in ATM confer increased risk of breast cancer. Am J Hum Genet. 2009;85:427–46.

Taylor MD, Gokgoz N, Andrulis IL, Mainprize TG, Drake JM, Rutka JT. Familial posterior fossa brain tumors of infancy secondary to germline mutation of the hSNF5 gene. Am J Hum Genet. 2000;66:1403–6.

Teh BT, Farnebo F, Kristoffersson U, et al. Autosomal dominant primary hyperparathyroidism and jaw tumor syndrome associated with renal hamartomas and cystic kidney disease: linkage to 1q21–q32 and loss of the wild type allele in renal hamartomas. J Clin Endocrinol Metab. 1996;81:4204–11.

Tello R, Blickman JG, Buonomo C, Herrin J. Meta analysis of the relationship between tuberous sclerosis complex and renal cell carcinoma. Eur J Radiol. 1998;27:131–8.

ten Bensel RW, Stadlan EM, Krivit W. The development of malignancy in the course of the Aldridge syndrome. J Pediatr. 1964;68:761–7.

ten Kate GL, Kleibeuker JH, Nagengast FM, Craanen M, Cats A, Menko FH, Vasen HF. Is surveillance of the small bowel indicated for Lynch syndrome families? Gut. 2007;56(9):1198–201. Epub 2007 Apr 4.

Thakker RV. Multiple endocrine neoplasia type 1. Endocrinol Metab Clin North Am. 2000;3:541–67. Review.

Theodoratou E, Campbell H, Tenesa A, McNeill G, Cetnarskyj R, Barnetson RA, et al. Modification of the associations between lifestyle, dietary factors and colorectal cancer risk by APC variants. Carcinogenesis. 2008;29(9):1774–80.

Thomson D, Duedal S, Kirner J, et al. Cancer risks and mortality in heterozygous ATM mutation carriers. J Natl Cancer Inst. 2005;97(11):813–22.

Thorensten YR, Roxas A, Kroiss R, et al. Contributions of ATM mutations to familial breast and ovarian cancer. Cancer Res. 2003;63:3325–33.

Thrasher AJ. New insights into the biology of Wiskott-Aldrich syndrome (WAS). American Society of Hematology Education Program. SH Education Book. January 1 2009 (1):132–8.

Tinat J, Bougeard G, Baert-Desurmont S, Vasseur S, Martin C, Bouvignies E, Caron O, Bressac-de PB, Berthet P, Dugast C, Bonaiti-Pellie C, Stoppa-Lyonnet D, Frebourg T. 2009 version of the Chompret criteria for Li Fraumeni syndrome. J Clin Oncol. 2009;27:e108–9.

Tischkowitz MD, Hodgson SV. Fanconi anaemia. J Med Genet. 2003;40:1–10.

Tischkowitz M, Xia B. PALB2/FANCN: recombining cancer and Fanconi anemia. Cancer Res. 2010;70:7353–9.

Tischkowitz M, Easton DF, Ball J, Hodgson SV, Mathew CG. Cancer incidence in relatives of British Fanconi Anaemia patients. BMC Cancer. 2008;8:257.

Tolmie JL, Boyd E, Batstone P, Ferguson-Smith ME, al Roomi L, Connor JM. Siblings with chromosome mosaicism, microcephaly, and growth retardation: the phenotypic expression of a human mitotic mutant? Hum Genet. 1988;80(2):197–200.

Tomanin R, Sarto F, Mazotti D, et al. Louis–Barr syndrome: spontaneous and induced chromosomal aberrations in lymphocytes and micronuclei in lymphocytes, oral mucosa and hair root cells. Hum Genet. 1989;85:31–8.

Tops CMJ, Vasen HFA, van Berge Henegouwen G, et al. Genetic evidence that Turcot syndrome is not allelic to familial adenomatous polyposis. Am Med Genet. 1992;43:888–93.

Toro JR, Glenn G, Duray P, Darling T, Weirich G, Zbar B, Linehan M, Turner ML. Birt–Hogg–Dube syndrome: a novel marker of kidney neoplasia. Arch Dermatol. 1999;135(10):1195–202.

Traverso G, Bettegowda C, Kraus J, Speicher MR, Kinzler KW, Vogelstein B, Lengauer C. Hyper-recombination and genetic instability in BLM-deficient epithelial cells. Cancer Res. 2003;63(24):8578–81.

Treem WR. Emerging concepts in celiac disease. Curr Opin Pediatr. 2004;16:552–9.

Trimbath JD, Petersen GM, Erdman SH, Ferre M, Luce MC, Giardiello FM. Café-au-lait spots and early onset colorectal neoplasia: a variant of HNPCC? Fam Cancer. 2001a;1(2):101–5.

Trimbath JD, Peterson GM, Erdman S, et al. Café – au-lait spots and early-onset colorectal neoplasia: a variant of HNPCC? Fam. Cancer. 2001b;1:101–5.

Trofatter JA, MacCollin MM, Rutter JL, Murrell JR, Duyao MP, Parry DM, Eldridge R, Kley N, Menon AG, Pulaski K, et al. A novel moesin-, ezrin-, radixin-like gene is a candidate for the neurofibromatosis 2 tumor suppressor. Cell. 1993;72:791–800.

Tuo J, Jaruga P, Rodriguez H, Bohr VA, Dizdaroglu M. Primary fibroblasts of Cockayne syndrome patients are defective in cellular repair of 8-hydroxyguanine and 8-hydroxyadenine resulting from oxidative stress. FASEB J. 2003;17(6):668–74.

Turcot J, Despres JP, St Pierre F. Malignant tumors of the central nervous sys-tem associated with familial polyposis of the colon. Dis Colon Rectum. 1959;2:465–8.

Uchino S, Noguchi S, Nagatomo M, et al. Screening of the Men1 gene and dis-covery of germ-line and somatic mutations in apparently sporadic parathyroid tumors. Cancer Res. 2000;60:5553–7.

Umar A, Boland CR, Terdiman JP, Syngal S, de La CA, Ruschoff J, Fishel R, Lindor NM, Burgart LJ, Hamelin R, Hamilton SR, Hiatt RA, Jass J, Lindblom A, Lynch HT, Peltomaki P, Ramsey SD, Rodriguez-Bigas MA, Vasen HF, Hawk ET, Barrett JC, Freedman AN, Srivastava S. Revised Bethesda guidelines for hereditary nonpolyposis colorectal cancer (Lynch syndrome) and microsatellite instability. J Natl Cancer Inst. 2004a;96:261–8.

Umar A, Risinger JI, Hawk ET, Barrett JC. Testing guidelines for hereditary non-polyposis colorectal cancer. Nat Rev Cancer. 2004b;4(2):153–8.

Van den Bos M, Van den Hoven M, Jongejan E, et al. More differences between HNPCC-related and sporadic carcinomas from the endometrium as compared to the colon. Am J Surg Path. 2004;28:706.

van den Munckhof P, Christiaans I, Kenter SB, Baas F, Hulsebos TJM. Germline SMARCB1 mutation predisposes to multiple meningiomas and schwannomas with preferential location of cranial meningiomas at the falx cerebri. Neurogenetics. 2012;13:1–7.

van der Horst GT, et al. UVB radiation-induced cancer predisposition in Cockayne syndrome group A (Csa) mutant mice. DNA Repair (Amsterdam). 2002;1(2):143–57.

van Slegtenhorst M, de Hoogt R, Hermans C, et al. Identification of the tuberous sclerosis gene TSC1 on chromosome 9q34. Science. 1997;277:805–8.

Varga EA, Pastore M, Prior T, Herman GE, McBride KL. The prevalence of PTEN mutations in a clinical pediatric cohort with autism spectrum disorders, developmental delay and macrocephaly. Genet Med. 2009;11:111–7.

Varley JM. Germline TP53 mutations and Li–Fraumeni syndrome. Hum Mutat. 2003;21:313–20.

Varley JM, McGown G, Thorncroft M, et al. Germ-line mutations of TP53 in Li–Fraumeni families: an extended study of 39 families. Cancer Res. 1997;57:3245–52.

Varon R, Vissinga C, Platzer M, Cerosaletti KM, Chrzanowska KH, Saar K, Beckmann G, Seemanova E, Cooper PR, Nowak NJ, Stumm M, Weemaes CMR, Gatti RA, Wilson RK,

Digweed M, Rosenthal A, Sperling K, Concannon P, Reis A. Nibrin, a novel DNA double-strand break repair protein, is mutated in Nijmegen breakage syndrome. Cell. 1998;93:467–76.

Vasen HF. Review article: The Lynch syndrome (hereditary nonpolyposis colorectal cancer). Aliment Pharmacol Ther. 2007;26 (Suppl 2):113–26.

Vasen HF, den Hartog Jager FC, Menko FH, et al. Screening for hereditary non-polyposis colorectal cancer: a study of 22 kindreds in the Netherlands. Am J Med. 1989;86:278–81.

Vasen HFA, Taal FM, Nagengast G, et al. Hereditary nonpolyposis colorectal cancer: results of long-term surveillance in 50 families. Eur J Cancer. 1995;31A:1145–8.

Vasen HF, Wijnen JT, Menko FH, et al. Cancer risk in families with hereditary nonpolyposis colorectal cancer diagnosed by mutation analysis. Gastroenterology. 1996;110:1020–7.

Vasen HF, Watson P, Mecklin JP, Lynch HT. New clinical criteria for hereditary nonpolyposis colorectal cancer (HNPCC, Lynch syndrome) proposed by the International Collaborative Group on HNPCC. Gastroenterology. 1999;116:1453–6.

Vasen HF, Stormorken A, Menko FH, Nagengast FM, Kleibeuker JH, Griffioen G, Taal BG, Moller P, Wijnen JT. Msh2 mutation carriers are at higher risk of cancer than Mlh1 mutation carriers: a study of hereditary nonpolyposis colorectal cancer families. J Clin Oncol. 2001;19(20):4074–80.

Vasen HF, Möslein G, Alonso A, Bernstein I, Bertario L, Blanco I, Burn J, Capella G, Engel C, Frayling I, Friedl W, Hes FJ, Hodgson S, Mecklin JP, Møller P, Nagengast F, Parc Y, Renkonen-Sinisalo L, Sampson JR, Stormorken A, Wijnen J. Guidelines for the clinical management of Lynch syndrome (hereditary non-polyposis cancer). J Med Genet. 2007;44:353–62. doi:10.1136/jmg.2007.048991.

Vasen HF, Möslein G, Alonso A, Aretz S, Bernstein I, Bertario L, Blanco I, Bülow S, Burn J, Capella G, Colas C, Engel C, Frayling I, Friedl W, Hes FJ, Hodgson S, Järvinen H, Mecklin JP, Møller P, Myrhøi T, Nagengast FM, Parc Y, Phillips R, Clark SK, de Leon MP, Renkonen-Sinisalo L, Sampson JR, Stormorken A, Tejpar S, Thomas HJ, Wijnen J. Guidelines for the clinical management of familial adenomatous polyposis (FAP). Gut. 2008;7(4):303–7. http://www.ncbi.nlm.nih.gov/pubmed/18194984.

Vasen HF, van der Meulen-de Jong AE, de Vos Tot Nederveen Cappel WH, Oliveira J. ESMO Guidelines Working Group. Familial colorectal cancer risk: ESMO clinical recommendations. Ann Oncol. 2009;20(4):51–3. doi:10.1093/annonc/mdp127. Review.

Vasen HF, Blanco I, Aktan-Collan K, Gopie JP, Alonso A, Aretz S, Bernstein I, Bertario L, Burn J, Capella G, Colas C, Engel C, Frayling IM, Genuardi M, Heinimann K, Hes FJ, Hodgson SV, Karagiannis JA, Lalloo F, Lindblom A, Mecklin JP, Møller P, Myrhoj T, Nagengast FM, Parc Y, Ponz de Leon M, Renkonen-Sinisalo L, Sampson JR, Stormorken A, Sijmons RH, Tejpar S, Thomas HJ, Rahner N, Wijnen JT, Järvinen HJ, Möslein G. Mallorca group. Revised guidelines for the clinical management of Lynch syndrome (HNPCC): recommendations by a group of European experts. Gut. 2013;62(6):812–23. doi:10.1136/gutjnl-2012-304356. Epub 2013 Feb 13.

Vaz F, Hanenberg H, Schuster B, Barker K, Wiek C, Erven V, Neveling K, Endt D, Kesterton I, Autore F, Fraternali F, Freund M, Hartmann L, Grimwade D, Roberts RG, Schaal H, Mohammed S, Rahman N, Schindler D, Mathew CG. Mutation of the RAD51C gene in a Fanconi anemia-like disorder. Nat Genet. 2010;42:406–9.

Venkitaraman AR. Tracing the network connecting brca and fanconi anaemia proteins. Nat Rev Cancer. 2004;4:266–76.

Versteege I, Sevenet N, Lange J, Rousseau-Merck MF, Ambros P, Handgretinger R, Aurias A, Delattre O. Truncating mutations of hSNF5/INI1 in aggressive paediatric cancer. Nature. 1998;394:203–6.

Vierimaa O, Georgitsi M, Lehtonen R, Vahteristo P, Kokko A, Raitila A, Tuppurainen K, Ebeling TM, Salmela PI, Paschke R, Gundogdu S, DeMenis E, Makinen MJ, Launonen V, Karhu A, Aaltonen LA. Pituitary adenoma predisposition caused by germline mutations in the AIP gene. Science. 2006;312:1228–30.

Viljeon D, Pearn J, Beighton P. Manifestations and natural history of idiopathic hemihypertrophy: a review of eleven cases. Clin Genet. 1984;26:81–6.

Villani A, Tabori U, Schiffman J, Shlien A, Beyene J, Druker H, Novokmet A, Finlay J, Malkin D. Biochemical and imaging surveillance in germline TP53 mutation carriers with Li-Fraumeni syndrome: a prospective observational study. Lancet Oncol. 2011;12:559–67.

Viniou N, Terpos E, Rombos J, et al. Acute myeloid leukaemia in a patient with ataxia telangiectasia: a case-report and review of the literature. Leukaemia. 2001;15:1668–70.

Viskochil D, Buchberg AM, Xu G, et al. Deletions and a translocation interrupt a cloned gene at the neurofibromatosis type 1 locus. Cell. 1990;62:187–92.

Vogt S, Jones N, Christian D, Engel C, Nielsen M, Kaufmann A, Steinke V, Vasen HF, Propping P, Sampson JR, Hes FJ, Aretz S. Expanded extracolonic tumor spectrum in MUTYH-associated polyposis. Gastroenterology. 2009;137(6):1976–85.e1–10.

Volikos E, Robinson J, Aittomäki K, Mecklin JP, Järvinen H, Westerman AM, de Rooji FW, Vogel T, Moeslein G, Launonen V, Tomlinson IP, Silver AR, Aaltonen LA. LKB1 exonic and whole gene deletions are a common cause of Peutz-Jeghers syndrome. J Med Genet. 2006;43(5):e18.

Wagner A, Barrows A, Wijnen JT, van der Klift H, Franken PF, Verkuijlen P, Nakagawa H, Geugien M, Jaghmohan-Changur S, Breukel C, Meijers-Heijboer H, Morreau H, van Puijenbroek M, Burn J, Coronel S, Kinarski Y, Okimoto R, Watson P, Lynch JF, de La CA, Lynch HT, Fodde R. Molecular analysis of hereditary nonpolyposis colorectal cancer in the United States: high mutation detection rate among clinically selected families and characterization of an American founder genomic deletion of the MSH2 gene. Am J Hum Genet. 2003;72(5):1088–100.

Wagner JE, Tolar J, Levran O, Scholl T, Deffenbaugh A, Satagopan J, Ben-Porat L, Mah K, Batish SD, Kutler DI, MacMillan ML, Hanenberg H, Auerbach AD. Germline mutations in BRCA2: shared genetic susceptibility to breast cancer, early onset leukemia and Fanconi anemia. Blood. 2004;103(7):2554–9.

Waite KA, Eng C. From developmental disorder to heritable cancer: it's all in the BMP/TGF-B family. Nat Rev Genet. 2003;4:763–73.

Wallace MR, Marchuk DA, Andersen LB, et al. Type 1 neurofibromatosis gene: identification of a large transcript disrupted in three NF1 patients. Science. 1990;249:181–6.

Walsh T, Casadei S, Lee MK, Pennil CC, Nord AS, Thornton AM, Roeb W, Agnew KJ, Stray SM, Wickramanayake A, Norquist B, Pennington KP, Garcia RL, King MC, Swisher EM. Mutations in 12 genes for inherited ovarian, fallopian tube, and peritoneal carcinoma identified by massively parallel sequencing. Proc Natl Acad Sci U S A. 2011;108(44):18032–7.

Walther MM, Choyke PL, Glenn G, Lyne JC, Rayford W, Venzon D, Linehan WM. Renal cancer in families with hereditary renal cancer: prospective analysis of a tumor size threshold for renal parenchymal sparing surgery. J Urol. 1999a;161:1475–9.

Walther MM, Herring J, Enquist E, Keiser HR, Linehan WM. von Recklinghausen's disease and pheochromocytomas. J Urol. 1999b;162:1582–6.

Wang J, German J, Ashby K, French SW. Ulcerative colitis complicated by dysplasia–adenoma–carcinoma in a man with Bloom's syndrome. J Clin Gastroenterol. 1999;28(4):380–2.

Wang LL, Levy ML, Lewis RA, et al. Clinical manifestations in a cohort of 41 Rothmund–Thomson syndrome patients. Am J Med Genet. 2001;102:11–7.

Wang LL, Gannavarapu A, Kozinetz CA, et al. Association between osteosarcoma and deleterious mutations in the RECQL4 gene in Rothmund–Thomson syndrome. J Natl Cancer Inst. 2003a;95:669–74.

Wang L, Cunningham JM, Winters JL, Guenther JC, French AJ, Boardman LA, Burgart LJ, McDonnell SK, Schaid DJ, Thibodeau SN. BRAF mutations in colon cancer are not likely attributable to defective DNA mismatch repair. Cancer Res. 2003b;63:5209–12.

Warburton D, Anyane-Yeboa K, Taterka P, Yu CY, Olsen D. Mosaic variegated aneuploidy with microcephaly: a new human mitotic mutant? Ann Genet. 1991;34(3–4):287–92.

Washecka R, Hanna M. Malignant renal tumors in tuberous sclerosis. Urology. 1991;37:340–3.

Watson P, Lynch HT. Cancer risk in mismatch repair gene mutation carriers. Fam Cancer. 2001;1:57–60.

Watson P, Lin KM, Rodruigez-Bigas MA, et al. Colorectal carcinoma survival among hereditary nonpolyposis colorectal cancer family members. Cancer. 1998;83:259–66.

Watson P, Vasen HF, Mecklin JP, et al. The risk of extra-colonic, extra-endometrial cancer in the Lynch syndrome. Int J Cancer. 2008;123(2):444–9.

Wautot V, Vercherat C, Lespinasse J, et al. Germline mutation profile of MEN1 in multiple endocrine neoplasia type 1: search for correlation between phenotype and the functional domains of the MEN1 protein. Hum Mutat. 2002;20:35–47.

Weber HC, Venzon DJ, Lin JT, et al. Determinants of metastatic rate and survival in patients with Zollinger–Ellison syndrome: a prospective long-term study. Gastroenterology. 1995;108:1637–49.

Weinstein LS, Shenker A, Geiman V, Merino MJ, Friedman E, Spiegel AM. Activating mutations of the stimulatory G protein in the McCune–Albright syndrome. New Engl J Med. 1991;325:1688–95.

Weinstein LS, Chen M, Liu J. Gs(alpha) mutations and imprinting defects in human disease. Ann NY Acad Sci. 2002;968:173–97.

Weirich G, Glenn G, Junker K, et al. Familial renal oncocytoma: clinicopatho-logical study of 5 families. J Urol. 1998;160:335–40.

Weksberg R, Smith AC, Squire J, Sadowski P. Beckwith–Wiedemann syndrome demonstrates a role for epigenetic control of normal development. Hum Mol Genet. 2003;12(Spec No 1):R61–8.

Wells SA, Baylin SB, Linehan WM, Farrell RE, Cox EB, Cooper CW. Provocative agents and the diagnosis of medullary carcinoma of the thyroid gland. Ann Surg. 1978;188:139–41.

Wells SA, Chi DD, Toshima D, et al. Predictive DNA testing and prophylactic thyroidectomy in patients at risk for multiple endocrine neoplasia type 2A. Ann Surg. 1994;200:237–50.

Whiteside D, McLeod R, Graham G, Steckley JL, Booth K, Somerville MJ, Andrew SE. A homozygous germ-line mutation in the human MSH2 gene predisposes to hematological malignancy and multiple cafe-au-lait spots. Cancer Res. 2002;62(2):359–62.

Wicking C, Shanlay S, Smyth I, Gillies S, Negus K, Graham S, Suthers G, Haites N, Edwards M, Wainwright B, Chenevix-Trench G. Most germ-line mutations in the nevoid basal cell carcinoma syndrome lead to a premature termination of the PATCHED protein, and no genotype-phenotype correlations are evident. Am J Hum Genet. 1997;60(1):21–6.

Wiedemann H-R. Tumors and hemihypertrophy associated with Wiedemann–Beckwith syndrome. Eur J Pediatr. 1983;141:129.

Wiedemann HR, Burgio GR, Aldenhoff P, Kunze J, Kaufmann HJ, Schirg E. The proteus syndrome. Partial gigantism of the hands and/or feet, nevi, hemihypertrophy, subcutaneous tumors, macrocephaly or other skull anomalies and possible accelerated growth and visceral affections. Eur J Pediatr. 1983;140:5–12.

Wiench M, Wygoda Z, Gubala E, et al. Estimation of risk of inherited medullary thyroid carcinoma in apparent sporadic patients. J Clin Oncol. 2001;19:1374–80.

Wijnen J, Khan PM, Vasen H, et al. Hereditary nonpolyposis colorectal cancer families not complying with the Amsterdam criteria show extremely low frequency of mismatch-repair gene mutations. Am J Hum Genet. 1997;61:329–35.

Wijnen J, et al. Clinical findings with implications for genetic testing in families with clustering of colorectal cancer. New Engl J Med. 1998;339:511–8.

Wijnen J, de Leew W, Nvasen H, et al. Familial endometrial cancer in female carriers of MSH6 germline mutations. Nat Genet. 1999;23:142–4.

Wilson BG, Roberts CW. SWI/SNF nucleosome remodellers and cancer. Nat Rev Cancer. 2011;11:481–92.

Wilson JR, Bateman AC, Hanson H, An Q, Evans G, Rahman N, Jones JL, Eccles DM. A novel HER2-positive breast cancer phenotype arising from germline TP53 mutations. J Med Genet. 2010;47:771–4.

Wimmer K, Etzler J. Constitutional mismatch repair-deficiency syndrome: have we so far seen only the tip of an iceberg? Hum Genet. 2008;124(2):105–22.

Win AK, Young JP, Lindor NM, et al. Colorectal and other cancer risks for carriers and noncarriers from families with a DNA mismatch repair gene mutation: a prospective cohort study. J Clin Oncol. 2012;30(9):958–64.

Wohlik N, Cote GJ, Bugalho MMJ, et al. Relevance of RET proto-oncogene mutations in sporadic medullary thyroid carcinoma. J Clin Endocrinol Metab. 1996;81:3740–5.

Wood NJ, Duffy SR. The outcome of endometrial carcinoma surveillance by ultrasound scan in women at risk of hereditary nonpolyposis colorectal carcinoma and familial colorectal carcinoma. Am Cancer Soc. 2003;1772:3.

Woods WG, Roloff JS, Lukens JN, Krivit W. The occurrence of leukemia in patients with the Shwachman syndrome. J Pediatr. 1981;90:425–9.

Woodward ER, Eng C, McMahon R, Voutilainen R, Affara NA, Ponder BAJ, Maher ER. Genetic predisposition to pheochromocytoma: analysis of candidate genes GDNF, RET and VHL. Hum Mol Genet. 1997;6:1051–6.

Woodward ER, Ricketts C, Killick P, Gad S, Morris MR, Kavalier F, Hodgson SV, Giraud S, Bressac-de Paillerets B, Chapman C, Escudier B, Latif F, Richard S, Maher ER. Familial non-VHL clear cell (conventional) renal cell carcinoma: clinical features, segregation analysis, and mutation analysis of FLCN. Clin Cancer Res. 2008;14(18):5925–30.

Xia B, Dorsman JC, Ameziane N, de Vries Y, Rooimans MA, Sheng Q, Pals G, Errami A, Gluckman E, Llera J, Wang W, Livingston DM, Joenje H, De Winter JP. Fanconi anemia is associated with a defect in the BRCA2 partner PALB2. Nat Genet. 2007;39:159–61.

Xia J, Bolyard AA, Rodger E, Stein S, Aprikyan AA, Dale DC, Link DC. Prevalence of mutations in ELANE, GFI1, HAX1, SBDS, WAS and G6PC3 in patients with severe congenital neutropenia. Br J Haematol. 2009;147:535–42.

Yang YJ, Han JW, Youn HD, Cho EJ. The tumor suppressor, parafibromin, mediates histone H3 K9 methylation for cyclin D1 repression. Nucl Acid Res. 2010;38:382–90.

Yart A, Gstaiger M, Wirbelauer C, Pecnik M, Anastasiou D, Hess D, Krek W. The HRPT2 tumor suppressor gene product parafibromin associates with human PAF1 and RNA polymerase II. Mol Cell Biol. 2005;25:5052–60.

Yee A, De Ravin SS, Elliott E, Ziegler JB. Severe combined immunodeficiency: a national surveillance study. Pediatr Allergy Immunol. 2008;19:298–302.

Yoneda Y, Saitsu H, Touyama M, Makita Y, Miyamoto A, Hamada K, Kurotaki N, Tomita H, Nishiyama K, Tsurusaki Y, Doi H, Miyake N, Ogata K, Naritomi K, Matsumoto N. Missense mutations in the DNA-binding/dimerization domain of NFIX cause Sotos-like features. J Hum Genet. 2012;57:207–11.

Yong D, Lim JG, Choi JR, et al. A case of Klinefelter syndrome with retroperitoneal teratoma. Yonsei Med J. 2000;41:136–9.

Yu CE, Oshima J, Fu YH, et al. Positional cloning of the Werner's syndrome gene. Science. 1996;272:258–62.

Zacharin M, Bajpai A, Chow CW, Catto-Smith A, Stratakis C, Wong MW, Scott R. Gastrointestinal polyps in McCune Albright syndrome. J Med Genet. 2011;48(7):458–61.

Zbar B, Alvord WG, Glenn G, Turner M, Pavlovich CP, Schmidt L, Walther M, Choyke P, Weirich G, Hewitt SM, Duray P, Gabril F, Greenberg C, Merino MJ, Toro J, Linehan WM. Risk of renal and colonic neoplasms and spontaneous pneumothorax in the Birt–Hogg–Dube syndrome. Cancer Epidemiol Biomark Prev. 2002;11(4):393–400.

Zbuk K, Eng C. Cancer phenomics: RET and PTEN as illustrative models. Nat Rev Cancer. 2007;7:35–45.

Zhou XP, Marsh DJ, Hampel H, Mulliken JB, Gimm O, Eng C. Germline and germline mosaic mutations associated with a Proteus-like syndrome of hemihypertrophy, lower limb asymmetry, arteriovenous malformations and lipomatosis. Hum Mol Genet. 2000;9:765–8.

Zhou XP, Hampel H, Thiele H, et al. Association of germline mutation in the *PTEN* tumor suppressor gene and a subset of Proteus sand Proteus-like syndromes. Lancet. 2001;358:210–1.

Zhou XP, Marsh DJ, Morrison CD, Maxwell M, Reifenberger G, Eng C. Germline and somatic PTEN mutations and decreased expression of PTEN protein and dysfunction of the PI3K/Akt pathway in Lhermitte-Duclos disease. Am J Hum Genet. 2003a;73:1191–8.

Zhou XP, Waite KA, Pilarski R, et al. Germline PTEN promoter mutations and deletions in Cowden/Bannayan–Riley–Ruvalcaba syndrome result in aberrant PTEN protein and dysregulation of the phosphoinositol-3-kinase/Akt pathway. Am J Hum Genet. 2003b;73:404–11.

Appendix
Genetic Differential Diagnoses by Organ System Neoplasms

Organ or neoplasia type	Histological type	Genetic differential diagnosis	Gene (if known)
Adrenal	Adrenocortical neoplasia	Li–Fraumeni syndrome (Latronico et al. 2001; Sameshima et al. 1992; Wagner et al. 1994; Varley et al. 1999; Hisada et al. 1998)	TP53
		Beckwith–Wiedemann syndrome	CDKN1C (p57KIP2), NSD1
		Carney complex (Stratakis et al. 2001; Watson et al. 2000; Ohara et al. 1993; Handley et al. 1992; Wallace et al. 1991; Cheung and Thompson 1989; Carney et al. 1985; Kirschner et al. 2000a)	PRKAR1A
		Multiple endocrine neoplasia type 1	MEN1
		McCune–Albright syndrome	GNAS1 (not germline)
	Adrenocortical hyperplasia	Site-specific adrenocortical hyperplasia	PDE11A
	Adrenocortical carcinoma	Li–Fraumeni syndrome	TP53
	Medulla– pheochromo- cytoma	von Hippel–Lindau disease (Neumann et al. 2002; Richard et al. 1994; Chen et al. 1995; Crossey et al. 1995; Gross et al. 1996; Glavac et al. 1996; Garcia et al. 1997; Atuk et al. 1998; Friedrich 2001; Eng et al. 1996)	VHL

(continued)

S.V. Hodgson et al., *A Practical Guide to Human Cancer Genetics,*
DOI 10.1007/978-1-4471-2375-0, © Springer-Verlag London 2014

Appendix (continued)

Organ or neoplasia type	Histological type	Genetic differential diagnosis	Gene (if known)
		Pheochromocytoma–paraganglioma syndrome (Neumann et al. 2002; Astuti et al. 2001; Gimm et al. 2000)	*SDHA, SDHB, SDHC, SDHD, SDHAF2, TMEM127, MAX*
		Multiple endocrine neoplasia (MEN) type 2 (Langer et al. 2002; Dotzenrath et al. 2001; Skogseid et al. 1995; Beckers et al. 1992)	*RET*
		Neurofibromatosis type 1 (Lima and Smith 1971; Takayama et al. 2001; Walther et al. 1999; Zoller et al. 1997; Sakaguchi et al. 1996; Ogawa et al. 1994; Chetty and Duhig 1993; Xu et al. 1992; Samuelsson and Samuelsson 1989; Kalff et al. 1982; Samuelsson and Axelsson 1981; Knight et al. 1973; Anneroth and Heimdahl 1978)	*NF1*
Bladder		Werner syndrome (Monnat 2002)	*WRN*
		Costello syndrome	*HRAS*
Brain	Glioma/ glioblastoma	Li–Fraumeni syndrome (Sameshima et al. 1992; Wagner et al. 1994; Varley et al. 1999; Hisada et al. 1998; Birch et al. 1994; Kleihues et al. 1997; Kyritsis et al. 1994; Li et al. 1995; Nichols et al. 2001; Vital et al. 1998; Zhou et al. 1999)	*TP53*
		Turcot syndrome (HNPCC) (Tamiya et al. 2000; Chan et al. 1999; Taylor et al. 1999; Leung et al. 1998; Van Meir 1998; Buerstedde et al. 1995; Hamilton et al. 1995)	*MLH1, MSH2, PMS1, PMS2*
		Hereditary retinoblastoma (Elias et al. 2001; Louis and von Deimling 1995; Taylor et al. 2000a)	*RB1*
	Optic glioma	Neurofibromatosis type 1 (Cnossen et al. 1997, 1998; Bilaniuk et al. 1997; McGaughran et al. 1999; Listernick et al. 1999; Faravelli et al. 1999; North 1998; Shah et al. 2000; Kornreich et al. 2001; Singhal et al. 2002)	*NF1*
	Trilateral retinoblastoma	Hereditary retinoblastoma (Elias et al. 2001; Louis and von Deimling 1995; Taylor et al. 2000a; Amoaku et al. 1996; Bader et al. 1980; Blach et al. 1994; De Potter et al. 1994; Holladay et al. 1991; Moll et al. 1997; Pesin and Shields 1989)	*RB1*

Appendix (continued)

Organ or neoplasia type	Histological type	Genetic differential diagnosis	Gene (if known)
	Astrocytoma	Neurofibromatosis type 1 (Bilaniuk et al. 1997; Kubo et al. 1996; Ito et al. 1997; Vinchon et al. 2000; Li et al. 2001; Perry et al. 2001; Gutmann et al. 2002)	*NF1*
		Tuberous sclerosis complex (O'Callaghan et al. 2000; Nabbout et al. 1999; Nishio et al. 2001; Torres et al. 1998; Turgut et al. 1996; Roszkowski et al. 1995)	*TSC1, TSC2*
		Melanoma-astrocytoma syndrome (Randerson-Moor et al. 2001; Bahuau et al. 1998; Greene 1999)	*CDKN2A/p16, p14ARF*
	Medulloblastoma/ NET	Turcot syndrome (FAP) (Van Meir 1998; Hamilton et al. 1995; Cohen 1982; Jarvis et al. 1988; Todd et al. 1981; Mastronardi et al. 1991)	*APC*
		Nevoid basal cell carcinoma syndrome (Neblett et al. 1971; Naguib et al. 1982; Lacombe et al. 1990; Kimonis et al. 1997; Taylor et al. 2002; Wolter et al. 1997; Minami et al. 2001)	*PTC*
		Rhabdoid predisposition syndrome (Sevenet et al. 1999)	*SNF5/INI1*
	Neurofibromas	Neurofibromatosis type 1 (Zoller et al. 1997; Carey et al. 1979; Riccardi et al. 1979; Sorensen et al. 1986; Szudek et al. 2000; North 2000; Rasmussen and Friedman 2000)	*NF1*
	Vestibular schwannomas	Neurofibromatosis type 2 (Parry et al. 1996; Kluwe et al. 1996; Welling 1998; Evans et al. 1998, 2000; Evans 1999; Baser et al. 2002)	*NF2*
	Meningioma	Neurofibromatosis type 2 (Evans 1999; Stemmer-Rachamimov et al. 1997; Antinheimo et al. 1997, 2000; Turgut et al. 1997; Caldemeyer and Mirowski 2001)	*NF2*
		Neurofibromatosis type 1 (Evans 1999)	*NF1*
		Cowden syndrome (Eng 2000; Starink et al. 1986; Lyons et al. 1993; Lindboe et al. 1995; Murata et al. 1999)	*PTEN*
		Werner syndrome (Monnat 2002)	*WRN*
	Ependymoma	Neurofibromatosis type 2 (Wertelecki et al. 1988)	*NF2*

(continued)

Appendix (continued)

Organ or neoplasia type	Histological type	Genetic differential diagnosis	Gene (if known)
	Hemangioma, hemangioblastoma	von Hippel–Lindau syndrome (Couch et al. 2000; Webster et al. 1998)	*VHL*
	Rhabdoid tumor/ atypical teratoid tumor	Rhabdoid predisposition syndrome (Sevenet et al. 1999; Taylor et al. 2000b)	*SNF5/INI1*
	Cerebellum, dysplastic gangliocytoma (Lhermitte– Duclos disease)	Cowden syndrome (Eng 2000; Starink et al. 1986; Lindboe et al. 1995; Murata et al. 1999; Nowak and Trost 2002; Nowak et al. 2001; Chapman et al. 1998; Thomas and Lewis 1995; Padberg et al. 1991; Robinson and Cohen 2000)	*PTEN, SDHB, SDH; KLLN* (epimutation)
	Choroid plexus tumors	Li–Fraumeni syndrome (Garber et al. 1990)	*TP53*
Breast, female	Carcinoma	Hereditary breast–ovarian cancer syndrome (HBOC) (Gayther et al. 1995, 1997; Couch et al. 1996; Neuhausen et al. 1996; Lancaster et al. 1996; Caligo et al. 1996; Agnarsson et al. 1998; Ligtenberg et al. 1999)	*BRCA1, BRCA2*
		Cowden syndrome/BRRS (Eng 2000; Starink et al. 1986; Schrager et al. 1998; Tsubosa et al. 1998; Marsh et al. 1998, 1999)	*PTEN, SDHB, SDH; KLLN* (epimutation)
		Li–Fraumeni syndrome (Hisada et al. 1998; Birch et al. 1994, 1998, 2001; Nichols et al. 2001; Bang et al. 1995; Varley et al. 1995; Huusko et al. 1999; Hung et al. 1999)	*TP53*
		Peutz–Jeghers syndrome (Boardman et al. 1998; Burdick and Prior 1982)	*LKB1/STK11*
		Ataxia-telangiectasia heterozygotes (Lavin 1998; Janin et al. 1999; Larson et al. 1997; Broeks et al. 2000; Sommer et al. 2002)	*ATM*
		Werner syndrome (Monnat 2002)	*WRN*
Breast, male	Carcinoma	HBOC (Schubert et al. 1997; Hakansson et al. 1997; Wolpert et al. 2000; Lobaccaro et al. 1993)	*BRCA2 (BRCA1)*
		Cowden syndrome (Eng 2000; Starink et al. 1986; Fackenthal et al. 2001)	*PTEN*
		Reifenstein syndrome (Wooster et al. 1992)	*AR*

Appendix (continued)

Organ or neoplasia type	Histological type	Genetic differential diagnosis	Gene (if known)
		Klinefelter syndrome (van Geel et al. 1985; Hultborn et al. 1997)	XXY
Colorectum	Adenocarcinoma	Hereditary non-polyposis colorectal cancer (HNPCC) syndrome (Lynch et al. 1985a; Lynch and Lynch 1995; Leach et al. 1993; Papadopoulos et al. 1994; Aaltonen and Peltomaki 1994; Froggatt et al. 1995; Akiyama et al. 1997; Berends et al. 2002)	*MLH1, MSH2, MSH6, PMS1, PMS2*
		Familial adenomatous polyposis (FAP) syndrome (Moisio et al. 2002; Presciuttini et al. 1994; Fodde and Khan 1995; Bunyan et al. 1995; Friedl et al. 1996; Armstrong et al. 1997; Eccles et al. 1997; Soravia et al. 1998; Heinimann et al. 1998)	*APC*
		Juvenile polyposis syndrome *SMAD4* (Zhou et al. 2001; Woodford-Richens et al. 2000, 2001; Howe et al. 2002)	*MADH4, BMPR1A*
		BMPR1A (Zhou et al. 2001; Friedl et al. 2002; Howe et al. 2001)	
		Peutz–Jeghers syndrome (Boardman et al. 1998; Burdick and Prior 1982; Giardiello et al. 1987; Linos et al. 1981)	*LKB1/STK11*
		Hereditary mixed polyposis syndrome(s) (Whitelaw et al. 1997; Thomas et al. 1996)	
		Autosomal recessive polyposis–colon cancer syndrome	*MYH*
		Birt–Hogg–Dubé syndrome	*BHD*
		Cowden syndrome	*PTEN*
	Polyp – adenoma	HNPCC (Watanabe et al. 1996; Watne 1997; Souza 2001; Cao et al. 2002)	*MLH1, MSH2, MSH6, PMS1, PMS2*
		FAP (Soravia et al. 1998; Wu et al. 1998; Brensinger et al. 1998; Wallis et al. 1999; Gebert et al. 1999; Giarola et al. 1999)	*APC*
		Hereditary mixed polyposis syndrome(s) (Whitelaw et al. 1997)	*PTEN*, Others
		Autosomal recessive polyposis-colon cancer syndrome (MYH-associated polyposis syndrome)	*MYH*

(continued)

Appendix (continued)

Organ or neoplasia type	Histological type	Genetic differential diagnosis	Gene (if known)
	Polyp – hamartoma	Juvenile polyposis syndrome (Zhou et al. 2001; Friedl et al. 2002; Entius et al. 1999; Sachatello and Griffen 1975; Howe et al. 1998a; Houlston et al. 1998)	MADH4, BMPR1A
		Peutz–Jeghers syndrome (Hanna et al. 1994)	LKB1/STK11
		Cowden syndrome/BRRS (Eng 2000; Starink et al. 1986; Marsh et al. 1998; Hanna et al. 1994; Hizawa et al. 1994)	PTEN
		Hereditary mixed polyposis syndrome(s) (Whitelaw et al. 1997; Thomas et al. 1996)	
		Tuberous sclerosis complex (Devroede et al. 1988)	TSC1, TSC2
		Gorlin syndrome	PTCH1
		Birt–Hogg–Dubé syndrome	BHD
Esophagus	Adenocarcinoma	Familial barrett esophagus–adenocarcinoma (Romero et al. 1997)	MSR1
	Squamous cell carcinoma	Familial esophageal squamous cell cancer (Hemminki and Jiang 2002)	
		Fanconi anemia (Linares et al. 1991; Gendal et al. 1988; Kozarek and Sanowski 1981)	FANC-X
		Tylosis and esophageal cancer (TOC) (Risk et al. 1999; Marger and Marger 1993; Ellis et al. 1994; Stevens et al. 1996; Maillefer and Greydanus 1999)	
Eye	Retinoblastoma, retinoma	Hereditary retinoblastoma (Cavenee et al. 1985; Goddard et al. 1990; Kratzke et al. 1994; Cowell and Cragg 1996; Harbour 1998; Lohmann 1999; Alonso et al. 2001)	RB1
	Angioma, hemangioblas-toma	von Hippel–Lindau syndrome (Glavac et al. 1996; Webster et al. 1998; Hes et al. 2000; Zbar et al. 1999)	VHL
	Melanoma	Li–Fraumeni syndrome (Hisada et al. 1998; Jay and McCartney 1993)	TP53
		Ocular melanocytosis (Singh et al. 1996, 1998)	
		Familial atypical mole melanoma (FAMMM)/P16 (Singh et al. 1995)	P16
		HBOC (Iscovich et al. 2002)	BRCA2

Appendix (continued)

Organ or neoplasia type	Histological type	Genetic differential diagnosis	Gene (if known)
		Site-specific/early onset, with or without cutaneous melanoma	*BAP1*
	Squamous cell carcinoma, anterior eye	Xeroderma pigmentosum (Goyal et al. 1994; Hertle et al. 1991; Sarma et al. 1973)	*XP-x*
	Hamartoma	Tuberous sclerosis complex (Gelisken et al. 1990; Kiribuchi et al. 1986)	*TSC1, TSC2*
		FAP (CHRPE)	*APC*
Head and neck	Squamous cell carcinomas	Fanconi anemia (Oksuzoglu and Yalcin 2002; Somers et al. 1995; Lustig et al. 1995; Kaplan et al. 1985)	*FANC-X*
		Bloom syndrome (Berkower and Biller 1988)	*BLM*
		Dyskeratosis syndrome (Drachtman and Alter 1995)	*TERC* (AD), *DKC1* (X-linked)
		Xeroderma pigmentosum (Kraemer et al. 1987; Patton and Valdez 1991; Shen et al. 2001)	*XP-x*
	Melanoma: nasal mucosa	Werner syndrome (Monnat 2002; Goto et al. 1996)	*WRN*
	Sebaceous carcinoma	Muir–Torre syndrome (40% eyelid) (Lynch et al. 1985b; Burgdorf et al. 1986; Cohen et al. 1995; Serleth and Kisken 1998; Coldron and Reid 2001)	*MSH2, MLH1*
Heart	Myxoma	Carney complex (Carney et al. 1985, 1986; Stratakis et al. 1996; Kirschner et al. 2000b; Edwards et al. 2002)	*PRKAR1A*
	Rhabdomyoma	Tuberous sclerosis complex (Nir et al. 1995; See et al. 1999; Jozwiak et al. 1994; Webb and Osborne 1992; Watson 1991)	*TSC1, TSC2*
Hematological	Leukemia, acute	Li–Fraumeni syndrome (Hisada et al. 1998; Birch et al. 1994; Kleihues et al. 1997; Imamura et al. 1994)	*TP53*
		Bloom syndrome (Passarge 1991; Gretzula et al. 1987; German et al. 1977; Poppe et al. 2001)	*BLM*
	Leukemia, acute myeloid	Fanconi anemia (Auerbach and Allen 1991; Faivre et al. 2000)	*FANC-x*
		Emberger syndrome[a]	*GATA2*
		Familial thrombocytopenia and predisposition to AML (Dowton et al. 1985; Arepally et al. 1998; Song et al. 1999; Michaud et al. 2002)	*RUNX1/AML1*

(continued)

Appendix (continued)

Organ or neoplasia type	Histological type	Genetic differential diagnosis	Gene (if known)
		Amegakaryocytic thrombocytopenia (Tonelli et al. 2000; Germeshausen et al. 2001)	*C-MPL*
		Diamond-Blackfan anemia (Janov et al. 1996; Krijanovski and Sieff 1997; Freedman 2000)	*RPS19*
		Shwachman–Diamond syndrome (Cipolli 2001; Smith et al. 1996; Woods et al. 1981)	*SBDS*
		Severe congenital neutropenia/ Kostmann syndrome (Li and Horwitz 2001; Welte and Dale 1996)	*ELA2, GFI1*
		Werner syndrome (Monnat 2002; Tao et al. 1971)	*WRN*
	Leukemia, acute lymphoid, PLL	Ataxia telangiectasia (Peterson et al. 1992; Taylor et al. 1996; Boultwood 2001)	*ATM*
		Nijmegen breakage syndrome (Varon et al. 2001)	*NBS1*
	Leukemia, juvenile chronic myeloid	Neurofibromatosis type 1 (Clark and Hutter 1982; Zvulunov et al. 1995; Hasle et al. 1995; Jang et al. 1999)	*NF1*
	Lymphoma, non-Hodgkin	Ataxia telangiectasia (Taylor et al. 1996; Stankovic et al. 1998; Murphy et al. 1999; Seidemann et al. 2000)	*ATM*
		Nijmegen breakage syndrome (Weemaes et al. 1994; Seidemann et al. 1999)	*NBS1*
		Bloom syndrome (Passarge 1991; Gretzula et al. 1987; Kaneko et al. 1997)	*BLM*
		Autoimmune lymphoproliferative syndrome/Canale–Smith syndrome (Peters et al. 1999; Straus et al. 1997, 2001; Vaishnaw et al. 1999; Jackson and Puck 1999; Rieux-Laucat et al. 1999; Drappa et al. 1996)	*FAS, FASL, CASP10*
		Chediak–Higashi syndrome (Argyle et al. 1982; Dent et al. 1966)	*LYST*
		Wiskott–Aldrich syndrome (Cotelingam et al. 1985)	*WAS*
		Duncan disease (X-linked lymphoproliferative disease) (Purtilo et al. 1977, 1982; Hamilton et al. 1980; Purtilo 1981)	*SH2D1A*

Appendix (continued)

Organ or neoplasia type	Histological type	Genetic differential diagnosis	Gene (if known)
	Hodgkin disease	Autoimmune lymphoproliferative syndrome/Canale–Smith syndrome (Peters et al. 1999; Straus et al. 1997, 2001; Rieux-Laucat et al. 1999; Drappa et al. 1996)	*FAS, FASL, CASP10*
		Ataxia telangiectasia (Boultwood 2001; Murphy et al. 1999; Seidemann et al. 2000; Harris and Seeler 1973; Frizzera et al. 1980; Hecht and Hecht 1990; Weyl Ben Arush et al. 1995; Olsen et al. 2001)	*ATM*
		Wiskott–Aldrich syndrome (Cotelingam et al. 1985; Frizzera et al. 1980)	*WAS*
		Nijmegen breakage syndrome (Seidemann et al. 2000)	*NBS*
		Emberger syndrome	*GATA2*
Intestine, small	Carcinoma (ampullary)	FAP (Ohsato et al. 1977; Norton and Gostout 1998; Sellner 1990)	*APC*
	Carcinoma (any location)	HNPCC (Watson and Lynch 1993; Bisgaard et al. 2002)	*MLH1, MSH2, MSH6, PMS1, PMS2*
		Peutz–Jeghers syndrome (Seidemann et al. 2000; Sellner 1990; Buckley et al. 1997; Luk 1995)	*LKB1/STK11*
		Juvenile polyposis syndrome (Luk 1995)	*MADH4, BMPR1A*
	Stromal tumor (GIST)	Hereditary gastrointestinal stromal tumor (Hirota et al. 2002; Handra-Luca et al. 2001; Maeyama et al. 2001; Isozaki et al. 2000; Nishida et al. 1998)	*KIT, PDGFA; SDHB/D* (in Carney Dyad)
	Carcinoid tumor	Neurofibromatosis type 1 (Chen et al. 1993; Benharroch et al. 1992; Stamm et al. 1986)	*NF1*
		MEN 1 (Carty et al. 1998; Bordi et al. 1997)	*MEN1*
Kidney	Renal cell carcinoma, clear cell	von Hippel–Lindau syndrome (Friedrich 2001; Maher et al. 1990, 1995, 1996; Walker 1998; Richards et al. 1998)	*VHL*
		Birt–Hogg–Dubé syndrome (Nickerson et al. 2002; Zbar et al. 2002; Toro et al. 1999)	*BHD*

(continued)

Appendix (continued)

Organ or neoplasia type	Histological type	Genetic differential diagnosis	Gene (if known)
		Cowden syndrome (Eng 2000; Starink et al. 1986; Haibach et al. 1992)	*PTEN, SDHB, SDHD; KLLN* (epimutation)
		Hereditary clear cell renal carcinoma (Woodward et al. 2000; Bodmer et al. 2002; Podolski et al. 2001; Druck et al. 2001; Eleveld et al. 2001; Kanayama et al. 2001)	
		Werner syndrome (Monnat 2002)	*WRN*
	Renal cell carcinoma, papillary	Familial papillary renal cell cancer (Malchoff et al. 2000; Olivero et al. 1999; Schmidt et al. 1997)	*MET*
		Multiple leiomyomatosis syndrome (Kiuru et al. 2001; Tomlinson et al. 2002)	*FH*
		Tuberous sclerosis complex (Sampson 1996; Al-Saleem et al. 1998)	*TSC1, TSC2*
		Hyperparathyroidism–jaw tumor syndrome (Haven et al. 2000)	*HRPT2*
		Birt–Hogg–Dube syndrome (Nickerson et al. 2002; Zbar et al. 2002; Toro et al. 1999; Khoo et al. 2001)	*BHD*
		Cowden syndrome	*PTEN, SDHB, SDHD; KLLN* (epimutation)
	Renal pelvis, transitional cell	HNPCC (Muir–Torre syndrome) (Lynch and Lynch 1994, 1995; Honchel et al. 1994)	*MSH2, MLH1*
	Angiomyolipoma	Tuberous sclerosis complex (Sampson 1996; Schillinger and Montagnac 1996; O'Hagan et al. 1996)	*TSC1, TSC2*
	Oncocytoma	Tuberous sclerosis complex (O'Hagan et al. 1996; Green 1987; Ruckle et al. 1993)	*TSC1, TSC2*
		Birt–Hogg–Dube (Nickerson et al. 2002)	*BHD*
		Cowden syndrome	*PTEN, SDHB, SDHD; KLLN* (epimutation)
	Wilms tumor	Hereditary Wilms tumor syndrome (Kaplinsky et al. 1996; Pelletier et al. 1991a; Little and Wells 1997; Dome and Coppes 2002)	*WT1*
		WAGR (Koufos et al. 1989; Grundy et al. 1995)	*WT1*, contiguous gene deletions
		Beckwith–Wiedemann syndrome (Koufos et al. 1989; Grundy et al. 1995; Cohen and Kurzrock 1995)	*CDKN1C* (*p57KIP2*), *NSD1*

Appendix (continued)

Organ or neoplasia type	Histological type	Genetic differential diagnosis	Gene (if known)
		Hyperparathyroidism–jaw tumor syndrome (Haven et al. 2000; Cavaco et al. 2001; Hobbs et al. 1999; Szabo et al. 1995)	*HRPT2*
		Denys–Drash syndrome (Little and Wells 1997; Pelletier et al. 1991b; Schumacher et al. 1998; Heathcott et al. 2002)	*WT1*
	Rhabdoid tumor/ atypical teratoid tumor	Rhabdoid predisposition syndrome (Sevenet et al. 1999)	*SNF5/INI1*
	Neuroblastoma	Site-specific neuroblastoma	*ALK, PHOX2B*
		Costello syndrome	*HRAS*
Liver	Hepatoblastoma	FAP (Garber et al. 1988; Hughes and Michels 1992; Giardiello et al. 1996; Gruner et al. 1998; Lynch et al. 2001)	*APC*
		Beckwith–Wiedemann syndrome (DeBaun and Tucker 1998)	*CDKN1C (p57KIP2), NSD1*
		Werner syndrome (Monnat 2002)	*WRN*
	Adenoma/ carcinoma	Fanconi anemia (Alter 1996)	*FANC-x*
		Beckwith–Wiedemann syndrome (DeBaun and Tucker 1998)	*CDKN1C (p57KIP2), NSD1*
Ovary	Carcinoma	HBOC (Meindl 2002; Sarantaus et al. 2001; Schoumacher et al. 2001; Pharoah et al. 1999)	*BRCA1, BRCA2*
		HNPCC (Brown et al. 2001; Watson et al. 2001; Cohn et al. 2000; Aarnio et al. 1999)	*MLH1, MSH2, MSH6, PMS1, PMS2*
	Germ cell	Dysgenetic gonads (XY karyotype) (Liu et al. 1995; Soh et al. 1992; Muller et al. 1992; Damjanov and Klauber 1980; Cussen and MacMahon 1979; Schellhas 1974; Teter 1970)	*DHH*
	Granulosa cell	Peutz–Jeghers syndrome (Rodu and Martinez 1984; Young et al. 1984; Clement et al. 1979; Christian 1971)	*LKB1/STK11*
		Ollier disease (Young et al. 1984; Asirvatham et al. 1991; Velasco-Oses et al. 1988)	*PTHR1*

(continued)

Appendix (continued)

Organ or neoplasia type	Histological type	Genetic differential diagnosis	Gene (if known)
		Maffucci syndrome (Young et al. 1984; Tanaka et al. 1992)	*PTHR1*
	Sertoli-Leydig cell	DICER1 syndrome	*DICER1*
Pancreas	Carcinoma	HNPCC (Yamamoto et al. 2001; Wei et al. 2002; Park et al. 1999)	*MLH1, MSH2, MSH6, PMS1, PMS2*
		Familial site-specific pancreatic cancer (Gates and Holladay 2002)	*BRCA2*
		Hereditary pancreatitis (Hengstler et al. 2000; O'Reilly and Kingsnorth 2000; Lowenfels et al. 1997)	*CFTR, SPINK, TRYP*
		HBOC (Murphy et al. 2002; Berman et al. 1996)	*BRCA2*
		Hereditary melanoma/FAMMM (Lynch et al. 2002; Vasen et al. 2000; Gruis et al. 1995; Lynch and Fusaro 1991)	*CDKN2A(p16)*
		von Hippel–Lindau syndrome (Libutti et al. 2000, 1998; Hammel et al. 2000)	*VHL*
		Peutz–Jeghers syndrome (Hemminki 1999)	*LKB1/STK11*
	Islet cell neoplasias	MEN 1 (Broughan et al. 1986; Dean et al. 2000; Lowney et al. 1998)	*MEN1*
		von Hippel–Lindau syndrome (Curley et al. 1998; Hough et al. 1994; Binkovitz et al. 1990)	*VHL*
		Neurofibromatosis type 1	*NF1*
Paraganglia	Paraganglioma	Hereditary pheochromocytoma–paraganglioma syndrome (Dannenberg et al. 2002; Cascon et al. 2002; Baysal et al. 2002)	*SDHA, SDHB, SDHC, SDHD, SDHAF2, TMEM127, MAX*
		von Hippel–Lindau syndrome (Reichardt et al. 2002; Baghai et al. 2002; Chew 2001)	*VHL*
		MEN 2 (Chew 2001)	*RET*
		Neurofibromatosis type 1 (Chew 2001)	*NF1*
		MEN 1	*MEN1*
Parathyroid	Adenoma/ hyperplasia	MEN 1 (Duh et al. 1987; Oberg et al. 1989; Sato et al. 2000)	*MEN1*
		MEN 2 (Eng et al. 1996; Duh et al. 1987; Howe et al. 1993; Kraimps et al. 1996)	*RET*
		Familial benign hypercalcemia (mild hyperparathyroidism)	*CASR*

Appendix   (continued)

Organ or neoplasia type	Histological type	Genetic differential diagnosis	Gene (if known)
		Hyperparathyroidism–jaw tumor syndrome (Haven et al. 2000; Cavaco et al. 2001)	*CDC73 (HRPT2)*
		Familial isolated hyperparathyroidism (FIHP)	*CDC73 (HRPT2)*
	Carcinoma	Hyperparathyroidism–jaw tumor syndrome	*CDC73 (HRPT2)*
Pituitary	Adenoma	MEN 1 (Carty et al. 1998; Oberg et al. 1989; Samaan et al. 1989; Wilkinson et al. 1993; Calender et al. 1995; Cebrian et al. 1999; Verges et al. 2002)	*MEN1*
		Carney complex (Carney et al. 1985; Kirschner et al. 2000a; Stratakis et al. 1996; Carney and Stratakis 1998; Stratakis 2001)	*PRKR1A*
		Site-specific pituitary adenoma	*AIP*
Prostate	Carcinoma	Hereditary prostate cancer syndromes (Wang et al. 2002; Simard et al. 2002)	
		HBOC (Gronberg et al. 2001; Sigurdsson et al. 1997; Tulinius et al. 2002)	*BRCA1, BRCA2*
Sarcoma	Osteosarcoma, soft tissue sarcoma	Li–Fraumeni syndrome (Hisada et al. 1998; Toguchida et al. 1992; Soussi et al. 1993)	*TP53*
		Werner syndrome (Goto et al. 1996; Bjornberg 1976)	*WRN*
		Hereditary retinoblastoma (Smith and Donaldson 1991; Wong et al. 1997)	*RB1*
		Neurofibromatosis type 1 (Zoller et al. 1997; Samuelsson and Axelsson 1981; Hayani et al. 1992)	*NF1*
		Rothmund–Thomson syndrome (Cumin et al. 1996; Lindor et al. 2000; Spurney et al. 1998; Wang et al. 2001)	*RECQL4*
		Werner syndrome (Monnat 2002)	*WRN*
	Soft tissue sarcoma (mainly rhabdomyo-sarcoma)	Costello syndrome	*HRAS*

(continued)

Appendix (continued)

Organ or neoplasia type	Histological type	Genetic differential diagnosis	Gene (if known)
	Malignant peripheral nerve sheath tumor (aka neurofibrosarcoma, malignant schwannoma)	Neurofibromatosis type 1 (Storm et al. 1980; Nambisan et al. 1984; Riccardi and Powell 1989; Rogalski and Louis 1991; Meis et al. 1992; Amir et al. 1993; Matsui et al. 1993)	*NF1*
	Gastrointestinal	Paraganglioma and gastric sarcoma (Carney and Stratakis 2002)	*SDHB/SDHD*
		Carney's triad (Valverde et al. 2001; Blei and Gonzalez-Crussi 1992)	
	GIST	GIST (Hirota et al. 2002; Isozaki et al. 2000; Nishida et al. 1998)	*KIT, PDGFA*
Skin	Melanoma	FAMMM (Lynch et al. 2002; Vasen et al. 2000; Gruis et al. 1995; Lynch and Fusaro 1991)	*CDKN2A/p16, CDK4*
		Xeroderma pigmentosum (English and Swerdlow 1987; Takebe et al. 1989)	*XP-x*
		Werner syndrome (Monnat 2002; Goto et al. 1996)	*WRN*
		Hereditary retinoblastoma (Moll et al. 1997; Eng et al. 1993)	*RB1*
		Melanoma-astrocytoma syndrome (Randerson-Moor et al. 2001; Bahuau et al. 1998)	*CDKN2A/p16, p14ARF*
		Uveal and cutaneous melanoma	*BAP1*
	Nonmelanoma carcinoma	Nevoid basal cell carcinoma (Gorlin) syndrome (Rayner et al. 1977; Gustafson et al. 1989; Gailani and Bale 1997)	*PTC*
		Xeroderma pigmentosum (Kraemer et al. 1987; Takebe et al. 1989; Cleaver et al. 1981)	*XP-x*
		Werner syndrome (Zalla 1980; Duvic and Lemak 1995)	*WRN*
		Fanconi anemia (Somers et al. 1995; Auerbach 1995)	*FANC-x*
		Bazex–Christol–Dupré syndrome (Gould and Barker 1978; Kidd et al. 1996)	
		Ferguson–Smith syndrome (Bale 1999; Richards et al. 1997; Chakrabarty and Perks 1996)	*TGFBR1*
	Squamous cell carcinoma	Dyskeratosis congenita (Bale 1999; Richards et al. 1997; Chakrabarty and Perks 1996)	*TERC* (AD), *DKC1* (X-linked)

Appendix (continued)

Organ or neoplasia type	Histological type	Genetic differential diagnosis	Gene (if known)
	Sebaceous carcinoma	Muir–Torre syndrome (Schwartz and Torre 1995; Rutten et al. 1999)	*MSH2, MLH1*
	Leiomyoma	Multiple leiomyomatosis syndrome (Tomlinson et al. 2002; Jozwiak et al. 1998)	*FH*
	Angiofibromas facial	Tuberous sclerosis complex (Webb et al. 1996; Sogut et al. 2002; Bellack and Shapshay 1986)	*TSC1, TSC2*
		MEN 1 (Darling et al. 1997; Marx et al. 1999; Sakurai et al. 2000)	*MEN1*
	Neurofibroma	Neurofibromatosis type 1 (Szudek et al. 2000; Chung et al. 1999; Friedman and Birch 1997; Goldberg et al. 1996)	*NF1*
	Trichilemmomas/ trichodiscomas/ folliculomas	Cowden syndrome (Eng 2000; Starink et al. 1986)	*PTEN*
		Birt–Hogg–Dube syndrome (Nickerson et al. 2002; Khoo et al. 2001; Ubogy-Rainey et al. 1987)	*BHD*
Stomach	Carcinoma	HNPCC (Lynch and Lynch 1995; Vasen et al. 1990; Watson and Lynch 1994; Cristofaro et al. 1987; Aarnio et al. 1995)	*MLH1, MSH2, MSH6, PMS1, PMS2*
		Hereditary diffuse gastric cancer syndrome (Shinmura et al. 1999; Guilford et al. 1999; Dunbier and Guilford 2001)	*CDH1*
		Ataxia telangiectasia (Haerer et al. 1969; Swift et al. 1976; Frais 1979)	*ATM*
		Li–Fraumeni syndrome (Hisada et al. 1998; Varley et al. 1995; Sugano et al. 1999)	*TP53*
		Juvenile polyposis syndrome (Yoshida et al. 1988; Sassatelli et al. 1993; Hofting et al. 1993; Howe et al. 1998b)	*MADH4, BMPR1A*
		FAP (Iwama et al. 1993)	*APC*
		Werner syndrome (Monnat 2002)	*WRN*
	Stromal tumors (GIST)	Hereditary gastrointestinal stromal tumor syndrome (Hirota et al. 2002; Isozaki et al. 2000; Nishida et al. 1998)	*KIT, PDGFRA*
Testis	Germ cell tumors	Klinefelter syndrome (Aizenstein et al. 1997; Simpson and Photopulos 1976)	XXY

(continued)

Appendix (continued)

Organ or neoplasia type	Histological type	Genetic differential diagnosis	Gene (if known)
		Familial testicular cancer (Cooper et al. 1994; Nicholson and Harland 1995; Heimdal et al. 1996; Rapley et al. 2000)	*KITLG, DMRT1*
		Carney complex (Carney et al. 1985; Kirschner et al. 2000a; Washecka et al. 2002)	*PRKAR1A*
		Androgen insensitivity (Gourlay et al. 1994; Rutgers and Scully 1991; Cassio et al. 1990; Chen et al. 1999)	*AR*
		Russell–Silver syndrome (Weiss and Garnick 1981)	
	Sertoli-Leydig cell	DICER syndrome	*DICER1*
	Gonadoblastoma	WAGR (Pelletier et al. 1991a; Mochon et al. 1987)	*WT1*, contiguous gene syndrome
Thyroid	Papillary	FAP (Lynch et al. 2001; Iwama et al. 1993; Bell and Mazzaferri 1993; van der Linde et al. 1998; Soravia et al. 1999; Cetta et al. 2000) (see text)	*APC*
		Cowden syndrome (Eng 2000; Starink et al. 1986; Nelen et al. 1996; Lee et al. 1997; Starink 1984)	*PTEN, SDHB, SDHD; KLLN* (epimutation)
		Carney complex (Kirschner et al. 2000a; Edwards et al. 2002; Stratakis et al. 1997, 1998)	*PRKAR1A*
		Familial non-medullary thyroid cancer syndromes (Loh 1997; Malchoff and Malchoff 1999; Uchino et al. 2002)	
		Familial papillary thyroid carcinoma (Malchoff et al. 1999; Lupoli et al. 1999; Musholt et al. 2000; Marchesi et al. 2000)	
	Follicular	Cowden syndrome (Eng 2000; Starink et al. 1986; Harach et al. 1999; Kameyama et al. 2001)	*PTEN*
		Werner syndrome (Monnat 2002; Ishikawa et al. 1999)	*WRN*
	Medullary	MEN 2 (Eng et al. 1996; Saad et al. 1984; Vasen et al. 1987; Calmettes 1989; Shimotake et al. 1990; Vasen et al. 1992; Iihara et al. 1997)	*RET*

Appendix (continued)

Organ or neoplasia type	Histological type	Genetic differential diagnosis	Gene (if known)
Uterus	Endometrial carcinoma	HNPCC (Watson and Lynch 1993; Brown et al. 2001; Vasen et al. 1990; Mecklin and Jarvinen 1991; Watson et al. 1994; Wijnen et al. 1998; Weber et al. 1999; Peel et al. 2000)	*MLH1, MSH2, MSH6, PMS1, PMS2*
		Cowden syndrome (Eng 2000; Starink et al. 1986; Marsh et al. 1998)	*PTEN*
	Myometrial leiomyoma	Cowden syndrome (Eng 2000; Starink et al. 1986; Marsh et al. 1998)	*PTEN*
		Multiple leiomyomatosis–renal cell cancer (Kiuru et al. 2001; Tomlinson et al. 2002; Launonen et al. 2001)	*FH*
Vulva	Squamous cell	Fanconi anemia (Wilkinson et al. 1984; Kennedy and Hart 1982)	*FANC-x*

[a]To add to Emberger Syndrome: Ostergaard et al. (2011)

References

Aaltonen LA, Peltomaki P. Genes involved in hereditary nonpolyposis colorectal carcinoma. Anticancer Res. 1994;14:1657–60.

Aarnio M, Mecklin JP, Aaltonen LA, Nystrom-Lahti M, Jarvinen HJ. Life-time risk of different cancers in hereditary non-polyposis colorectal cancer (HNPCC) syndrome. Int J Cancer. 1995;64:430–3.

Aarnio M, Sankila R, Pukkala E, et al. Cancer risk in mutation carriers of DNA-mismatch-repair genes. Int J Cancer. 1999;81:214–8.

Agnarsson BA, Jonasson JG, Bjornsdottir IB, Barkardottir RB, Egilsson V, Sigurdsson H. Inherited BRCA2 mutation associated with high grade breast cancer. Breast Cancer Res Treat. 1998;47:121–7.

Aizenstein RI, Hibbeln JF, Sagireddy B, Wilbur AC, O'Neil HK. Klinefelter's syndrome associated with testicular microlithiasis and mediastinal germ-cell neoplasm. J Clin Ultrasound. 1997;25:508–10.

Akiyama Y, Sato H, Yamada T, et al. Germ-line mutation of the hMSH6/GTBP gene in an atypical hereditary nonpolyposis colorectal cancer kindred. Cancer Res. 1997;57:3920–3.

Alonso J, Garcia-Miguel P, Abelairas J, et al. Spectrum of germline RB1 gene mutations in Spanish retinoblastoma patients: phenotypic and molecular epidemiological implications. Hum Mutat. 2001;17:412–22.

Al-Saleem T, Wessner LL, Scheithauer BW, et al. Malignant tumors of the kidney, brain, and soft tissues in children and young adults with the tuberous sclerosis complex. Cancer. 1998;83:2208–16.

Alter BP. Fanconi's anemia and malignancies. Am J Hematol. 1996;53:99–110.

Amir H, Moshi E, Kitinya JN. Neurofibromatosis and malignant schwannomas in Tanzania. East Afr Med J. 1993;70:650–3.

Amoaku WM, Willshaw HE, Parkes SE, Shah KJ, Mann JR. Trilateral retinoblastoma. A report of five patients. Cancer. 1996;78:858–63.

Anneroth G, Heimdahl A. Syndrome of multiple mucosal neurofibromas, pheochromocytoma and medullary thryoid carcinoma. Report of a case. Int J Oral Surg. 1978;7:126–31.

Antinheimo J, Haapasalo H, Haltia M, et al. Proliferation potential and histological features in neurofibromatosis 2-associated and sporadic meningiomas. J Neurosurg. 1997;87:610–4.

Antinheimo J, Sankila R, Carpen O, Pukkala E, Sainio M, Jaaskelainen J. Population-based analysis of sporadic and type 2 neurofibromatosis- associated meningiomas and schwannomas. Neurology. 2000;54:71–6.

Arepally G, Rebbeck TR, Song W, Gilliland G, Maris JM, Poncz M. Evidence for genetic homogeneity in a familial platelet disorder with predisposition to acute myelogenous leukemia (FPD/AML). Blood. 1998;92:2600–2.

Argyle JC, Kjeldsberg CR, Marty J, Shigeoka AO, Hill HR. T-cell lymphoma and the Chediak-Higashi syndrome. Blood. 1982;60:672–6.

Armstrong JG, Davies DR, Guy SP, Frayling IM, Evans DG. APC mutations in familial adenomatous polyposis families in the Northwest of England. Hum Mutat. 1997;10:376–80.

Asirvatham R, Rooney RJ, Watts HG. Ollier's disease with secondary chondrosarcoma associated with ovarian tumour. A case report. Int Orthop. 1991;15:393–5.

Astuti D, Latif F, Dallol A, et al. Gene mutations in the succinate dehydrogenase subunit SDHB cause susceptibility to familial pheochromocytoma and to familial paraganglioma. Am J Hum Genet. 2001;69:49–54.

Atuk NO, Stolle C, Owen Jr JA, Carpenter JT, Vance ML. Pheochromocytoma in von Hippel-Lindau disease: clinical presentation and mutation analysis in a large, multigenerational kindred. J Clin Endocrinol Metab. 1998;83:117–20.

Auerbach AD. Fanconi anemia. Dermatol Clin. 1995;13:41–9.

Auerbach AD, Allen RG. Leukemia and preleukemia in Fanconi anemia patients. A review of the literature and report of the International Fanconi Anemia Registry. Cancer Genet Cytogenet. 1991;51:1–12.

Bader JL, Miller RW, Meadows AT, Zimmerman LE, Champion LA, Voute PA. Trilateral retinoblastoma. Lancet. 1980;2:582–3.

Baghai M, Thompson GB, Young Jr WF, Grant CS, Michels VV, van Heerden JA. Pheochromocytomas and paragangliomas in von Hippel-Lindau disease: a role for laparoscopic and cortical-sparing surgery. Arch Surg. 2002;137:682–8; discussion 688–9.

Bahuau M, Vidaud D, Jenkins RB, et al. Germ-line deletion involving the INK4 locus in familial proneness to melanoma and nervous system tumors. Cancer Res. 1998;58:2298–303.

Bale SJ. The "sins" of the fathers: self-healing squamous epithelioma in Scotland. J Cutan Med Surg. 1999;3:207–10.

Bang YJ, Kang SH, Kim TY, et al. The first documentation of Li-Fraumeni syndrome in Korea. J Korean Med Sci. 1995;10:205–10.

Baser ME, Makariou EV, Parry DM. Predictors of vestibular schwannoma growth in patients with neurofibromatosis Type 2. J Neurosurg. 2002;96:217–22.

Baysal BE, Willett-Brozick JE, Lawrence EC, et al. Prevalence of SDHB, SDHC, and SDHD germline mutations in clinic patients with head and neck paragangliomas. J Med Genet. 2002;39:178–83.

Beckers A, Abs R, Willems PJ, et al. Aldosterone-secreting adrenal adenoma as part of multiple endocrine neoplasia type 1 (MEN1): loss of heterozygosity for polymorphic chromosome 11 deoxyribonucleic acid markers, including the MEN1 locus. J Clin Endocrinol Metab. 1992;75:564–70.

Bell B, Mazzaferri EL. Familial adenomatous polyposis (Gardner's syndrome) and thyroid carcinoma. A case report and review of the literature. Dig Dis Sci. 1993;38:185–90.

Bellack GS, Shapshay SM. Management of facial angiofibromas in tuberous sclerosis: use of the carbon dioxide laser. Otolaryngol Head Neck Surg. 1986;94:37–40.

Benharroch D, Sion-Vardi N, Goldstein J. Neurofibromatosis involving the small bowel associated with adenocarcinoma of the ileum with a neuroendocrine component. Pathol Res Pract. 1992;188:959–63.

Berends MJ, Wu Y, Sijmons RH, et al. Molecular and clinical characteristics of MSH6 variants: an analysis of 25 index carriers of a germline variant. Am J Hum Genet. 2002;70:26–37.

Berkower AS, Biller HF. Head and neck cancer associated with Bloom's syndrome. Laryngoscope. 1988;98:746–8.

Berman DB, Costalas J, Schultz DC, Grana G, Daly M, Godwin AK. A common mutation in BRCA2 that predisposes to a variety of cancers is found in both Jewish Ashkenazi and non-Jewish individuals. Cancer Res. 1996;56:3409–14.

Bilaniuk LT, Molloy PT, Zimmerman RA, et al. Neurofibromatosis type 1: brain stem tumours. Neuroradiology. 1997;39:642–53.

Binkovitz LA, Johnson CD, Stephens DH. Islet cell tumors in von Hippel-Lindau disease: increased prevalence and relationship to the multiple endocrine neoplasias. AJR Am J Roentgenol. 1990;155:501–5.

Birch JM, Hartley AL, Tricker KJ, et al. Prevalence and diversity of constitutional mutations in the p53 gene among 21 Li-Fraumeni families. Cancer Res. 1994;54:1298–304.

Birch JM, Blair V, Kelsey AM, et al. Cancer phenotype correlates with constitutional TP53 genotype in families with the Li-Fraumeni syndrome. Oncogene. 1998;17:1061–8.

Birch JM, Alston RD, McNally RJ, et al. Relative frequency and morphology of cancers in carriers of germline TP53 mutations. Oncogene. 2001;20:4621–8.

Bisgaard ML, Jager AC, Myrhoj T, Bernstein I, Nielsen FC. Hereditary non-polyposis colorectal cancer (HNPCC): phenotype-genotype correlation between patients with and without identified mutation. Hum Mutat. 2002;20:20–7.

Bjornberg A. Werner's syndrome and malignancy. Acta Derm Venereol. 1976;56:149–50.

Blach LE, McCormick B, Abramson DH, Ellsworth RM. Trilateral retinoblastoma–incidence and outcome: a decade of experience. Int J Radiat Oncol Biol Phys. 1994;29:729–33.

Blei E, Gonzalez-Crussi F. The intriguing nature of gastric tumors in Carney's triad. Ultrastructural and immunohistochemical observations. Cancer. 1992;69:292–300.

Boardman LA, Thibodeau SN, Schaid DJ, et al. Increased risk for cancer in patients with the Peutz-Jeghers syndrome. Ann Intern Med. 1998;128:896–9.

Bodmer D, Eleveld M, Kater-Baats E, et al. Disruption of a novel MFS transporter gene, DIRC2, by a familial renal cell carcinoma-associated t(2;3)(q35;q21). Hum Mol Genet. 2002;11:641–9.

Bordi C, Falchetti A, Azzoni C, et al. Aggressive forms of gastric neuroendocrine tumors in multiple endocrine neoplasia type I. Am J Surg Pathol. 1997;21:1075–82.

Boultwood J. Ataxia telangiectasia gene mutations in leukaemia and lymphoma. J Clin Pathol. 2001;54:512–6.

Brensinger JD, Laken SJ, Luce MC, et al. Variable phenotype of familial adenomatous polyposis in pedigrees with 3′ mutation in the APC gene. Gut. 1998;43:548–52.

Broeks A, Urbanus JH, Floore AN, et al. ATM-heterozygous germline mutations contribute to breast cancer- susceptibility. Am J Hum Genet. 2000;66:494–500.

Broughan TA, Leslie JD, Soto JM, Hermann RE. Pancreatic islet cell tumors. Surgery. 1986;99:671–8.

Brown GJ, St John DJ, Macrae FA, Aittomaki K. Cancer risk in young women at risk of hereditary nonpolyposis colorectal cancer: implications for gynecologic surveillance. Gynecol Oncol. 2001;80:346–9.

Buckley JA, Siegelman SS, Jones B, Fishman EK. The accuracy of CT staging of small bowel adenocarcinoma: CT/pathologic correlation. J Comput Assist Tomogr. 1997;21:986–91.

Buerstedde JM, Alday P, Torhorst J, Weber W, Muller H, Scott R. Detection of new mutations in six out of 10 Swiss HNPCC families by genomic sequencing of the hMSH2 and hMLH1 genes. J Med Genet. 1995;32:909–12.

Bunyan DJ, Shea-Simonds J, Reck AC, Finnis D, Eccles DM. Genotype-phenotype correlations of new causative APC gene mutations in patients with familial adenomatous polyposis. J Med Genet. 1995;32:728–31.

Burdick D, Prior JT. Peutz-Jeghers syndrome. A clinicopathologic study of a large family with a 27-year follow-up. Cancer. 1982;50:2139–46.

Burgdorf WH, Pitha J, Fahmy A. Muir-Torre syndrome. Histologic spectrum of sebaceous proliferations. Am J Dermatopathol. 1986;8:202–8.

Caldemeyer KS, Mirowski GW. Neurofibromatosis type 2. J Am Acad Dermatol. 2001;45:744–5.

Calender A, Giraud S, Cougard P, et al. Multiple endocrine neoplasia type 1 in France: clinical and genetic studies. J Intern Med. 1995;238:263–8.

Caligo MA, Ghimenti C, Cipollini G, et al. BRCA1 germline mutational spectrum in Italian families from Tuscany: a high frequency of novel mutations. Oncogene. 1996;13:1483–8.

Calmettes C. Multiple endocrine neoplasia type II: clinical, biological and epidemiological features. French Medullary Study Group. Horm Res. 1989;32:41–6.

Cao Y, Pieretti M, Marshall J, et al. Challenge in the differentiation between attenuated familial adenomatous polyposis and hereditary nonpolyposis colorectal cancer: case report with review of the literature. Am J Gastroenterol. 2002;97:1822–7.

Carey JC, Laub JM, Hall BD. Penetrance and variability in neurofibromatosis: a genetic study of 60 families. Birth Defects Orig Artic Ser. 1979;15:271–81.

Carney JA, Stratakis CA. Epithelioid blue nevus and psammomatous melanotic schwannoma: the unusual pigmented skin tumors of the Carney complex. Semin Diagn Pathol. 1998; 15:216–24.

Carney JA, Stratakis CA. Familial paraganglioma and gastric stromal sarcoma: a new syndrome distinct from the Carney triad. Am J Med Genet. 2002;108:132–9.

Carney JA, Gordon H, Carpenter PC, Shenoy BV, Go VL. The complex of myxomas, spotty pigmentation, and endocrine overactivity. Medicine (Baltimore). 1985;64:270–83.

Carney JA, Hruska LS, Beauchamp GD, Gordon H. Dominant inheritance of the complex of myxomas, spotty pigmentation, and endocrine overactivity. Mayo Clin Proc. 1986;61:165–72.

Carty SE, Helm AK, Amico JA, et al. The variable penetrance and spectrum of manifestations of multiple endocrine neoplasia type 1. Surgery. 1998;124:1106–13; discussion 1113–4.

Cascon A, Ruiz-Llorente S, Cebrian A, et al. Identification of novel SDHD mutations in patients with phaeochromocytoma and/or paraganglioma. Eur J Hum Genet. 2002;10:457–61.

Cassio A, Cacciari E, D'Errico A, et al. Incidence of intratubular germ cell neoplasia in androgen insensitivity syndrome. Acta Endocrinol (Copenh). 1990;123:416–22.

Cavaco BM, Barros L, Pannett AA, et al. The hyperparathyroidism-jaw tumour syndrome in a Portuguese kindred. QJM. 2001;94:213–22.

Cavenee WK, Hansen MF, Nordenskjold M, et al. Genetic origin of mutations predisposing to retinoblastoma. Science. 1985;228:501–3.

Cebrian A, Herrera-Pombo JL, Diez JJ, et al. Genetic and clinical analysis in 10 Spanish patients with multiple endocrine neoplasia type 1. Eur J Hum Genet. 1999;7:585–9.

Cetta F, Montalto G, Gori M, Curia MC, Cama A, Olschwang S. Germline mutations of the APC gene in patients with familial adenomatous polyposis-associated thyroid carcinoma: results from a European cooperative study. J Clin Endocrinol Metab. 2000;85:286–92.

Chakrabarty KH, Perks AG. Ferguson-Smith syndrome: the importance of long term follow-up. Br J Plast Surg. 1996;49:497–8.

Chan TL, Yuen ST, Chung LP, et al. Germline hMSH2 and differential somatic mutations in patients with Turcot's syndrome. Genes Chromosomes Cancer. 1999;25:75–81.

Chapman MS, Perry AE, Baughman RD. Cowden's syndrome, Lhermitte-Duclos disease, and sclerotic fibroma. Am J Dermatopathol. 1998;20:413–6.

Chen CH, Lin JT, Lee WY, et al. Somatostatin-containing carcinoid tumor of the duodenum in neurofibromatosis: report of a case. J Formos Med Assoc. 1993;92:900–3.

Chen F, Kishida T, Yao M, et al. Germline mutations in the von Hippel-Lindau disease tumor suppressor gene: correlations with phenotype. Hum Mutat. 1995;5:66–75.

Chen CP, Chern SR, Wang TY, Wang W, Wang KL, Jeng CJ. Androgen receptor gene mutations in 46, XY females with germ cell tumours. Hum Reprod. 1999;14:664–70.

Chetty R, Duhig JD. Bilateral pheochromocytoma-ganglioneuroma of the adrenal in type 1 neurofibromatosis. Am J Surg Pathol. 1993;17:837–41.

Cheung PS, Thompson NW. Carney's complex of primary pigmented nodular adrenocortical disease and pigmentous and myxomatous lesions. Surg Gynecol Obstet. 1989;168:413–6.

Chew SL. Paraganglioma genes. Clin Endocrinol (Oxf). 2001;54:573–4.

Christian CD. Ovarian tumors: an extension of the Peutz-Jeghers syndrome. Am J Obstet Gynecol. 1971;111:529–34.

Chung CJ, Armfield KB, Mukherji SK, Fordham LA, Krause WL. Cervical neurofibromas in children with NF-1. Pediatr Radiol. 1999;29:353–6.

Cipolli M. Shwachman-Diamond syndrome: clinical phenotypes. Pancreatology. 2001;1:543–8.

Clark RD, Hutter Jr JJ. Familial neurofibromatosis and juvenile chronic myelogenous leukemia. Hum Genet. 1982;60:230–2.

Cleaver JE, Zelle B, Hashem N, El-Hefnawi MH, German J. Xeroderma pigmentosum patients from Egypt: II. Preliminary correlations of epidemiology, clinical symptoms and molecular biology. J Invest Dermatol. 1981;77:96–101.

Clement S, Efrusy ME, Dobbins 3rd WO, Palmer RN. Pelvic neoplasia in Peutz-Jeghers syndrome. J Clin Gastroenterol. 1979;1:341–3.

Cnossen MH, Stam EN, Cooiman LC, et al. Endocrinologic disorders and optic pathway gliomas in children with neurofibromatosis type 1. Pediatrics. 1997;100:667–70.

Cnossen MH, de Goede-Bolder A, van den Broek KM, et al. A prospective 10 year follow up study of patients with neurofibromatosis type 1. Arch Dis Child. 1998;78:408–12.

Cohen SB. Familial polyposis coli and its extracolonic manifestations. J Med Genet. 1982;19:193–203.

Cohen PR, Kurzrock R. Miscellaneous genodermatoses: Beckwith-Wiedemann syndrome, Birt-Hogg- Dube syndrome, familial atypical multiple mole melanoma syndrome, hereditary tylosis, incontinentia pigmenti, and supernumerary nipples. Dermatol Clin. 1995;13:211–29.

Cohen PR, Kohn SR, Davis DA, Kurzrock R. Muir-Torre syndrome. Dermatol Clin. 1995;13:79–89.

Cohn DE, Babb S, Whelan AJ, et al. Atypical clustering of gynecologic malignancies: a family study including molecular analysis of candidate genes. Gynecol Oncol. 2000;77:18–25.

Coldron J, Reid I. Muir-Torre syndrome. J R Coll Surg Edinb. 2001;46:178–9.

Cooper MA, Fellows J, Einhorn LH. Familial occurrence of testicular cancer. J Urol. 1994;151:1022–3.

Cotelingam JD, Witebsky FG, Hsu SM, Blaese RM, Jaffe ES. Malignant lymphoma in patients with the Wiskott-Aldrich syndrome. Cancer Invest. 1985;3:515–22.

Couch FJ, Farid LM, DeShano ML, et al. BRCA2 germline mutations in male breast cancer cases and breast cancer families. Nat Genet. 1996;13:123–5.

Couch V, Lindor NM, Karnes PS, Michels VV. von Hippel-Lindau disease. Mayo Clin Proc. 2000;75:265–72.

Cowell JK, Cragg H. Constitutional nonsense germline mutations in the RB1 gene detected in patients with early onset unilateral retinoblastoma. Eur J Cancer. 1996;32A:1749–52.

Cristofaro G, Lynch HT, Caruso ML, et al. New phenotypic aspects in a family with Lynch syndrome II. Cancer. 1987;60:51–8.

Crossey PA, Eng C, Ginalska-Malinowska M, et al. Molecular genetic diagnosis of von Hippel-Lindau disease in familial pheochromocytoma. J Med Genet. 1995;32:885–6.

Cumin I, Cohen JY, David A, Mechinaud F, Avet-Loiseau H, Harousseau JL. Rothmund-Thomson syndrome and osteosarcoma. Med Pediatr Oncol. 1996;26:414–6.

Curley SA, Lott ST, Luca JW, Frazier ML, Killary AM. Surgical decision-making affected by clinical and genetic screening of a novel kindred with von Hippel-Lindau disease and pancreatic islet cell tumors. Ann Surg. 1998;227:229–35.

Cussen LJ, MacMahon RA. Germ cells and ova in dysgenetic gonads of a 46-XY female dizygotic twin. Am J Dis Child. 1979;133:373–5.

Damjanov I, Klauber G. Microscopic gonadoblastoma in dysgenetic gonad of an infant: an ultrastructural study. Urology. 1980;15:605–9.

Dannenberg H, Dinjens WN, Abbou M, et al. Frequent germ-line succinate dehydrogenase subunit D gene mutations in patients with apparently sporadic parasympathetic paraganglioma. Clin Cancer Res. 2002;8:2061–6.

Darling TN, Skarulis MC, Steinberg SM, Marx SJ, Spiegel AM, Turner M. Multiple facial angiofibromas and collagenomas in patients with multiple endocrine neoplasia type 1. Arch Dermatol. 1997;133:853–7.

De Potter P, Shields CL, Shields JA. Clinical variations of trilateral retinoblastoma: a report of 13 cases. J Pediatr Ophthalmol Strabismus. 1994;31:26–31.

Dean PG, van Heerden JA, Farley DR, et al. Are patients with multiple endocrine neoplasia type I prone to premature death? World J Surg. 2000;24:1437–41.

DeBaun MR, Tucker MA. Risk of cancer during the first four years of life in children from The Beckwith-Wiedemann Syndrome Registry. J Pediatr. 1998;132:398–400.

Dent PB, Fish LA, White LG, Good RA. Chediak-Higashi syndrome. Observations on the nature of the associated malignancy. Lab Invest. 1966;15:1634–42.

Devroede G, Lemieux B, Masse S, Lamarche J, Herman PS. Colonic hamartomas in tuberous sclerosis. Gastroenterology. 1988;94:182–8.

Dome JS, Coppes MJ. Recent advances in Wilms tumor genetics. Curr Opin Pediatr. 2002;14:5–11.

Dotzenrath C, Goretzki PE, Cupisti K, Yang Q, Simon D, Roher HD. Malignant endocrine tumors in patients with MEN 1 disease. Surgery. 2001;129:91–5.

Dowton SB, Beardsley D, Jamison D, Blattner S, Li FP. Studies of a familial platelet disorder. Blood. 1985;65:557–63.

Drachtman RA, Alter BP. Dyskeratosis congenita. Dermatol Clin. 1995;13:33–9.

Drappa J, Vaishnaw AK, Sullivan KE, Chu JL, Elkon KB. Fas gene mutations in the Canale-Smith syndrome, an inherited lymphoproliferative disorder associated with autoimmunity. N Engl J Med. 1996;335:1643–9.

Druck T, Podolski J, Byrski T, et al. The DIRC1 gene at chromosome 2q33 spans a familial RCC-associated t(2;3)(q33;q21) chromosome translocation. J Hum Genet. 2001; 46:583–9.

Duh QY, Hybarger CP, Geist R, et al. Carcinoids associated with multiple endocrine neoplasia syndromes. Am J Surg. 1987;154:142–8.

Dunbier A, Guilford P. Hereditary diffuse gastric cancer. Adv Cancer Res. 2001;83:55–65.

Duvic M, Lemak NA. Werner's syndrome. Dermatol Clin. 1995;13:163–8.

Eccles DM, Lunt PW, Wallis Y, et al. An unusually severe phenotype for familial adenomatous polyposis. Arch Dis Child. 1997;77:431–5.

Edwards A, Bermudez C, Piwonka G, et al. Carney's syndrome: complex myxomas. Report of four cases and review of the literature. Cardiovasc Surg. 2002;10:264–75.

Eleveld MJ, Bodmer D, Merkx G, et al. Molecular analysis of a familial case of renal cell cancer and a t(3;6)(q12;q15). Genes Chromosomes Cancer. 2001;31:23–32.

Elias WJ, Lopes MB, Golden WL, Jane Sr JA, Gonzalez-Fernandez F. Trilateral retinoblastoma variant indicative of the relevance of the retinoblastoma tumor-suppressor pathway to medulloblastomas in humans. J Neurosurg. 2001;95:871–8.

Ellis A, Field JK, Field EA, et al. Tylosis associated with carcinoma of the oesophagus and oral leukoplakia in a large Liverpool family – a review of six generations. Eur J Cancer B Oral Oncol. 1994;2:102–12.

Eng C. Will the real Cowden syndrome please stand up: revised diagnostic criteria. J Med Genet. 2000;37:828–30.

Eng C, Li FP, Abramson DH, et al. Mortality from second tumors among long-term survivors of retinoblastoma. J Natl Cancer Inst. 1993;85:1121–8.

Eng C, Clayton D, Schuffenecker I, et al. The relationship between specific RET proto-oncogene mutations and disease phenotype in multiple endocrine neoplasia type 2. International RET mutation consortium analysis. JAMA. 1996;276:1575–9.

English JS, Swerdlow AJ. The risk of malignant melanoma, internal malignancy and mortality in xeroderma pigmentosum patients. Br J Dermatol. 1987;117:457–61.

Entius MM, Westerman AM, van Velthuysen ML, et al. Molecular and phenotypic markers of hamartomatous polyposis syndromes in the gastrointestinal tract. Hepatogastroenterology. 1999;46:661–6.

Evans DG. Neurofibromatosis type 2: genetic and clinical features. Ear Nose Throat J. 1999;78:97–100.

Evans DG, Trueman L, Wallace A, Collins S, Strachan T. Genotype/phenotype correlations in type 2 neurofibromatosis (NF2): evidence for more severe disease associated with truncating mutations. J Med Genet. 1998;35:450–5.

Evans DG, Sainio M, Baser ME. Neurofibromatosis type 2. J Med Genet. 2000;37:897–904.

Fackenthal JD, Marsh DJ, Richardson AL, et al. Male breast cancer in Cowden syndrome patients with germline PTEN mutations. J Med Genet. 2001;38:159–64.

Faivre L, Guardiola P, Lewis C, et al. Association of complementation group and mutation type with clinical outcome in fanconi anemia. European Fanconi Anemia Research Group. Blood. 2000;96:4064–70.

Faravelli F, Upadhyaya M, Osborn M, Huson SM, Hayward R, Winter R. Unusual clustering of brain tumours in a family with NF1 and variable expression of cutaneous features. J Med Genet. 1999;36:893–6.

Fodde R, Khan PM. Genotype-phenotype correlations at the adenomatous polyposis coli (APC) gene. Crit Rev Oncog. 1995;6:291–303.

Frais MA. Gastric adenocarcinoma due to ataxia-telangiectasia (Louis-Bar syndrome). J Med Genet. 1979;16:160–1.

Freedman MH. Diamond-Blackfan anaemia. Baillieres Best Pract Res Clin Haematol. 2000;13:391–406.

Friedl W, Meuschel S, Caspari R, et al. Attenuated familial adenomatous polyposis due to a mutation in the 3′ part of the APC gene. A clue for understanding the function of the APC protein. Hum Genet. 1996;97:579–84.

Friedl W, Uhlhaas S, Schulmann K, et al. Juvenile polyposis: massive gastric polyposis is more common in MADH4 mutation carriers than in BMPR1A mutation carriers. Hum Genet. 2002;111:108–11.

Friedman JM, Birch PH. Type 1 neurofibromatosis: a descriptive analysis of the disorder in 1,728 patients. Am J Med Genet. 1997;70:138–43.

Friedrich CA. Genotype-phenotype correlation in von Hippel-Lindau syndrome. Hum Mol Genet. 2001;10:763–7.

Frizzera G, Rosai J, Dehner LP, Spector BD, Kersey JH. Lymphoreticular disorders in primary immunodeficiencies: new findings based on an up-to-date histologic classification of 35 cases. Cancer. 1980;46:692–9.

Froggatt NJ, Koch J, Davies R, et al. Genetic linkage analysis in hereditary non-polyposis colon cancer syndrome. J Med Genet. 1995;32:352–7.

Gailani MR, Bale AE. Developmental genes and cancer: role of patched in basal cell carcinoma of the skin. J Natl Cancer Inst. 1997;89:1103–9.

Garber JE, Li FP, Kingston JE, et al. Hepatoblastoma and familial adenomatous polyposis. J Natl Cancer Inst. 1988;80:1626–8.

Garber JE, Burke EM, Lavally BL, et al. Choroid plexus tumors in the breast cancer-sarcoma syndrome. Cancer. 1990;66:2658–60.

Garcia A, Matias-Guiu X, Cabezas R, et al. Molecular diagnosis of von Hippel-Lindau disease in a kindred with a predominance of familial phaeochromocytoma. Clin Endocrinol (Oxf). 1997;46:359–63.

Gates Jr LK, Holladay DV. A syndrome of hereditary pancreatic adenocarcinoma and cysts of the liver and kidneys. Gastroenterology. 2002;122:796–9.

Gayther SA, Warren W, Mazoyer S, et al. Germline mutations of the BRCA1 gene in breast and ovarian cancer families provide evidence for a genotype-phenotype correlation. Nat Genet. 1995;11:428–33.

Gayther SA, Mangion J, Russell P, et al. Variation of risks of breast and ovarian cancer associated with different germline mutations of the BRCA2 gene. Nat Genet. 1997;15:103–5.

Gebert JF, Dupon C, Kadmon M, et al. Combined molecular and clinical approaches for the identification of families with familial adenomatous polyposis coli. Ann Surg. 1999;229:350–61.

Gelisken F, Gelisken O, Sadikoglu Y. Tuberous sclerosis: ocular findings and their correlation with cranial computed tomography. Bull Soc Belge Ophtalmol. 1990;238:111–21.

Gendal ES, Mendelson DS, Janus CL, Schlossberg I, Vogel JM. Squamous cell carcinoma of the esophagus in Fanconi's anemia. Dysphagia. 1988;2:178–9.

German J, Bloom D, Passarge E. Bloom's syndrome. V. Surveillance for cancer in affected families. Clin Genet. 1977;12:162–8.

Germeshausen M, Ballmaier M, Welte K. Implications of mutations in hematopoietic growth factor receptor genes in congenital cytopenias. Ann N Y Acad Sci. 2001;938:305–20; discussion 320–1.

Giardiello FM, Welsh SB, Hamilton SR, et al. Increased risk of cancer in the Peutz-Jeghers syndrome. N Engl J Med. 1987;316:1511–4.

Giardiello FM, Petersen GM, Brensinger JD, et al. Hepatoblastoma and APC gene mutation in familial adenomatous polyposis. Gut. 1996;39:867–9.

Giarola M, Stagi L, Presciuttini S, et al. Screening for mutations of the APC gene in 66 Italian familial adenomatous polyposis patients: evidence for phenotypic differences in cases with and without identified mutation. Hum Mutat. 1999;13:116–23.

Gimm O, Armanios M, Dziema H, Neumann HP, Eng C. Somatic and occult germ-line mutations in SDHD, a mitochondrial complex II gene, in nonfamilial pheochromocytoma. Cancer Res. 2000;60:6822–5.

Glavac D, Neumann HP, Wittke C, et al. Mutations in the VHL tumor suppressor gene and associated lesions in families with von Hippel-Lindau disease from central Europe. Hum Genet. 1996;98:271–80.

Goddard AD, Phillips RA, Greger V, et al. Use of the RB1 cDNA as a diagnostic probe in retinoblastoma families. Clin Genet. 1990;37:117–26.

Goldberg Y, Dibbern K, Klein J, Riccardi VM, Graham Jr JM. Neurofibromatosis type 1 – an update and review for the primary pediatrician. Clin Pediatr (Phila). 1996;35:545–61.

Goto M, Miller RW, Ishikawa Y, Sugano H. Excess of rare cancers in Werner syndrome (adult progeria). Cancer Epidemiol Biomark Prev. 1996;5:239–46.

Gould DJ, Barker DJ. Follicular atrophoderma with multiple basal cell carcinomas (Bazex). Br J Dermatol. 1978;99:431–5.

Gourlay WA, Johnson HW, Pantzar JT, McGillivray B, Crawford R, Nielsen WR. Gonadal tumors in disorders of sexual differentiation. Urology. 1994;43:537–40.

Goyal JL, Rao VA, Srinivasan R, Agrawal K. Oculocutaneous manifestations in xeroderma pigmentosa. Br J Ophthalmol. 1994;78:295–7.

Green JA. Renal oncocytoma and tuberous sclerosis. A case report. S Afr Med J. 1987;71:47–8.

Greene MH. The genetics of hereditary melanoma and nevi. 1998 update. Cancer. 1999;86:2464–77.

Gretzula JC, Hevia O, Weber PJ. Bloom's syndrome. J Am Acad Dermatol. 1987;17:479–88.

Gronberg H, Ahman AK, Emanuelsson M, Bergh A, Damber JE, Borg A. BRCA2 mutation in a family with hereditary prostate cancer. Genes Chromosomes Cancer. 2001;30:299–301.

Gross DJ, Avishai N, Meiner V, Filon D, Zbar B, Abeliovich D. Familial pheochromocytoma associated with a novel mutation in the von Hippel-Lindau gene. J Clin Endocrinol Metab. 1996;81:147–9.

Gruis NA, Sandkuijl LA, van der Velden PA, Bergman W, Frants RR. CDKN2 explains part of the clinical phenotype in Dutch familial atypical multiple-mole melanoma (FAMMM) syndrome families. Melanoma Res. 1995;5:169–77.

Grundy P, Coppes MJ, Haber D. Molecular genetics of Wilms tumor. Hematol Oncol Clin North Am. 1995;9:1201–15.

Gruner BA, DeNapoli TS, Andrews W, Tomlinson G, Bowman L, Weitman SD. Hepatocellular carcinoma in children associated with Gardner syndrome or familial adenomatous polyposis. J Pediatr Hematol Oncol. 1998;20:274–8.

Guilford PJ, Hopkins JB, Grady WM, et al. E-cadherin germline mutations define an inherited cancer syndrome dominated by diffuse gastric cancer. Hum Mutat. 1999;14:249–55.

Gustafson G, Lindahl B, Dahl E, Svensson A. The nevoid basal cell carcinoma syndrome–Gorlin's syndrome. Multiple jaw cysts and skin cancer. Swed Dent J. 1989;13:131–9.

Gutmann DH, Hedrick NM, Li J, Nagarajan R, Perry A, Watson MA. Comparative gene expression profile analysis of neurofibromatosis 1- associated and sporadic pilocytic astrocytomas. Cancer Res. 2002;62:2085–91.

Haerer AF, Jackson JF, Evers CG. Ataxia-telangiectasia with gastric adenocarcinoma. JAMA. 1969;210:1884–7.

Haibach H, Burns TW, Carlson HE, Burman KD, Deftos LJ. Multiple hamartoma syndrome (Cowden's disease) associated with renal cell carcinoma and primary neuroendocrine carcinoma of the skin (Merkel cell carcinoma). Am J Clin Pathol. 1992;97:705–12.

Hakansson S, Johannsson O, Johansson U, et al. Moderate frequency of BRCA1 and BRCA2 germ-line mutations in Scandinavian familial breast cancer. Am J Hum Genet. 1997;60:1068–78.

Hamilton JK, Paquin LA, Sullivan JL, et al. X-linked lymphoproliferative syndrome registry report. J Pediatr. 1980;96:669–73.

Hamilton SR, Liu B, Parsons RE, et al. The molecular basis of Turcot's syndrome. N Engl J Med. 1995;332:839–47.

Hammel PR, Vilgrain V, Terris B, et al. Pancreatic involvement in von Hippel-Lindau disease. The Groupe Francophone d'Etude de la Maladie de von Hippel-Lindau. Gastroenterology. 2000;119:1087–95.

Handley J, Carson D, Sloan J, et al. Multiple lentigines, myxoid tumours and endocrine overactivity; four cases of Carney's complex. Br J Dermatol. 1992;126:367–71.

Handra-Luca A, Flejou JF, Molas G, et al. Familial multiple gastrointestinal stromal tumours with associated abnormalities of the myenteric plexus layer and skeinoid fibres. Histopathology. 2001;39:359–63.

Hanna RM, Dahniya MH, Seddiq MA, Kamel H. Case report: a case of solitary Peutz-Jegher's hamartoma in the small bowel with angiographic evaluation. Br J Radiol. 1994;67:897–9.

Harach HR, Soubeyran I, Brown A, Bonneau D, Longy M. Thyroid pathologic findings in patients with Cowden disease. Ann Diagn Pathol. 1999;3:331–40.

Harbour JW. Overview of RB gene mutations in patients with retinoblastoma. Implications for clinical genetic screening. Ophthalmology. 1998;105:1442–7.

Harris VJ, Seeler RA. Ataxia-telangiectasia and Hodgkin's disease. Cancer. 1973;32:1415–20.

Hasle H, Kerndrup G, Jacobsen BB. Childhood myelodysplastic syndrome in Denmark: incidence and predisposing conditions. Leukemia. 1995;9:1569–72.

Haven CJ, Wong FK, van Dam EW, et al. A genotypic and histopathological study of a large Dutch kindred with hyperparathyroidism-jaw tumor syndrome. J Clin Endocrinol Metab. 2000;85:1449–54.

Hayani A, Mahoney Jr DH, Hawkins HK, Steuber CP, Hurwitz R, Fernbach DJ. Soft-tissue sarcomas other than rhabdomyosarcoma in children. Med Pediatr Oncol. 1992;20:114–8.

Heathcott RW, Morison IM, Gubler MC, Corbett R, Reeve AE. A review of the phenotypic variation due to the Denys-Drash syndrome- associated germline WT1 mutation R362X. Hum Mutat. 2002;19:462.

Hecht F, Hecht BK. Cancer in ataxia-telangiectasia patients. Cancer Genet Cytogenet. 1990;46:9–19.

Heimdal K, Olsson H, Tretli S, Flodgren P, Borresen AL, Fossa SD. Familial testicular cancer in Norway and southern Sweden. Br J Cancer. 1996;73:964–9.

Heinimann K, Mullhaupt B, Weber W, et al. Phenotypic differences in familial adenomatous polyposis based on APC gene mutation status. Gut. 1998;43:675–9.

Hemminki A. The molecular basis and clinical aspects of Peutz-Jeghers syndrome. Cell Mol Life Sci. 1999;55:735–50.

Hemminki K, Jiang Y. Familial and second esophageal cancers: a nation-wide epidemiologic study from Sweden. Int J Cancer. 2002;98:106–9.

Hengstler JG, Bauer A, Wolf HK, et al. Mutation analysis of the cationic trypsinogen gene in patients with pancreatic cancer. Anticancer Res. 2000;20:2967–74.

Hertle RW, Durso F, Metzler JP, Varsa EW. Epibulbar squamous cell carcinomas in brothers with Xeroderma pigmentosa. J Pediatr Ophthalmol Strabismus. 1991;28:350–3.

Hes F, Zewald R, Peeters T, et al. Genotype-phenotype correlations in families with deletions in the von Hippel-Lindau (VHL) gene. Hum Genet. 2000;106:425–31.

Hirota S, Nishida T, Isozaki K, et al. Familial gastrointestinal stromal tumors associated with dysphagia and novel type germline mutation of KIT gene. Gastroenterology. 2002;122:1493–9.

Hisada M, Garber JE, Fung CY, Fraumeni Jr JF, Li FP. Multiple primary cancers in families with Li-Fraumeni syndrome. J Natl Cancer Inst. 1998;90:606–11.

Hizawa K, Iida M, Matsumoto T, et al. Gastrointestinal manifestations of Cowden's disease. Report of four cases. J Clin Gastroenterol. 1994;18:13–8.

Hobbs MR, Pole AR, Pidwirny GN, et al. Hyperparathyroidism-jaw tumor syndrome: the HRPT2 locus is within a 0.7-cM region on chromosome 1q. Am J Hum Genet. 1999;64:518–25.

Hofting I, Pott G, Schrameyer B, Stolte M. Familial juvenile polyposis with predominant stomach involvement. Z Gastroenterol. 1993;31:480–3.

Holladay DA, Holladay A, Montebello JF, Redmond KP. Clinical presentation, treatment, and outcome of trilateral retinoblastoma. Cancer. 1991;67:710–5.

Honchel R, Halling KC, Schaid DJ, Pittelkow M, Thibodeau SN. Microsatellite instability in Muir-Torre syndrome. Cancer Res. 1994;54:1159–63.

Hough DM, Stephens DH, Johnson CD, Binkovitz LA. Pancreatic lesions in von Hippel-Lindau disease: prevalence, clinical significance, and CT findings. AJR Am J Roentgenol. 1994;162:1091–4.

Houlston R, Bevan S, Williams A, et al. Mutations in DPC4 (SMAD4) cause juvenile polyposis syndrome, but only account for a minority of cases. Hum Mol Genet. 1998;7:1907–12.

Howe JR, Norton JA, Wells Jr SA. Prevalence of pheochromocytoma and hyperparathyroidism in multiple endocrine neoplasia type 2A: results of long-term follow-up. Surgery. 1993;114:1070–7.

Howe JR, Roth S, Ringold JC, et al. Mutations in the SMAD4/DPC4 gene in juvenile polyposis. Science. 1998a;280:1086–8.

Howe JR, Mitros FA, Summers RW. The risk of gastrointestinal carcinoma in familial juvenile polyposis. Ann Surg Oncol. 1998b;5:751–6.

Howe JR, Bair JL, Sayed MG, et al. Germline mutations of the gene encoding bone morphogenetic protein receptor 1A in juvenile polyposis. Nat Genet. 2001;28:184–7.

Howe JR, Shellnut J, Wagner B, et al. Common deletion of SMAD4 in juvenile polyposis is a mutational hotspot. Am J Hum Genet. 2002;70:1357–62.

Hughes LJ, Michels VV. Risk of hepatoblastoma in familial adenomatous polyposis. Am J Med Genet. 1992;43:1023–5.

Hultborn R, Hanson C, Kopf I, Verbiene I, Warnhammar E, Weimarck A. Prevalence of Klinefelter's syndrome in male breast cancer patients. Anticancer Res. 1997;17:4293–7.

Hung J, Mims B, Lozano G, et al. TP53 mutation and haplotype analysis of two large African American families. Hum Mutat. 1999;14:216–21.

Huusko P, Castren K, Launonen V, et al. Germ-line TP53 mutations in Finnish cancer families exhibiting features of the Li-Fraumeni syndrome and negative for BRCA1 and BRCA2. Cancer Genet Cytogenet. 1999;112:9–14.

Iihara M, Yamashita T, Okamoto T, et al. A nationwide clinical survey of patients with multiple endocrine neoplasia type 2 and familial medullary thyroid carcinoma in Japan. Jpn J Clin Oncol. 1997;27:128–34.

Imamura J, Miyoshi I, Koeffler HP. p53 in hematologic malignancies. Blood. 1994;84:2412–21.

Iscovich J, Abdulrazik M, Cour C, Fischbein A, Pe'er J, Goldgar DE. Prevalence of the BRCA2 6174 del T mutation in Israeli uveal melanoma patients. Int J Cancer. 2002;98:42–4.

Ishikawa Y, Sugano H, Matsumoto T, Furuichi Y, Miller RW, Goto M. Unusual features of thyroid carcinomas in Japanese patients with Werner syndrome and possible genotype-phenotype relations to cell type and race. Cancer. 1999;85:1345–52.

Isozaki K, Terris B, Belghiti J, Schiffmann S, Hirota S, Vanderwinden JM. Germline-activating mutation in the kinase domain of KIT gene in familial gastrointestinal stromal tumors. Am J Pathol. 2000;157:1581–5.

Ito Y, Oki S, Mikami T, et al. Familial astrocytoma associated with von Recklinghausen's disease: report of two cases. No Shinkei Geka. 1997;25:283–8.

Iwama T, Mishima Y, Utsunomiya J. The impact of familial adenomatous polyposis on the tumorigenesis and mortality at the several organs. Its rational treatment. Ann Surg. 1993;217:101–8.

Jackson CE, Puck JM. Autoimmune lymphoproliferative syndrome, a disorder of apoptosis. Curr Opin Pediatr. 1999;11:521–7.

Jang KA, Choi JH, Sung KJ, Moon KC, Koh JK, Im DJ. Juvenile chronic myelogenous leukemia, neurofibromatosis 1, and xanthoma. J Dermatol. 1999;26:33–5.

Janin N, Andrieu N, Ossian K, et al. Breast cancer risk in ataxia telangiectasia (AT) heterozygotes: haplotype study in French AT families. Br J Cancer. 1999;80:1042–5.

Janov AJ, Leong T, Nathan DG, Guinan EC. Diamond-Blackfan anemia. Natural history and sequelae of treatment. Medicine (Baltimore). 1996;75:77–8.

Jarvis L, Bathurst N, Mohan D, Beckly D. Turcot's syndrome. A review. Dis Colon Rectum. 1988;31:907–14.

Jay M, McCartney AC. Familial malignant melanoma of the uvea and p53: a Victorian detective story. Surv Ophthalmol. 1993;37:457–62.

Jozwiak S, Kawalec W, Dluzewska J, Daszkowska J, Mirkowicz-Malek M, Michalowicz R. Cardiac tumours in tuberous sclerosis: their incidence and course. Eur J Pediatr. 1994;153:155–7.

Jozwiak S, Schwartz RA, Janniger CK, Michalowicz R, Chmielik J. Skin lesions in children with tuberous sclerosis complex: their prevalence, natural course, and diagnostic significance. Int J Dermatol. 1998;37:911–7.

Kalff V, Shapiro B, Lloyd R, et al. The spectrum of pheochromocytoma in hypertensive patients with neurofibromatosis. Arch Intern Med. 1982;142:2092–8.

Kameyama K, Takami H, Miyajima K, Mimura T, Hosoda Y, Ito K. Papillary carcinoma occurring within an adenomatous goiter of the thyroid gland in Cowden's disease. Endocr Pathol. 2001;12:73–6.

Kanayama H, Lui WO, Takahashi M, et al. Association of a novel constitutional translocation t(1q;3q) with familial renal cell carcinoma. J Med Genet. 2001;38:165–70.

Kaneko H, Inoue R, Fukao T, et al. Two Japanese siblings with Bloom syndrome gene mutation and B-cell lymphoma. Leuk Lymphoma. 1997;27:539–42.

Kaplan MJ, Sabio H, Wanebo HJ, Cantrell RW. Squamous cell carcinoma in the immunosuppressed patient: Fanconi's anemia. Laryngoscope. 1985;95:771–5.

Kaplinsky C, Ghahremani M, Frishberg Y, Rechavi G, Pelletier J. Familial Wilms' tumor associated with a WT1 zinc finger mutation. Genomics. 1996;38:451–3.

Kennedy AW, Hart WR. Multiple squamous-cell carcinomas in Fanconi's anemia. Cancer. 1982;50:811–4.

Khoo SK, Bradley M, Wong FK, Hedblad MA, Nordenskjold M, Teh BT. Birt-Hogg-Dube syndrome: mapping of a novel hereditary neoplasia gene to chromosome 17p12-q11.2. Oncogene. 2001;20:5239–42.

Kidd A, Carson L, Gregory DW, et al. A Scottish family with Bazex-Dupre-Christol syndrome: follicular atrophoderma, congenital hypotrichosis, and basal cell carcinoma. J Med Genet. 1996;33:493–7.

Kimonis VE, Goldstein AM, Pastakia B, et al. Clinical manifestations in 105 persons with nevoid basal cell carcinoma syndrome. Am J Med Genet. 1997;69:299–308.

Kiribuchi K, Uchida Y, Fukuyama Y, Maruyama H. High incidence of fundus hamartomas and clinical significance of a fundus score in tuberous sclerosis. Brain Dev. 1986;8:509–17.

Kirschner LS, Sandrini F, Monbo J, Lin JP, Carney JA, Stratakis CA. Genetic heterogeneity and spectrum of mutations of the PRKAR1A gene in patients with the carney complex. Hum Mol Genet. 2000a;9:3037–46.

Kirschner LS, Carney JA, Pack SD, et al. Mutations of the gene encoding the protein kinase A type I-alpha regulatory subunit in patients with the Carney complex. Nat Genet. 2000b;26:89–92.

Kiuru M, Launonen V, Hietala M, et al. Familial cutaneous leiomyomatosis is a two-hit condition associated with renal cell cancer of characteristic histopathology. Am J Pathol. 2001;159:825–9.

Kleihues P, Schauble B, zur Hausen A, Esteve J, Ohgaki H. Tumors associated with p53 germline mutations: a synopsis of 91 families. Am J Pathol. 1997;150:1–13.

Kluwe L, Bayer S, Baser ME, et al. Identification of NF2 germ-line mutations and comparison with neurofibromatosis 2 phenotypes. Hum Genet. 1996;98:534–8.

Knight 3rd WA, Murphy WK, Gottlieb JA. Neurofibromatosis associated with malignant neurofibromas. Arch Dermatol. 1973;107:747–50.

Kornreich L, Blaser S, Schwarz M, et al. Optic pathway glioma: correlation of imaging findings with the presence of neurofibromatosis. AJNR Am J Neuroradiol. 2001;22:1963–9.

Koufos A, Grundy P, Morgan K, et al. Familial Wiedemann-Beckwith syndrome and a second Wilms tumor locus both map to 11p15.5. Am J Hum Genet. 1989;44:711–9.

Kozarek RA, Sanowski RA. Carcinoma of the esophagus associated with Fanconi's anemia. J Clin Gastroenterol. 1981;3:171–4.

Kraemer KH, Lee MM, Scotto J. Xeroderma pigmentosum. Cutaneous, ocular, and neurologic abnormalities in 830 published cases. Arch Dermatol. 1987;123:241–50.

Kraimps JL, Denizot A, Carnaille B, et al. Primary hyperparathyroidism in multiple endocrine neoplasia type IIa: retrospective French multicentric study. Groupe d'Etude des Tumeurs a Calcitonine (GETC, French Calcitonin Tumors Study Group), French Association of Endocrine Surgeons. World J Surg. 1996;20:808–12; discussion 812–3.

Kratzke RA, Otterson GA, Hogg A, et al. Partial inactivation of the RB product in a family with incomplete penetrance of familial retinoblastoma and benign retinal tumors. Oncogene. 1994;9:1321–6.

Krijanovski OI, Sieff CA. Diamond-Blackfan anemia. Hematol Oncol Clin North Am. 1997;11:1061–77.

Kubo O, Sasahara A, Tajika Y, Kawamura H, Kawabatake H, Takakura K. Pleomorphic xanthoastrocytoma with neurofibromatosis type 1: case report. Noshuyo Byori. 1996;13:79–83.

Kyritsis AP, Bondy ML, Xiao M, et al. Germline p53 gene mutations in subsets of glioma patients. J Natl Cancer Inst. 1994;86:344–9.

Lacombe D, Chateil JF, Fontan D, Battin J. Medulloblastoma in the nevoid basal-cell carcinoma syndrome: case reports and review of the literature. Genet Couns. 1990;1:273–7.

Lancaster JM, Wooster R, Mangion J, et al. BRCA2 mutations in primary breast and ovarian cancers. Nat Genet. 1996;13:238–40.

Langer P, Cupisti K, Bartsch DK, et al. Adrenal involvement in multiple endocrine neoplasia type 1. World J Surg. 2002;26:891–6.

Larson GP, Zhang G, Ding S, et al. An allelic variant at the ATM locus is implicated in breast cancer susceptibility. Genet Test. 1997;1:165–70.

Latronico AC, Pinto EM, Domenice S, et al. An inherited mutation outside the highly conserved DNA-binding domain of the p53 tumor suppressor protein in children and adults with sporadic adrenocortical tumors. J Clin Endocrinol Metab. 2001;86:4970–3.

Launonen V, Vierimaa O, Kiuru M, et al. Inherited susceptibility to uterine leiomyomas and renal cell cancer. Proc Natl Acad Sci U S A. 2001;98:3387–92.

Lavin M. Role of the ataxia-telangiectasia gene (ATM) in breast cancer. A-T heterozygotes seem to have an increased risk but its size is unknown. BMJ. 1998;317:486–7.

Leach FS, Nicolaides NC, Papadopoulos N, et al. Mutations of a mutS homolog in hereditary nonpolyposis colorectal cancer. Cell. 1993;75:1215–25.

Lee HR, Moon YS, Yeom CH, et al. Cowden's disease – a report on the first case in Korea and literature review. J Korean Med Sci. 1997;12:570–5.

Leung SY, Chan TL, Chung LP, et al. Microsatellite instability and mutation of DNA mismatch repair genes in gliomas. Am J Pathol. 1998;153:1181–8.

Li FQ, Horwitz M. Characterization of mutant neutrophil elastase in severe congenital neutropenia. J Biol Chem. 2001;276:14230–41.

Li YJ, Sanson M, Hoang-Xuan K, et al. Incidence of germ-line p53 mutations in patients with gliomas. Int J Cancer. 1995;64:383–7.

Li J, Perry A, James CD, Gutmann DH. Cancer-related gene expression profiles in NF1-associated pilocytic astrocytomas. Neurology. 2001;56:885–90.

Libutti SK, Choyke PL, Bartlett DL, et al. Pancreatic neuroendocrine tumors associated with von Hippel Lindau disease: diagnostic and management recommendations. Surgery. 1998;124:1153–9.

Libutti SK, Choyke PL, Alexander HR, et al. Clinical and genetic analysis of patients with pancreatic neuroendocrine tumors associated with von Hippel-Lindau disease. Surgery. 2000;128:1022–7; discussion 1027–8.

Ligtenberg MJ, Hogervorst FB, Willems HW, et al. Characteristics of small breast and/or ovarian cancer families with germline mutations in BRCA1 and BRCA2. Br J Cancer. 1999;79:1475–8.

Lima JB, Smith PD. Sipple's syndrome (pheochromocytoma and thyroid carcinoma) with bilateral breast carcinoma. Am J Surg. 1971;121:732–5.

Linares M, Pastor E, Gomez A, Grau E. Hepatocellular carcinoma and squamous cell carcinoma in a patient with Fanconi's anemia. Ann Hematol. 1991;63:54–5.

Lindboe CF, Helseth E, Myhr G. Lhermitte-Duclos disease and giant meningioma as manifestations of Cowden's disease. Clin Neuropathol. 1995;14:327–30.

Lindor NM, Furuichi Y, Kitao S, Shimamoto A, Arndt C, Jalal S. Rothmund-Thomson syndrome due to RECQ4 helicase mutations: report and clinical and molecular comparisons with Bloom syndrome and Werner syndrome. Am J Med Genet. 2000;90:223–8.

Linos DA, Dozois RR, Dahlin DC, Bartholomew LG. Does Peutz-Jeghers syndrome predispose to gastrointestinal malignancy? A later look. Arch Surg. 1981;116:1182–4.

Listernick R, Charrow J, Gutmann DH. Intracranial gliomas in neurofibromatosis type 1. Am J Med Genet. 1999;89:38–44.

Little M, Wells C. A clinical overview of WT1 gene mutations. Hum Mutat. 1997;9:209–25.

Liu YC, Wei TC, Hsu YH, Fang JS, Lee ML. Gonadoblastoma and chroiocarcinoma in dysgenic gonads: report of a case. J Formos Med Assoc. 1995;94:568–71.

Lobaccaro JM, Lumbroso S, Belon C, et al. Androgen receptor gene mutation in male breast cancer. Hum Mol Genet. 1993;2:1799–802.

Loh KC. Familial nonmedullary thyroid carcinoma: a meta-review of case series. Thyroid. 1997;7:107–13.

Lohmann DR. RB1 gene mutations in retinoblastoma. Hum Mutat. 1999;14:283–8.

Louis DN, von Deimling A. Hereditary tumor syndromes of the nervous system: overview and rare syndromes. Brain Pathol. 1995;5:145–51.

Lowenfels AB, Maisonneuve P, DiMagno EP, et al. Hereditary pancreatitis and the risk of pancreatic cancer. International Hereditary Pancreatitis Study Group. J Natl Cancer Inst. 1997;89:442–6.

Lowney JK, Frisella MM, Lairmore TC, Doherty GM. Pancreatic islet cell tumor metastasis in multiple endocrine neoplasia type 1: correlation with primary tumor size. Surgery. 1998;124:1043–8, discussion 1048–9.

Luk GD. Diagnosis and therapy of hereditary polyposis syndromes. Gastroenterologist. 1995;3:153–67.

Lupoli G, Vitale G, Caraglia M, et al. Familial papillary thyroid microcarcinoma: a new clinical entity. Lancet. 1999;353:637–9.

Lustig JP, Lugassy G, Neder A, Sigler E. Head and neck carcinoma in Fanconi's anaemia–report of a case and review of the literature. Eur J Cancer B Oral Oncol. 1995;31B:68–72.

Lynch HT, Fusaro RM. Pancreatic cancer and the familial atypical multiple mole melanoma (FAMMM) syndrome. Pancreas. 1991;6:127–31.

Lynch HT, Lynch JF. 25 years of HNPCC. Anticancer Res. 1994;14:1617–24.

Lynch HT, Lynch J. Genetics, natural history, surveillance, management, and gene mapping in the Lynch syndrome. Pathol Biol (Paris). 1995;43:151–8.

Lynch HT, Kimberling W, Albano WA, et al. Hereditary nonpolyposis colorectal cancer (Lynch syndromes I and II). I. Clinical description of resource. Cancer. 1985a;56:934–8.

Lynch HT, Fusaro RM, Roberts L, Voorhees GJ, Lynch JF. Muir-Torre syndrome in several members of a family with a variant of the Cancer Family Syndrome. Br J Dermatol. 1985b;113:295–301.

Lynch HT, Thorson AG, McComb RD, Franklin BA, Tinley ST, Lynch JF. Familial adenomatous polyposis and extracolonic cancer. Dig Dis Sci. 2001;46:2325–32.

Lynch HT, Brand RE, Hogg D, et al. Phenotypic variation in eight extended CDKN2A germline mutation familial atypical multiple mole melanoma-pancreatic carcinoma-prone families: the familial atypical mole melanoma-pancreatic carcinoma syndrome. Cancer. 2002;94:84–96.

Lyons CJ, Wilson CB, Horton JC. Association between meningioma and Cowden's disease. Neurology. 1993;43:1436–7.

Maeyama H, Hidaka E, Ota H, et al. Familial gastrointestinal stromal tumor with hyperpigmentation: association with a germline mutation of the c-kit gene. Gastroenterology. 2001;120:210–5.

Maher ER, Yates JR, Harries R, et al. Clinical features and natural history of von Hippel-Lindau disease. Q J Med. 1990;77:1151–63.

Maher ER, Webster AR, Moore AT. Clinical features and molecular genetics of Von Hippel-Lindau disease. Ophthalmic Genet. 1995;16:79–84.

Maher ER, Webster AR, Richards FM, et al. Phenotypic expression in von Hippel-Lindau disease: correlations with germline VHL gene mutations. J Med Genet. 1996;33:328–32.

Maillefer RH, Greydanus MP. To B or not to B: is tylosis B truly benign? Two North American genealogies. Am J Gastroenterol. 1999;94:829–34.

Malchoff CD, Malchoff DM. Familial nonmedullary thyroid carcinoma. Semin Surg Oncol. 1999;16:16–8.

Malchoff CD, Sarfarazi M, Tendler B, Forouhar F, Whalen G, Malchoff DM. Familial papillary thyroid carcinoma is genetically distinct from familial adenomatous polyposis coli. Thyroid. 1999;9:247–52.

Malchoff CD, Sarfarazi M, Tendler B, et al. Papillary thyroid carcinoma associated with papillary renal neoplasia: genetic linkage analysis of a distinct heritable tumor syndrome. J Clin Endocrinol Metab. 2000;85:1758–64.

Marchesi M, Biffoni M, Biancari F, et al. Familial papillary carcinoma of the thyroid: a report of nine first- degree relatives of four families. Eur J Surg Oncol. 2000;26:789–91.

Marger RS, Marger D. Carcinoma of the esophagus and tylosis. A lethal genetic combination. Cancer. 1993;72:17–9.

Marsh DJ, Coulon V, Lunetta KL, et al. Mutation spectrum and genotype-phenotype analyses in Cowden disease and Bannayan-Zonana syndrome, two hamartoma syndromes with germline PTEN mutation. Hum Mol Genet. 1998;7:507–15.

Marsh DJ, Kum JB, Lunetta KL, et al. PTEN mutation spectrum and genotype-phenotype correlations in Bannayan-Riley-Ruvalcaba syndrome suggest a single entity with Cowden syndrome. Hum Mol Genet. 1999;8:1461–72.

Marx SJ, Agarwal SK, Kester MB, et al. Multiple endocrine neoplasia type 1: clinical and genetic features of the hereditary endocrine neoplasias. Recent Prog Horm Res. 1999;54:397–438.

Mastronardi L, Ferrante L, Lunardi P, Cervoni L, Fortuna A. Association between neuroepithelial tumor and multiple intestinal polyposis (Turcot's syndrome): report of a case and critical analysis of the literature. Neurosurgery. 1991;28:449–52.

Matsui I, Tanimura M, Kobayashi N, Sawada T, Nagahara N, Akatsuka J. Neurofibromatosis type 1 and childhood cancer. Cancer. 1993;72:2746–54.

McGaughran JM, Harris DI, Donnai D, et al. A clinical study of type 1 neurofibromatosis in north west England. J Med Genet. 1999;36:197–203.

Mecklin JP, Jarvinen HJ. Tumor spectrum in cancer family syndrome (hereditary nonpolyposis colorectal cancer). Cancer. 1991;68:1109–12.

Meindl A. Comprehensive analysis of 989 patients with breast or ovarian cancer provides BRCA1 and BRCA2 mutation profiles and frequencies for the German population. Int J Cancer. 2002;97:472–80.

Meis JM, Enzinger FM, Martz KL, Neal JA. Malignant peripheral nerve sheath tumors (malignant schwannomas) in children. Am J Surg Pathol. 1992;16:694–707.

Michaud J, Wu F, Osato M, et al. In vitro analyses of known and novel RUNX1/AML1 mutations in dominant familial platelet disorder with predisposition to acute myelogenous leukemia: implications for mechanisms of pathogenesis. Blood. 2002;99:1364–72.

Minami M, Urano Y, Ishigami T, Tsuda H, Kusaka J, Arase S. Germline mutations of the PTCH gene in Japanese patients with nevoid basal cell carcinoma syndrome. J Dermatol Sci. 2001;27:21–6.

Mochon MC, Blanc JF, Plauchu H, Philip T. WAGR syndrome, Wilms' tumor, aniridia, gonado-blastoma, mental retardation: a review apropos of 2 cases. Pediatrie. 1987;42:249–52.

Moisio AL, Jarvinen H, Peltomaki P. Genetic and clinical characterisation of familial adenomatous polyposis: a population based study. Gut. 2002;50:845–50.

Moll AC, Imhof SM, Bouter LM, Tan KE. Second primary tumors in patients with retinoblastoma. A review of the literature. Ophthalmic Genet. 1997;18:27–34.

Monnat JRJ. Werner syndrome. In: Fletcher C, Mertens F, editors. Pathology and genetics of tumours of soft tissue and bone. London: WHO/IARC; 2002.

Muller J, Visfeldt J, Philip J, Skakkebaek NE. Carcinoma in situ, gonadoblastoma, and early invasive neoplasia in a nine-year-old girl with 46, XY gonadal dysgenesis. APMIS. 1992;100:170–4.

Murata J, Tada M, Sawamura Y, Mitsumori K, Abe H, Nagashima K. Dysplastic gangliocytoma (Lhermitte-Duclos disease) associated with Cowden disease: report of a case and review of the literature for the genetic relationship between the two diseases. J Neurooncol. 1999;41:129–36.

Murphy RC, Berdon WE, Ruzal-Shapiro C, et al. Malignancies in pediatric patients with ataxia telangiectasia. Pediatr Radiol. 1999;29:225–30.

Murphy KM, Brune KA, Griffin C, et al. Evaluation of candidate genes MAP2K4, MADH4, ACVR1B, and BRCA2 in familial pancreatic cancer: deleterious BRCA2 mutations in 17%. Cancer Res. 2002;62:3789–93.

Musholt TJ, Musholt PB, Petrich T, Oetting G, Knapp WH, Klempnauer J. Familial papillary thyroid carcinoma: genetics, criteria for diagnosis, clinical features, and surgical treatment. World J Surg. 2000;24:1409–17.

Nabbout R, Santos M, Rolland Y, Delalande O, Dulac O, Chiron C. Early diagnosis of subependy-mal giant cell astrocytoma in children with tuberous sclerosis. J Neurol Neurosurg Psychiatry. 1999;66:370–5.

Naguib MG, Sung JH, Erickson DL, Gold LH, Seljeskog EL. Central nervous system involvement in the nevoid basal cell carcinoma syndrome: case report and review of the literature. Neurosurgery. 1982;11:52–6.

Nambisan RN, Rao U, Moore R, Karakousis CP. Malignant soft tissue tumors of nerve sheath origin. J Surg Oncol. 1984;25:268–72.

Neblett CR, Waltz TA, Anderson DE. Neurological involvement in the nevoid basal cell carcinoma syndrome. J Neurosurg. 1971;35:577–84.

Nelen MR, Padberg GW, Peeters EA, et al. Localization of the gene for Cowden disease to chro-mosome 10q22-23. Nat Genet. 1996;13:114–6.

Neuhausen S, Gilewski T, Norton L, et al. Recurrent BRCA2 6174delT mutations in Ashkenazi Jewish women affected by breast cancer. Nat Genet. 1996;13:126–8.

Neumann HP, Bausch B, McWhinney SR, et al. Germ-line mutations in nonsyndromic pheochro-mocytoma. N Engl J Med. 2002;346:1459–66.

Nichols KE, Malkin D, Garber JE, Fraumeni Jr JF, Li FP. Germ-line p53 mutations predispose to a wide spectrum of early-onset cancers. Cancer Epidemiol Biomarkers Prev. 2001;10:83–7.

Nicholson PW, Harland SJ. Inheritance and testicular cancer. Br J Cancer. 1995;71:421–6.

Nickerson M, Warren M, Toro J, et al. Mutations in a novel gene lead to kidney tumors, lung wall defects, and benign tumors of the hair follicle in patients with the Birt-Hogg-Dube syndrome. Cancer Cell. 2002;2:157.

Nir A, Tajik AJ, Freeman WK, et al. Tuberous sclerosis and cardiac rhabdomyoma. Am J Cardiol. 1995;76:419–21.

Nishida T, Hirota S, Taniguchi M, et al. Familial gastrointestinal stromal tumours with germline mutation of the KIT gene. Nat Genet. 1998;19:323–4.

Nishio S, Morioka T, Suzuki S, Kira R, Mihara F, Fukui M. Subependymal giant cell astrocytoma: clinical and neuroimaging features of four cases. J Clin Neurosci. 2001;8:31–4.

North KN. Clinical aspects of neurofibromatosis 1. Eur J Paediatr Neurol. 1998;2:223–31.

North K. Neurofibromatosis type 1. Am J Med Genet. 2000;97:119–27.

Norton ID, Gostout CJ. Management of periampullary adenoma. Dig Dis. 1998;16:266–73.

Nowak DA, Trost HA. Lhermitte-Duclos disease (dysplastic cerebellar gangliocytoma): a malformation, hamartoma or neoplasm? Acta Neurol Scand. 2002;105:137–45.

Nowak DA, Trost HA, Porr A, Stolzle A, Lumenta CB. Lhermitte-Duclos disease (Dysplastic gangliocytoma of the cerebellum). Clin Neurol Neurosurg. 2001;103:105–10.

O'Callaghan FJ, Lux A, Osborne J. Early diagnosis of subependymal giant cell astrocytoma in children with tuberous sclerosis. J Neurol Neurosurg Psychiatry. 2000;68:118.

O'Hagan AR, Ellsworth R, Secic M, Rothner AD, Brouhard BH. Renal manifestations of tuberous sclerosis complex. Clin Pediatr (Phila). 1996;35:483–9.

O'Reilly DA, Kingsnorth AN. Hereditary pancreatitis and mutations of the cationic trypsinogen gene. Br J Surg. 2000;87:708–17.

Oberg K, Skogseid B, Eriksson B. Multiple endocrine neoplasia type 1 (MEN-1). Clinical, biochemical and genetical investigations. Acta Oncol. 1989;28:383–7.

Ogawa T, Mitsukawa T, Ishikawa T, Tamura K. Familial pheochromocytoma associated with von Recklinghausen's disease. Intern Med. 1994;33:110–4.

Ohara N, Komiya I, Yamauchi K, et al. Carney's complex with primary pigmented nodular adrenocortical disease and spotty pigmentations. Intern Med. 1993;32:60–2.

Ohsato K, Yao T, Watanabe H, Iida M, Itoh H. Small-intestinal involvement in familial polyposis diagnosed by operative intestinal fiberscopy: report of four cases. Dis Colon Rectum. 1977;20:414–20.

Oksuzoglu B, Yalcin S. Squamous cell carcinoma of the tongue in a patient with Fanconi's anemia: a case report and review of the literature. Ann Hematol. 2002;81:294–8.

Olivero M, Valente G, Bardelli A, et al. Novel mutation in the ATP-binding site of the MET oncogene tyrosine kinase in a HPRCC family. Int J Cancer. 1999;82:640–3.

Olsen JH, Hahnemann JM, Borresen-Dale AL, et al. Cancer in patients with ataxia-telangiectasia and in their relatives in the nordic countries. J Natl Cancer Inst. 2001;93:121–7.

Ostergaard P, Simpson MA, Connell FC, Steward CG, Brice G, Woollard WJ, Dafou D, Kilo T, Smithson S, Lunt P, Murday VA, Hodgson S, Keenan R, Pilz DT, Martinez-Corral I, Makinen T, Mortimer PS, Jeffery S, Trembath RC, Mansour S. Mutations in GATA2 cause primary lymphedema associated with a predisposition to acute myeloid leukemia (Emberger syndrome). Nat Genet. 2011;43(10):929–31.

Padberg GW, Schot JD, Vielvoye GJ, Bots GT, de Beer FC. Lhermitte-Duclos disease and Cowden disease: a single phakomatosis. Ann Neurol. 1991;29:517–23.

Papadopoulos N, Nicolaides NC, Wei YF, et al. Mutation of a mutL homolog in hereditary colon cancer. Science. 1994;263:1625–9.

Park JG, Park YJ, Wijnen JT, Vasen HF. Gene-environment interaction in hereditary nonpolyposis colorectal cancer with implications for diagnosis and genetic testing. Int J Cancer. 1999;82:516–9.

Parry DM, MacCollin MM, Kaiser-Kupfer MI, et al. Germ-line mutations in the neurofibromatosis 2 gene: correlations with disease severity and retinal abnormalities. Am J Hum Genet. 1996;59:529–39.

Passarge E. Bloom's syndrome: the German experience. Ann Genet. 1991;34:179–97.

Patton LL, Valdez IH. Xeroderma pigmentosum: review and report of a case. Oral Surg Oral Med Oral Pathol. 1991;71:297–300.

Peel DJ, Ziogas A, Fox EA, et al. Characterization of hereditary nonpolyposis colorectal cancer families from a population-based series of cases. J Natl Cancer Inst. 2000;92:1517–22.

Pelletier J, Bruening W, Li FP, Haber DA, Glaser T, Housman DE. WT1 mutations contribute to abnormal genital system development and hereditary Wilms' tumour. Nature. 1991a;353:431–4.

Pelletier J, Bruening W, Kashtan CE, et al. Germline mutations in the Wilms' tumor suppressor gene are associated with abnormal urogenital development in Denys-Drash syndrome. Cell. 1991b;67:437–47.

Perry A, Giannini C, Raghavan R, et al. Aggressive phenotypic and genotypic features in pediatric and NF2- associated meningiomas: a clinicopathologic study of 53 cases. J Neuropathol Exp Neurol. 2001;60:994–1003.

Pesin SR, Shields JA. Seven cases of trilateral retinoblastoma. Am J Ophthalmol. 1989;107:121–6.

Peters AM, Kohfink B, Martin H, et al. Defective apoptosis due to a point mutation in the death domain of CD95 associated with autoimmune lymphoproliferative syndrome, T-cell lymphoma, and Hodgkin's disease. Exp Hematol. 1999;27:868–74.

Peterson RD, Funkhouser JD, Tuck-Muller CM, Gatti RA. Cancer susceptibility in ataxia-telangiectasia. Leukemia. 1992;6:8–13.

Pharoah PD, Easton DF, Stockton DL, Gayther S, Ponder BA. Survival in familial, BRCA1-associated, and BRCA2-associated epithelial ovarian cancer. United Kingdom Coordinating Committee for Cancer Research (UKCCCR) Familial Ovarian Cancer Study Group. Cancer Res. 1999;59:868–71.

Podolski J, Byrski T, Zajaczek S, et al. Characterization of a familial RCC-associated t(2;3) (q33;q21) chromosome translocation. J Hum Genet. 2001;46:685–93.

Poppe B, Van Limbergen H, Van Roy N, et al. Chromosomal aberrations in Bloom syndrome patients with myeloid malignancies. Cancer Genet Cytogenet. 2001;128:39–42.

Presciuttini S, Varesco L, Sala P, et al. Age of onset in familial adenomatous polyposis: heterogeneity within families and among APC mutations. Ann Hum Genet. 1994;58:331–42.

Purtilo DT. Immunopathology of the X-linked lymphoproliferative syndrome. Hamatol Bluttransfus. 1981;26:207–14.

Purtilo DT, DeFlorio Jr D, Hutt LM, et al. Variable phenotypic expression of an X-linked recessive lymphoproliferative syndrome. N Engl J Med. 1977;297:1077–80.

Purtilo DT, Sakamoto K, Barnabei V, et al. Epstein-Barr virus-induced diseases in boys with the X-linked lymphoproliferative syndrome (XLP): update on studies of the registry. Am J Med. 1982;73:49–56.

Randerson-Moor JA, Harland M, Williams S, et al. A germline deletion of p14(ARF) but not CDKN2A in a melanoma-neural system tumour syndrome family. Hum Mol Genet. 2001;10:55–62.

Rapley EA, Crockford GP, Teare D, et al. Localization to Xq27 of a susceptibility gene for testicular germ-cell tumours. Nat Genet. 2000;24:197–200.

Rasmussen SA, Friedman JM. NF1 gene and neurofibromatosis 1. Am J Epidemiol. 2000; 151:33–40.

Rayner CR, Towers JF, Wilson JS. What is Gorlin's syndrome? The diagnosis and management of the basal cell naevus syndrome, based on a study of thirty-seven patients. Br J Plast Surg. 1977;30:62–7.

Reichardt P, Apel TW, Domula M, et al. Recurrent polytopic chromaffin paragangliomas in a 9-year-old boy resulting from a novel germline mutation in the von Hippel-Lindau gene. J Pediatr Hematol Oncol. 2002;24:145–8.

Riccardi VM, Powell PP. Neurofibrosarcoma as a complication of von Recklinghausen neurofibromatosis. Neurofibromatosis. 1989;2:152–65.

Riccardi VM, Kleiner B, Lubs ML. Neurofibromatosis: variable expression is not intrinsic to the mutant gene. Birth Defects Orig Artic Ser. 1979;15:283–9.

Richard S, Beigelman C, Duclos JM, et al. Pheochromocytoma as the first manifestation of von Hippel-Lindau disease. Surgery. 1994;116:1076–81.

Richards FM, Goudie DR, Cooper WN, et al. Mapping the multiple self-healing squamous epithelioma (MSSE) gene and investigation of xeroderma pigmentosum group A (XPA) and PATCHED (PTCH) as candidate genes. Hum Genet. 1997;101:317–22.

Richards FM, Webster AR, McMahon R, Woodward ER, Rose S, Maher ER. Molecular genetic analysis of von Hippel-Lindau disease. J Intern Med. 1998;243:527–33.

Rieux-Laucat F, Blachere S, Danielan S, et al. Lymphoproliferative syndrome with autoimmunity: a possible genetic basis for dominant expression of the clinical manifestations. Blood. 1999;94:2575–82.

Risk JM, Mills HS, Garde J, et al. The tylosis esophageal cancer (TOC) locus: more than just a familial cancer gene. Dis Esophagus. 1999;12:173–6.

Robinson S, Cohen AR. Cowden disease and Lhermitte-Duclos disease: characterization of a new phakomatosis. Neurosurgery. 2000;46:371–83.

Rodu B, Martinez Jr MG. Peutz-Jeghers syndrome and cancer. Oral Surg Oral Med Oral Pathol. 1984;58:584–8.

Rogalski RP, Louis DS. Neurofibrosarcomas of the upper extremity. J Hand Surg [Am]. 1991;16:873–6.

Romero Y, Cameron AJ, Locke 3rd GR, et al. Familial aggregation of gastroesophageal reflux in patients with Barrett's esophagus and esophageal adenocarcinoma. Gastroenterology. 1997;113:1449–56.

Roszkowski M, Drabik K, Barszcz S, Jozwiak S. Surgical treatment of intraventricular tumors associated with tuberous sclerosis. Childs Nerv Syst. 1995;11:335–9.

Ruckle HC, Torres VE, Richardson RL, Zincke H. Renal tumors. Curr Opin Nephrol Hypertens. 1993;2:201–10.

Rutgers JL, Scully RE. The androgen insensitivity syndrome (testicular feminization): a clinicopathologic study of 43 cases. Int J Gynecol Pathol. 1991;10:126–44.

Rutten A, Burgdorf W, Hugel H, et al. Cystic sebaceous tumors as marker lesions for the Muir-Torre syndrome: a histopathologic and molecular genetic study. Am J Dermatopathol. 1999;21:405–13.

Saad MF, Ordonez NG, Rashid RK, et al. Medullary carcinoma of the thyroid. A study of the clinical features and prognostic factors in 161 patients. Medicine (Baltimore). 1984;63:319–42.

Sachatello CR, Griffen Jr WO. Hereditary polypoid diseases of the gastrointestinal tract: a working classification. Am J Surg. 1975;129:198–203.

Sakaguchi N, Sano K, Ito M, Baba T, Fukuzawa M, Hotchi M. A case of von Recklinghausen's disease with bilateral pheochromocytoma- malignant peripheral nerve sheath tumors of the adrenal and gastrointestinal autonomic nerve tumors. Am J Surg Pathol. 1996; 20:889–97.

Sakurai A, Matsumoto K, Ikeo Y, et al. Frequency of facial angiofibromas in Japanese patients with multiple endocrine neoplasia type 1. Endocr J. 2000;47:569–73.

Samaan NA, Ouais S, Ordonez NG, Choksi UA, Sellin RV, Hickey RC. Multiple endocrine syndrome type I. Clinical, laboratory findings, and management in five families. Cancer. 1989;64:741–52.

Sameshima Y, Tsunematsu Y, Watanabe S, et al. Detection of novel germ-line p53 mutations in diverse-cancer-prone families identified by selecting patients with childhood adrenocortical carcinoma. J Natl Cancer Inst. 1992;84:703–7.

Sampson JR. The kidney in tuberous sclerosis: manifestations and molecular genetic mechanisms. Nephrol Dial Transplant. 1996;11:34–7.

Samuelsson B, Axelsson R. Neurofibromatosis. A clinical and genetic study of 96 cases in Gothenburg, Sweden. Acta Derm Venereol Suppl. 1981;95:67–71.

Samuelsson B, Samuelsson S. Neurofibromatosis in Gothenburg, Sweden. I. Background, study design and epidemiology. Neurofibromatosis. 1989;2:6–22.

Sarantaus L, Vahteristo P, Bloom E, et al. BRCA1 and BRCA2 mutations among 233 unselected Finnish ovarian carcinoma patients. Eur J Hum Genet. 2001;9:424–30.

Sarma CC, Ghose B, Saikia TC. Xeroderma pigmentosa with ocular involvement (two case reports with discussion on the subject). Indian J Dermatol. 1973;18:47–50.

Sassatelli R, Bertoni G, Serra L, Bedogni G, Ponz de Leon M. Generalized juvenile polyposis with mixed pattern and gastric cancer. Gastroenterology. 1993;104:910–5.

Sato M, Miyauchi A, Takahara J. Clinical aspects of hyperparathyroidism in Japanese multiple endocrine neoplasia type 1. Biomed Pharmacother. 2000;54 Suppl 1:86s–9.

Schellhas HF. Malignant potential of the dysgenetic gonad. II. Obstet Gynecol. 1974;44:455–62.

Schillinger F, Montagnac R. Chronic renal failure and its treatment in tuberous sclerosis. Nephrol Dial Transplant. 1996;11:481–5.

Schmidt L, Duh FM, Chen F, et al. Germline and somatic mutations in the tyrosine kinase domain of the MET proto-oncogene in papillary renal carcinomas. Nat Genet. 1997;16:68–73.

Schoumacher F, Glaus A, Mueller H, Eppenberger U, Bolliger B, Senn HJ. BRCA1/2 mutations in Swiss patients with familial or early-onset breast and ovarian cancer. Swiss Med Wkly. 2001;131:223–6.

Schrager CA, Schneider D, Gruener AC, Tsou HC, Peacocke M. Clinical and pathological features of breast disease in Cowden's syndrome: an underrecognized syndrome with an increased risk of breast cancer. Hum Pathol. 1998;29:47–53.

Schubert EL, Lee MK, Mefford HC, et al. BRCA2 in American families with four or more cases of breast or ovarian cancer: recurrent and novel mutations, variable expression, penetrance, and the possibility of families whose cancer is not attributable to BRCA1 or BRCA2. Am J Hum Genet. 1997;60:1031–40.

Schumacher V, Scharer K, Wuhl E, et al. Spectrum of early onset nephrotic syndrome associated with WT1 missense mutations. Kidney Int. 1998;53:1594–600.

Schwartz RA, Torre DP. The Muir-Torre syndrome: a 25-year retrospect. J Am Acad Dermatol. 1995;33:90–104.

See JS, Shen EY, Chiu NC, et al. Tuberous sclerosis with visceral organ involvement. Acta Paediatr Taiwan. 1999;40:305–8.

Seidemann K, Tiemann M, Henze G, Sauerbrey A, Muller S, Reiter A. Therapy for non-Hodgkin lymphoma in children with primary immunodeficiency: analysis of 19 patients from the BFM trials. Med Pediatr Oncol. 1999;33:536–44.

Seidemann K, Henze G, Beck JD, et al. Non-Hodgkin's lymphoma in pediatric patients with chromosomal breakage syndromes (AT and NBS): experience from the BFM trials. Ann Oncol. 2000;11:141–5.

Sellner F. Investigations on the significance of the adenoma-carcinoma sequence in the small bowel. Cancer. 1990;66:702–15.

Serleth HJ, Kisken WA. A Muir-Torre syndrome family. Am Surg. 1998;64:365–9.

Sevenet N, Sheridan E, Amram D, Schneider P, Handgretinger R, Delattre O. Constitutional mutations of the hSNF5/INI1 gene predispose to a variety of cancers. Am J Hum Genet. 1999;65:1342–8.

Shah JR, Patkar DP, Pungavkar SA, Parmer H. Extensive gliomas of visual tract in a patient of neurofibromatosis-I. Indian J Pediatr. 2000;67:939–40.

Shen H, Sturgis EM, Khan SG, et al. An intronic poly (AT) polymorphism of the DNA repair gene XPC and risk of squamous cell carcinoma of the head and neck: a case-control study. Cancer Res. 2001;61:3321–5.

Shimotake T, Iwai N, Yanagihara J, Suzuki G, Takai S. The natural history of multiple endocrine neoplasia type 2A – a clinical analysis. Jpn J Surg. 1990;20:290–3.

Shinmura K, Kohno T, Takahashi M, et al. Familial gastric cancer: clinicopathological characteristics, RER phenotype and germline p53 and E-cadherin mutations. Carcinogenesis. 1999;20:1127–31.

Sigurdsson S, Thorlacius S, Tomasson J, et al. BRCA2 mutation in Icelandic prostate cancer patients. J Mol Med. 1997;75:758–61.

Simard J, Dumont M, Soucy P, Labrie F. Perspective: prostate cancer susceptibility genes. Endocrinology. 2002;143:2029–40.

Simpson JL, Photopulos G. The relationship of neoplasia to disorders of abnormal sexual differentiation. Birth Defects Orig Artic Ser. 1976;12:15–50.

Singh AD, Shields CL, Shields JA, Eagle RC, De Potter P. Uveal melanoma and familial atypical mole and melanoma (FAM-M) syndrome. Ophthalmic Genet. 1995;16:53–61.

Singh AD, Shields CL, Shields JA, De Potter P. Bilateral primary uveal melanoma. Bad luck or bad genes? Ophthalmology. 1996;103:256–62.

Singh AD, De Potter P, Fijal BA, Shields CL, Shields JA, Elston RC. Lifetime prevalence of uveal melanoma in white patients with oculo(dermal) melanocytosis. Ophthalmology. 1998;105:195–8.

Singhal S, Birch JM, Kerr B, Lashford L, Evans DG. Neurofibromatosis type 1 and sporadic optic gliomas. Arch Dis Child. 2002;87:65–70.

Skogseid B, Rastad J, Gobl A, et al. Adrenal lesion in multiple endocrine neoplasia type 1. Surgery. 1995;118:1077–82.

Smith LM, Donaldson SS. Incidence and management of secondary malignancies in patients with retinoblastoma and Ewing's sarcoma. Oncology (Huntingt). 1991;5:135–41; discussion 142, 147–8.

Smith OP, Hann IM, Chessells JM, Reeves BR, Milla P. Haematological abnormalities in Shwachman-Diamond syndrome. Br J Haematol. 1996;94:279–84.

Sogut A, Ozmen M, Sencer S, et al. Clinical features of tuberous sclerosis cases. Turk J Pediatr. 2002;44:98–101.

Soh LT, Ang PT, Lim-Tan SK. Embryonal carcinoma arising in Turner's syndrome. Ann Acad Med Singap. 1992;21:386–9.

Somers GR, Tabrizi SN, Tiedemann K, Chow CW, Garland SM, Venter DJ. Squamous cell carcinoma of the tongue in a child with Fanconi anemia: a case report and review of the literature. Pediatr Pathol Lab Med. 1995;15:597–607.

Sommer SS, Buzin CH, Jung M, et al. Elevated frequency of ATM gene missense mutations in breast cancer relative to ethnically matched controls. Cancer Genet Cytogenet. 2002;134:25–32.

Song WJ, Sullivan MG, Legare RD, et al. Haploinsufficiency of CBFA2 causes familial thrombocytopenia with propensity to develop acute myelogenous leukaemia. Nat Genet. 1999;23:166–75.

Soravia C, Berk T, Madlensky L, et al. Genotype-phenotype correlations in attenuated adenomatous polyposis coli. Am J Hum Genet. 1998;62:1290–301.

Soravia C, Sugg SL, Berk T, et al. Familial adenomatous polyposis-associated thyroid cancer: a clinical, pathological, and molecular genetics study. Am J Pathol. 1999;154:127–35.

Sorensen SA, Mulvihill JJ, Nielsen A. Long-term follow-up of von Recklinghausen neurofibromatosis. Survival and malignant neoplasms. N Engl J Med. 1986;314:1010–5.

Soussi T, Leblanc T, Baruchel A, Schaison G. Germline mutations of the p53 tumor-suppressor gene in cancer-prone families: a review. Nouv Rev Fr Hematol. 1993;35:33–6.

Souza RF. A molecular rationale for the how, when and why of colorectal cancer screening. Aliment Pharmacol Ther. 2001;15:451–62.

Spurney C, Gorlick R, Meyers PA, Healey JH, Huvos AG. Multicentric osteosarcoma, Rothmund-Thomson syndrome, and secondary nasopharyngeal non-Hodgkin's lymphoma: a case report and review of the literature. J Pediatr Hematol Oncol. 1998;20:494–7.

Stamm B, Hedinger CE, Saremaslani P. Duodenal and ampullary carcinoid tumors. A report of 12 cases with pathological characteristics, polypeptide content and relation to the MEN I syndrome and von Recklinghausen's disease (neurofibromatosis). Virchows Arch A Pathol Anat Histopathol. 1986;408:475–89.

Stankovic T, Kidd AM, Sutcliffe A, et al. ATM mutations and phenotypes in ataxia-telangiectasia families in the British Isles: expression of mutant ATM and the risk of leukemia, lymphoma, and breast cancer. Am J Hum Genet. 1998;62:334–45.

Starink TM. Cowden's disease: analysis of fourteen new cases. J Am Acad Dermatol. 1984;11:1127–41.

Starink TM, van der Veen JP, Arwert F, et al. The Cowden syndrome: a clinical and genetic study in 21 patients. Clin Genet. 1986;29:222–33.

Stemmer-Rachamimov AO, Horgan MA, Taratuto AL, et al. Meningioangiomatosis is associated with neurofibromatosis 2 but not with somatic alterations of the NF2 gene. J Neuropathol Exp Neurol. 1997;56:485–9.

Stevens HP, Kelsell DP, Bryant SP, et al. Linkage of an American pedigree with palmoplantar keratoderma and malignancy (palmoplantar ectodermal dysplasia type III) to 17q24. Literature survey and proposed updated classification of the keratodermas. Arch Dermatol. 1996;132:640–51.

Storm FK, Eilber FR, Mirra J, Morton DL. Neurofibrosarcoma. Cancer. 1980;45:126–9.

Stratakis CA. Clinical genetics of multiple endocrine neoplasias, Carney complex and related syndromes. J Endocrinol Invest. 2001;24:370–83.

Stratakis CA, Carney JA, Lin JP, et al. Carney complex, a familial multiple neoplasia and lentiginosis syndrome. Analysis of 11 kindreds and linkage to the short arm of chromosome 2. J Clin Invest. 1996;97:699–705.

Stratakis CA, Courcoutsakis NA, Abati A, et al. Thyroid gland abnormalities in patients with the syndrome of spotty skin pigmentation, myxomas, endocrine overactivity, and schwannomas (Carney complex). J Clin Endocrinol Metab. 1997;82:2037–43.

Stratakis CA, Kirschner LS, Taymans SE, et al. Carney complex, Peutz-Jeghers syndrome, Cowden disease, and Bannayan-Zonana syndrome share cutaneous and endocrine manifestations, but not genetic loci. J Clin Endocrinol Metab. 1998;83:2972–6.

Stratakis CA, Kirschner LS, Carney JA. Clinical and molecular features of the Carney complex: diagnostic criteria and recommendations for patient evaluation. J Clin Endocrinol Metab. 2001;86:4041–6.

Straus SE, Lenardo M, Puck JM. The Canale-Smith syndrome. N Engl J Med. 1997;336:1457; discussion 1457–8.

Straus SE, Jaffe ES, Puck JM, et al. The development of lymphomas in families with autoimmune lymphoproliferative syndrome with germline Fas mutations and defective lymphocyte apoptosis. Blood. 2001;98:194–200.

Sugano K, Taniguchi T, Saeki M, Tsunematsu Y, Tomaru U, Shimoda T. Germline p53 mutation in a case of Li-Fraumeni syndrome presenting gastric cancer. Jpn J Clin Oncol. 1999;29:513–6.

Swift M, Sholman L, Perry M, Chase C. Malignant neoplasms in the families of patients with ataxia- telangiectasia. Cancer Res. 1976;36:209–15.

Szabo J, Heath B, Hill VM, et al. Hereditary hyperparathyroidism-jaw tumor syndrome: the endocrine tumor gene HRPT2 maps to chromosome 1q21-q31. Am J Hum Genet. 1995;56:944–50.

Szudek J, Birch P, Riccardi VM, Evans DG, Friedman JM. Associations of clinical features in neurofibromatosis 1 (NF1). Genet Epidemiol. 2000;19:429–39.

Takayama T, Kato Y, Tsuru N, et al. A case of pheochromocytoma with von Recklinghausen's and review of 67 Japanese cases. Nippon Hinyokika Gakkai Zasshi. 2001;92:479–83.

Takebe H, Nishigori C, Tatsumi K. Melanoma and other skin cancers in xeroderma pigmentosum patients and mutation in their cells. J Invest Dermatol. 1989;92:236S–8.

Tamiya T, Hamazaki S, Ono Y, et al. Ganglioglioma in a patient with Turcot syndrome. Case report. J Neurosurg. 2000;92:170–5.

Tanaka Y, Sasaki Y, Nishihira H, Izawa T, Nishi T. Ovarian juvenile granulosa cell tumor associated with Maffucci's syndrome. Am J Clin Pathol. 1992;97:523–7.

Tao LC, Stecker E, Gardner HA. Werner's syndrome and acute myeloid leukemia. Can Med Assoc J. 1971;105:951 passim.

Taylor AM, Metcalfe JA, Thick J, Mak YF. Leukemia and lymphoma in ataxia telangiectasia. Blood. 1996;87:423–38.

Taylor MD, Perry J, Zlatescu MC, et al. The hPMS2 exon 5 mutation and malignant glioma. Case report. J Neurosurg. 1999;90:946–50.

Taylor MD, Mainprize TG, Rutka JT. Molecular insight into medulloblastoma and central nervous system primitive neuroectodermal tumor biology from hereditary syndromes: a review. Neurosurgery. 2000a;47:888–901.

Taylor MD, Gokgoz N, Andrulis IL, Mainprize TG, Drake JM, Rutka JT. Familial posterior fossa brain tumors of infancy secondary to germline mutation of the hSNF5 gene. Am J Hum Genet. 2000b;66:1403–6.

Taylor MD, Liu L, Raffel C, et al. Mutations in SUFU predispose to medulloblastoma. Nat Genet. 2002;31:306–10.

Teter J. Prognosis, malignancy, and curability of the germ-cell tumor occurring in dysgenetic gonads. Am J Obstet Gynecol. 1970;108:894–900.

Thomas DW, Lewis MA. Lhermitte-Duclos disease associated with Cowden's disease. Int J Oral Maxillofac Surg. 1995;24:369–71.

Thomas HJ, Whitelaw SC, Cottrell SE, et al. Genetic mapping of hereditary mixed polyposis syndrome to chromosome 6q. Am J Hum Genet. 1996;58:770–6.

Todd DW, Christoferson LA, Leech RW, Rudolf L. A family affected with intestinal polyposis and gliomas. Ann Neurol. 1981;10:390–2.

Toguchida J, Yamaguchi T, Dayton SH, et al. Prevalence and spectrum of germline mutations of the p53 gene among patients with sarcoma. N Engl J Med. 1992;326:1301–8.

Tomlinson IP, Alam NA, Rowan AJ, et al. Germline mutations in FH predispose to dominantly inherited uterine fibroids, skin leiomyomata and papillary renal cell cancer. Nat Genet. 2002;30:406–10.

Tonelli R, Scardovi AL, Pession A, et al. Compound heterozygosity for two different amino-acid substitution mutations in the thrombopoietin receptor (c-mpl gene) in congenital amegakaryocytic thrombocytopenia (CAMT). Hum Genet. 2000;107:225–33.

Toro JR, Glenn G, Duray P, et al. Birt-Hogg-Dube syndrome: a novel marker of kidney neoplasia. Arch Dermatol. 1999;135:1195–202.

Torres OA, Roach ES, Delgado MR, et al. Early diagnosis of subependymal giant cell astrocytoma in patients with tuberous sclerosis. J Child Neurol. 1998;13:173–7.

Tsubosa Y, Fukutomi T, Tsuda H, et al. Breast cancer in Cowden's disease: a case report with review of the literature. Jpn J Clin Oncol. 1998;28:42–6.

Tulinius H, Olafsdottir GH, Sigvaldason H, et al. The effect of a single BRCA2 mutation on cancer in Iceland. J Med Genet. 2002;39:457–62.

Turgut M, Akalan N, Ozgen T, Ruacan S, Erbengi A. Subependymal giant cell astrocytoma associated with tuberous sclerosis: diagnostic and surgical characteristics of five cases with unusual features. Clin Neurol Neurosurg. 1996;98:217–21.

Turgut M, Ozcan OE, Bertan V. Meningiomas in childhood and adolescence: a report of 13 cases and review of the literature. Br J Neurosurg. 1997;11:501–7.

Ubogy-Rainey Z, James WD, Lupton GP, Rodman OG. Fibrofolliculomas, trichodiscomas, and acrochordons: the Birt-Hogg-Dube syndrome. J Am Acad Dermatol. 1987;16:452–7.

Uchino S, Noguchi S, Kawamoto H, Yamashita H, Watanabe S, Shuto S. Familial nonmedullary thyroid carcinoma characterized by multifocality and a high recurrence rate in a large study population. World J Surg. 2002;26:897–902.

Vaishnaw AK, Toubi E, Ohsako S, et al. The spectrum of apoptotic defects and clinical manifestations, including systemic lupus erythematosus, in humans with CD95 (Fas/APO-1) mutations. Arthritis Rheum. 1999;42:1833–42.

Valverde K, Henderson M, Smith CR, Tallett S, Chan HS. Typical and atypical Carney's triad presenting with malignant hypertension and papilledema. J Pediatr Hematol Oncol. 2001;23:519–24.

van der Linde K, Vasen HF, van Vliet AC. Occurrence of thyroid carcinoma in Dutch patients with familial adenomatous polyposis. An epidemiological study and report of new cases. Eur J Gastroenterol Hepatol. 1998;10:777–81.

van Geel AN, van Slooten EA, Mavrunac M, Hart AA. A retrospective study of male breast cancer in Holland. Br J Surg. 1985;72:724–7.

Van Meir EG. "Turcot's syndrome": phenotype of brain tumors, survival and mode of inheritance. Int J Cancer. 1998;75:162–4.

Varley JM, McGown G, Thorncroft M, et al. An extended Li-Fraumeni kindred with gastric carcinoma and a codon 175 mutation in TP53. J Med Genet. 1995;32:942–5.

Varley JM, McGown G, Thorncroft M, et al. Are there low-penetrance TP53 Alleles? Evidence from childhood adrenocortical tumors. Am J Hum Genet. 1999;65:995–1006.

Varon R, Reis A, Henze G, von Einsiedel HG, Sperling K, Seeger K. Mutations in the Nijmegen Breakage Syndrome gene (NBS1) in childhood acute lymphoblastic leukemia (ALL). Cancer Res. 2001;61:3570–2.

Vasen HF, Nieuwenhuijzen Kruseman AC, Berkel H, et al. Multiple endocrine neoplasia syndrome type 2: the value of screening and central registration. A study of 15 kindreds in The Netherlands. Am J Med. 1987;83:847–52.

Vasen HF, Offerhaus GJ, den Hartog Jager FC, et al. The tumour spectrum in hereditary nonpolyposis colorectal cancer: a study of 24 kindreds in the Netherlands. Int J Cancer. 1990;46:31–4.

Vasen HF, van der Feltz M, Raue F, et al. The natural course of multiple endocrine neoplasia type IIb. A study of 18 cases. Arch Intern Med. 1992;152:1250–2.

Vasen HF, Gruis NA, Frants RR, van Der Velden PA, Hille ET, Bergman W. Risk of developing pancreatic cancer in families with familial atypical multiple mole melanoma associated with a specific 19 deletion of p16 (p16-Leiden). Int J Cancer. 2000;87:809–11.

Velasco-Oses A, Alonso-Alvaro A, Blanco-Pozo A, Nogales Jr FF. Ollier's disease associated with ovarian juvenile granulosa cell tumor. Cancer. 1988;62:222–5.

Verges B, Boureille F, Goudet P, et al. Pituitary disease in MEN type 1 (MEN1): data from the France-Belgium MEN1 multicenter study. J Clin Endocrinol Metab. 2002;87:457–65.

Vinchon M, Soto-Ares G, Ruchoux MM, Dhellemmes P. Cerebellar gliomas in children with NF1: pathology and surgery. Childs Nerv Syst. 2000;16:417–20.

Vital A, Bringuier PP, Huang H, et al. Astrocytomas and choroid plexus tumors in two families with identical p53 germline mutations. J Neuropathol Exp Neurol. 1998;57:1061–9.

Wagner J, Portwine C, Rabin K, Leclerc JM, Narod SA, Malkin D. High frequency of germ-line p53 mutations in childhood adrenocortical cancer. J Natl Cancer Inst. 1994; 86:1707–10.

Walker C. Molecular genetics of renal carcinogenesis. Toxicol Pathol. 1998;26:113–20.

Wallace TM, Levin HS, Ratliff NB, Hobbs RE. Evaluation and management of Carney's complex: an illustrative case. Cleve Clin J Med. 1991;58(248–50):255–6.

Wallis YL, Morton DG, McKeown CM, Macdonald F. Molecular analysis of the APC gene in 205 families: extended genotype- phenotype correlations in FAP and evidence for the role of APC amino acid changes in colorectal cancer predisposition. J Med Genet. 1999;36:14–20.

Walther MM, Herring J, Enquist E, Keiser HR, Linehan WM. von Recklinghausen's disease and pheochromocytomas. J Urol. 1999;162:1582–6.

Wang LL, Levy ML, Lewis RA, et al. Clinical manifestations in a cohort of 41 Rothmund-Thomson syndrome patients. Am J Med Genet. 2001;102:11–7.

Wang L, McDonnell SK, Elkins DA, et al. Analysis of the RNASEL gene in familial and sporadic prostate cancer. Am J Hum Genet. 2002;71:116–23.

Washecka R, Dresner MI, Honda SA. Testicular tumors in Carney's complex. J Urol. 2002;167:1299–302.

Watanabe T, Muto T, Sawada T, Miyaki M. Flat adenoma as a precursor of colorectal carcinoma in hereditary nonpolyposis colorectal carcinoma. Cancer. 1996;77:627–34.

Watne AL. Colon polyps. J Surg Oncol. 1997;66:207–14.

Watson GH. Cardiac rhabdomyomas in tuberous sclerosis. Ann N Y Acad Sci. 1991;615:50–7.

Watson P, Lynch HT. Extracolonic cancer in hereditary nonpolyposis colorectal cancer. Cancer. 1993;71:677–85.

Watson P, Lynch HT. The tumor spectrum in HNPCC. Anticancer Res. 1994;14:1635–9.

Watson P, Vasen HF, Mecklin JP, Jarvinen H, Lynch HT. The risk of endometrial cancer in heredi-tary nonpolyposis colorectal cancer. Am J Med. 1994;96:516–20.

Watson JC, Stratakis CA, Bryant-Greenwood PK, et al. Neurosurgical implications of Carney complex. J Neurosurg. 2000;92:413–8.

Watson P, Butzow R, Lynch HT, et al. The clinical features of ovarian cancer in hereditary nonpol-yposis colorectal cancer. Gynecol Oncol. 2001;82:223–8.

Webb DW, Osborne JP. Incidence of tuberous sclerosis in patients with cardiac rhabdomyoma. Am J Med Genet. 1992;42:754–5.

Webb DW, Clarke A, Fryer A, Osborne JP. The cutaneous features of tuberous sclerosis: a popula-tion study. Br J Dermatol. 1996;135:1–5.

Weber TK, Chin HM, Rodriguez-Bigas M, et al. Novel hMLH1 and hMSH2 germline mutations in African Americans with colorectal cancer. JAMA. 1999;281:2316–20.

Webster AR, Richards FM, MacRonald FE, Moore AT, Maher ER. An analysis of phenotypic variation in the familial cancer syndrome von Hippel-Lindau disease: evidence for modifier effects. Am J Hum Genet. 1998;63:1025–35.

Weemaes CM, Smeets DF, van der Burgt CJ. Nijmegen Breakage syndrome: a progress report. Int J Radiat Biol. 1994;66:S185–8.

Wei SC, Wang MH, Shieh MC, Wang CY, Wong JM. Clinical characteristics of Taiwanese heredi-tary non-polyposis colorectal cancer kindreds. J Formos Med Assoc. 2002;101:206–9.

Weiss GR, Garnick MB. Testicular cancer in a Russell-Silver dwarf. J Urol. 1981;126:836–7.

Welling DB. Clinical manifestations of mutations in the neurofibromatosis type 2 gene in vestibu-lar schwannomas (acoustic neuromas). Laryngoscope. 1998;108:178–89.

Welte K, Dale D. Pathophysiology and treatment of severe chronic neutropenia. Ann Hematol. 1996;72:158–65.

Wertelecki W, Rouleau GA, Superneau DW, et al. Neurofibromatosis 2: clinical and DNA linkage studies of a large kindred. N Engl J Med. 1988;319:278–83.

Weyl Ben Arush M, Rosenthal J, Dale J, et al. Ataxia telangiectasia and lymphoma: an indication for individualized chemotherapy dosing-report of treatment in a highly inbred Arab family. Pediatr Hematol Oncol. 1995;12:163–9.

Whitelaw SC, Murday VA, Tomlinson IP, et al. Clinical and molecular features of the hereditary mixed polyposis syndrome. Gastroenterology. 1997;112:327–34.

Wijnen JT, Vasen HF, Khan PM, et al. Clinical findings with implications for genetic testing in families with clustering of colorectal cancer. N Engl J Med. 1998;339:511–8.

Wilkinson EJ, Morgan LS, Friedrich Jr EG. Association of Fanconi's anemia and squamous-cell carcinoma of the lower female genital tract with condyloma acuminatum. A report of two cases. J Reprod Med. 1984;29:447–53.

Wilkinson S, Teh BT, Davey KR, McArdle JP, Young M, Shepherd JJ. Cause of death in multiple endocrine neoplasia type 1. Arch Surg. 1993;128:683–90.

Wolpert N, Warner E, Seminsky MF, Futreal A, Narod SA. Prevalence of BRCA1 and BRCA2 mutations in male breast cancer patients in Canada. Clin Breast Cancer. 2000;1:57–63; discussion 64–5.

Wolter M, Reifenberger J, Sommer C, Ruzicka T, Reifenberger G. Mutations in the human homologue of the Drosophila segment polarity gene patched (PTCH) in sporadic basal cell carcinomas of the skin and primitive neuroectodermal tumors of the central nervous system. Cancer Res. 1997;57:2581–5.

Wong FL, Boice Jr JD, Abramson DH, et al. Cancer incidence after retinoblastoma. Radiation dose and sarcoma risk. JAMA. 1997;278:1262–7.

Woodford-Richens K, Bevan S, Churchman M, et al. Analysis of genetic and phenotypic heterogeneity in juvenile polyposis. Gut. 2000;46:656–60.

Woodford-Richens KL, Rowan AJ, Poulsom R, et al. Comprehensive analysis of SMAD4 mutations and protein expression in juvenile polyposis: evidence for a distinct genetic pathway and polyp morphology in SMAD4 mutation carriers. Am J Pathol. 2001;159:1293–300.

Woods WG, Roloff JS, Lukens JN, Krivit W. The occurrence of leukemia in patients with the Shwachman syndrome. J Pediatr. 1981;99:425–8.

Woodward ER, Clifford SC, Astuti D, Affara NA, Maher ER. Familial clear cell renal cell carcinoma (FCRC): clinical features and mutation analysis of the VHL, MET, and CUL2 candidate genes. J Med Genet. 2000;37:348–53.

Wooster R, Mangion J, Eeles R, et al. A germline mutation in the androgen receptor gene in two brothers with breast cancer and Reifenstein syndrome. Nat Genet. 1992;2:132–4.

Wu JS, Paul P, McGannon EA, Church JM. APC genotype, polyp number, and surgical options in familial adenomatous polyposis. Ann Surg. 1998;227:57–62.

Xu W, Mulligan LM, Ponder MA, et al. Loss of NF1 alleles in phaeochromocytomas from patients with type I neurofibromatosis. Genes Chromosomes Cancer. 1992;4:337–42.

Yamamoto H, Itoh F, Nakamura H, et al. Genetic and clinical features of human pancreatic ductal adenocarcinomas with widespread microsatellite instability. Cancer Res. 2001;61:3139–44.

Yoshida T, Haraguchi Y, Tanaka A, et al. A case of generalized juvenile gastrointestinal polyposis associated with gastric carcinoma. Endoscopy. 1988;20:33–5.

Young RH, Dickersin GR, Scully RE. Juvenile granulosa cell tumor of the ovary. A clinicopathological analysis of 125 cases. Am J Surg Pathol. 1984;8:575–96.

Zalla JA. Werner's syndrome. Cutis. 1980;25:275–8.

Zbar B, Kaelin W, Maher E, Richard S. Third International Meeting on von Hippel-Lindau disease. Cancer Res. 1999;59:2251–3.

Zbar B, Alvord WG, Glenn G, et al. Risk of renal and colonic neoplasms and spontaneous pneu-mothorax in the Birt-Hogg-Dube syndrome. Cancer Epidemiol Biomark Prev. 2002;11:393–400.

Zhou XP, Sanson M, Hoang-Xuan K, et al. Germline mutations of p53 but not p16/CDKN2 or PTEN/MMAC1 tumor suppressor genes predispose to gliomas. The ANOCEF Group. Association des NeuroOncologues d'Expression Francaise. Ann Neurol. 1999;46:913–6.

Zhou XP, Woodford-Richens K, Lehtonen R, et al. Germline mutations in BMPR1A/ALK3 cause a subset of cases of juvenile polyposis syndrome and of Cowden and Bannayan-Riley-Ruvalcaba syndromes. Am J Hum Genet. 2001;69:704–11.

Zoller ME, Rembeck B, Oden A, Samuelsson M, Angervall L. Malignant and benign tumors in patients with neurofibromatosis type 1 in a defined Swedish population. Cancer. 1997;79:2125–31.

Zvulunov A, Barak Y, Metzker A. Juvenile xanthogranuloma, neurofibromatosis, and juvenile chronic myelogenous leukemia. World statistical analysis. Arch Dermatol. 1995;131:904–8.

Index